# A

# CONSUMER'S

# DICTIONARY OF

# FOOD ADDITIVES

# A

# CONSUMER'S

# DICTIONARY OF

# FOOD ADDITIVES

## COMPLETELY REVISED AND UPDATED
## SIXTH EDITION

*Descriptions in Plain English of More Than*

*12,000 Ingredients Both Harmful and Desirable Found in Foods*

# RUTH WINTER, M.S.

THREE RIVERS PRESS
NEW YORK

This book provides general information about food additives. If you have particular questions or concerns about any food additive and your personal health or if you believe you are reacting to a food additive, you should consult your physician.

Published by Three Rivers Press, New York, New York.
Member of the Crown Publishing Group, a division of Random House, Inc.
www.crownpublishing.com

THREE RIVERS PRESS and the Tugboat design are registered trademarks of Random House, Inc.

Printed in the United States of America

Library of Congress Cataloging-in-Publication Data

Winter, Ruth, 1930–
A consumer's dictionary of food additives : descriptions in plain English of more than 12,000 ingredients both harmful and desirable found in foods / Ruth Winter.—
6th ed.
1. Food additives—Dictionaries.   I. Title.
TX553.A3W55 2004
664'.06'03—dc22      2004005062

ISBN 1-4000-5232-7

10  9  8  7  6  5  4  3  2  1

Sixth Edition

*To my husband, Arthur Winter, M.D.,*
*my daughter, Robin Winter-Sperry, M.D.,*
*my sons, Craig and Grant,*
*my son-in-law, Jonathan Sperry,*
*and my grandchildren, Samantha, Hunter, and Katelynd*

# CONTENTS

# A

# CONSUMER'S

# DICTIONARY OF

# FOOD ADDITIVES

# DO YOU WANT TO KNOW WHAT IS ADDED TO YOUR FOOD?

Are you worried about additives in your food that may be:

- allergens?
- antibiotics?
- cancer-causing agents?
- digestion disrupters?
- hormones?
- pesticides?
- untested new chemical compounds?

This sixth edition of *A Consumer's Dictionary of Food Additives* is your guide to gaining insight into additives—direct and indirect—that you and your loved ones may be eating and drinking regularly without your knowledge! Thousands of chemicals are added to our food. Many are beneficial but a number may be harmful or even lethal.

Additives are substances, or a mixture of substances, other than basic foodstuffs, that are present in food as a result of any aspect of production, processing, storage, or packaging. BHT, for example, is a preservative, stabilizer, and antioxidant added in many foods. It is used as a chewing-gum base, added to potato and sweet potato flakes and dry breakfast cereals, an emulsion stabilizer for shortenings used in enriched rice, animal fats, and shortenings containing animal fats. BHA is a preservative, stabilizer, and antioxidant in many products, including beverages, ice cream, ices, candy, baked goods, chewing gum, gelatin desserts, soup bases, potatoes, and in emulsions for stabilizers for shortenings. Some substances, vitamins E and C, for example, are considered both nutrients and additives. The two vitamins are sometimes added for their ability to retard rancidity. Red No. 3 and annatto are examples of colorings. The majority of food additives have nothing to do with nutritional value, as you will see from the contents of this dictionary—most are added to feed our illusions. All our lives we are subjected to beautiful pictures of foods in our magazines and on television. We have come to expect an advertiser's concept of perfection in color and texture, even though Mother Nature may not turn out all her products that way. As a result, the skins of the oranges we eat are dyed bright orange to match our mental image of an ideal orange. Our poultry is fed a chemical to color the meat yellow to look more appetizing, and our fruits and vegetables are kept unblemished by fungicides, pesticides, herbicides, and other antispoilants.

We are very busy. We want our meals to be easy to prepare, but still tasty. One of the quotes used most often by food experts is that "the consuming public will not buy food products on the basis of their nutritional profile/clinical benefits—taste is the key!" No wonder then that the biggest category of food additives is flavorings and flavor enhancers, a growing market which is expected to top $1.46 billion in 2006.

At the time of the first edition of this book, food additives were a $1.3 billion a year business in the United States. The number increased to more than $4.73 billion a year when the fifth edition was published. With this sixth edition, the total U.S. market for food additives is an estimated $5.8 billion. The European Parliament, in fact, issued the following statement in 2003: "The ever increasing number of food additives leads to a cumulation of a large number of small risks for food safety, which are not easily evaluable, and which might create synergy effects between different substances. The total number of authorized food additives should therefore be limited, so that the industry, when applying for a new authorization, has to make a proposal for withdrawing an additive of little use."

Food sellers also know that if they put "new" on the package, we are almost always tempted to buy it. They spend, therefore, $1.4 billion annually to introduce ten thousand new food products, some with novel additives and many with new combinations of additives.[1] The danger in this is that food additives are rarely used individually in foods, so one meal may contain many different additives that can interact with one another. In addition, additives can change or react during cooking or processing. When this book was first published in 1978, there were thirty-five widely used additives that had been approved as safe for food use then but have since been removed as unsafe, most because they were found to be capable of causing cancer.

Two major positive changes have occurred since the first edition was published in 1978:

1. The U.S. Food and Drug Administration (FDA) has increased its computerization of information about food additives so regulators, scien-

---

[1]BUSINESS COMMUNICATIONS COMPANY, INC., 25 Van Zant Street, Norwalk, CT 06855, Telephone: (203) 853-4266, ext. 309; e-mail: publisher@bccresearch.com

tists, and manufacturers have better access to what is known and unknown about these chemicals.

2. The evaluation of food additives has become international and scientists and regulators from other countries can provide additional input about the use and safety of substances added to foods.

## Persistent Problems

However, there are some problems mentioned in all five previous editions that haven't gone away. For example:

- Enforcement of the Delaney Amendment that mandated that no cancer-causing additive could be added to food continues to be lax and known carcinogens are in what we eat and drink.

- Antibiotic and hormonal residues still contaminate our food.

- The determination that a food additive is generally recognized as safe (GRAS) is largely left up to the manufacturer.

- Some unidentified additives are listed as "natural" flavorings or colorings—a potentially dangerous situation for a number of allergic individuals.

- More than forty percent of the 50 million pounds of antibiotics produced in the United States are used for farm animals and crops. The inability to control the residues of more than 101 antibiotics[2] in meat, poultry, and vegetable crops may be contributing to the increasingly alarming antibiotic-resistant bacteria. In fact, in 2000 the FDA's Center for Veterinary Medicine (CVM) proposed withdrawing approval of the use of fluoroquinolone antibiotics in poultry because chickens and turkeys develop fluoroquinolone-resistant bacterial infections, campylobacter, the most common bacterial cause of diarrheal illness in approximately 2 million Americans a year. It is usually just uncomfortable but it can be fatal. Eating poultry with fluoroquinolone-resistant bacteria may lead to the development of fluoroquinolone-resistant campylobacter infections in humans.[3] We could then develop cross-resistance to all fluoroquinolone drugs. Cipro®, prescribed for the bioterrorism bacterial weapon anthrax (and for many other infections) is a fluoroquinolone. The European

---

[2]FDA Approved Animal Drug Products, Online Database System, September 8, 2003.
[3]Linda Bren, "Antibiotic Resistance from Down on the Chicken Farm," *FDA Consumer* January–February 2001, pp. 10–11.

Union has banned most antibiotics in feed as growth promoters and intends to ban the remining four by 2006.

- Eighty percent of U.S. livestock and poultry are treated with animal drugs.

- The continued use of pesticides, many of which are known cancer-causing agents or toxins that contaminate food crops and animals. In fact, the attorneys general of Connecticut, Massachusetts, New Jersey, and New York sued the federal Environmental Protection Agency on September 15, 2003, contending that it is allowing unacceptably high levels of pesticide residues in some foods favored by children.

- Only a minuscule fraction of the food that enters our country by land, sea, and air is ever checked by our guardian agencies. Nearly two-thirds of the fish, almost half the fruits, and more than 10 percent of the vegetables we eat are imported. This means that of the more than 20 billion pounds of produce we import per year, only 2 to 3 percent undergoes FDA inspection.

You, therefore, must be the primary gatekeeper to protect your family's health by being a conscientious and informed consumer. What do you want from your food? You are part of the market force. By using this book to understand the labels and by selecting wisely, you can affect the sales of more wholesome foods and protect the health of your family. With this book, you will be better able to:

- evaluate foods
- read labels
- identify nutritious foods
- understand what labels do not reveal
- avoid salt
- avoid hidden sugars
- avoid allergens
- find foods abundant in desirable ingredients
- plan a healthier diet

The first place to begin is with the food label.

## Take Time to Read the Label

A food label is a contract between you and the manufacturer. Like most contracts, it may be difficult to understand—what is not included may be just as important as what is. The government estimates that over the next twenty years, labels will reduce national health care costs substantially by making it easier for the public to choose more healthful diets.

Newer regulations give more down-to-earth serving sizes (see page 23). Instead of a food manufacturer presenting a calorie or fat count for half a teaspoonful they give the count for half a cup—the realistic serving size.

Can you decipher the chemicals on the label? How do you know which ones are good, bad, or unnecessary? You can look them up in this dictionary and you can check with the sources listed at the end of this chapter.

## Who Is in the Mix?

Below is the sometimes confusing alphabet soup of agencies involved with food additives.

The FDA's list is called **EFAUS** for **Every Food Additive Added in the United States.** This is a great start, but far from complete. In fact, the list does not even have the synthetic flavorings in use that are determined Generally Recognized As Safe (GRAS) by the Expert Panel of the Flavor and Extract Manufacturers Association (FEMA), a trade organization. The sixth edition of *A Consumer's Dictionary of Food Additives* has scores of substances—some of them quite unappetizing—that may be on your plate but not listed by EFAUS. This dictionary also describes the benefits and potential harm of food additives, which the EFAUS list does not.

The **Joint FAO/WHO Expert Committee on Food Additives (JECFA)** is an international expert scientific committee that is administered jointly by the **Food and Agriculture Organization of the United Nations (FAO)** and the **World Health Organization (WHO).** It has been meeting since 1956, initially to evaluate the safety of food additives. Its work now also includes the evaluation of contaminants, naturally occurring toxicants, and residues of veterinary drugs in food. To date, JECFA has evaluated more than 1,500 food additives, approximately 40 contaminants and naturally occurring toxicants, and residues of approximately 90 veterinary drugs. The committee has also developed principles for the safety assessment of chemicals in food that are consistent with current thinking on risk assessment and take into account recent developments in toxicology and other relevant sciences.

JECFA normally meets twice a year with individual agendas covering either food additives, contaminants, and naturally occurring toxicants in food or residues of veterinary drugs in food. The membership of the meetings varies accordingly, with different sets of experts being called on depending on the subject matter of the meeting.

**Codex Alimentarius Commission (CAC)** is an international government body formed to protect the health of the consumer and facilitate international trade in food. In the 1960s, JECFAC began to provide expert advice to CAC.

The **European Union (EU)** has created a list of approved food additives. EU legislation requires that most additives used in foods be labeled clearly in the list of ingredients, either by name or by an E number. This sixth edition of *A Consumer's Dictionary of Food Additives* is the first edition that presents evaluations by foreign agencies.

These organizations are doing a painstaking job of evaluating research on substances in our foods and estimating the average daily intake (ADI) of such chemicals. It is not realistic to use animals or humans to test every combination of additives and every chemical that is produced during processing and cooking. Decisions are made based upon information gleaned from published studies and from the advice of experts. Progress is slow because the agencies meet infrequently. In some instances, an additive is approved and even listed as **Generally Recognized As Safe (GRAS)** such as in the classic case of cyclamates and more recently glycine. The artificial sweeteners known as cyclamates listed as GRAS were removed from the food market in 1969 because they were found to cause bladder cancer in rats. At that time, 175 million Americans—including young children— were swallowing cyclamates in significant doses in many products ranging from chewing gum to soft drinks. In April 2003, the FDA rescinded its GRAS status for the amino acid additive glycine because "reports in scientific literature indicate that adverse effects were found in cases where high levels of glycine were administered in diets of experimental animals and current usage information indicates that the daily dietary intake of glycine by humans may be substantially increasing due to changing use patterns in food technology." Glycine, according to the FDA, is a masking agent for saccharin in beverages and bases. It is also used by food producers to improve protein.

The FAO/WHO and FDA do have lists of current additives slated for top priority evaluation and you will read about these substances in the dictionary portion of this book. You will also discover these major organizations—the FAO/WHO, FDA, and EU—do not always agree on the safety of a particular additive. Take stevioside, for example, a sweetener about 300 times as sweet as sugar derived from a South American plant, *Stevia rebaudiana*. Stevioside is allowed in food in Japan, South Korea, Brazil, and seven other countries. In 1999, the Joint Expert Committee on Food Additives of the World Health Organization (JECFA) and the Scientific Committee for Food of the European Union (EU) reviewed stevioside and determined that on the basis of the scientific data available, stevioside was not acceptable as a sweetener because no adequate reports on its potential mutagenicity, carcinogenicity, and toxicity were available. Stevioside was on the U.S. market in the 1980s and then banned in 1991 because the FDA said that it had not seen studies concluding stevioside was a safe food additive. The FDA, nevertheless, does allow stevioside to be used today as a dietary supplement. (Dietary supplements are not subject to FDA regulations as of this writing.) The agency, however, seizes any food products with stevioside as a food additive including drinks, seafood, fruits, vegetables, and candies. To complicate things further, new studies in the scientific literature conclude that stevioside may lower blood pressure and has potential as a drug for Type II diabetes.[4] Is stevioside a safe food additive or not? How much is genuine worry about its safety and how much is pressure by producers of competitive sweeteners to keep it off the market? Stay tuned.

The case of hexadienal, on the other hand, is an example of one U.S. agency not knowing what the other is doing. This food additive is a synthetic chemical with a "green" or "citrus odor" used in flavorings. A relative, trans, trans-2, 4-hexidienal occurs naturally in a wide variety of foods, including kiwifruit and peanuts. The National Cancer Institute asked the National Toxicology Program (NTP)—which actually does laboratory tests for government agencies—to test hexadienal because of the chemical's cancer-causing potential based on its structure and its potential link to oxidized dietary fats and human malignancies. The NTP informed the National Cancer Institute of its findings. On October 18, 2001, its studies showed that hexadienal was indeed carcinogenic in rats and mice causing oral and forestomach malignancies. The FDA, however, still lists hexadienal as ASP, meaning the agency has sought "fully updated toxicology information" and hexadienal remains as an approved food additive in several different compounds. The FAO/WHO also says of hexadienal that there is "No safety concern at current levels of intake when used as a flavoring agent." Should we be concerned about the use of this unnecessary chemical that has been found in actual testing to have potential cancer-causing properties?

Does the FDA list of ingredients designated as Generally Recognized As Safe (GRAS) mean they are really safe?

---

[4]P. B. Jeppesen, S. Gregersen, and S. E. Rolfsen, et al. "Antihyperglycemic and Blood Pressure-Reducing Effects of Stevioside in the Diabetic Goto-Katizak Rat," *Metabolism* (United States), March 2003, 52(3): 372–78; J. C. Liu, P. K. Kao, and P. Chan, et al. "Mechanism of the Antihypertensive Effect of Stevioside in Anesthetized Dogs, *Pharmacology* (Switzerland), January 2003, 67(1): 14–20; C. N. Lee, K. L. Wong, and J. C. Liu, et al. "Inhibitory Effect of Stevioside on Calcium Influx to Produce Antihypertension, *Planta Med* (Germany), December 2001, 67(9): 796–99.

# *Generally Recognized As Safe (GRAS) List*

Congress established the GRAS list in 1958. These substances that had been added to food over a long time, and which under the conditions of their intended use were generally recognized as safe by qualified scientists, would be exempt from premarket clearance. At that point, Congress had acted on a very marginal response—of returns from those scientists sent questionnaires. Approximately 355 out of 900 responded, and only about 100 of those responses had substantive comments. Three items were removed from the originally published list. Two groups of substances were designated exempt from the Food Additives Amendment:

- Substances sanctioned by the FDA or USDA prior to 1958.
- Substances classified by the FDA as generally recognized as safe (GRAS) such as salt, sugar, spices, caffeine, vitamins, monosodium glutamate, and several hundred other food ingredients. Since 1958, the FDA and USDA claim to monitor all prior sanctioned and GRAS substances in response to new scientific information and evidence on the safety of these substances.

Needless to say, in recent years, developments in the scientific fields and in consumer awareness brought to light the inadequacies in food additive testing. So did the discovery that some additives listed as GRAS did not have adequate testing at all. As a result of these inadequacies, in 1969 President Richard Nixon directed the FDA to reevaluate all of the items on the GRAS list. By 1980, 415 substances that had been in use prior to the 1958 Food Additives Amendment to the Food, Drug and Cosmetic Act were reviewed. The committee's evaluations were based on review of medical and scientific literature and unpublished reports. In some cases the research extended back sixty years. The number of references obtained for a given GRAS substance ranged from twenty-three reports for carnauba wax to two thousand for vitamin A. Then in the late 1990s, the federal government further enfeebled the Generally Recognized As Safe food additive category. Instead of petitioning the FDA for affirmation, manufacturers simply have to notify the FDA of their additive's GRAS status and provide some evidence to support it. The FDA says that letting the manufacturer determine what is Generally Recognized As Safe and making it simpler to obtain FDA approval allows the FDA to "gain increased awareness of ingredients in the nation's food supply and the cumulative dietary exposure to GRAS substances" and, of course, save money. Despite this backtracking, most of the ingredients that appear on the GRAS list are safe and many are desirable. Those entries that have been generally recognized as safe have the designation GRAS at the end of their listing in this dictionary. In this edition you will also note an E at the end of some listings, signifying the additive has been approved by the European Union.

The Color Additive Amendment to the Food, Drug and Cosmetic Act was passed in 1960. Both the Food Additives Amendment and the Color Additive Amendment include a provision which prohibits the approval of an additive if it is found to cause cancer in humans or animals. This amendment is often referred to as the Delaney Amendment, named for its congressional sponsor, Rep. James Delaney (D-NY). Regulations known as Good Manufacturing Practices (GMP) limit the amount of food and color additives used in food to achieve their desired effect.

Manufacturers do have to present a petition to sell a new food additive. Approximately one hundred new food and color additive petitions are submitted to the FDA annually. A food or color additive petition is supposed to provide convincing evidence that the proposed additive performs as it is intended and is safe for human consumption. Upon approval, the FDA issues regulations including the types of foods in which an additive can be used, the maximum amounts to be used, and how they must be identified on food labels. Additives proposed for use in meat and poultry products must also receive specific authorization by U.S. Department of Agriculture (USDA); where evidence is submitted that justifies use of a different standard, a safety factor in applying animal experimentation data to man of 100 to 1, is used; that is, a food additive for use by man will not be granted a tolerance that exceeds one one-hundredth of the maximum amount demonstrated to be without harm to experimental animals. Don't blame me for using "man" and leaving out women and children. That's the way the rule reads and that may be one of its weaknesses. Children and pregnant women, for example, may not be protected by the 100 to 1 safety factor the same way that a healthy young male may be. This disparity has been recognized in drug testing but not in additive testing at this writing.

## New Problem— Potential Food Bioterrorism

We want fresh strawberries in winter and tomatoes all year round yet we have replaced many of our farms with housing and roadways and our edibles are increasingly being grown in other countries. Only a tiny fraction of the food that enters our ports is checked by our guardian agencies. Not only do we have to worry about foreign foods with undesirable additives and residues, we now have to be protected against terroristic tampering. In 2003, the FDA announced publication of proposed regulations required by the Public Health Security and Bioterrorism Preparedness and Response Act of 2002. Two regulations deal with establishing and maintaining records among food firms and the administrative detention of foods that may pose a risk to public health. Two regulations concern the registration of food facilities and prior notice of imported foods. These regulations further bolster the FDA's ability to protect the more than 400,000 domestic and foreign facilities that deal with food within our country, according to former FDA Commissioner Dr. Mark B. McClellan, M.D., Ph.D. Under the rule, manufacturers, processors, packers, distributors, receivers, holders, and importers of food must keep records identifying the immediate source from which they received the food, as well as the immediate subsequent recipient to whom they sent it. This requirement applies to almost all foreign and domestic food sources and almost all recipients of food destined for consumption in the United States. It would assist the FDA in addressing credible threats of serious adverse health consequences or death to humans or animals. It is unbelievable that record keeping for tracking foods—such as those including illegal additives and contaminants—has not been required before! As a side benefit for all, an additional $20.5 million was given for Counter Terrorism–Food Safety. The increase is supposed to provide grants to states, increased laboratory preparedness, and funds to develop the foods registration system. The grants to the states are meant to be used to build states' infrastructure to enable them to become part of the Laboratory Response Network and conduct direct federal food inspections. Increased laboratory preparedness should theoretically allow the agency's laboratory accreditation program to continue and to develop uniform scientific practices.

There are loopholes, however. "To minimize the economic burden on food companies affected" by the rule, the FDA allows companies to keep the required information in any form they prefer. The proposed rule also states that existing records can be used to satisfy the requirements of the regulations if those records contain all the required information. With respect to the immediate previous source, the specific source of each ingredient that was used to make every lot of finished food product would have to be identified if this information is reasonably available. What is reasonably available may vary from case to case, according to the FDA. If an article of food is reasonably believed to be adulterated and presents a threat of serious adverse health consequence or death to humans or animals, firms are required to provide these and other records to the FDA within four hours during certain business hours, or eight hours at other times. Transporters (e.g., trucking companies, private delivery carriers, railroads, and airlines) are also required to keep similar documentation, including information about all means of transportation used.

Farms, restaurants (including all operations that prepare food for, or serve food directly to, consumers), fishing vessels not engaged in processing, and firms regulated exclusively by the U.S. Department of Agriculture, are exempted from the new record-keeping requirements. With some exceptions, foreign facilities are excluded if their food products undergo further manufacturing/processing, including packaging, by another facility outside the United States. Retail food operations are exempted from maintaining records on immediate subsequent recipients of foods sold directly to consumers.

The FDA's Center for Food Safety and Applied Nutrition has set priorities not only emphasizing the prevention of terrorism on the food supply and handling transmissible diseases from food to humans, they have also added emphasis on food additives, dietary supplements, and food biotechnology and increased their attention on food allergens. Twenty cents out of every dollar we spend goes toward a product under the jurisdiction of the FDA. There are 1,900 field operatives in the FDA workforce who also have responsibility for the multibillion-dollar drug and cosmetic industries. The FDA's Center for Food Safety has 904 full-time employees, including office personnel, down from 924 in 2001. They are dedicated public servants but they must deal with the fact that some contaminated, diseased food such as listeria-tainted cheeses can kill quickly and the FDA can react rapidly, but cancer-causing or neurotoxic additives may cause damage and kill slowly over twenty years or more.

## BIOTECH FOODS

Biotechnology is an umbrella term covering a vast variety of processes for using living organisms (such as plants, animals, and microbes) or any part of these organisms to create new or improved products. It includes the newer forms of genetic engineering, which offer a faster and more precise and controllable means to manipulate genes than traditional breeding and selection techniques. The science has been applied to plants, animals, and foods. Genetic engineering may genuinely alarm countries to which we export our products or be used as an excuse to ban imports competitive with national producers. Although the idea of genetic manipulation frightens a lot of consumers, biotechnology is not really new. For thousands of years humans have used bacteria and yeast to produce foods such as cheese and bread. In the 1860s, the scientist Gregor Mendel discovered the genetic principles of selective and crossbreeding. Using Mendelian genetics, the agricultural community bred hybrid forms of many crops, selecting traits that made them more resilient and otherwise desirable. Such breeding methods largely accounted for the phenomenal gains in productivity during the twentieth century.

The most common goals of biotechnology today are to create a longer shelf life, expand the ability to grow and ship perishable products, and to make produce and animals more productive and disease resistant. Biotechnology is often divided into old and new varieties. The older forms include plant and animal breeding and fermentation, which are based on the use of whole living organisms. The newer biotechnologies use parts of living organisms, manipulating the chromosomes or DNA strands or the genetic sequences that control specific traits. Biotech tomatoes, for example, travel better, look very appealing, and reportedly have more resistance to fungus and insects. Biotech canola oil has more unsaturated fats while biotech soybeans reportedly have more nutritive value.

Questions have been raised about whether genetic manipulation may introduce toxins and allergens into foods. Naturally occurring toxins are present at low levels in many foods. Although they have seldom posed a safety problem, they could cause illness if concentrated at high levels and consumed in large quantities. The introduction of allergens creates hazards for sensitive individuals, which has prompted the Food and Drug Administration to require special labeling for such products. Indeed, there may be changes in some products but producers claim that in many cases these alterations improve nutritive value.

The FDA says that it will review genetically altered foods if:

- the concentration of any naturally occurring toxins in the plant has been increased.
- an allergen not commonly found in the plant has been introduced.
- the levels of important nutrients have changed.
- new substances have been introduced into food that raise safety questions.
- if there is a problem with an environmental effect.
- if accepted, established scientific practices have not been followed.

The U.S. Department of Agriculture regulates the products of biotechnology but not the process itself. It requires notification for genetically engineered crops that are field-tested in accordance with specific safety criteria. In addition it has special requirements that companies have to satisfy before slaughtering transgenic animals. They must describe any drugs or chemicals given to the animals, along with the biological techniques and products used. Before granting approval for slaughter, the USDA tries to scrutinize safety on three levels:

1. Any hazards introduced by the transgene, that is, the genetic material introduced into the animal.

2. The safety of the final food product.

3. Any secondary changes in the animal caused by the insertion of new DNA.

Some consumer and environmental groups believe that the FDA's approach fails to protect public health because, in their view, genetic engineering poses unique food and environmental safety risks that warrant premarket testing and review. These groups contend that the FDA's policy allows manufacturers too much discretion in determining the safety of new food products before marketing them. Some believe that genetic engineering is a radical new technology—not an extension of traditional breeding—and will introduce products that have not been a part of the food supply. Some argue that the new techniques allow genetic modifications that were not possible with traditional breeding methods.

Other countries have been developing biotechnology products: Japan and China have created many products similar to those under development in the United States and are actively working on more. Japan, for example, has produced a low-allergen variety of rice. China currently has many test plots of transgenic plants under cultivation. Europe is actively exploring biotechnology. The nations of Europe, however, have been unable to reach a uniform agreement on the regulations governing biotechnology. As a result, the research remains mostly in the laboratory with few field studies under way. In 2004, U.S. Agriculture Secretary Ann Veneman said her agency is studying whether to adopt a risk-based system to protect the environment and food supply. She said the agency aims to protect conventional plants and to ease requirements for monitoring long-term environmental effects of genetically engineered plants. The department issued a statement saying it also may use the process for allowing products onto the market "to provide flexibility for long-term marketing."

There is also an entity known as the Precautionary Principle (PP) that was introduced into the United Nations in 1972. It has been an object of debate ever since. Basically, it was intended to provide environmental risk managers with a tool for decision making about extraordinary environmental threats, such as ship bilge dumping and chemical spills. Since its introduction, it has expanded to a wide base of environmental concerns including genetically modified foods and food additives including the bovine growth hormone (BST) *(see)*. Supplementing cows' natural levels of BST reportedly improves their efficiency as milk producers by 5 to 10 percent without proportionally increasing production costs. PP is not recognized in the United States but the European Union, Canada, and the

World Health Organization have adopted it. Many in the United States and elsewhere feel that the PP is sometimes just used as an excuse to prevent competitive imports of food products. Still, those who favor the PP say that people have a duty to take anticipatory action to prevent harm. The burden of proof of the harmlessness of a new technology, process, activity, or chemical lies with the proponents, not with the general public. Before using a new technology, process, or chemical, or starting a new activity, people have an obligation to examine "a full range of alternatives" including the alternative of doing nothing and decisions applying the precautionary principle must be "open, informed, and democratic" and "must include affected parties."

Organic Consumers Association is a grassroots nonprofit organization concerned with food safety, organic farming, sustainable agricultural, fair trade, and genetic engineering (biotech, biotechnology, transgenic). Keyword issues: genetically engineered food, Genetically Modified Organism (GMO), mad cow, CJD, BSE (mad cow disease), organic food, permaculture, BGH, genetically engineered, bovine growth hormone, animal cloning, plant cloning, food labeling, food contamination, pesticide, animal feed, organic farms, food safety, food irradiation, activism, anti-globalization, grassroots, fair trade, and fair trade coffee. The OCA believes that consumers will have no way of knowing which whole and processed foods are genetically engineered. Vegetarians and religious groups with dietary restrictions could unwittingly eat fruits and vegetables that contain unlabeled genetic material from insects, fish, fowl, pigs, and other animals. This consumer group is also concerned that bioengineered plants may have elevated levels of allergens or toxins. The European Parliament approved legislation on July 3, 2003, to require labels for food and feed made with genetically altered ingredients, a move that was hailed by environmentalists but pilloried by U.S. farmers. Intended to inform European consumers, the legislation requires supermarkets to label all foods containing more than 0.9 percent of genetically modified organisms. The legislation also requires genetically modified foods like grains to be traced from their creation to the EU through the processing stage and into the supermarket.

The FDA does not require special labeling for foods to indicate whether or not a food or food ingredient is a bioengineered product.

## Identifying Nutritious Foods

The goal of this dictionary is not only to help you find foods that use safe ingredients but also nutritious foods that will aid your family's health. Again the label is the best tool for locating and evaluating the nutritional content of foods. The key here is the nutritional chart required on almost every foodstuff since the middle of the 1990s. It provides very valuable information but can be somewhat confusing. The following are explanations that will make it clearer and more useful for you.

Daily values (DV) comprise two sets of references for nutrients:

1. Daily Reference Values (DRVs)
2. Reference Daily Intakes (RDIs)

## DAILY REFERENCE VALUES (DRVs)

These designations are for nutrients for which no set of standards previously existed, such as fat, cholesterol, carbohydrates, proteins, and fibers. DRVs for these energy-producing nutrients are based on the number of calories consumed per day. For labeling purposes, 2,000 calories has been established for calculations. This level was chosen, in part, because many health experts say it approximates the maintenance calorie requirements of the group most often targeted for weight reduction: postmenopausal women.

DRVs for the energy-producing nutrients are calculated as follows:

- Fat based on 30 percent of calories.
- Saturated fat based on 10 percent of calories.
- Carbohydrates based on 60 percent of calories.
- Protein based on 10 percent of calories.
- Fiber based on 11.5 grams of fiber per 1,000 calories.

The DRVs for cholesterol, sodium, and potassium, which do not contribute calories, remain the same no matter what the calorie level. Because of the links between certain nutrients and specific diseases, DRVs for some nutrients represent the uppermost limit considered desirable. Eating too much fat or cholesterol, for example, has been linked to heart disease and too much sodium to the risk of high blood pressure. Therefore, the label shows you a product has less than the uppermost limits of DRVs for fats, cholesterol, and sodium which are:

- total fat: less than 65 g
- saturated fat: less than 20 g (total saturated fat now includes trans fats *(see)*
- cholesterol: less than 300 mg
- sodium: less than 2,400 mg

## REFERENCE DAILY INTAKES (RDIs)

A set of dietary references based on and replacing the Recommended Dietary Allowances (RDAs) for essential vitamins and minerals and, in selected groups, protein. You will continue to see vitamins and minerals expressed as percentages on the label but these figures now refer to the Daily Values.

Here are the RDIs—once familiar to us as RDAs:

| Nutrient | Amount |
|---|---|
| vitamin A | 5,000 International Units (IU) |
| vitamin C | 60 milligrams (mg) |
| thiamin | 1.5 mg |
| riboflavin | 1.7 mg |
| niacin | 20 mg |
| calcium | 1.0 gram (g) |
| iron | 18 mg |
| vitamin D | 400 IU |
| vitamin E | 30 IU |
| vitamin $B_6$ | 2.0 mg |
| folic acid | 0.4 mg |
| vitamin $B_{12}$ | 6 micrograms (mcg) |
| phosphorus | 1.0 g |
| iodine | 150 mcg |
| magnesium | 5 mg |
| copper | 2 mg |
| biotin | 0.3 mg |
| pantothenic acid | 10 mg |

The mandatory and voluntary dietary components on the label and order in which they must appear are:

- total calories
- calories from fat
- calories from saturated fat (including trans fats)
- stearic acid (on meat and poultry products only)

- polyunsaturated fat
- monounsaturated fats
- cholesterol
- sodium
- potassium
- dietary fiber
- soluble fiber
- insoluble fiber
- sugars
- sugar alcohol (for example, the sugar substitutes xylitol, mannitol, and sorbitol)
- other carbohydrates (the difference between total carbohydrates and the sum of dietary fiber, sugars, and sugar alcohol if declared)
- protein
- vitamin A
- percent of vitamin A present as beta-carotene
- vitamin C
- calcium
- iron
- other essential vitamins and minerals

If a food is fortified or enriched with any of the optional components, or a claim is made about any of them, pertinent additional nutrition information becomes mandatory. These mandatory and voluntary components are the only ones allowed on the nutrition panel.

When a caloric value for a serving of food is fewer than 5 calories, the FDA allows the label to read "zero" calories. If a fat calorie is less than 0.5 grams, it can be listed as "calories from fat zero."

# Guiding Principles for Nutrition Labeling and Fortification (2004)

Government agencies are not satisfied with the information on food labels. One of the major problems is that they do not know how much we read the labels. Another is that as new scientific information about the effects of what we eat on our health becomes available, recommendations should change. The current percent Daily Values (%DV) that appear on your food labels are partly based on 1968 RDA *(see)* and in Canada, the nutrient information is from that nation's 1983 Recommended Nutrient Intakes (RNIs). The U.S. Institute of Medicine has been working to develop four more categories:

1. The Estimated Average Requirement (EAR): The average daily nutrient intake level estimated to meet the requirement of half the healthy individuals in a particular life stage and gender group.

2. The Adequate Intake (AI): The recommended average daily intake level based on observed or experimentally determined approximations or estimates of nutrient intake by a group (or groups) of apparently healthy people that are assumed to be adequate—used when an RDA cannot be determined.

3. The Recommended Dietary Allowances (RDAs): The average daily dietary nutrient intake level sufficient to meet the nutrient requirement of 97–98 percent of healthy individuals in a particular life stage and gender group.

4. Tolerable Upper Intake Levels (UL): The highest average daily nutrient intake level that is likely to pose no risk of adverse health effects to almost all in the general population. As intake increases above the UL, the potential risk of adverse effects may increase.

These reference values are replacements for the former RDAs in the United States and the RNIs in Canada, harmonizing the recommendations of both.

The nutrition label experts are also working on the acceptable macronutrient distribution range (AMDR): a range of intakes of a particular energy source (nutrient) associated with a reduced risk of chronic disease.

## No Nutrition Information

Some foods are exempt from nutrition labeling. Due to space limitations, small packages such as a candy bar do NOT have to provide nutrition information on the label. However, an address or telephone number must be provided for shoppers who wish to obtain this material. It is important for consumers to realize that products produced and sold in the same state and not shipped interstate, or that do not have ingredients that move interstate, are not subject to FDA regulations. Other foods that do not have to provide nutrition labeling include:

- Food produced by small businesses. The FDA defines a small business as one with food sales of less than $50,000 a year or total sales of less than $500,000. The Food Safety and Inspection Service of the U.S. Department of Agriculture (FSIS) defines a small business as one employing five hundred or fewer employees and producing no more than a certain amount of product per year.
- Food served for immediate consumption, such as that served in restaurants and hospital cafeterias, on airplanes, and by food service vendors (such as mall cookie counters, sidewalk vendors, and vending machines).
- Ready-to-eat foods that are not for immediate consumption, as long as the food is primarily prepared on site, for example, many bakery, deli, and candy store items.
- Food shipped in bulk, as long as it is not for sale in that form to consumers.
- Medical foods.
- Plain coffee and tea, flavor extracts, food colors, some spices, and other foods that contain no significant amounts of any nutrients.
- Donated foods.
- Products intended for export.
- Individually wrapped U.S.-Department-of-Agriculture's-Food-and-Safety-Inspection-Service-regulated products weighing less than half an ounce and making no nutrient content claims.

Although these foods are exempt, they are free to carry nutrition information when appropriate as long as it complies with the new regulations.

Bioengineered food such as "Flavr Savr" tomato and milk produced with bovine somatotropin (BST) *(see)* are not listed on labels. Government agencies, in fact, forbid dairy food producers to say that no BST was used in their products.[5]

Besides the panel giving specific information about the nutritional value (or lack thereof) of foods, there are other terms that indicate nutritional value:

---

[5]Keith Schneider, "FDA Warns the Dairy Industry Not to Label Milk Hormone-Free," *New York Times,* February 8, 1994, p. 1.

## Food Grade

The USDA has established grades for more than three hundred food products. Grading for most products is done voluntarily at the manufacturer's request (and expense) by a USDA inspector, and a USDA grade symbol may then appear on the package; lack of a symbol does not mean substandard product. Unfortunately, these grades lack continuity among product categories (Grade AA is the highest grade for eggs; Grade A is the highest for milk). Meat and poultry, however, whether fresh or processed and packaged, must be inspected and carry an inspection stamp.

## Special Dietary Information or Disinformation

- *Low calorie* . . . fewer than 40 calories per serving.
- *Low sodium* . . . 140 mg or fewer per serving.
- *Very low sodium* . . . fewer than 35 mg per serving.
- *Sodium free* . . . fewer than 5 mg per serving.
- *Low fat* . . . 3 g or fewer per serving.
- *Low saturated fat* . . . means 1 g or fewer per serving.
- *Low cholesterol* . . . signifies 20 mg or fewer per serving.
- *High or source of* . . . denotes the beneficial presence of a nutrient such as fiber or vitamins.
- *High or excellent source of* . . . contains 20 percent or more of the Daily Value *(see)* for a particular nutrient in a serving.
- *Good source of* . . . supplies 10 to 19 percent of the Daily Value *(see)* for a particular nutrient.
- *Reduced* . . . means a product has been nutritionally altered and contains at least 25 percent less of a nutrient (such as fat) or 25 percent fewer calories than the regular product.
- *Less* . . . means a product contains 25 percent less of a nutrient or 25 percent fewer calories than the reference food. For example, pretzels that have 25 percent less fat than potato chips could carry a "less" claim.
- *Light or lite* . . . signifies a product contains one-third fewer calories or half the fat of the comparison food. "Light in sodium" may be used on

food in which the sodium content has been reduced by at least 50 percent.

- *More* . . . means a product contains at least 10 percent more of the Daily Value *(see)* for a desirable nutrient, such as fiber, than the regular food.
- *Fresh* . . . signifies a food that has not been heat processed or frozen and supposedly contains no preservatives.
- *Lean and extra lean* . . . describes the fat content of meats, poultry, seafood, and game meats. Lean = fewer than 10 g fat per serving. Extra lean = fewer than 5 g fat per serving.
- *Percent fat free* . . . used only to describe foods that qualify as low fat.
- *High potency* . . . describes a nutrient in a food that is 100 percent or more of the RDI *(see)* established for that product. The term may also be used with multi-ingredient products if two-thirds of the nutrients are present at 100 percent of the RDI.
- *Antioxidant* . . . may be used in conjunction with currently defined claims for "good source" and "high" to describe a nutrient scientifically shown to be absorbed in a sufficient quantity such as vitamin E to inactivate free radicals *(see)* or prevent free radical–initiated chemical reactions in the food.

Sometimes, you have to learn to read between the lines. There are terms on packages that may be misleading. For example "unsalted," "processed without salt," or "no salt added" may signify that the producer didn't put any additional salt in during processing but the food may still be naturally high in sodium. For example, a low sodium soy sauce has 390 mg of sodium per teaspoon (who can use only a teaspoon of soy sauce on a dish?) and a popular tomato-vegetable drink with "no salt added" has 90 milligrams per 4.5 fluid ounces. Salt can also be listed under dozens of "sodium" designations such as monosodium glutamate and sodium caseinate adding additional salt to your diet. Sugar labeling, like salt, can be deceptive. A food can be labeled "sugar free" or "sugar-less" and still contain calories from sugar alcohols *(see)* such as xylitol, sorbitol, and mannitol.

## *Organic, Natural, or What?*

The purchase of "organic foods" has reportedly been increasing by 20 percent a year since 1990, even though they are usually more expensive than nonorganic products. Organic purports that animals and crops are grown without additives including pesticides, antibiotics, and hormones. How do you know a product is really organic? Government organic food labeling regulations went into effect in 2002. The USDA put in place a set of national standards that foods labeled "organic" must meet, whether grown in the United States or imported. If growers do not follow the regulations, they can be fined up to $10,000 for each violation. A government-approved certifier inspects the farm where organic food is grown to make sure the farmer is following all the necessary rules. If you see the USDA Organic seal, the item is at least 95 percent organic. If the label says "made with organic ingredients," the product must contain at least 70 percent and up to 95 percent organic ingredients, excluding water and salt. The USDA seal cannot be used on these. For products with less than 70 percent organic ingredients, labels are allowed to list the organic items in the ingredient panel only, but not display the word "organic" on front. In 2003, however, four months after the standards took effect, Congress passed legislation permitting "organic" livestock to be fed nonorganic feed (which may include antibiotics and pesticides) when organic feed is twice the price of conventional feed. It took ten years of hard-fought negotiations to get the USDA standards passed but it took just some backroom time to weaken the regulations.

Natural and organic are not interchangeable. Other truthful claims, such as free-range, hormone-free, and natural, can still appear on food labels. However, don't confuse these terms with "organic." Only food labeled "organic" has been certified as meeting USDA organic standards, according to the USDA.

## *Pesticides*

When pesticide chemical residues occur in processed foods due to the use of raw agricultural commodities that bore or contained a pesticide chemical in conformity with an exemption granted or a tolerance prescribed by American or European agencies, the processed food will not be regarded as adulterated so long as good manufacturing practice has been followed in removing any residue from the raw agricultural commodity in the processing (such as by peeling or washing) and so long as the concentration of the residue in the processed food when ready to eat is not greater than the tolerance prescribed for the raw agricultural commodity. But if the residue in the processed food we are ready to eat is higher than the tolerance prescribed for the raw agricultural stuff from which it was made, the processed food is adulterated. How can we know how much of the pesticide remains in what we are eating? Unfortunately, we can't, especially if it comes from a country with unskilled and sometimes illegal application of chemicals.

# Who Checks
# the Nutritional Analysis of a Product?

Being on a low salt diet, I have often wondered who checks the analysis of a product for the amount of sodium or any other ingredient. The FDA does not approve, and is not in a position to endorse or recommend, specific laboratories. The FDA tells food processors: "assistance may be available through the following sources: trade and professional associations, trade publications, colleges and universities, and by looking in local phone books under testing or analytical laboratories. For compliance purposes, FDA uses appropriate methods published by the Association of Analytical Chemists in Official Methods of Analysis of the AOAC International."

When researchers at Columbia University, in New York City, checked the calorie content of packaged foods, they found the actual calories as much as three and a half times higher than the labels indicated. The blatant underestimations occurred with regionally sold foods rather than with national brands.[6] See Appendix A "What Counts as a Serving?"

# Fighting Obesity

The federal government wants to reduce the huge number of Americans who are obese, so the FDA is looking for ways to revise labeling on food packages to help you count calories. At this writing, the rules have not been set but are likely to include the percentage of the recommended daily calorie intake a product contains. The Agency, recognizing that most people consume a whole snack package and/or soda at once, proposes that the labels list the total calories instead of just a theoretical "serving." The FDA is also proposing that restaurants provide calorie and other health information on their menus. The government agency is recommending increased enforcement to ensure accurate labeling and research on healthier foods and better weight-loss drugs.

In the meantime, could a food additive other than sugar be, in large part, responsible for the current increase in obesity? Fructose *(see)* has been used to sweeten food and soft drinks since the 1970s. The introduction of the high-fructose, corn-based sweetener dovetailed with the beginning of the sharp rise in obesity rates, which has set alarm bells ringing among public

---

[6]Roger Field, "Calorie Counts on Food Labels Can Be Misleading," *Medical Tribune,* October 21, 1993, p. 3.

health officials. Consumption of high-fructose corn sweeteners increased more than 1,000 percent between 1970 and 1990, far exceeding changes in intake of any other food or food group. The corn fructose additives account for 40 percent of all sweeteners added to food and drink and are the only sweeteners used in the production of U.S. soft drinks. George Bray, a professor at the Louisiana State University System's Pennington Biomedical Research Center pointed out in 2004 that body weights rose slowly for most of the twentieth century until the late 1980s. Since that time, many countries showed a sudden increase in the rate at which obesity has been galloping forward and Bray and other academic and government scientists believe that high-fructose sweetened foods may be a major cause.

## LOW-CARB

The newest craze, quickly taken up by food producers, is the low-carb diet. Books such as those by the late Robert Atkins, M.D., and the newer *The South Beach Diet* by Arthur Agatston, M.D., have promoted meat, eggs, and other fatty foods over carbohydrates *(see)*. While the phenomenon may not last too long, the shelves of the supermarkets are increasingly filled with products containing fewer carbohydrates. They achieve the "low-carbs" by doing such manipulations as replacing wheat flour with soy flour; adding extra fiber and high-fat ingredients, and replacing sugar with sugar alcohols *(see)*. The FDA as of this writing has not set standards for labeling products as "low-carb."

# Avoiding Certain Additives

Contrary to public belief, food additives are not a modern innovation. Adding chemicals to food began in the dawn of civilization when man first discovered that by adding salt to meat, the meat would last longer.

The father of modern food additives laws was Dr. Harvey W. Wiley, who in the early 1900s led the fight against chemical preservatives such as boric acid, formaldehyde, and salicylic acid. He dramatized the problem by his famous "Poison Squad" comprised of young men willing to be guinea pigs, which meant eating measured amounts of these chemicals to determine toxicity. As a result of Dr. Wiley's pioneering work, the first Federal Food and Drug Act was passed in 1906.

The FDA operates the Adverse Reaction Monitoring System (ARMS) to help serve as an ongoing safety check of all additives. The system monitors and investigates complaints by individuals or their physicians that are believed to be related to specific foods, food and color additives, or vitamin and mineral supplements. The ARMS computerized database helps officials decide whether reported adverse reactions represent a real public health risk associated with food so that appropriate action can be taken. You and your loved one are unique, however. An additive that may not bother someone else at your table may be upsetting and in rare cases extremely serious to you and/or yours. Below are some of the major potential problems, especially if you suffer from allergies, food sensitivities, a compromised immune system, diabetes, high blood pressure, heart problems, or a genetic susceptibility to cancer.

## AVOIDING SALT

The basic sources of cereals are salt free—wheat, corn, rice, and oats. Yet instant oatmeal may contain 360 mg per serving, instant corn grits 590 mg, and instant cream of wheat 180 mg. If you're willing to cook the noninstant cereals, you can avoid the high salt. It's providing the "instant" that dishes out the sodium. Some seventy sodium compounds are used in foods, as you will see in this book. The National Academy of Sciences, whose experts establish dietary guidelines, recommends that we ingest no more than 2,400 milligrams of sodium for the entire day. The average American ingests 3,500 to 7,000 milligrams. (A teaspoon of salt has about 2,000 milligrams of sodium.) If the numbers for sodium look very low on a label, look again and be aware of the difference between milligrams (mg) and grams (g). Some companies make you think there is less by saying 2 grams of sodium, for example, which is really 2,000 milligrams.

## AVOIDING SUGAR

Sugar, as you may recall, also masquerades under a variety of names and can be difficult to avoid. Common names such as sucrose, fructose, and corn syrup may be familiar to readers but a food can be labeled "sugar free" or "sugar-less" and still contain calories from sugar alcohols such as xylitol, sorbitol, and mannitol. Saccharin is a nonnutritive sweetener—that is, it has no calories. Aspartame has the same calories as sugar, but is so much sweeter that only small amounts are needed to provide the desired sweetness in a product.

We may even be getting more than we bargained for when we get our sweets from fruit juice. A popular brand of diet fruit juice has a beautiful picture of an open pineapple and a cut orange on its label proclaiming it to be "sugar free" and "low sodium." It is, however, artificially colored with FD and C Yellow No. 5 and No. 6, both recognized allergens, flavored with benzoate of soda—a flavoring agent and also a common allergen—and sweetened with saccharin and aspartame. Now from what tree was that concoction harvested?

## AVOIDING ALLERGENS

Seven million Americans are estimated to have food allergies and even minuscule amounts of allergens can cause severe reactions and may even be lethal. But under the current law, manufacturers can add small amounts of allergens as incidental ingredients without mentioning them on packaging, listing them instead as "natural flavors." According to the American Academy of Allergy, Asthma, and Immunology, more than thirty thousand people a year are rushed to emergency rooms in the United States because of food allergies.

An allergic reaction to certain food additives may range from an itchy, runny nose or sore throat to indigestion and even death. Any food may cause an allergic reaction, but the eight most common offenders identified are milk, fish, wheat, peanuts, eggs, soybeans, tree nuts, shellfish, rice, and corn.

Food allergens—those parts of foods that cause allergic reactions—are usually proteins. Most of these allergens can still cause reactions even after they are cooked or have undergone digestion in the intestines. Numerous food proteins have been studied to establish allergen content. In some food groups, especially tree nuts and seafood, an allergy to one member of a food family may result in the person being allergic to all the members of the same group. This is known as cross-reactivity. However, some people may be allergic to both peanuts and walnuts, which are from different food families; these allergies are called coincidental allergies, because they are not related. Within animal groups of foods, cross-reactivity is not as common. For example, people allergic to cow's milk can usually eat beef, and patients allergic to eggs can usually eat chicken.

The only specific treatment for food allergy is avoidance but escaping a food allergen in the form of a hidden additive is not simple. For example, if you were allergic to corn, you would have to try and avoid corn sugar, dextrose, and corn syrup. You would have to know that they are used in maple, nut, and root beer flavorings for beverages, ice cream, ices, candy, and baked goods. The syrup is also used in bacon, baking mixes, powders, beers, bourbon, breads, cheese, cereals, chop suey, chow mein, confectioners' sugar, cream puffs, fish products, ginger ale, hams, jellies, processed meats, peanut butters, canned peas, plastic food wrappers, sherbets, whiskeys, and American wines. It may also be found in corn chips, fritters, frostings, canned or frozen fruit, graham crackers, gravies, grits, gum, monosodium glutamate, oleomargarine, pablum, tortillas, vinegar, yeasts, bologna, baking powder, bath powder, frying fats, and fruit juices. Sulfites and peanuts (*see* both), which may be in foods as additives, are among the most common causes of the life-threatening allergic reaction, anaphylaxis *(see)*.

As pointed out, it is difficult to avoid certain allergenic food additives but it can help if you read the listings for the additive to which you know you are allergic and note the foods to which it may be added. By reading the dictionary, you will learn about various names for an additive you may want to avoid. For example, milk may not be listed as an ingredient on a label; rather, the label may list casein (a milk protein), sodium caseinate, or milk solids. Not every food that contains wheat identifies it as such; sometimes wheat is listed as gluten. Similarly, egg white is frequently listed as albumin. The FDA is moving toward requiring the most common food allergens—peanuts, soybeans, milk, eggs, fish, crustaceans, tree nuts, and wheat—to be listed on the label if a product contains them: a benefit, if it comes to fruition.

Food intolerance is sometimes confused with food allergy. Food intolerance refers to an abnormal response to a food or food additive. It differs from an allergy in that it does not involve the immune system. For instance, you may have uncomfortable abdominal symptoms after consuming milk. This reaction is most likely caused by a milk sugar (lactose) intolerance in which you may lack the enzymes to break down milk sugar for proper digestion. Other food intolerance reactions may be triggered by druglike chemicals in some foods. Symptoms can include nervousness after consuming caffeine in coffee or soft drinks, headaches triggered by chemicals in cheese and chocolate, or various adverse reactions to chemicals and preservatives added to food, called food additives. The most common food additives that may cause sensitivity reactions include aspartame, benzoates, BHA and BHT, FD and C dyes Yellow No. 5 and Red No. 3, monosodium glutamate (MSG), nitrates/nitrites, parabens and sulfites *(see* all). Your allergist/immunologist can help you determine the difference between intolerance and allergy and help you in establishing a management plan.

## AVOIDING HYPERACTIVITY

In the 1970s, some scientists suggested that food additives or colors may be linked to childhood hyperactivity. Since that time, well-controlled studies have been conducted and have produced no evidence that food additives or colors cause hyperactivity or learning disabilities in children. In 1982, the Consensus Development Panel of the National Institutes of Health (NIH) concluded that there was no scientific evidence to support the claim that additives or colorings cause hyperactivity. Subsequent scientific studies continue to support the NIH panel's conclusion. I suspect parents of hyperactive children who eat sugar or colored foods and become wild may believe differently. The Feingold Program has a great deal of information on this topic (see page 46).

## AVOIDING SUSPECTED CANCER-CAUSING ADDITIVES

A major report on the relationship between nutrition and the development of cancer concludes that 3 to 4 million cases of cancer per year could be prevented by appropriate diet.[7]

# The Delaney Amendment

Written by Congressman James Delaney, the amendment was part of the 1958 law requested by the Food and Drug Administration. The law stated that food and chemical manufacturers had to test additives before they were put on the market and the results had to be submitted to the FDA. Delaney's amendment specifically states that "no additive may be permitted in any amount if the tests show that it produces cancer when fed to man or animals or by other appropriate tests." Ever since it was enacted, it has been severely attacked by food and chemical manufacturers, the Nutrition Council of the American Medical Association, and several FDA commissioners. The FDA commissioners claim it is unenforceable.

The Food and Drug Administration amended its regulations regarding carcinogenic compounds used in food production in 2003 and revised the definition of the term "No Residue" in the New Animal Drug Regulations.[8] The original rule was put in place in 1985 to protect against the known carcinogen diethylstibesterol (DES) *(see)* given to animals to make them put on weight. The DES proviso provided that the FDA could approve an animal feed additive or a new animal drug that induces cancer if there were "no residue" of such additive or drug found after slaughter. The FDA also revised in the definition of "Preslaughter withdrawal period or milk discard time" the phrase "for the residue of carcinogenic concern in the edible product to deplete to the concentration that will satisfy the operational definition of 'no residue'" by adding in its place "at which no residue is detectable in the edible product using the approved regulatory method (i.e., the marker residue is below the the Level of Detection (LOD)." This LOD is defined as the amount that might cause a cancer in one out of a million animals and since animals are not the whole human diet, the FDA and the producers' lawyers who forced this issue maintain the risk is slight or

---

[7]John R. Seffrin, Ph.D., CEO of the American Cancer Society and American Association for Health Educators School, "Personal Behaviors Are What Really Matters When It Comes to Avoiding Cancer," presented to the American Association for Health Educators, St. Louis, March 22, 1997.
[8]"Revision of the Definition of the Term 'No Residue' in the New Animal Drug Regulations," Federal Register, December 23, 2002, 67(246), Rules and Regulations.

nonexistent if we eat meat or drink milk from an animal with a minuscule bit of a carcinogen present.

The problems with identifying exposure to a cancer-causing additive are:

- In most instances exposure to cancer-causing agents (carcinogens) takes place twenty to thirty years before a statistically significant increase in cancer can be detected. Only then can it be adduced that the increase in cancer may have been caused by exposure to specific cancer-causing agents.

- Animal studies may give clues, but laboratory conditions and the bodies of other creatures may not result in valid conclusions for humans.

- Each of us is unique in the way our bodies process chemicals based on our age, sex, heredity, medical history, diet, and behavior. Epidemiologists estimate that approximately one-third of all cancer deaths can be attributed to diet.[9]

- No one can definitively say how much of a carcinogen causes cancer.

The Delaney Amendment, as pointed out, is being essentially ignored. The listings in this dictionary site the known or suspected additives that can be carcinogenic. There are well-known ones such as nitrates and nitrites *(see)*. If you can't resist bacon and processed meats that contain them, then you can reduce their effects by eating or drinking something high in vitamin C. If you want to avoid other additives such as saccharin or vinyl chlorides, you can by not buying products containing them.

While the testing of additives in our food for carcinogenicity may be imperfect, even less testing is being done to determine if food additives may be toxic to the brain and nerves, although a number of scientists believe that neurotoxins are even more of a problem in food than carcinogens.[10]

## *Avoiding Neurotoxins*

In humans, neurotoxicants can adversely affect a broad spectrum of behavioral functions, including the ability to learn, to interact appropriately with others,

---

[9]Robert J. Scheuplein, "Perspectives on Toxicological Risk—An Example: Food-borne Carcinogenic Risk," *Critical Reviews in Food Science and Nutrition,* 32(2): 105–21.

[10]Bernard Weiss, Ph.D., University of Rochester School of Medicine, *Nutrition Update* 1, 1983, pp. 21–38; Charles Vorhees and R. E. Butcher, *Developmental Toxicology,* ed. K. Snell (London: Croom Helm, 1982), 247–98.

and to perceive and respond to environmental stimuli; basically these represent everyday functions that enable people to live productive lives. The FDA is now focusing on neurotoxicity and is trying to develop more relevant information about the potential adverse effects of chemicals on the structural and functional integrity of the nervous system and should help obtain the information needed for a reasonable assessment of potential neurotoxic hazard."[11]

In the meantime, the dictionary cites those chemicals, such as monosodium glutamate and Red No. 3 (*see* both) that have been found to be suspected neurotoxins. Most of the chemicals identified as neurotoxins in the dictionary are pesticides, since they have long been identified with nerve damage. They are difficult to avoid unless you grow your own food without chemicals and don't buy processed edibles. You can reduce your intake by avoiding those additives listed in the dictionary that have been cited as potential neurotoxins such as glutamates used in flavorings, butyl phosphorotrithioate used in animal feed and the food coloring Red No. 3 (*see* all).

## What About Health Claims?

When you look at the shelves in a supermarket today, it's hard to determine whether you are buying cereal or a drink or a medicine with a breakfast food or fruit juice added. In fact, there is a whole category unofficially called nutraceuticals. Snapple's Fire claims it well help you keep your energy going with ginkgo biloba, ginseng, and guarana (*see* all) and if you feel stressed, Celestial Seasonings sells a brew that contains valerian, spearmint leaves, lemongrass, hawthorn berries, and orange blossoms (*see* all). Joint Juice contains glucosamine, a nutritional supplement believed to help rejuvenate joints and treat arthritis. Mott's Clamato Energgia, according to the company, is claimed to be the first vegetable juice–based energy drink geared toward the Latino market. It contains "energy-releasing herbs" like taurine, ginseng, guarana, and B vitamins (*see* all). If you need to stay awake, you may opt for Jolt Caffeine-Energy Gum. It contains guarana and ginseng (*see* both in the dictionary). Two pieces are claimed to contain the same amount of caffeine as one cup of coffee. It comes in spearmint and ice mint flavors. Dasani, owned by Coca-Cola, promotes a "7-Day Refresh Drink" that will make you "feel great about yourself" Dasani is, according to its promotion, "purified water with a unique blend of minerals." Another company, Provexis, at this writing, is hoping to put a "clot busting" health drink, CardioFlow, on the market. It contains an extract from tomatoes

---

[11]Thomas J. Sobotka, Ph.D., "Revisions to the FDA's Redbook Guidelines for Toxicity Testing: Neurotoxicity," *Critical Reviews in Food Science and Nutrition,* 32(2): 165–71.

which is said to have a beneficial effect in reducing the tendency for excessive blood clotting, which in some circumstances can lead to heart attacks, stroke, and deep vein thrombosis.

What about the health claims for everyday foods like cereals and vegetables? This is an area that has really burgeoned since the last edition of this book and the FDA is still struggling with it.

On December 18, 2002, the FDA announced a new initiative to encourage the flow of high quality, science-based information regarding the health benefits of conventional foods and dietary supplements to consumers.[12] In the last edition of this book, the FDA had approved only the following health claims on food labels:

- calcium and osteoporosis
- fat and cancer
- saturated fat and cholesterol and coronary heart disease (CHD)
- fiber-containing grain products, fruits and vegetables and cancer
- fruits, vegetables, and grain products that contain fiber, particularly soluble fiber, and coronary heart disease (CHD)
- sodium and hypertension
- oats and oat flour and cholesterol

In 2004, the FDA allowed the claim that walnuts lower HDL "bad" cholesterol. The U.S. Court of Appeals for the D.C. Circuit, however, ruled that the First Amendment does not permit the FDA to reject health claims that the agency determines to be potentially misleading unless the agency also reasonably determines that no disclaimer would eliminate the potential deception. The court ruled that a complete ban would be appropriate only when the government could demonstrate with empirical evidence that "those disclaimers" would bewilder consumers and fail to correct for deceptiveness. In the Federal Register of December 20, 2002, the FDA announced that it would apply this ruling to health claims in the labeling of conventional foods as well as dietary supplements.

The FDA will review all qualified health claims before they are used on a food label. This process will involve a full review of the available scientific evidence, and may include a detailed assessment by experts on scientific evidence affiliated with the Agency for Healthcare Quality Research or by other independent experts in addition to FDA staff as appropriate. The agency began applying these interim guidelines to health claim petitions submitted on or after September 1, 2003. In many of these activities, the FDA

---

[12]Pearson, 164 F.3d at 659–60.

announced that it is working closely with the Federal Trade Commission, the agency that helps regulate advertising.

One of the first health claims under the new rules is walnuts being helpful in warding off heart disease. Similar claims for other nuts are being evaluated at this writing.

While the FDA is struggling to identify false health claims, so are the members of the European Union. Researchers in Britain, however, have figuratively thrown in the towel. They have shown that consumers are prone to be misled by some health claims and thus proposed that only foods meeting a certain nutritional profile—those low in salt, sugars, or fat—be allowed to make a health claim.

The aim of this dictionary is to help you cut through the burgeoning health claim hype presented to you in the media and in the store.

## Understanding Additive Uses

Today, food processors have in their repository an estimated three thousand chemicals they can add to what we eat. Some are deleterious, some are harmless, and some are beneficial.

Every one of those chemicals used in food processing is supposed to serve one or more of the following purposes:[13]

- improve nutritional value
- enhance quality or consumer acceptability
- improve the keeping quality
- make the food more readily available
- facilitate its preparation

Other chemicals are added to improve the keeping quality of some products, processes that embalm them. Bread has sixteen chemicals to keep it feeling "fresh." One type of bread, balloon bread, undergoes rigor mortis thanks to its additive, plaster of paris. Ironically, when nothing is added to the foods, they cost us considerably more. Unbleached flour costs four times as much as bleached; untreated tomatoes five times as much as regular canned tomatoes, and unsulfured raisins are six times the cost of treated ones.

The purpose of this dictionary is to enable you to look up any additive under its alphabetical listing to determine whether this is something you want to be eating so you can reject cancer-causing agents or toxins.

---

[13]Food Protection Committee of the National Academy of Sciences, which evaluates the safety of additives, 1998.

This dictionary includes almost all the food additives in common use. For the sake of clarity and ease of use, I have grouped their nearly fifty functions under the following broad categories:

## PRESERVATIVES

These "antispoilants" are used to help prevent microbiological spoilage and chemical deterioration. There are many different types, of which about one hundred are in common use. Preservatives for fatty products are called antioxidants, which prevent the production of off-flavors and off-odors. Some common antioxidants include benzoic acid used in margarine and butylated hydroxyanisole (BHA) used in lard, shortenings, crackers, soup bases, and potato chips.

In bread, preservatives are usually "mold" inhibitors. They include sodium and calcium propionate, sodium diacetate, and such acetic substances as acetic acid and lactic acid. Sorbic acid and sodium and potassium salts are preservatives used in cheeses, syrups, and pie fillings.

Preservatives used to prevent mold and fungus growth on citrus fruits are called "fungicides." Sequestering agents, still another type of preservative, prevent physical or chemical changes that affect color, flavor, texture, or appearance. Ethylenediaminetetraacetic acid (EDTA) and its salts, for instance, are used to prevent the adverse effects of the presence of metals in such products as soft drinks where metal ions can cause clouding. Sequestrants used in dairy products to keep them "fresh and sweet" include sodium, calcium, and potassium salts of citric, tartaric, and pyrophosphoric acids. Other common multipurpose preservatives are the gas sulfur dioxide, propyl gallate, and, of course, sugar, salt, and vinegar.

Food processors have explored some novel food preservation systems. Consumers evidently prefer a preservative from a "natural source" which enables the processors to use the word "natural" on the label. Bacteriocins are not new; however, like nisin—derived from the starter bacteria for yogurt—they are now being employed to extend shelf life in a variety of food products. The use of bacteriocins is likely to be expanded in the future, especially in dairy and refrigerated foods.

## NONCHEMICAL PRESERVATION

- Modified and controlled atmosphere packaging relies on inhibiting microbial growth by excluding oxygen or by inhibitory concentrations of carbon dioxide. Expected to increase in use, particularly with fresh fruits and vegetables sold at retail.

- Irradiated food. When food is irradiated, it is loaded onto a conveyor belt and passed through a radiation cell where it is showered with beams of ionizing radiation produced by high radioactive isotopes. The radiation can inhibit ripening and kill certain bacteria and molds that induce spoilage, so that food looks and tastes fresh for up to several weeks. The process does not make food radioactive and does not change the food's color or texture in most cases. Does it destroy nutrients? Does it create radiolytic products in food after exposure that may cause genetic damage? Is irradiation less dangerous than some of the other chemicals added to foods as preservatives? These questions are being hotly debated. The FDA requires foods that have been irradiated to reveal that on the label and to display an international logo, a flower in a circle so you will be able to decide for yourself.

• Ohmic heating. An electric current is passed through the food to create heat from the electrical resistance within the food. This technology is used for heat-sensitive foods, but some enzymes are difficult to inactivate with high-pressure processing.

• Pulsed electric field processing uses a very strong pulsed electric current to disrupt microbial cells and pasteurize foods with little or no heating.

• Bright light processing uses an intense white light to kill bacteria on the surface of foods; this light does not penetrate deeply into foods and can be used only for surface pasteurization.

• Aseptic processing. The aseptic filler is a highly specialized piece of equipment designed to sterilize the packaging material, pack the sterile product into its container in a sterile environment, and then seal the package.

• Microwave pasteurization. Microwave Technologies, Inc., in Sayerville, New Jersey, announced in 2003 the effectiveness of its microwave pasteurization technology for extending the shelf life of packaged fresh waffles at room temperature and of packaged French toast at refrigerated temperatures. The company claims that its technology to pasteurize freshly made packaged breakfast foods will enable manufacturers to extend shelf life up to six times longer than current shelf life without the use of any chemical preservatives. Ready to heat and serve breakfast foods have become a substantial part of the over $3 billion breakfast foods category.

• Fresh refrigerated products have grown along with busy households. They may have chemical preservatives but are designed to offer the convenience of frozen and canned foods while providing homemade taste and appearance. Typically, they are cooked just enough to ward off spoilage for a short period of time. As a further aid to freshness, they are often sealed in packaging that contains little or no oxygen that can extend shelf life for several weeks. Scientists, however, are concerned that some dangerous bacteria may not be killed during the minimal precooking and those microorganisms that cause botulism can flourish in an oxygen-free environment. One publicized outbreak of botulism associated with this category could devastate it.

# More Conventional Methods of Adding Additives Directly to Food for Various Purposes:

## ACIDS, ALKALIES, BUFFERS, NEUTRALIZERS

The degree of acidity or alkalinity is important in many processed foods. An acid such as potassium acid tartrate, sodium aluminum phosphate, or tartaric acid acts on the leavening agent in baked goods and releases the gas that causes the desired "rising." The flavor of many soft drinks, other than cola types, is modified by the use of an acid such as citric acid from citrus fruits, malic acid from apples, or tartaric acid, a component of grapes. Phosphoric acid is used to give colas the "tangy" taste. The same acids that are used in soft drinks are also used in churning cream to help preserve the flavor and keeping quality of butter. Alkalies such as ammonium hydroxide in cocoa products and ammonium carbonate in candy, cookies, and crackers are used to make the products more alkaline. Buffers and neutralizing agents are chemicals added to foods to control acidity or alkalinity, just as acids and alkalies are added directly. Some common chemicals in this class are ammonium bicarbonate, calcium carbonate, potassium acid tartrate, sodium aluminum phosphate, and tartaric acid.

## MOISTURE CONTENT CONTROLS

Humectants are necessary in the production of some types of confections and candy to prevent drying out. Without a humectant, shredded coconut, for example, would not remain soft and pliable. Substances used for this purpose include glycerin, which retains the soft, moist texture of marshmallows, propylene glycol, and sorbitol. On the other hand, calcium silicate is used to prevent table salt from caking due to moisture absorption from the air.

## PHYSIOLOGIC ACTIVITY CONTROLS

The chemicals in this group are added to fresh foods to serve as ripeners or antimetabolic agents. For instance, ethylene gas is used to hasten the ripening of bananas and maleic hydrazide is used to prevent potatoes from sprouting. Coming into increasing use are enzymes that are of natural origin and generally believed to be nontoxic. Of all food enzyme additives, amylases that act on starch have the most numerous applications. Various amylases from plant, animal, fungal, and bacterial sources have been used to break down the components of starch to make it more digestible. Enzymes are also used in the fermentation of sugar to make candy, in the brewing industry, and in the manufacture of artificial honey, bread, and frozen milk concentrates.

## BLEACHING AND MATURING AGENTS/BREAD IMPROVERS

Fresh ground flour is pale yellow. Upon storage, it slowly becomes white and undergoes an aging process that improves its baking qualities. For more than fifty years, processors have added oxidizing agents to the flour to accelerate this process, thus reducing storage costs, spoilage, and the opportunity for insect infestation. Compounds such as benzoyl peroxide bleach the flour without effect on baking qualities. Other compounds, such as oxides of nitrogen, chlorine dioxide, nitrosyl chloride, and chlorine have both a bleaching and maturing or "improving" ability. Bread improvers used by the baking industry contain oxidizing substances such as potassium bromate, potassium iodate, and calcium peroxide. They also contain inorganic salts such as ammonium or calcium sulfate and ammonium phosphates, which serve as yeast foods and dough conditioners. The quantities used are relatively small as these can easily result in an inferior product. Bleaching agents may also be used in other foods such as cheese to improve the appearance of the finished product.

## PROCESSING AIDS

Many chemicals fall into this category. Sanitizing agents, for instance, to clean bacteria and debris from products, are considered such aids. So are clarifying agents which remove extraneous materials. Tannin, for instance, is used for clarifying liquids in the wine and brewing industries. Gelatin and albumin remove small particles and minute traces of copper and iron in the production of vinegar and some beverages. Emulsifiers and emulsion stabilizers help to maintain a mixture and ensure consistency. They affect characteristics such as volume, uniformity, and fineness of grain (bakery products have a softer "crumb" and slower "firming" rate). They influence the ease of mixing and smoothness, such as the whipping property of frozen desserts and the smoothness of cake mixes. They help maintain homogeneity and keeping quality in such products as mayonnaise, candy, and salad dressing. Some common emulsifiers are lecithin, the monoglycerides and diglycerides, and propylene glycol alginate. Sorbitan derivatives are used to retard "bloom," the whitish deposits of high-melting components of cocoa butter that occasionally appear on the surface of chocolate candy. Food chemists sometimes call emulsifiers "surfactants" or "surface active-agents."

## TEXTURIZERS OR STABILIZERS

These are added to products to give them "body" and maintain a desired texture. For instance, calcium chloride or some other calcium salt is added to canned tomatoes and canned potatoes to keep them from falling apart. Sodium nitrate and sodium nitrite are used in curing meats to develop and stabilize the pink color. Nitrogen, carbon dioxide, and nitrous oxide are used in pressure-packed containers of certain foods to act as whipping agents or as propellants. The texture of ice cream and other frozen desserts is dependent on the size of the ice crystals in the product. By the addition of agar-agar, gelatin, cellulose gum, or some other gum, the size of the ice crystals is stabilized. Texturizer gums are also used in chocolate milk to increase the viscosity of the product and to prevent the settling of cocoa particles at the bottom of the container. Gelatin pectin and starch are used in confectionery products to give a desired texture. Artificially sweetened beverages also need bodying agents because they do not contain the "thickness" normally contributed by sugar. The thickeners employed include such natural gums as sodium alginate and pectins. The foaming properties of brewed beer can also be improved by the addition of texturizers.

## COLORING AGENTS

Food colors of both natural and synthetic origin are extensively used in processed foods and they play a major role in increasing the acceptability and attractiveness of these products. However, the indiscriminate use of color can conceal damage or inferiority, or make the product appear better than it actually is. The World Health Organization in delineating some 140 different kinds of colorants found many to be unsafe. Coal-tar colors were subject to a special provision in a 1938 law that required every coal-tar color used in food to be listed with the government as "harmless and suitable for use" and every batch of the color intended for use in food had to be certified by a government agency as safe. Some of the colors originally listed as "harmless" were found to produce injury when fed to animals and were removed from the list. In 1960, the federal government required manufacturers to retest all artificial colors to determine safety. At present there are nine permanently listed as safe. Among them FD and C Blue No. 1 and FD and C Citrus Red No. 2 have been shown to cause tumors at the site of injection in animals but the FDA does not consider this significant because the experiment concerned injection by needle and not by ingestion in food or application on the skin. FD and C Red No. 40, one of the most widely used colorings, is also being questioned because it is made from a base known to be carcinogenic and because many scientists feel that it should not have been given permanent listing based solely on the manufacturer's tests.

Among the natural colors used in foods are annatto, carotene, chlorophyll, cochineal, saffron, and turmeric (*see* all). Just because a color is natural doesn't necessarily mean it is completely safe. Annatto *(see),* for example, is being studied for toxicity. Foods that are frequently colored include candies, baked goods, soft drinks, and such dairy products as butter, cheese, and cream.

## FLAVORINGS

A wide variety of spices, natural extractives, oleoresins, and essential oils are used in processed foods. In fact, of the three thousand food additives known to be added to our food supply, two thousand are flavorings used to replace the flavors lost during processing. In addition, the modern flavor chemist has produced many synthetic flavors. Flavoring agents are the most numerous additive and they are increasing all the time with the influx of immigrants. The buying power of ethnic consumers in the United States is believed to have reached $1 trillion and ethnic foods are growing 9 percent annually. As the popularity of ethnic-type foods continues to grow and diversify, so do the new flavorings added to foods including natural and synthetic flavorings such as hibiscus, jalapeño, green chilies, coconut curry, beef bourguignon, hot peanut spice, teriyaki, guanabana, and tamarind.

About five hundred flavorings are natural and the remainder synthetic. They are usually employed in amounts ranging from a few to three hundred parts per million. Amyl acetate, benzaldehyde, carvone, ethyl acetate, ethyl butyrate, and methyl salicylate are typical compounds employed in the preparation of flavoring materials. However, many of the compounds used in synthetic flavorings are also found in natural products or derive from natural acids. Essential oils, such as oil of lemon and oil of orange, are natural flavors made by extraction of the fruit rind. There are also flavor enhancers, the commonest being monosodium glutamate (MSG) and maltol.

## NUTRITION SUPPLEMENTS

Enrichment of food means that the natural nutrients have been removed during processing and then replaced. Enrichment of cereal foods, much touted by the big producers, is supposed to provide 12 to 23 percent of the daily supply of thiamin, niacin, and iron, and 10 percent of the riboflavin recommended for human consumption.

Fortification of food means that additional nutrients are added to the product to make it more nutritious than it was before. For instance, vitamin C is added to orange drinks and vitamin A to margarine. Vitamin D is used to fortify milk to prevent rickets and potassium iodide is added to iodized salt to prevent goiter, a thyroid tumor caused by iodine deficiency. Some processors add certain amino acids, the building blocks of protein, to increase the protein component of their product.

## MISCELLANEOUS ADDITIVES

A number of additional substances are employed for various purposes. Certain sugar substitutes are used in food for persons who must restrict their intake of ordinary sweets. Saccharin and sorbitol are commonly used for this purpose. Glazes and polishes such as waxes and gum benzoin are used on coated confections to give luster to an otherwise dull surface. Magnesium carbonate and tricalcium phosphate are employed as anticaking agents in table salt, and calcium stearate is used for a similar purpose in garlic salt.

# More Information Is Needed on Food Additives

Although officially the FDA claims to know what additives are being used in food, FDA researchers report that it is impossible to check small manufacturers. Efforts have been made through the years to have food manufacturers register and provide the information. Ironically, thanks to the new bioterrorism threat, the FDA is asking food processors to register (see pages 9–11).

There is still much to learn about additives. Animal studies usually rely on feeding rats or mice with much higher levels of an additive than a human would be expected to eat, so that ill effects seen at such high doses may not occur at normal levels of consumption.

- Animal studies cannot model the effects of variation in amounts of additives eaten by people of all ages. For example, young children might eat large amounts of food colorings in sweets.
- Food additives might cause effects in humans that cannot be recognized in animals, for example, feeling sick or headaches.
- Animal studies are not likely to show whether an additive will cause an allergic reaction in humans.

• It is still uncertain that the safety of an additive that might be eaten by humans all their lives can be predicted by using animals which are given the additive for only up to two years. As you may conclude when you read the entries in this book, many additives are beneficial and necessary and others should be removed from our food supply as soon as possible.

# HOW TO USE THIS BOOK

While unique in content, this dictionary follows the format of most standard dictionaries. The following are sample entries with any explanatory notes that may be necessary.

**MARJORAM, POT** • Sweet Marjoram. The natural extract of the flowers and leaves of two varieties of the fragrant marjoram plant. The oleoresin *(see)* is used in sausage and spice flavorings for condiments and meats (3,500 ppm). The seed is used in sausage and spice flavorings for meats and condiments. Sweet marjoram is used in sausage and spice flavorings for beverages, baked goods, condiments, meats, and soups. The sweet oil is used in vermouth, wine, and spice flavorings for beverages, ice cream, ices, candy, baked goods, and condiments. Also used in hair preparations, perfumes, and soaps. Can irritate the skin. The redness, itching, and warmth experienced when applied to the skin are caused by local dilation of the blood vessels or by local reflex. May produce allergic reactions. Essential oils such as marjoram are believed to penetrate the skin easily and produce systemic effects. GRAS.

This entry says that pot marjoram is a natural flavoring extract, that there are two kinds of marjoram—pot and sweet. Both are utilized as an oleoresin, a seed, and as sweet oil. By looking up "oleoresin" we learn that it means a natural plant product consisting of essential oil and resin extracted from a substance, such as ginger, by means of alcohol, ether, or acetone and that oleoresins are usually more uniform and more potent than the original product. The "ppm" figures stand for "parts per million," that is, 3,500 parts of marjoram is added to a million parts of meat. However, because ppm amounts (they do not appear on labels) represent maximum rather than actual usage, they are not reliable estimates of consumption, and are included here only to show how amounts can be relatively large or small. GRAS means, of course, that the item is on the government's generally recognized as safe list although it may not have undergone laboratory testing. "GRAS in packaging" means that even though substances from the containers may migrate into the food, they are assumed not harmful.

**WORMWOOD** • Absinthium. A European woody herb with a bitter taste, used in bitters and liquor flavoring for beverages and liquors. The extract is used in bitters, liquor, and vermouth flavorings for beverages, ice cream, candy, and liquors, and in making absinthe. The oil is a dark green to brown and a narcotic substance. Used in bitters, apple, vermouth, and wine flavorings for beverages, ice cream, ices, candy, baked goods, and liquors. In large doses or frequently repeated doses, it is a narcotic poison, causing headache, trembling, and convulsions. Ingestion of the volatile oil or of the liquor, absinthe, may cause gastrointestinal symptoms, nervousness, stupor, coma, and death.

"Absinthium" is another name for wormwood (which is cross-referenced in the dictionary.) A similar example is the entry for lye.

**SODIUM SESQUICARBONATE** • Lye. White crystals, flakes, or powder produced from sodium carbonate. Soluble in water. Used as a neutralizer for butter, cream, fluid milk, ice cream, in the processing of olives before canning, cacao products, and canned peas. Used as an alkalizer in bath salts, shampoos, tooth powders, and soaps. Irritating to the skin and mucous membranes. May cause allergic reaction in the hypersensitive. The final report to the FDA of the Select Committee on GRAS Substances stated in 1980 that it should continue its GRAS status with no limitations other than good manufacturing practices.

Terminology generally has been kept to a middle road between technician and average interested citizen, while at the same time avoiding oversimplification of data. If in doubt, look up any term. Isolate (used in its chemical context), extract, or anhydride, for example, are in the entries describing chemicals but also have their own entries to help you clarify them. Many abbreviations have been used to save space but their definitions are listed in the dictionary and the major ones are right at the beginning of the text. With *A Consumer's Dictionary of Food Additives* you will be able to work with the current labels to determine the purpose and the desirability or toxicity of the additives listed. You will be able to assert your right to wholesome food along with a wholesome environment. By having options in the marketplace and by rejecting those products that are needlessly costly or unsafe or unpalatable in favor of "clean" food, you strike back at greed and ignorance as practiced by too many in the food industry. More importantly, you reward those manufacturers who deserve your purchases.

There is little doubt that what we eat affects our health. Our bodies are wonderful machines that can detoxify and render harmless many poisons we ingest, and we don't want to overburden them by taking unnecessary chances. Certainly, not all food additives are harmful. Some, in fact, are greatly beneficial. I hope this book will allow you to make wiser choices.

# If You Need More Information
# or Have a Problem

## UNITED STATES

A number of agencies offer information about food additives and benefits and difficulties they may cause.

If you have a problem that you think or know may be due to a food additive, the FDA, in particular, wants to know about it because that is how it discovers something may be wrong. The widespread distribution of food additives and consequent public safety concerns necessitate timely and reliable evaluation of suspected adverse reactions. Currently, consumer complaints related to food additives as well as other food products, are monitored by passive surveillance, carried out primarily by the Food and Drug Administration. Therefore, it is very important that should you have had an adverse reaction to a food product, you report it. To report an incident or to ask a question about a processed food ingredient, contact:

Consumer Inquiries: 888-INFO-FDA
The Office of Consumer Affairs
Food and Drug Administration, HFE-88
5600 Fishers Lane
Rockville, MD 20857

The FDA Food and Seafood Information Line is at 1-800-FDA-4010 (1-800-332-4010). Reports relating to dietary supplements appear on the FDA website but are updated only four time a year. This creates substantial delay between the time the FDA learns of an adverse reaction and others learn about it. Ideally, they should appear on the net as soon as the FDA learns about it. The FDA website is: http://www.FDA.gov.

Reporting Adverse Events
You can play an important public health role by reporting to the Food and Drug Administration any adverse events or other problems with FDA-regulated products. Timely reporting allows the agency to take prompt action. Report what happened as soon as possible. Have the following information ready:

- Description of the adverse event
- Name, address, and phone number of the doctor or hospital if emergency treatment was provided

- Name of product and manufacturer
- Any codes or identifying marks on the product label or container
- Name and address of the store where you purchased the product and the date of purchase.

To report an emergency that requires immediate action, such as a case of food-borne illness, call the FDA's main emergency number, staffed twenty-four hours a day: 301-443-1240.

To report a nonemergency adverse event, contact the FDA district office nearest you. Look up the FDA's phone number under the Department of Health and Human Services in the blue U.S. government section of the telephone directory. Or check the phone numbers listed by state at: www.fda.gov/opacom/backgrounders/complain.html.

If the problem involves meat or poultry, which are regulated by the U.S. Department of Agriculture, call the USDA hotline at 1-800-535-4555. Operates toll free weekdays 10–4 EST.

The USDA Center for Nutrition Policy and Promotion (CNPP) was created on December 1, 1994, and is the focal point within the USDA where scientific research is linked with the nutritional needs of the public. http://www.fns.usda.gov/fncs

USDA Organic Standards, National Organic Program
202-720-3252
USDA-AMS-TM-NOP, Room 4008 S. Bldg., Ag Stop 0268
1400 Independence SW
Washington, DC 20250
http://www.ams.usda.gov/nop

Integrated Risk Information System (IRIS), prepared and maintained by the U.S. Environmental Protection Agency (U.S. EPA)
Health assessment information on a chemical substance is included in IRIS only after a comprehensive review of chronic toxicity data by U.S. EPA health scientists from several program offices and the Office of Research and Development. For technical questions about the scientific information content in IRIS contact:

U.S. EPA Risk Information Hotline 301-345-2870
Fax: 301-345-2876; e-mail: Hotline.IRIS@epamail.epa.gov
http://www.epa.gov/iris/intro.htm

By regular mail:
IRIS
c/o ASRC
6301 Ivy Lane, Suite 300
Greenbelt, MD 20770

National Toxicology Program
The National Toxicology Program (NTP), within the U.S. Department of Health and Human Services, is an interagency program headquartered at the National Institutes of Health's National Institute of Environmental Health Sciences (NIEHS) located in Research Triangle Park, North Carolina.

Please send queries, comments, and suggestions to: ntpwm@niehs.nih.gov

If you want regulations strengthened and agencies such as the FDA and USDA well funded so they can more adequately protect our food supply, contact your senators and representatives. The phone number for the House and Senate office buildings is 202-224-3121.
If you want any federal agency, including the White House, the Federal Information Center (FIC) is 800-688-9889.

It can be frustrating trying to report something to agencies, especially if they have a push-this-number type system. Eventually, with persistence, you will be able to not only make yourself feel better, you will be protecting the rest of us from a similar adverse experience.

More consumer information:
If you have food allergies or think you might, you may contact:

American Academy of Allergy, Asthma and Immunology (AAAAI)
611 East Wells Street
Milwaukee, WI 53202
AAAAI Physician Referral and
Information Line
800-822-2762
www.aaaai.org

Allergy and Asthma Network: Mothers of Asthmatics
2751 Prosperity Avenue, Suite 150
Fairfax, VA 22031
800-878-4403
703-641-9595
http://www.aanma.org

Food Allergy and Anaphylaxis Network (FAAN)
10400 Eaton Place, Suite 107
Fairfax, VA 22030
703-691-3179 or 800-929-4040
http://www.foodallergy.org

Asthma and Allergy Foundation of America
1125 15th Street NW, Suite 502
Washington, DC 20036
800-7-ASTHMA
202-466-7643
http://www.aafa.org

American Dietetic Association
(answers questions about nutrition)
216 West Jackson Boulevard
Chicago, IL 60606-6995
312-899-0040 or 800-877-1600
http://www.EatRight.org

CSPI Center for Science in the Public Interest
(publishes *Nutrition Action Healthletter;* often petitions the FDA about
actual and potential problems with food additives)
1875 Connecticut Avenue NW, Suite 300
Washington, DC 20009-5728
http://www.cspinet.org/

Organic Consumers Association
6101 Cliff Estate Road
Little Marais, MN 55614
Activist or media inquiries: 218-226-4164; Fax: 218-353-7652
Información en Español: 415-271-6833
http://www.organicconsumers.org/index.htm

The Feingold® Program
The Dietary Connection to Better Behavior, Learning & Health
127 East Main Street, Suite 106
Riverhead, NY 11901
Contact: 800-321-3287 (U.S. only)
631-369-9340; Fax: 631-369-2988
http://www.feingold.org
e-mail: Help@feingold.org

Canadian Food Inspection Agency Headquarters
59 Camelot Drive
Ottawa, Ontario K1A 0Y9
613-225-2342; Fax: 613-228-6601
1-800-442-2342
http://www.inspection.gc.ca/english/directory/maindire.shtml

## EUROPEAN UNION

http://www.eurunion.org/legislat/Foodstuffs/FoodAdditivs.htm
European Union
Delegation of the European Commission to the United States
2300 M Street NW
Washington, DC 20037
Tel: 202-862-9500; Fax: 202-429-1766

## WORLD HEALTH ORGANIZATION INFORMATION SOURCES

Global Environment Monitoring System—Food Contamination Monitoring and Assessment Programme (GEMS/Food)
Food additives and contaminants resulting from food manufacturing and processing can also adversely affect health. Since 1976, WHO has implemented the Global Environment Monitoring System—Food Contamination Monitoring and Assessment Programme (GEMS/Food), which has informed governments, the Codex Alimentarius Commission, and other relevant institutions, as well as the public, on levels and trends of contaminants in food, their contribution to total human exposure, and their significance with regard to public health and trade.
Mail address:
WHO European Centre for Environment and Health, Rome Division
via Francesco Crispi
10-00187 Rome, Italy
Tel.: 0039 06 487751; Fax: 0039 06 4877599
www.who.int/fsf/gems.htm

FAO/WHO food additive evaluations can be searched at:
http://www.who.int/health_topics/food_additives/en/
http://www.who.int/foodsafety/chem/en/
e-mail: foodsafety@who.int

Joint FAO/WHO Expert Committee on Food Additives (JECFA)
http://www.who.int/pcs/jecfa/jecfa.htm

## Abbreviations Frequently Used in This Book

| | |
|---|---|
| **ASP** | The FDA's full up-to-date toxicology information has been sought. |
| **EAF** | There is reported use of the substance, but the FDA has not yet been assigned it for toxicology literature search. |
| **NEW** | There is reported use of the substance, and the FDA has an initial toxicology literature search in progress. |
| **NIL** | Although listed as added to food, the FDA has no current reported use of the substance, and therefore although toxicology information may be available in PAFA, it is not being updated. |
| **NUL** | The FDA has no reported use of the substance and there is no toxicology information available in PAFA. |
| **BAN** | The substance was formerly approved as a food additive but is now banned; there may be some toxicology data available. |
| **PAFA** | Priority-based Assessment of Food Additives. |
| **FDA** | United States Food and Drug Administration. |
| **GRAS** | Generally Recognized As Safe. |
| **USDA** | United States Department of Agriculture. |
| **E** | Approved by the European Union. |
| **FAO\WHO** | An international group of experts from the World Health Organization and the Food and Agriculture Organization of the United Nations. |

# A

**ABEYANCE** • The term used by the FDA that includes petitions that were filed and were found after detailed review by the Office of Food Additives (OFAS) to be deficient. The OFAS does not actively work on petitions in abeyance. When all the information required to address the deficiency or deficiencies is provided, a petition can be refiled with the FDA and assigned a new filing date.

**ABIES ALBA MILL** • *See* Pine Needle Oil.

**ABIETIC ACID** • Sylvic Acid. Chiefly a texturizer in the making of soaps. A widely available natural acid, water insoluble, prepared from pine rosin, usually yellow and composed of either glassy or crystalline particles. Employed to carry nutrients that are added to enriched rice in amounts up to .0026 percent of the weight of the nutrient mixture. Used also in the manufacture of vinyls, lacquers, and plastics. Little is known about abietic acid toxicity; it is harmless when injected into mice but causes paralysis in frogs and is slightly irritating to human skin and mucous membranes. May cause allergic reactions.

**ABSINTHIUM** • Extract or Oil. *See* Wormwood.

**ABSOLUTE** • The term refers to a plant-extracted material that has been concentrated but that remains essentially unchanged in its original taste and odor. Often called "natural perfume materials" because they are not subjected to heat and water as are distilled products. *See* Distilled.

**AC** • Abbreviation for Anticaking Agent.

**ACACIA** • *Acacia vera. Acacia senegal.* Gum Arabic. Egyptian Thorn. Catechu (from the Latin *Acacia catechu,* which is interchangeable with acacia). Acacia is the odorless, colorless, tasteless dried exudate from the trunk of the acacia tree grown in Africa, the Near East, India, and the southern United States. Its most distinguishing quality among the natural gums is its ability to dissolve rapidly in water. The use of acacia dates back four thousand years to when the Egyptians employed it in paints. Its principal use in the confectionery industry is to retard sugar crystallization and as a thickener for candies, jellies, glazes, and chewing gum. As a stabilizer, it prevents chemical breakdown in food mixtures. Gum acacia is a foam stabilizer in the soft drink and brewing industries. Other uses are for mucilage, and the gum gives form and shape to tablets. In 1976, the FDA placed acacia in the GRAS category as an emulsifier, flavoring additive, processing aid, and stabilizer in beverages at 2.0 percent, chewing gum at 5.6 percent; as a formulation aid, stabilizer, and humectant in confections and frostings at 12.4 percent; as a humectant stabilizer and formulation aid in hard candy at 46.5 percent; in soft candy at 85 percent; in nut formulations at 1.0 percent; and in all other food categories at 8.3 percent of the product. Medically, it is used as a demulcent to soothe irritations, particularly of the mucous membranes. It slightly reduces cholesterol in the blood. It can cause allergic reactions such as skin rash and asthmatic attacks. Oral toxicity is low. *See also* Vegetable Gums and Catechu Extract. GRAS. ASP. E

**ACCEPTABLE DAILY INTAKE (ADI)** • An estimate of the amount of a food additive, expressed on a body-weight basis, that can be ingested daily over a lifetime without appreciable health risk, according to the World Health Organization (1987).

**ACE K** • *See* Acesulfame Potassium.

**ACENAPHTHENE** • 1,2-Dihydroacenaphthylene. 1,8-Ethylenenaphthalene. Derived from coal tar, it is used as a dye intermediate in pharmaceuticals, insecticides, fungicides, and plastics. No absorption data are available for acenaphthene; however, by analogy to structurally related polycyclic aromatic hydrocarbons (PAHs), it would be expected to be absorbed from the gastrointestinal tract and lungs. The anhydride of naphthalic acid was identified as a urinary metabolite in rats treated orally with acenaphthene. Although a large body of literature exists on the toxicity and carcinogenicity of PAHs, primarily benzo[a]pyrene, toxicity data for acenaphthene are very limited. *See* coal tar.

**ACEPHATE (0-S-DIMETHYL ACETYLPHOSPHERAMIDOTHIOATE and 0-S-DIMETHYL PHOSPHORAMIDO THIOATE)** • A contact and systemic pesticide found in cottonseed meal resulting from application to growing crops. The FDA permits a tolerance of 8 ppm in cottonseed and 4 ppm in soybean meal resulting from application to growing crops.

**ACER SPICATUM LAM** • *See* Mountain Maple Extract.

**ACEROLA** • Used as an antioxidant. Derived from the ripe fruit of the West Indian or Barbados cherry grown in Central America and the West Indies. A rich source of ascorbic acid. Used in vitamin C.

**ACESULFAME POTASSIUM** • Acesulfame K. Sunette. Ace K. In a petition filed in September 1982, the American Hoechst Corporation asked for approval to make this nonnutritive sweetener two hundred times sweeter than table sugar for use in chewing gum, dry beverage mixes, confections, canned fruit, gelatins, puddings, custards, and as a tabletop sweetener. The petition, including fifteen volumes of research studies, said the sweetener is not metabolized and would not add calories to the diet. The FDA approved acesulfame K on July 27, 1988, for use in dry food products and for sale in powder form or tablets that can be applied directly by the consumer. It has about the same sweetening power as aspartame *(see),* but unlike aspartame, has no calories. Hoechst obtained approval to use acesulfame K as an ingredient in liquids and baked goods and candies. The sweetener had previously been approved for use in twenty countries including France and Britain. Pepsi and Coca-Cola use it in Europe and Canada in their diet drinks. The Food and Drug Administration said that four long-term animal studies in dogs, mice, and rats had not shown any toxic effects that could be pinned on the sweetener. However, the Center for Science in the Public Interest, a Washington, D.C.–based consumer group, sent a warning to the FDA more than six months before the sweetener's approval saying that animals fed acesulfame K in two different studies suffered more tumors than others that did not receive the compound. In another study cited by CSPI, diabetic rats had a higher blood level of cholesterol when fed the sweetener. The FDA said in a press release that it had considered the Center's concerns and concluded that "any tumors found were typical of what could routinely be expected and were not due to feeding with acesulfame K." Hoechst said that acesulfame is not metabolized by the body and is excreted unchanged by humans and animals. When heated to decomposition emits toxic fumes. ASP. E

**ACETAL** • A volatile liquid derived from acetaldehyde *(see)* and alcohol. Used in fruit flavorings (it has a nutlike aftertaste) and as a hypnotic in medicine. It is a central nervous system depressant, similar in action to paraldehyde but more toxic. Paraldehyde is a hypnotic and sedative whose side effects are respiratory depression, cardiovascular collapse, and possible high blood pressure reactions. No known skin toxicity. ASP

**ACETALDEHYDE** • Ethanal. Occurs naturally in apples, broccoli, cheese, coffee, grapefruit, and other vegetables and fruit. Used as a solvent. It is irritating to the mucous membranes. Its ability to depress the central nervous system is greater than that of formaldehyde *(see),* and ingestion produces symptoms of "drunkenness." Acetaldehyde is thought to be a factor in the toxic effect caused by drinking alcohol after taking the antialcohol drug Antabuse. Inhalation usually limited by intense irritation of lungs. Ingestion of large doses may cause death by respiratory paralysis. Skin toxicity not identified. GRAS. ASP

**ACETALDEHYDE DIISOAMYL ACETYAL** • Flavoring. Labeled GRAS by the Expert Panel of the Flavor and Extract Manufacturers Association in 2003.

**ACETALDEHYDE ETHYL CIS-3-HEXENYL ACETAL** • A synthetic flavoring. The FDA has as of this writing not yet done a thorough toxicology search. *See* Acetaldehyde.

**ACETALDEHYDE PHENETHYL PROPYL ACETAL** • Petital. A synthetic fruit flavoring additive for beverages, ice cream, ices, candy, and baked goods. *See* Acetaldehyde for toxicity. ASP

***p*-ACETAMIDOBENZOIC ACID** • *See* Benzoic Acid.

**ACETANISOLE** • A synthetic flavoring additive, colorless to pale yellow solid, with an odor of hawthorn or hay, moderately soluble in alcohol and most fixed oils. Acetanisole is used in butter, caramel, chocolate, fruit, nut, and vanilla flavorings, which go into beverages, ice cream, ices, candy, baked goods, and chewing gum.

**ACETATE** • Salt of acetic acid *(see)* used in liquor, nut, coffee, vanilla, honey, pineapple, and cheese flavorings for beverages, ice cream, sherbets, cakes, cookies, pastries, and candy. May be irritating to the stomach if consumed in large quantities.

**ACETIC ACID** • Occurs naturally in apples, cheese, cocoa, coffee, grapes, skim milk, oranges, peaches, pineapples, strawberries, and a variety of other fruits and plants. Vinegar is about 4 to 6 percent acetic acid and essence of vinegar is about 14 percent. It is used in cheese, baked goods, and animal feeds. Solvent for gums, resins, and volatile oils. Styptic, it stops bleeding when applied to a cut on the skin. Potential adverse skin reactions include irritation or itching, hives, and overgrowth of organisms that do not respond to germ-killers. In its glacial form (without much water) it is highly corrosive and its vapors are capable of producing lung obstruction. Less than 5 percent acetic acid in solution is mildly irritating to the skin. It caused cancer in rats and mice when given orally or by injection. GRAS. ASP. E

**ACETIC ACID, CITRONELLYL ESTER** • A flavoring additive found in oils of citronella geranium, and about twenty other oils. Colorless liquid; fruity odor. Used as a flavoring additive in mayonnaise, salad dressings, and sauces. Mildly toxic by ingestion. A human skin irritant.

**ACETIC ANHYDRIDE** • Acetyl Oxide. Acetic Oxide. Colorless liquid with a strong odor, it is derived from oxidation of acetaldehyde *(see)*. It is used as a dehydrating and acetylating additive (*see* Dehydrated and Acetylated) and in the production of dyes, perfumes, plastics, food starch, and aspirin. It is a strong irritant and may cause burns and eye damage. The FDA says there is no reported use of the chemical and no toxicology information is available. NUL

**ACETIC ETHER** • A synthetic additive, transparent, colorless liquid with a fragrant, refreshing odor, used in butter, butterscotch, fruit, nut, and spice flavorings for beverages, ice cream, ices, candy, baked goods (1,000 ppm), and chewing gum (4,000 ppm). Also used to coat vegetables.

**ACETISOEUGENOL** • White crystals with a clove odor, used as a flavoring additive. It is moderately toxic by ingestion. When heated to decomposition, it emits acrid smoke and irritating fumes. The FDA permits its use at a level not to exceed an amount reasonably required to accomplish the intended effect.

**ACETOACETIC ESTER** • *See* Ethyl Acetoacetate.

**ACETOIN** • Acetyl Methyl Carbinol. A flavoring additive and aroma carrier used in perfumery, it occurs naturally in broccoli, grapes, pears, cultured dairy products, cooked beef, and cooked chicken. As a product of fermentation and of cream ripened for churning, it is a colorless or pale yellow liquid or a white powder, has a buttery odor, and must be stored in a light-resistant container. It is used in raspberry, strawberry, butter, butterscotch, caramel, coconut, coffee, fruit, liquor, rum, nut, walnut, vanilla, cream soda, and cheese flavorings for beverages, ice cream, ices, candy, baked goods, margarine, gelatin desserts, cottage cheese, and shortenings. Mildly toxic by injection under the skin. A moderate skin irritant. When heated to decomposition it emits acrid smoke and fumes. GRAS. ASP

**2-ACETONAPHTHONE** • Orange Crystals. 2-Naphthyl Ketone. White crystalline solid with an orange blossom odor. Used as a flavoring additive. Moderately toxic by ingestion. A human skin irritant. When heated to decomposition it emits acrid smoke and fumes.

**ACETONE** • A colorless ethereal liquid derived by oxidation or fermentation and used as a solvent for spices. Not more than 30 ppm may be a residual in the product. It is also frequently used in nail polish removers and nail finishes and as a solvent for airplane dope, fats, oils, and waxes. Inhalation may irritate the lungs, and in large amounts it is narcotic, causing symptoms of drunkenness similar to ethanol *(see)*. In 1992, the FDA proposed a ban on acetone in astringent *(see)* products because it had not been shown to be safe and effective as claimed.

**ACETONE PEROXIDE** • Acetone *(see)* to which an oxygen-containing compound has been added. A maturing additive for bleaching flour and dough, it has a sharp, acrid odor similar to hydrogen peroxide. The food additive acetone peroxide may be safely used in flour, and in bread and rolls where standards of identity do not preclude its use. A strong oxidizing additive, it can be damaging to the skin and eyes. The Internet is full of instructions on how to make a bomb out of this additive. NIL

**ACETOPHENONE** • Acetyl Benzene. Benzoyl Methide. A synthetic additive derived from coal tar, with an odor of bitter almonds, used in strawberry, floral, fruit, cherry, almond, walnut, tobacco, vanilla, and tonka bean flavorings for beverages, ice cream, ices, candy, baked goods, gelatin desserts, and chewing gum. It occurs naturally in strawberries and tea and may cause allergic reactions. Poisonous by injection. Moderately toxic by ingestion. A skin and severe eye irritant. Narcotic in high concentrations. When heated to decomposition it emits acrid smoke and fumes. ASP

**ACETOSTEARIN** • Obtained from fats and oils, it is a glyceride *(see)* that the Select Committee on GRAS Substances stated in 1980 should be GRAS with no limitations. It is used as a protective coating for food and as a plasticizer. NUL *See also* Stearic Acid.

**ACETOXYDIHYDROTHEASPIRANE** • Flavoring from tobacco used in baked goods, instant coffee/tea, snacks, soups, seasonings, meat products, and tobacco. FEMA GRAS; used in cigarettes. EAF

**4-ACETYOXY-2,5-DIMETHYL-3(2H)FURANONE** • Synthetic balsam-like flavor. EAF

**4(*p*-ACETOXYPHENYL)-2-BUTANONE** • Synthetic flavoring. NIL

**ACETYL ACETONE** • Acetoacetone. Diacetyl Methane. Colorless to slightly yellow liquid with a pleasant odor. Used as a flavoring additive in food. The FDA requires it not be used in excess of the amount reasonably required to accomplish the intended effect. Moderately toxic if ingested, injected, or inhaled.

**ACETYL BENZENE** • *See* Acetophenone.

**ACETYLAMINO-5-NITROTHIAZOLE** • Acinitrazole. Trichloral. Tritheom. An animal drug used in turkeys and limited to 0.1 ppm in the bird's flesh by the FDA. When heated to decomposition emits toxic fumes.

**ACETYL BENZOYL PEROXIDE** • White crystals decomposed by water and organic matter. Used in medicine as a germicide and disinfectant. It is used to bleach flour. Toxic when ingested.

**ACETYL BUTYRYL** • *See* 2,3-Hexanedione.

**ACETYL-*o*-CREOSOL** • *See* *o*-Tolyl Acetate.

**3-ACETYL-2,5-DIMETHYL FURAN** • Yellow liquid with a strong roasted-nut odor, it is used as a flavoring additive. When heated to decomposition it emits acrid smoke and irritating fumes. The FDA has toxicology information on this food additive. GRAS. ASP

**2-ACETYL;-3,(5 or 6)-DIMETHYLPYRAZINE, MIXTURE OF ISO-MERS** • Flavoring additive used in baked goods, beverages, breakfast cereal, chewing gum, confectionery frostings, egg products, fats, fish products, frozen dairy, fruit ices, gelatins, gravies, hard candies, instant coffee and tea, jams, meat products, milk products, seasonings, snack foods, soft candy, and soups. ASP

**3-ACETYL-2,5-DIMETHYLTHIOPHENE** • A flavoring additive. ASP

**2-ACETYL-3-ETHYLPYRAZINE** • A flavoring additive. ASP

**ACETYL EUGENOL** • *See* Eugenyl Acetate.

**ACETYL FORMALDEHYDE** • *See* Pyruvaldehyde.

**ACETYL FORMIC ACID** • *See* Pyruvaldehyde.

**ACETYL HEXAMETHYL TETRALIN** • Synthetic musk used mostly in cosmetics but in some food additives. It is closely related to acetyl ethyl tetramethyl tetralin, which was voluntarily removed from perfumes when it was reported to cause nerve damage in animals. The "hexa" component was inserted to make the fragrances less volatile and less allergenic.

**ACETYLMERCAPTOHEXYL ACETATE** • Synthetic flavoring. EAF

***n*-ACETYL-L-METHIONINE** • Nutrient in foods except infant foods and products containing added nitrites/nitrates *(see both)*. Limited to 3.1 percent by weight of the total protein in the food. When heated to decomposition emits toxic fumes. ASP

**ACETYL METHYL CARBINYL ACETATE** • *See* Acetoin. ASP

**2-ACETYL-5-METHYLFURAN** • A synthetic flavoring. ASP

**2-ACETYL-3-METHYLPYRAZINE** • Synthetic flavoring used in baked goods, beverages, breakfast cereals, chewing gum, confectionery frostings, egg products, fats/oils, fish products, frozen dairy, fruit ices, gelatins, gravies, hard candy, instant coffee/tea, jams, meat products, milk products, seasonings, snack foods, soft candy, and soups. Declared GRAS by FEMA *(see)*. EAF

**4-ACETYL-2-METHYLPYRIMIDINE** • A flavoring, a nitrogen substance. NIL

**ACETYL-(*p*-NITROPHENYL)-SULFANILAMIDE** • A feed additive. *See* Sulfanitran.

**ACETYL NONYRYL** • *See* 2,3-Undecadione.

**ACETYL PELARGONYL** • *See* 2,3-Undecadione.

**ACETYL PENTANOYL** • *See* 2,3-Heptanedione.

**ACETYL PROPIONYL** • Yellow liquid. Soluble in water. Used as a butterscotch or chocolate-type flavoring. *See* 2,3-Pentanedione.

**2-ACETYL PYRAZINE** • Colorless to pale yellow crystals or liquid with a sweet popcornlike odor. Used as a flavoring additive. Skin and eye irritant. When heated to decomposition emits toxic fumes. GRAS. EAF

**2-ACETYLPYRIDINE** • Synthetic flavoring that is said to require in-depth toxicology studies by FEMA *(see)*. ASP

**2-ACETYL PYRROLE** • Light beige to yellow crystals with a breadlike odor used as a flavoring additive. When heated to decomposition emits toxic fumes. GRAS when used at a level not in excess of the amount reasonably required.

**4-ACETYL-6-TERT-BUTYL-1,1-DIMETHYL-INDANE** • A synthetic flavoring. ASP

**2-ACETYLTHIAZOLE** • Used in the manufacture of fungicides and dyes. ASP

**2-ACETYL-2-THIAZOLINE** • Flavoring isolated from lychee, a Chinese tropical fruit. EAF

**3-(ACETYLTHIO)-2-METHYLFURAN** • Intermediate used in the manufacture of food additives. EAF

***p*-ACETYL TOLUENE** • *See* 4-Methyl Acetophenone.

**ACETYL-*p*-TOLYL ACETATE** • *See p*-Tolyl Acetate.

**ACETYL TRIBUTYL CITRATE** • *See* Citric Acid.

**ACETYL TRIETHYL CITRATE** • A clear, oily, essentially odorless liquid used as a solvent and plasticizer. Moderately toxic by ingestion. When heated to decomposition it emits acrid smoke and fumes. *See* Citric Acid.

**ACETYL TRIOCETYL CITRATE PECTIN** • Citrus Pectin. A jelly-forming powder obtained from citrus peel and used as a texturizer and thickening additive to form gels with sugars and acids. Light in color. It has no known toxicity.

**ACETYL VALERYL** • Yellow liquid used as cheese, butter, and miscellaneous flavorings. *See* 2,3-Heptanedione.

**ACETYL VANILLIN** • *See* Vanillin Acetate.

**ACETYLATED** • Any organic compound that has been heated with acetic anhydride or acetyl chloride to remove its water. Acetylation is used to coat candy and other foods to hold in moisture. Acetic anhydride produces irritation and necrosis of tissues in vapor state and carries a warning against contact with skin and eyes.

**ACETYLATED DISTARCH ADIPATE and PHOSPHATE** • Starches *(see)* that have been modified to change their solubility and digestibility. The Select Committee on GRAS Substances stated in 1980 that there is no available evidence that demonstrates or suggests a hazard to the public when they are used at levels now current and in the manner now practiced. However, it is not possible to determine, without additional data, whether a significant increase in consumption would constitute a dietary hazard. They can continue GRAS with limitations on amounts that can be added to food. E

**ACETYLATED DISTARCH PROPANOL** • A starch *(see)* that has been modified to change its solubility and digestibility. The final report to the FDA of the Select Committee on GRAS Substances stated in 1980 that although no evidence in the available information on it demonstrates a hazard to the public at current use levels, uncertainties exist requiring that additional studies be conducted. GRAS status is continued while tests are being completed and evaluated, the FDA said in 1980. Since then, no action has been reported.

**ACETYLATED HYDROGENATED COTTONSEED GLYCERIDE** • *See* Cottonseed Oil and Acetylated.

**ACETYLATED HYDROGENATED LARD GLYCERIDE** • *See* Lard and Lard Oils.

**ACETYLATED HYDROGENATED VEGETABLE GLYCERIDE** • *See* Vegetable Oils.

**ACETYLATED MONOGLYCERIDES** • Acetylated mono- and diglyceride esters *(see)* of glycerin with acetic acid and edible fat-forming fatty acids. May be white to pale yellow liquids or solids. Bland tasting. Used as coating additives, emulsifiers, lubricants, solvents, and texture-modifying additives in baked goods, cake shortening, desserts, fruits, ice creams, margarines, meat products, nuts, oleomargarine, peanut butter, puddings, shortening, and whipped toppings. Use permitted by the FDA at a level not in excess of the amount reasonably required to accomplish the intended effects. When heated to decomposition it emits acrid smoke and irritating fumes.

**ACETYLATED OXIDIZED STARCH** • Thickener; stabilizer; binder; emulsifier. E

**ACETYLATED STARCH** • Acetate *(see)* is used to make the starch more digestible. The statement "ADI not specified" means that, on the basis of the available data (toxicological, biochemical, and other), the total daily intake of the substance, arising from its use or uses at the levels necessary to achieve the desired effect and from its acceptable background in food, does not, in the opinion of the FAO/WHO Committee, represent a hazard to health. For this reason, and for the reasons stated in individual evaluations, the establishment of an acceptable daily intake (ADI) is deemed unnecessary. E

**ACETYLATED SUCROSE DISTEARATE** • The acetyl ester of sucrose distearate. *See* Ester and Sucrose Distearate.

**ACETYLISOEUGENOL** • Isoeugenol Acetate. White crystals with a spicy, clovelike odor, it is used as an aroma and flavor carrier in foods. In perfumery, it is used especially for carnation-type odors.

**ACETYLMETHYL CARBINOL** • Slightly yellow liquid or crystals used as an aroma and flavor carrier. *See* Acetoin.

**2- or 3-ACETYLPYRIDINE** • Additives used in making synthetic food additives.

**2-ACETYLTHIAZOLE** • Found in beans, potatoes, artichokes, asparagus, beef, beer, brazil nuts, rice, boiled shrimp; synthetic flavoring used in snack foods. Also used in the manufacture of fungicides and dye. FEMA GRAS

**ACHILLEIC ACID** • *See* Aconitic Acid.

**ACID** • An acid is a substance capable of turning blue litmus paper red and of forming hydrogen ions when dissolved in water. An acid aqueous solution is one that has a pH *(see)* of less than 7. Citric acid *(see)* is an example of a widely used acid in foods.

**ACID HYDROLYZED PROTEINS** • Acid Hydrolyzed Milk Protein. Hydrolyzed Plant Protein (HPP). Hydrolyzed Vegetable Protein (HVP). Hydrolyzed (Source) Protein Extract. Composed mainly of amino acids, small peptides, and salts resulting from almost complete hydrolysis *(see)* of peptide bones in edible protein materials treated with heat or food-grade acids. The edible proteins used as raw materials are derived from corn, soy, wheat, yeast, peanuts, rice, or other suitable vegetable or plant sources, or from milk. Products may be in liquid, paste, powder, or granular form. Used as a flavoring additive or flavor enhancer in bologna, salami, sauces, and stuffing. Use at level not in excess of the amount reasonably required to accomplish the intended effect. When heated to decomposition it emits acrid smoke and irritating fumes.

**ACID-MODIFIED STARCHES** • Usually made by mixing an acid—such as hydrochloric or sulfuric—water, and starch at temperatures too low for gelatinization. When the starch has been reduced in viscosity to the degree desired, the acid is neutralized and the starch is filtered, washed, and dried. It is done so that starches can be cooked and used at higher concentrations than unmodified starches. Acid-modified starches are often used for salad dressings and puddings and as inexpensive thickening additives. The final report to the FDA of the Select Committee on GRAS Substances stated in 1980 that acid-modified starches are GRAS with no limitations.

**ACIDOPHILUS** • A type of bacteria that ferments milk and has been used medically to treat intestinal disorders.

**ACID POTASSIUM SULFITE** • *See* Sulfites.

**ACIDS** • *See* Acidulants.

**ACIDULANTS** • Acids. An acid is a substance capable of turning blue litmus paper red and of forming hydrogen ions when dissolved in water. An acid aqueous solution is one with a pH less than 7 (*see* pH). Acidulants are acids that make a substance more acid and function as flavoring additive to acidify taste, to blend unrelated flavoring characteristics, and to mask any undesirable aftertaste. Acidulants are also used as preservatives to prevent germ and spore growths that spoil foods. Acidulants control the acid-alkali (pH) balance and are used in meat curings to enhance color and flavor and as a preservative. Among the most common acids added to foods are acetic, propionic, and sorbic (*see all*).

**ACIFLUOREN, SODIUM** • Herbicide. FDA tolerances are 0.02 ppm residues in cattle and sheep, kidney and liver. Residues in rice, milk, and eggs is tolerated at 0.1 ppm.

**ACIMETON** • Lobamine. Banthionine. Cynaron. Methilanin. Neston. White crystalline platelets with a characteristic odor. Used as a dietary supplement and nutrient. Moderately toxic by ingestion and other routes. When heated to decomposition it emits toxic fumes. *See* Methionine.

**ACONITIC ACID** • Citridic Acid. Equisetic Acid. Achilic Acid. A flavoring additive found in beetroot and cane sugar. Most of the commercial aconitic acids, however, are manufactured by sulfuric acid dehydration of citric acid. It is used in fruit, brandy, and rum flavorings for beverages, ice cream, ices, candy, baked goods, liquors, and chewing gum. Also used in the manufacture of plastics and buna rubber. GRAS

**ACROLEIN** • A yellow, transparent liquid byproduct of petroleum produced by the oxidation of propylene. Sources include combustion of wood, paper, cotton, petroleum products, and polyolefins. Used in modifying food starch. Used in making plastics and metal products. Toxic, causes tearing and intense irritation of the upper respiratory tract. It is also a skin irritant and a fire hazard from heat and flame. The FDA says there is no reported use of the chemical and there is no toxicology information available. The latest IRIS (*see*) evaluation says that it may interfere with vitamin metabolism and may be why animals in studies have shortened longevity. It is also listed as a cancer-causing agent by Environmental Defense. NUL

**ACRYLAMIDE** • Colorless, odorless crystals soluble in water and derived from acrylonitrile and sulfuric acid. It is used in clarifying beet sugar or cane sugar juice and in cornstarch. It is also used as a thickener and suspending additive in nonmedicated animal feeds. It is toxic by skin absorption. On

April 24, 2002, researchers at the Swedish National Food Administration and Stockholm University reported finding the chemical acrylamide in a variety of fried and oven-baked foods. The initial Swedish research indicates that acrylamide formation is particularly associated with traditional high-temperature cooking processes for certain carbohydrate-rich foods. Since the Swedish report, similar findings have been reported by Norway, the United Kingdom, and Switzerland. Preliminary analysis by the FDA suggests that U.S. results will be in basic agreement with these findings. The discovery of acrylamide in foods is a concern because acrylamide is a potential human carcinogen and damaging to genes. Acrylamide appears to form as a by-product of high-temperature cooking processes (greater than 120°C/248°F). It does not appear to be present in food before cooking. Research to date suggests that acrylamide formation is particularly likely in carbohydrate-rich foods. However, tests on carbohydrate-rich foods cooked at lower temperatures (e.g., by boiling) have shown much lower acrylamide levels. The FDA says at this time not enough is known about acrylamide formation to identify safe modifications to food processing techniques that will clearly prevent or reduce formation. Identifying mechanisms of formation will ultimately be an important step in identifying ways to reduce or prevent acrylamide formation during cooking. Acrylamide causes cancer in laboratory animals and therefore is considered a potential human carcinogen. Scientists have conducted epidemiological studies of people exposed to acrylamide in the workplace. The studies did not show increased cancer risk with acrylamide exposure. However, these studies do not rule out the possibility that acrylamide in food can cause cancer, both because of the limited number of people in the studies and because the route of exposure for the workers was not through food. In June 2002, the World Health Organization (WHO) and the Food and Agriculture Organization (FAO) convened an expert consultation on acrylamide. The consultation, which was attended by three FDA experts, concluded that the presence of acrylamide in food is a major concern, and recommended more research on mechanisms of formation and toxicity. Both the WHO/FAO consultation and the FDA have recommended that people continue to eat a balanced diet rich in fruits and vegetables. The WHO/FAO consultation advised that food should not be cooked excessively, that is, for too long or at too high a temperature, but also advised that it is important to cook all food thoroughly—particularly meat and meat products—to destroy food-borne pathogens (bacteria, viruses, etc.) that might be present. As for acrylamides used in food processing, no emphasis was placed on them and the residues that we may be eating. Acrylamide is in a number of food additives used in processing and added to food products such as polyacrylamide *(see)* used as a thickener.

**ACRYLAMIDE-SODIUM ACRYLATE RESIN** • Used to dilute pesticides for application. NIL

**ACRYLATE-ACRYLAMIDE RESIN** • Acrylic Acid. Colorless, odorless crystals soluble in water and derived from acrylonitrile and sulfuric acid. It is used as a clarifying additive in beet sugar and cane sugar juice and liquor or corn starch hydrolysate (5 ppm by weight of juice, 10 ppm by weight of liquor or hydrolysate). It is also used in the manufacture of dyes, adhesives. It is toxic by skin absorption. ASP

**ACRYLIC ACID** • Colorless liquid with an acrid odor, it is derived by condensing ethylene oxide with hydrocyanic acid followed by reaction with sulfuric acid. It is used for making plastics and resins.

**ACRYLIC ACID-2-ACRYLAMIDO-2-METHYL PROPANE SUL-FONIC ACID COPOLYMER** • Used as a coating for film in contact with food or drinks. *See* Acrylic Acid. NUL

**ACRYLIC RESINS** • Polymers *(see)* of acrylics. Used in waxy oils, base coats, protective coatings, and waterproofing. Acrylates *(see)*, if inhaled, can cause allergic reactions in humans.

**ACRYLONITRILE COPOLYMERS** • Used in packaging materials. When heated to decomposition it emits acrid smoke and irritating fumes.

**ACRYLONITRILE POLYMER WITH STYRENE** • Used in coatings and films in packaging materials. No restrictions, but cyanide and its compounds are on the Community Right-to-Know List *(see)*. *See also* Styrene.

**ACTADECYLSILOXYDIMETHYLSIOLOXYPOLYSILOXANE** • A component of defoaming additives *(see)* used in processing beets and yeast.

**ACTIVATED CHARCOAL (CARBON)** • Charcoal is obtained by destructive distillation of organic material such as vegetables or animal bones and is activated by heating with steam or carbon dioxide, which results in a porous material. Used to remove impurities that cause undesirable color, taste, or odor in liquid. The major sources are lignite, coal, and coke. The Select Committee of the Federation of American Societies for Experimental Biology (FASEB), under contract to the FDA, concluded that it is not a hazard to human health at current or possible future use levels. However, the Committee said because the substance is extensively used in the food industry, it would be prudent to have purity specifications for food-grade activated carbon to assure the absence of any cancer-causing hydrocarbons in food. It can cause a dust irritation, particularly to the eyes and mucous membranes. It is used to relieve intestinal discomfort and diarrhea and to counteract poisons. It adheres to many drugs and chemicals inhibiting their absorption from the GI tract. Potential adverse reactions include black stools and nausea. ASP

**ACTIVATED 7-DEHYDROCHOLESTEROL** • *See* Vitamin $D_3$.

**ADENOSINE** • White crystalline powder with mild saline or bitter taste. It is isolated by the hydrolysis of yeast nucleic acid.

**ADENOSINE PHOSPHATE** • *See* Adenosine Triphosphate.

**ADENOSINE TRIPHOSPHATE** • Adenylic Acid. An organic compound that is derived from adenosine *(see)*. A fundamental unit of nucleic acid, it serves as a source of energy for biochemical transformation in plants, photosynthesis, and also for many chemical reactions in the body, especially those associated with muscular activity.

**ADI** • Abbreviation for Acceptable Daily Intake *(see)*.

**ADIPATES** • The salts of adipic acid *(see)* used in food packaging. Some are suspected cancer-causing additives.

**ADIPIC ACID** • Hexanedioic Acid. Colorless needlelike formations, fairly insoluble in water; found in beets. A buffering and neutralizing additive impervious to humidity. Used in flavorings for baked goods, baking powder, condiments, dairy products, meat products, oils, oleomargarine, relishes, snack foods, canned vegetables, beverages, and gelatin desserts (5,000 ppm) to impart a smooth, tart taste. Also used as a buffer and neutralizing additive in confections, but limited to 3 percent of contents and in the manufacture of plastics and nylons, and as a substitute for tartaric acid *(see)* in baking powders because it is impervious to humidity. The final report to the FDA of the Select Committee on GRAS Substances stated in 1980 that it should continue its GRAS status with no limitations other than good manufacturing practices. Poison by injection and moderately toxic by other routes. A severe eye irritant. ASP. E

**ADIPIC ANHYDRIDE** • A starch-modifying additive, not to exceed 0.12 percent of the starch compound. *See* Modified Starch. ASP

**ADSORBATE** • A powdered flavor made by coating liquid flavoring on the surface of a powder such as cornstarch, salt, or maltodextrin *(see all)*.

**AEROSOL** • Small particles of material suspended in gas.

**AFLATOXIN** • A mold that contaminates corn and peanuts. Poisonous by ingestion and moderately toxic by other routes. Carcinogenic and mutagenic.

**AGAR-AGAR** • Gelidium. Japanese Isinglass. A stabilizer and thickener, it is transparent, odorless, and tasteless, and obtained from various seaweed found in the Pacific and Indian Oceans and the Sea of Japan. Agar was the first seaweed to be extracted, purified, and dried. Discovered by a Japanese innkeeper around 1658 and introduced in Europe and the United States by visitors from China in the 1800s as a substitute for gelatin, it goes into beverages, ice cream, ices, frozen custard, sherbet, meringue, baked goods, jelly, frozen candied sweet potatoes, icings, confections, artificially sweetened jellies and preserves. It can be 1.2 percent of candy and 0.25 percent of frozen desserts, jelly, and preserves. Agar serves as a substitute for gelatin and is used for thickening milk and cream. It is also a bulk laxative, and aside from causing an occasional allergic reaction is nontoxic. The final report to the FDA of the Select Committee on GRAS Substances stated in 1980 that there is no evidence in the available information that it is a hazard to the public when used as it is now, and it should continue its GRAS status with limitations on amounts that can be added to food. Mildly toxic by ingestion. ASP. E

**AGAVE LECHUGUILLA** • American Aloe. Native to the warm part of the United States and known by its heavy, stiff leaf and tall panicle or spike of candelabralike flowers. The leaves are used for a juice employed in cosmetics as an adhesive and in medicines as a diuretic. The fermented juice is popular in Mexico for its distilled spirit (mescal).

**AGRIMONY EXTRACT** • An extract of *Agrimonia eupatoria,* an herb found in north temperate regions. It has yellow flowers and bristly fruit.

**AI** • Abbreviation for Adequate Intake. A value based on observed or experimentally determined approximations of nutrient intake by a group of healthy people. It is used when the RDA *(see)* cannot be determined.

**AKLOMIDE** • Gray scales from alcohol, it is used as an animal drug to combat fungus infections in chickens. The FDA residue tolerances are: 4.5 ppm in liver and muscle of uncooked edible tissue of chickens and 3 ppm in skin and fat.

**ALACHLOR** • Lasso. Alanex. A preemergent herbicide. The FDA permits its use. The EPA has determined it is a cancer-causing additive in rats and mice.

**ALANEX** • *See* Alachlor.

**ALANINE (B-, L-, and DL-)** • Colorless crystals derived from protein. A nonessential amino acid, it is used in microbiological research and as a dietary supplement in the L and DL forms. It is used as a flavor enhancer at 1 percent for pickling spice. It is now GRAS for addition to food. It caused cancer of the skin in mice and tumors when injected into their abdomens. ASP

**ALAR** • *See* Daminozide.

**ALBENDAZOLE** • Zental. Valbazen. A worm medicine given to cattle. The FDA tolerances for residues are: 0.2 ppm in uncooked edible cattle tissue; 0.6 ppm in muscle; 1.2 ppm in liver; 1.8 ppm in kidney; 2.4 ppm in fat.

**ALBUMEN** • *See* Albumin.

**ALBUMIN** • Albumen. A group of simple proteins composed of nitrogen, carbon, hydrogen, oxygen, and sulfur that are soluble in water. Albumin is usually derived from egg white and employed as an emulsifier in foods and cosmetics. May cause a reaction in those allergic to eggs. In large amounts can produce symptoms of lack of biotin, a growth factor in the lining of the cells. ASP

**ALBUMIN MACRO AGGREGATES** • Used as a binder and firming additive in sausage, soups, stews, and wine. Poisonous by injection.

**ALCOHOL** • Ethyl Alcohol. Ethanol. Alcohol is widely used as a solvent in the cosmetic and food fields. Alcohol is manufactured by the fermentation of starch, sugar, and other carbohydrates. It is clear, colorless, and flammable, with a somewhat pleasant odor and a burning taste. Medicinally used externally as an antiseptic and internally as a stimulant and hypnotic. Absolute alcohol is ethyl alcohol to which a substance has been added to make it unfit for drinking. Rubbing Alcohol contains not less than 68.5 percent and not more than 71.5 percent by volume of absolute alcohol and a remainder of denaturants, such as perfume oils. Toxic in large doses. *See also* Anisyl Alcohol.

**ALCOHOL, DENATURED** • This refers to ethyl alcohol, which is deliberately made unfit for drinking.

**ALCOHOL DENATURED FORMULA 23A** • Used as a diluent in color additive mixtures for coloring eggshells. NUL

**ALCOHOL, SDA-3A** • Diluent in color additive for marking food. *See* Alcohol, Denatured. NUL

**ALCOHOLS/PHOSPHATE ESTERS** • May be used at a level not to exceed 0.2 percent to assist in the lye peeling of fruit and vegetables.

**ALDEHYDE** • Used to flavor certain cherry ice creams and candy and snacks. *See* Aldehyde, Alipahatic.

**ALDEHYDE, ALIPHATIC** • A class of organic chemical compounds intermediate between acids and alcohols. Aldehydes contain less oxygen than acids and less hydrogen than alcohols. Most aldehydes are irritating to the skin and gastrointestinal tract.

**ALDICARB** • Temik. Crystals from isopropyl ether used as an insecticide, spider killer, and worm killer on citrus pulp in the growing crop. FDA tolerance is 0.6 ppm, 0.3 ppm in cottonseed hulls, and 0.5 ppm in sorghum.

**ALDRIN** • Aldrex. Altox. Drinox. A pesticide. Poison by ingestion, skin contact, intravenous, intraperitoneal, and other routes. Causes tumors, cancer, and birth defects. Human systemic effects by ingestion: excitement, tremors, and nausea or vomiting. Continued acute exposure causes liver damage.

**ALFALFA** • *Medicago sativa.* Herb and Seed. Lucerne. A natural cola, liquor, and maple flavoring additive for beverages and cordials. Alfalfa is widely cultivated for forage and is a commercial source of chlorophyll. GRAS. EAF

**ALGAE, BROWN** • Kelp. Ground, dried seaweed used to carry natural spices, seasonings, and flavorings. A source of alginic acid *(see).* Also used in chewing-gum base. All derivatives of alginic acid are designated "algin." The food industry is one of the major users of alginates *(see)* along with the pharmaceutical, cosmetic, rubber, and paper industries. The United States is the largest producer of alginates. The final report to the FDA of the Select Committee on GRAS Substances stated in 1980 that it should continue its GRAS status with no limitations other than good manufacturing practices. Nontoxic. NUL

**ALGAE MEAL, DRIED** • Permanently listed to be used in chicken feed to enhance color of chicken skin and egg yolks. NUL

**ALGANET** • Coloring additive used in casings and rendered fats. *See* Algae, Brown.

**ALGIN** • The sodium salt of alginic acid *(see)*, it is used in cheeses, frozen desserts, soda water, jellies, and preserves as a stabilizer. GRAS

**ALGINATES** • Ammonium, Calcium, Potassium, and Sodium. All derivatives of alginic acid are designated "algin." Gelatinous substances obtained from certain seaweed and used as stabilizers and water retainers in beverages, ice cream, ices, frozen custard, emulsions, desserts, baked goods, and confectionery ingredients. A clarifying additive for wine, chocolate milk, meat, toppings, cheeses, cheese spreads, cheese snacks, salad dressings, and artificially sweetened jelly and jam ingredients. Alginates are used also as stabilizers in gassed cream (pressure-dispensed whipped cream). The alginates assure a creamy texture and prevent formation of ice crystals in ice creams. Alginates have been used in the making of ice pops to impart smoothness of texture by ensuring that the fruit flavors are uniformly distributed throughout the ice crystals during freezing, helping the pops retain flavor and color, and to stop dripping. The final report to the FDA of the Select Committee on GRAS Substances stated in 1980 that there is no evidence in the available information that calcium, sodium, or potassium alginates are a hazard to the public when used as they are now, and their GRAS status will continue with limitations on the amounts that can be added to food. Alginates are also used as emulsifiers in hand lotions obtained from certain seaweeds and used as emulsifiers in creams, as thickening additives in shampoos, wave sets, and lotions. Ammonium alginate is used in boiler water and is not GRAS. ASP

**ALGINIC ACID** • Obtained as a highly gelatinous precipitate from seaweed. It is odorless and tasteless and is used as a stabilizer in ice cream, frozen custard, ice milk, fruit, sherbet, water ices, beverages, icings, cheeses, cheese spreads, cheese snacks, French dressing, and salad dressing. It is also used as a defoaming additive in processed foods. Capable of absorbing two hundred to three hundred times its weight of water and salts. The sodium carbonate *(see)* extracts of brown dried seaweed are treated with acid to achieve the result. Resembles albumin or gelatin *(see both)*. Alginic acid is slowly soluble in water, forming a thick liquid. WHO/FAO *(see)* observed that in a ninety-day study in rats, 15 percent alginate in the diet resulted in an enlarged, distended, heavy lower intestine, bumpy urinary bladder, and calcium deposits in the renal pelvis. A slight decrease in growth was also seen. The FAO/WHO Committee noted that alginic acid and its salts have a laxative effect at high level of intake. The committee did not set an ADI *(see)* for alginic acid. GRAS. EAF. E

**ALITAME** • A candidate for approval as an artificial sweetener, it has two thousand times the sweetness of sugar and no calories. Its potential use is in all areas requiring sweetening. It is derived from the amino acid alanine *(see)* and is related to aspartame *(see)*. The benefits include a clean, sweet taste, good stability at high temperatures, broad pH *(see)* range, and high water solubility. The drawbacks are the off-flavor from prolonged storage in some acidic solutions.

**ALKALI** • The term originally covered the caustic and mild forms of potash and soda. Now a substance is regarded as an alkali if it gives hydroxyl ions in solution. An alkaline aqueous solution is one with a pH *(see)* greater than 7. Sodium bicarbonate is an example of an alkali that is used to neutralize excess acidity.

**ALKALOID** • A compound of vegetable origin. Usually derived from a nitrogen compound such as pyridine, quinoline, isoquinoline, or pyrrole, designated by the ending -ine. Examples are atropine, morphine, nicotine, quinine, codeine, caffeine, cocaine, and strychnine. The alkaloids are potent and include the hallucinogen mescaline and the deadly poison brucine. There are alkaloids that act on the liver, nerves, lungs, and digestive systems.

**ALKANE** • *See* Alkanet Root.

**ALKANET ROOT** • Alkane Ferrous Sulfate. A red coloring obtained from extraction of the herblike tree root grown in Asia Minor and the Mediterranean. Used as a copper or blue coloring (when combined with metals) for hair oils and other cosmetics. It was also used as a coloring for wines, inks, and sausage casings. The FDA withdrew the authorization for use in 1988. NUL

**ALKANNIN** • A red powder and the principal ingredient of alkanet root *(see)*.

**ALKYL** • Meaning "from alcohol," usually derived from alkane. Any one of a series of saturated hydrocarbons such as methane. The introduction of one or more alkyls into a compound is to make the product more soluble. The mixture is usually employed with surfactants *(see),* which have a tendency to float when not alkylated.

**ALKYL BETAINES** • *See* Alkyl Sulfates.

**ALKYL ETHER SULFATES** • *See* Alkyl Sulfates.

*n*-**ALKYL (C12-C18) BENZYLDIMETHYL-AMMONIUM CHLORIDE** • A quaternary ammonium compound *(see)*.

*n*-**ALKYL (C12-C14) DIMETHYLETHYLBENZYL AMMONIUM CHLORIDE** • A quaternary ammonium compound *(see)*.

*n*-**ALKYL-HYDROXY-POLY(OXYETHYLENE)** • Quaternary ammonium compound used to wash sugar beets prior to slicing.

**ALKYL SULFATES** • Surfactants *(see)* used in foods, drugs, and cosmetics. The Germans during World War II developed these compounds when vegetable fats and oils were scarce. A large number of alkyl sulfates have been prepared from primary alcohols by treatment with sulfuric acid; the alcohols are usually prepared from fatty acids *(see)*. Alkyl sulfates are low in acute and chronic toxicity but may cause skin irritation.

**ALKYLENE OXIDE ADDUCTS OF ALKYL ALCOHOLS** • Used to assist in lye peeling of fruits and vegetables. FDA permits less than 0.2 percent in lye. NIL

**ALLERGEN** • A substance that provokes an allergic reaction in the susceptible but does not normally affect other people. Plant pollens, fungi spores, and animal danders are some of the common allergens.

**ALLERGIC CONTACT DERMATITIS** • ACD. Skin rash caused by direct contact with a substance to which the skin is sensitive. Symptoms include a red rash, swelling, and intense itching. Blisters may develop and break open, forming a crust. ACD may develop at any age and may be acute or chronic. Symptoms may appear seven to ten days after the first exposure to an allergen. More often, the allergic reaction doesn't develop for many years and may require many repeated low-level exposures. Once the sensitivity does develop, however, contact with the triggering allergen will produce symptoms within twenty-four to forty-eight hours. An attack builds in severity from one to seven days. Even without treatment, healing often occurs in one or two weeks, though it may take a month or longer.

**ALLERGIC REACTION** • An adverse immune response following repeated contact with otherwise harmless substances such as pollens, molds, foods, cosmetics, and drugs.

**ALLERGY** • An altered immune response to a specific substance, such as ragweed, pollen, on reexposure to it.

**ALLOMALEIC ACID** • *See* Fumaric Acid.

**ALLSPICE** • A natural flavoring from the dried berries of the allspice tree. Allspice is used in liquor, meat, and spice flavorings for beverages, ice cream, ices, candy, baked goods (1,400 ppm), chewing gum, condiments (1,000 ppm), and meats. Allspice oleoresin (a natural mixture of oil and resin) is used in sausage flavoring for baked goods, meat, and condiments. Allspice oil is used in sausage, berry cola, peach, rum, nut, allspice, cinnamon, ginger, nutmeg, and eggnog flavorings for beverages, ice cream, ices, candy, baked goods, chewing gum (1,700 ppm), condiments, pickles, meats, liquors, and soups. A weak sensitizer that may cause skin rash on contact. GRAS. ASP

**ALLURA RED** • *See* FD and C Red No. 40. E

**ALLYIC SULFIDES** • Found in garlic and onions, these compounds may protect against cancer-causing additives by stimulating production of a detoxification enzyme, glutathione-S-transferase.

**ALLYL-** • Prefix meaning, "derived from allyl alcohol" *(see)*.

**ALLYL ALCOHOL** • A colorless, pungent liquid made chiefly from allyl chloride heated to a thick substance in the presence of oxygen. It is used to make resins and plasticizers and as the basis for many synthetic flavorings.

*p***-ALLYL ANISOLE** • Esdragol. Isoanethole. Tarragon. Isolated from the rind of *Persea gratissima*, and from oil of estragon, found in oils of Russian anise, basil, fennel, turpentine, and others. A flavoring additive used in bakery products, both alcoholic and nonalcoholic beverages, chewing gum, confections, fish, ice cream, salads, sauces, and vinegar.

**ALLYL ANTHRANILATE** • A synthetic citrus fruit and grape flavoring additive for beverages, ice cream, ices, candy, baked goods, and gelatin desserts. ASP

**ALLYL BUTYRATE** • A synthetic butter, fruit, and pineapple flavoring additive for beverages, ice cream, ices, candy, baked goods, and gelatin desserts. ASP

**ALLYL CAPROATE** • 2-Propenyl-N-Hexanoate. Flavoring additive used in candy, gelatin desserts, puddings. Poison by ingestion and skin contact. An irritant to human skin.

**ALLYL CINNAMATE** • A light to yellow liquid with a cherry odor, it is used as a synthetic fruit and grape flavoring additive for beverages, ice cream, ices, candy, baked goods. Moderately toxic by ingestion. Human skin irritant. ASP

**ALLYL CROTONATE** • Used in the manufacture of vitamins and flavorings. ASP

**ALLYL CYCLOHEXANE ACETATE** • A synthetic pineapple flavoring additive for beverages, ice cream, ices, candy, baked goods. ASP

**ALLYL CYCLOHEXANE BUTYRATE** • A synthetic pineapple flavoring additive for beverages, ice cream, ices, candy, baked goods. ASP

**ALLYL CYCLOHEXANE HEXANOATE** • A synthetic fruit flavoring additive for beverages, ice cream, ices, candy, baked goods. ASP

**ALLYL CYCLOHEXANE PROPIONATE** • A synthetic, liquid and colorless with a pineapplelike odor, used in pineapple flavorings for beverages, ice cream, ices, candy, baked goods, gelatin desserts, puddings, chewing gum, and icings. Poisonous by ingestion. When heated to decomposition it emits acrid smoke and irritating fumes. ASP

**ALLYL DISULFIDE** • Found naturally in garlic and leeks but considered a synthetic flavoring. It is used in garlic, onion, and spice flavorings for meats and condiments. ASP

**ALLYL ENANTHATE** • *See* Allyl Heptanoate.

**AL1YL 2-ETHYLBUTYRATE** • A synthetic berry, fruit, and brandy flavoring additive for beverages, ice cream, ices, candy, baked goods, gelatin desserts, and puddings. GRAS. ASP

**ALLYL 2-FUROATE** • A synthetic coffee and pineapple flavoring additive for beverages, ice cream, ices, candy, baked goods, and gelatin desserts. GRAS. ASP

**ALLYL HEPTANOATE** • A synthetic berry, fruit, and brandy flavoring additive for beverages, ice cream, ices, candy, baked goods, gelatin desserts, and chewing gum. Moderately toxic by ingestion and skin contact. A human skin irritant. Combustible liquid. When heated to decomposition it emits acrid smoke and irritating fumes. GRAS

**ALLYL HEXANOATE** • A synthetic orange, strawberry, apple, apricot, peach, pineapple, and tutti-frutti flavoring additive for beverages, ice cream, ices, candy, baked goods, gelatin desserts, and toppings. GRAS. ASP

**ALLYL a-IONONE** • Cetone V. A synthetic additive, yellow, with a strong fruity, pineapplelike odor, used in fruit flavorings for beverages, ice cream, ices, candy, baked goods, gelatin desserts, and toppings. A skin irritant. GRAS

**ALLYL ISOTHIOCYANATE** • Mustard Oil. A naturally occurring additive in mustard, horseradish, and onion used in meat and spice flavorings for beverages, ice cream, ices, candy, condiments, meat, and pickles. Colorless or pale yellow with a pungent, irritating odor and acrid taste. It is used also in the manufacture of war gas. Can cause blisters and other skin problems. Toxic. ASP

**ALLYL ISOVALERATE** • Derived from valeric acid *(see)*, it is used as a flavoring. Listed as a cancer-causing agent by Environmental Defense. ASP

**ALLYL MERCAPTAN** • A synthetic spice flavoring additive for beverages, ice cream, ices, candy, baked goods, and meats. Poison by inhalation and ingestion. Strong irritant to the skin and mucous membranes. Dangerous fire hazard. ASP

**4-ALLYL-2-METHOXY PHENOL** • *See* Eugenol.

**ALLYL METHYL DISULFIDE** • A synthetic flavoring. *See* Allyl Alcohol and Sulfides. ASP

**ALLYL METHYL TRISULFIDE** • *See* Allyl Alcohol and Sulfides. NIL

**ALLYL NONANOATE** • A synthetic fruit and wine flavoring additive for beverages, ice cream, ices, candy, baked goods, and meats. ASP

**ALLYL OCTANOATE** • A synthetic pineapple flavoring additive for beverages, ice cream, ices, candy, baked goods, and gelatin desserts. Moderately toxic by ingestion. A skin irritant. ASP

**ALLYL PELARGONATE** • Liquid, fruity odor used in flavors and perfumes.

**ALLYL PHENOXYACETATE** • Acetate PA. A synthetic fruit and grape flavoring additive for beverages, ice cream, ices, candy, baked goods, and gelatin desserts. Moderately toxic by ingestion and skin contact. ASP

**ALLYL PHENYLACETATE** • A synthetic pineapple and honey flavoring additive for beverages, ice cream, ices, candy, baked goods. ASP

**ALLYL PROPIONATE** • A synthetic pineapple flavoring additive for beverages, ice cream, ices, candy, baked goods. ASP

**ALLYL SORBATE** • A synthetic fruit and grape flavoring additive for beverages, ice cream, ices, candy, baked goods, and gelatin desserts. ASP

**ALLYL SULFHYDRATE** • *See* Allyl Mercaptan.

**ALLYL SULFIDE** • A synthetic fruit and grape flavoring additive for beverages, ice cream, ices, candy, baked goods, condiments, and meats. Occurs naturally in garlic and horseradish. Irritates the eyes and respiratory tract. Readily absorbed through the skin. Acute exposure can cause unconsciousness. Long-term exposure can cause liver and kidney damage. ASP

**ALLYL THIOPROPIONATE** • A flavoring derived from the onion. ASP

**ALLYL TIGLATE** • A synthetic fruit and grape flavoring additive for beverages, ice cream, ices, candy, baked goods. ASP

**ALLYL 10-UNDECENOATE** • A synthetic fruit flavoring additive for beverages, ice cream, ices, candy, baked goods. ASP

**ALLYL UNDECYLENATE** • *See* Allyl 10-Undecenoate.

***p*-ALLYLANISOLE** • *See* Estragole.

**ALLYL THIOL** • *See* Allyl Mercaptan.

**4-ALLYLVERATROLE** • *See* Eugenyl Methyl Ether.

**ALMOND OIL** • Bitter Almond Oil. A flavoring additive from the ripe seed of a small tree grown in Italy, Spain, and France. Colorless or slightly yellow, strong almond odor, and mild taste. Used in cherry and almond flavorings for beverages, ice cream, ices, candy, baked goods, chewing gums, maraschino cherries, and gelatin desserts. Used also in the manufacture of liqueurs and perfumes. It is distilled to remove hydrocyanic acid (prussic acid), which is toxic. Nontoxic without the hydrocyanic acid. GRAS. ASP

**ALOE VERA** • A compound expressed from the aloe plant leaf from a South African lilylike plant. Used in bitters, vermouth, and spice flavorings for beverages (2,000 ppm) and alcoholic drinks. It contains 99.5 percent water, with the remaining 0.5 percent composed of some twenty amino acids *(see)* and carbohydrates. It has been used as a cathartic but was found to cause severe intestinal cramps and sometimes kidney damage. Cross-reacts with benzoin and balsam Peru in those who are allergic to these ingredients. EAF

**ALPHA-ACETOLACTATE DECARBOXYLASE** • An enzyme prepration derived from *Bacillus subtillis* modified by recombinant methods to contain gene coding for enzyme from *B.brevis*. Used as a processing aid in the production of alcoholic malt beverages and distilled liquors. EAF

**ALPHA-AMYLASE ENZYME PREPARATION FROM BACILLUS STEAROTHERMOPHILUS** • An enzyme used to modify food starch. (*See* Modified Starch) GRAS. EAF. *See* Bacillus Stearothermophilus.

**ALPHA-GALACTOSIDASE FROM MORTIERELLA VINACEAE** • An enzyme used in the production of sugar from sugar beets to increase sugar yield. No residue is permitted in finished product.

**(ALPHA RS, 2R)-FLUVALINATE (RS)-ALPHA-CYANO-3-PHEN-OXYBEN-ZYL(R)-2[2-CHLORO-4-TRIFLUOROMETHYL)ANILINO]-3-METHYLBU-TONATE** • An insecticide. FDA residue tolerances are 1 ppm as a residue on cottonseed; 1 ppm as a residue in cottonseed oil; 0.3 ppm in cottonseed hulls; 0.05 ppm as a residue in meat by-products and fat of cattle, goats, hogs, poultry, and sheep; 0.01 ppm as residues in milk, eggs, fat, meat of cattle, goats, hogs, poultry, and sheep. Contains cyanide *(see)*.

**ALPHA TOCOPHEROL** • There is reported use of the chemical; it has not yet been assigned for toxicology literature. GRAS. E. *See* Tocopherols and Vitamin E.

**ALTHEA FLOWERS or ROOT** • Marshmallow Root. A natural flavoring substance from a plant grown in Europe, Asia, and the United States. The dried root is used in strawberry, cherry, and root beer flavorings for beverages. The boiled root is used as a demulcent in ointments to soothe mucous membranes. The roots, flowers, and leaves are used externally as a poultice. There is reported use of the chemical; it has not yet been assigned for toxicology literature. NUL for flowers. EAF for root

**ALUM** • Potash Alum. Aluminum Ammonium. Potassium Sulfate. A colorless, odorless, crystalline, water-soluble solid used as a styptic (stops bleeding). A double sulfate of aluminum and ammonium potassium, it is also employed to harden gelatin. Has produced gum damage and fatal intestinal hemorrhages. It has a low toxicity in experimental animals but ingestion of thirty grams (an ounce) has killed an adult human. In concentrated solutions alum is also known to cause kidney and gum damage. GRAS when used in packaging only. NUL

**ALUMINUM** • Silvery white, crystalline solid. It is frequently used in food additives. Ingestion or inhalation of aluminum can aggravate kidney and lung disorders. Aluminum deposits have been found in the brains of Alzheimer's victims but its part, if any, in this degenerative brain disorder is not clear. The European Parliament in 2003 said these aluminum-containing additives set free aluminium, which can lead to intoxications and which seem to contribute to Alzheimer's disease. People suffering from certain kidney disfunctions can accumulate aluminium in their organism. Therefore, the Parliament said these additives should be banned. On the other hand at this writing, it is approved by the European Union (E).

**ALUMINUM AMMONIUM SULFATE** • Odorless, colorless crystals with a strong astringent taste. Used in purifying drinking water, in baking powders, as a buffer and neutralizing additive in milling, and in the cereal industries. Used also for fireproofing and in the manufacture of vegetable glue and artificial gems. In medicine, it is an astringent and styptic (stops bleeding). Ingestion of large amounts may cause burning in mouth and pharynx, vomiting, and diarrhea. The final report to the FDA of the Select Committee on GRAS Substances stated in 1980 that it should continue its GRAS status with no limitations other than good manufacturing practice. ASP. E

**ALUMINUM CALCIUM SILICATE** • Anticaking additive used so that it is 2 percent of table salt. Used also in vanilla powder to prevent caking. Essentially harmless when given orally. GRAS. NIL

**ALUMINUM CAPRATE** • Salt of aluminum used in processing food. *See* Caprylic Acid and Aluminum Salts. NUL

**ALUMINUM CAPRYLATE** • Salt used in processing. *See* Caprylic Acid and Aluminum Salts. NUL

**ALUMINUM DISTEARATE** • A binder that holds loose powders together when compressed into a solid cake form. *See* Aluminum Stearates.

**ALUMINUM HYDROXIDE** • An alkali used as a leavening additive in the production of baked goods. Also used as a gastric antacid in medicine. Practically insoluble in water but not in alkaline solutions. Aluminum hydroxide has a low toxicity but may cause constipation if ingested. The final report to the FDA of the Select Committee on GRAS Substances stated in 1980 that it should continue its GRAS status for packaging only, with no limitations other than good manufacturing practices. ASP

**ALUMINUM ISOSTEARATES / LAURATES / STEARATES** • The aluminum salt of a mixture of isostearic acid, lauric acid, and stearic acid *(see all)*. Used as a gelling additive.

**ALUMINUM ISOSTEARATES / MYRISTATES** • Myristates is the aluminum salt of a mixture of isostearic acid and myristic acid *(see both)*. Used as a gelling additive.

**ALUMINUM ISOSTEARATES/PALMITATES** • Palmitate is the aluminum salt of palmitic acid *(see)* and isostearic acid *(see)*. Used as a gelling additive.

**ALUMINUM LACTATE** • The aluminum salts of lactic acid *(see both)*.

**ALUMINUM LAURATE** • Used as anticaking additive or free-flow additive, emulsifier or emulsifier salt. NUL

**ALUMINUM MONOSTEARATE** • Anticaking additive, binder, emulsifier, and stabilizer used in packaging materials and various foods. Must conform to FDA specifications for salts, fats, or fatty acids derived from edible oils.

**ALUMINUM MYRISTATES / PALMITATES** • Myristates is the aluminum salt of a mixture of palmitic acid and isostearic acid *(see both)*. Used as a gelling additive. NUL

**ALUMINUM NICOTINATE** • Used as a source of niacin in special diet foods, also as a medication to dilate blood vessels and to combat fat. Tablets of 625 milligrams are a complex of aluminum nicotinate, nicotinic acid, and aluminum hydroxide. Side effects are flushing, rash, and gastrointestinal distress when taken in large doses. NIL

**ALUMINUM OLEATE** • A yellow, thick, acidic mass practically insoluble in water. Used in packaging, as lacquer for metals, in waterproofing, and for thickening lubricating oils. Low toxicity. The final report to the FDA of the Select Committee on GRAS Substances stated in 1980 that it should continue its GRAS status for packaging only, with no limitations other than good manufacturing practices. NUL

**ALUMINUM PALMITATE** • White granules, insoluble in water, used as a lubricant and waterproofing and packaging material. Also used to thicken petroleum and as an antiperspirant. The final report to the FDA of the Select Committee on GRAS Substances stated in 1980 that it should continue its GRAS status for packaging only, with no limitations other than good manufacturing practices. NUL

**ALUMINUM PHOSPHIDE** • Used to fumigate processed foods including corn grits, brewers' malt, and brewers' rice. The FDA requires that processors aerate the finished food for forty-eight hours before it is offered to the consumer. It further warns that under no conditions should the formulation containing aluminum phosphide be used so that it or its unreacted residues will come into contact with any processed food. Reacts with moist air to produce the highly toxic phosphine. Residues of phosphine in or on processed food may not exceed .01 parts per million, according to the FDA. Phosphine may cause pain in the region of the diaphragm, a feeling of coldness, weakness, vertigo, shortness of breath, bronchitis, edema, lung damage, convulsions, coma, and death.

**ALUMINUM POTASSIUM SULFATE** • Colorless, odorless, hard, transparent crystals or powder with a sweet antiseptic taste used for clarifying sugar and as a firming additive and carrier for leaching additives. It is used in the production of sweet and dill pickles, cereal, flours, bleached flours, and cheese. Ingestion of large quantities may cause burning in the mouth and throat and stomach distress. The final report to the FDA of the Select Committee on GRAS Substances stated in 1980 that it should continue its GRAS status with no limitations other than good manufacturing practices. ASP

**ALUMINUM SALTS** • Aluminum Acetate. Aluminum Caprate. Aluminum Caprylate. Aluminum Chloride. Aluminum Chlorohydrate. Aluminum Diacetate. Aluminum Distearate. Aluminum Glycinate. Aluminum Hydroxide. Aluminum Lanolate. Aluminum Methionate. Aluminum Phenolsulfonate. Aluminum Silicate. Aluminum Stearate. Aluminum Sulfate. Aluminum Tristearate. These are both the strong and weak acids of aluminum used in food processing. The strong salts may cause skin irritation.

**ALUMINUM SALTS OF FATTY ACIDS** • Used as binders, emulsifiers, and anticaking additives. Regulated and used according to good manufacturing practices. *See* Aluminum Sodium Sulfate. NIL

**ALUMINUM SILICATE** • Kaolin. Obtained naturally from clay or synthesized, used as an anticaking and coloring ingredient. Essentially harmless when given orally. E

**ALUMINUM SODIUM SULFATE** • Colorless crystals used as a buffer, firming additive, neutralizing additive, and carrier for bleaching additives. For other uses, see Aluminum Potassium Sulfate. The final report to the FDA of the Select Committee on GRAS Substances stated in 1980 that it should continue its GRAS status with no limitations other than good manufacturing practices. A weak sensitizer. Local contact may cause skin rash. ASP. E

**ALUMINUM STEARATES** • Hard, plasticlike materials used in waterproofing fabrics, thickening lubricating oils, and as a chewing-gum base component and a defoamer component used in processing beet sugar and yeast. Aluminum tristearate is a hard plastic material used as a thickener and coloring in cosmetics. NUL

**ALUMINUM SULFATE** • Cake Alum. Patent Alum. Colorless crystals, soluble in water. Odorless, with a sweet, mildly astringent taste. Used in producing sweet and dill pickles and as a modifier for starch. It is used in packaging materials, pickle relish, potatoes, and shrimp packages. Moderately toxic by ingestion and injection. May affect reproduction. The final report to the FDA of the Select Committee on GRAS Substances stated in 1980 that it should continue its GRAS status with no limitations other than good manufacturing practices. ASP. E

**AMARANTH** • Red No. 2, banned by the FDA in 1976 and reaffirmed in 1980. E

**AMARANTH FLOUR** • A grain grown in Central and South America for thousands of years, it is high in protein and fiber. Because it costs more than other grains, it is usually found only in health food stores.

**AMBERGRIS** • Concretion from the intestinal tract of the sperm whale found in tropical seas. About 80 percent cholesterol, it is a gray to black waxy mass used for fixing delicate odors in perfumery. It is also used in a flavoring for food and beverages. GRAS. EAF

**AMBRETTE** • A natural flavoring additive from the seed of the hibiscus plant, clear yellow to amber as a liquid, with a musky odor. Seed used in berry and floral flavorings for beverages, ice cream, ices, candy, baked goods. The tincture is used in black walnut and vanilla flavorings for the same products and in cordials. The seed oil is used in fruit flavoring for beverages, ice cream, candy, and baked goods. GRAS. EAF

**AMBRETTOLID** • Formed in ambrette seed oil. Used as a flavoring, perfume fixative. EAF.

**AMBUSH** • Ectiban. Exmin. Permethrin. A pesticide, poisonous by inhalation and injection. Moderately toxic by ingestion. May be mutagenic. A skin irritant.

**AMDR** • Acceptable macronutrient distribution range (*see* page 18).

**AMERICAN DILLSEED OIL** • *See* Dill.

**AMES TEST** • Dr. Bruce Ames, a biochemist at the University of California, developed a simple, inexpensive test in the early 1970s using bacteria that reveals whether a chemical is a mutagen. Almost all chemicals that are known carcinogens have also been shown to be mutagenic on the Ames Test. Whether the test can identify carcinogens is still controversial.

**AMINE OXIDES** • Surfactants derived from ammonia *(see both)*.

**2-AMINOACETOPHENONE** • Used in flavorings particularly in beer and wines. EAF

**AMINO ACIDS** • The body's building blocks, from which proteins are constructed. Of the twenty-two known amino acids, eight cannot be manufactured in the body in sufficient quantities to sustain healthy growth. These eight are called "essential" because they are necessary to maintain good health. A ninth, histidine, is thought to be necessary for growth only in childhood. Widely used in moisturizers and emollients because they are thought to help penetrate the skin. Certain amino acid deficiencies appear to have tumor-suppressing action. The amino acids of protein foods are separated by digestion and go into a general pool from which the body takes the ones it needs to synthesize its own personal proteins.

**4-AMINO-6-tert-BUTYL-3-(METHYL THIO)-1,2,4-TRIAZIN-5-ONE** • Sencoral. Secorex. An herbicide used on barley and sugarcane and in potato chips, processed potatoes, molasses, and wheat, except flour. Under the EPA Genetic Toxicology Program. Poison by ingestion. A selective residue herbicide.

**DL-(3-AMINO-3-CARBOXYPROPYL)DIMETHYLSULFONIUM CHLORIDE** • Flavoring. ASP

**4-AMINO-6-(1,1-DIMETHYL-ETHYL)-3-(METHYLTHIO)-1,2,4-TRIAZINE-5 (4H)-ONE** • Metribuzin. Herbicide found in processed potatoes, including potato chips. Herbicide is applied on the raw agricultural commodity. The FDA tolerances are 3 ppm in processed potatoes and potato chips; 3 ppm in animal feed using wheat; 2 ppm in animal feed using tomato pomace; 0.3 ppm in animal feed using sugarcane molasses; and 0.5 ppm in animal feed using sugarcane bagasse. Toxic.

**AMINOGLYCOSIDE 3′-PHOSPHOTRANSFERASE II** • An enzyme implicated in antibiotic resistance. Bacterial resistance to antibiotics is an increasing concern. By evolving characteristics such as altered antibiotic targets, or enzymes able to chemically modify antibiotics, bacteria are increasingly able to evade their effects. Aminoglycosides are a class of antibiotic commonly used in the treatment of nosocomial infections. This enzyme is used to combat antibiotics in food. ASP

**AMINO TRI(METHYLENE PHOSPHONIC ACID), SODIUM SALT** • Corrosion and scale inhibitor, water softening additive. NUL

**1-AMINO-2-PROPANOL** • Used in processing some food additives such as vitamins and fats and beverages, confectionery frostings, frozen dairy, gelatins, hard candies, and instant coffee. Corrosive, causes burns. Harmful by inhalation, ingestion, and through skin absorption. Causes severe eye irritation, with possible burns. Very destructive of mucous membranes. EAF

**4-AMINO-3,5,6-TRICHLOROPICOLINIC ACID** • Amdon Grazon. Borolin. Chloramp. An herbicide and defoliant used on barley, oats, and wheat. An experimental cancer-causing additive and teratogen. Moderately toxic by ingestion.

*p*-AMINOBENZOIC ACID • *See* para-Aminobenzoic Acid.

*para*-AMINOBENZOIC ACID • The colorless or yellowish acid found in vitamin B complex. Miscellaneous uses. The FDA has said it should be used at less than 30 milligrams per day as a food additive. In an alcohol and water solution plus a little light perfume, it is sold under a wide variety of names as a sunscreen lotion. It is also used as a local anesthetic in sunburn products. It is used medicinally to treat arthritis. However, it can cause eczema *(see)* and a sensitivity to light in susceptible people whose skin may react to sunlight by erupting with a rash, sloughing, and/or swelling. GRAS. NUL

AMINOBENZYLPENICILLIN • Acillin. Ado Bacillin. Alpen. Penbritin. Vicilin. Animal drug used in beef, milk, and pork. Under the EPA Genetic Toxicology Program. Moderately toxic by injection. Human systemic effects by ingestion: fever, agranulocytosis, and other blood effects. May be mutagenic.

6-AMINOCAPROIC ACID • *See* Amino Acids and Caproic Acid.

AMINOGLYCOSIDE 3′-PHOPHOTRANS FERASE II • There is reported use of the chemical; it has not yet been assigned for toxicology literature.

AMINOMETHYL PROPANEDIOL • Crystals made from nitrogen compounds that are soluble in alcohol and mixable with water. Used as an emulsifying ingredient in mineral oils.

AMINOMETHYL PROPANOL • An alcohol made from nitrogen compounds; mixes with water. Soluble in alcohol and used as an emulsifying ingredient. Used in medicines that reduce body water. Prolonged skin exposure may cause irritation due to alkalinity, but in most commercial products the alkalinity is neutralized. It is used in cosmetics up to 10 percent.

AMINOPEPTIDASE FROM LACTOCOCCUS LACTIS • Enzyme used to make cheddar cheese and protein hydrolysates. There is reported use of the chemical; it has not yet been assigned for toxicology literature. GRAS. EAF

AMITRAZ • A pesticide that is tolerated in 7 ppm in citrus pulp for use in animal feeds. The toleration in milk is 0.03 ppm and in the fat of cattle and hogs, 0.1 ppm. As residues in kidney and liver of hogs, 0.2 ppm, and in meat by-products of cattle and hogs, 0.03 ppm.

AMMONIA • Used as a pesticide exempt from requirement of tolerance. Liquid used in permanent wave (cold) and hair bleaches. Obtained by blowing steam through incandescent coke. Ammonia is also used in the manufacture of explosives and synthetic fabrics. It is extremely toxic when inhaled in concentrated vapors and is irritating to the eyes and mucous membranes.

**AMMONIATED COTTONSEED MEAL** • As a source of protein for ruminants and chickens and nonprotein nitrogen.

**AMMONIATED GLYCYRRHIZIN** • *See* Licorice. GRAS

**AMMONIATED RICE HULLS** • Used in feed for beef cattle as a source of crude fiber and sole source of nonprotein nitrogen.

**AMMONIUM ACETATE** • Ammonium Salt of Acetic Acid *(see* Acetic Acid*).* A buffer for protein and nucleic acid purifications. Used as a preservative for meats. The weight-of-evidence judgment supports the likelihood that the substance is a human carcinogen.

**AMMONIUM ALGINATE** • A stabilizer and water retainer. The report to the FDA of the Select Committee on GRAS Substances stated in 1980 that there is no evidence in the available information that it is a hazard to the public when used as it is now, and it should continue its GRAS status with limitation on amounts that can be added to food. *See* Alginates. E

**AMMONIUM BICARBONATE** • An alkali used as a leavening additive in the production of baked goods, confections, and cocoa products. Usually prepared by passing carbon dioxide gas through concentrated ammonia water. Shiny, hard, colorless or white crystals; faint odor of ammonia. Used also in powder formulas in cooling baths. Used medicinally as an expectorant and to break up intestinal gas. Also used in compost heaps to accelerate decomposition. The final report to the FDA of the Select Committee on GRAS Substances stated in 1980 that it should continue its GRAS status with no limitations other than good manufacturing practices. ASP

**AMMONIUM BITARTRATE** • White crystals, soluble in water, derived from tartaric acid. Used in baking powder.

**AMMONIUM CARBONATE** • A white solid alkali derived partly from ammonium bicarbonate *(see)* and used as a neutralizer and buffer in permanent wave solutions and creams. It decomposes when exposed to air. Also used in baking powders and for defatting woolens. Ammonium carbonate can cause skin rashes on the scalp, forehead, or hands. The final report to the FDA of the Select Committee on GRAS Substances stated in 1980 that it should continue its GRAS status with no limitations other than good manufacturing practices. *See* Ammonium Bicarbonate. ASP. E

**AMMONIUM CASEINATE** • The ammonium salt of casein, a protein occurring in milk and cheese. *See* Casein. NUL

**AMMONIUM CHLORIDE** • Ammonium salt that occurs naturally. Colorless, odorless crystals or white powder, saline in taste, and incompatible with alkalies. Used as a dough conditioner and a yeast food in bread, rolls, buns, and so on. Saline in taste. If ingested, can cause nausea, vomiting, and acidosis in doses of 0.5 to 1 gram. Lethal as an intramuscular dose in rats and guinea pigs. As with any ammonia compound, concentrated solutions can be irritating to the skin. The final report to the FDA of the Select Committee on GRAS Substances stated in 1980 that it should continue GRAS status for packaging only with no limitations other than good manufacturing practices. ASP

**AMMONIUM CITRATE** • The salt of citric acid *(see)*, it is a natural constituent of plants and animals and dissolves easily in water, releasing free acid. Used as a sequestrant, flavor enhancer, and as a firming additive. The final report to the FDA of the Select Committee on GRAS Substances stated in 1980 that it should continue its GRAS status with no limitations other than good manufacturing practices. ASP

**AMMONIUM GLUCONATE** • Prepared from gluconic acid with ammonia, it is used as an emulsifying additive for cheese and salad dressings. NUL

**AMMONIUM HYDROXIDE** • Ammonium Bicarbonate. Ammonia Water. A weak alkali formed when ammonia dissolves in water; exists only in solution. A clear colorless liquid with an extremely pungent odor. Used as a buffer and neutralizer in cocoa products and in animal feeds. Also used in detergents and for removing stains. It is irritating to the eyes and mucous membranes. A human poison by ingestion. A severe eye irritant. The final report to the FDA of the Select Committee on GRAS Substances stated in 1980 that it should continue its GRAS status for packaging only, with no limitations other than good manufacturing practices. GRAS. ASP. E

**AMMONIUM ISOVALERATE** • *See* Isovaleric Acid. ASP

**AMMONIUM OLEATE** • The ammonium salt of oleic acid *(see)* used as an emulsifying additive.

**AMMONIUM PECTINATE** • Used in the production of beer. *See* Pectin and Ammonium. EAF

**AMMONIUM PERSULFATE** • Ammonium Peroxydisulfate. Odorless crystals or white powder. Used as an oxidizer and bleacher and as a modifier for food starches. *See* Modified Starch. ASP

**AMMONIUM PHOSPHATE** • Monobasic and Dibasic. Ammonium Salt. An odorless, white or colorless crystalline powder with a cooling taste used in mouthwashes. They are used as acidic constituents of baking powder. They are used as buffers, leavening additives, and bread, roll, and bun improvers up to 10 percent of product. Used in brewing industry. They are also used in fireproofing textiles, paper, and wood, for purifying sugar, and in yeast cultures and fertilizers. Monobasic is used as baking powder with sodium bicarbonate. Medically used for their saline action. They have a diuretic effect (reducing body water) and they make urine more acid. The final report to the FDA of the Select Committee on GRAS Substances stated in 1980 that it should continue its GRAS status with no limitations other than good manufacturing practices. ASP

**AMMONIUM PHOSPHATIDES** • Manufactured either synthetically or from a mixture of glycerol and partially hardened rape seed oil *(see both)*. Used mainly as an emulsifier, to lower the surface tension of water thus allowing the better combining of oils, fats, and water, and as a stabilizer, to prevent separation. Similar in use to lecithin *(see)*. Limited use as an antioxidant. Vegetarians should note that although industrial manufacturing based on propylene or sugar accounts for a large percentage of glycerol production, it can be obtained as a by-product in making soap from animal and vegetable fats and oils.

**AMMONIUM POTASSIUM HYDROGEN** • A stabilizer used in packaging.

**AMMONIUM SACCHARIN** • *See* Saccharin.

**AMMONIUM SULFATE** • Ammonium salt. A yeast food, dough conditioner, and buffer in bakery products. Colorless, odorless, white crystals or powder. A neutralizer in permanent wave lotions. Industrially used in freezing mixtures, fireproofing fabrics, and tanning. Used medicinally to prolong analgesia. Fatal to rats in large doses. The final report to the FDA of the Select Committee on GRAS Substances stated in 1980 that it should continue its GRAS status with no limitations other than good manufacturing practices. *See* uses for Ammonium Phosphate. ASP. E

**AMMONIUM SULFIDE** • A salt derived from sulfur and ammonia used as a synthetic spice flavoring additive for baked foods and condiments. ASP

**AMMONIUM SULFITE** • A processing additive in foods, medicines, and cosmetics. EAF

**AMOXICILLIN TRIHYDRATE** • An animal drug used in meat and milk. Tolerance is 0.01 ppm in milk and uncooked edible tissues of meat. Moderately toxic.

**AMP** • The abbreviation for aminomethyl propanol *(see)*.

**AMPD** • The abbreviation for aminomethyl propanediol *(see)*.

**AMPHO** • Means double or both.

**AMPHOTERIC** • A material that can display both acid and basic properties. Used primarily in surfactants *(see)* and contains betaines and imidazoles *(see both)*.

**AMPICILLIN TRIHYDRATE** • Amcill. Princillin. Vidopen. Animal drug used in meat. FDA tolerance is 0.01 ppm residue in uncooked tissue of cattle and swine and in milk.

**AMPROLIUM** • Crystals from methanol and ethanol *(see both)* used as an animal drug in beef, chicken, eggs, pheasants, and turkey. Limitation in chickens and turkeys of 1 ppm in liver and kidney, 0.5 ppm in muscle. Limitation of 8 ppm in egg yolks, 4 ppm in whole eggs.

**AMYL** • Prefix meaning derived from amyl alcohol *(see)*.

**AMYL ACETATE** • Banana Oil. Pear Oil. Obtained from amyl alcohol, with a strong fruity odor. Used in nail finishes and nail polish remover as a solvent, and as an artificial fruit essence in perfume. Also used in food and beverage flavoring and for perfuming shoe polish. Amyl acetate is a skin irritant and causes central nervous system depression when ingested.

Exposure of 950 ppm for one hour has caused headache, fatigue, chest pain, and irritation of the mucous membranes.

**AMYL ALCOHOL** • A synthetic berry, chocolate, apple, banana, pineapple, liquor, and rum flavoring additive for beverages, ice cream, ices, candy, baked goods, gelatin desserts, and chewing gum. Used as a solvent in nail polish. It occurs naturally in cocoa and oranges and smells like camphor. Highly toxic and narcotic; ingestion of as little as 30 milligrams has killed humans. Inhalation causes violent coughing. ASP

**AMYL ALDEHYDE** • *See* Valeraldehyde.

**AMYL BUTYRATE** • A synthetic flavoring additive, colorless, with a strong apricot odor. Occurs naturally in cocoa. Used in raspberry, strawberry, butter, butterscotch, fruit, apple, apricot, banana, cherry, grape, peach, pineapple, and vanilla flavorings for beverages, ice cream, ices, candy, baked goods, cherry syrup, and chewing gum. Used in some perfume formulas for its apricotlike odor. ASP

**AMYL CAPRATE** • *See* Cognac Oil.

**AMYL CINNAMIC ALDEHYDE** • Liquid with a strong floral odor in perfumes and flavorings. *See* Cinnamic Acid.

**AMYL DECANOATE** • Approved as a synthetic flavoring, but there is no current reported use of the chemical, and therefore, although toxicology information may be available, it is not being updated by the FDA. NIL

**AMYL FORMATE** • A synthetic flavoring. ASP

**AMYL 2-FUROATE** • A synthetic rum and maple flavoring additive for beverages, candy, baked goods, and condiments. ASP

**AMYL GALLATE** • An antioxidant obtained from nutgalls and from molds. *See* Gallates.

**AMYL HEPTANOATE** • A synthetic lemon, coconut, fruit, and nut flavoring additive for beverages, ice cream, ices, candy, baked goods, gelatin desserts, puddings, and chewing gum. ASP

**AMYL HEXANOATE** • A synthetic citrus, chocolate, fruit, and liquor flavoring additive for beverages, ice cream, ices, candy, baked goods, and gelatin desserts. ASP

**2-AMYL-59 or 60-KETO-1, 4-DIOXANE** • A synthetic fruit flavoring additive for beverages, ice cream, ices, candy, baked goods, and shortening. ASP

**AMYL METHYL DISULFIDE** • A flavoring determined GRAS by the Expert Panel of the Flavor and Extract Manufacturers Association.

**AMYL OCTANOATE** • Occurs naturally in apples. A synthetic chocolate, fruit, and liquor flavoring additive for beverages, ice cream, ices, candy, baked goods, and gelatin desserts. ASP

*a*-**AMYL-B-PHENYL ACROLEIN BUXINE** • *See a*-Amylcinnamaldehyde.

**AMYL PROPIONATE** • Colorless liquid with a fruity, applelike odor used in perfumes, flavors, and in lacquers. When heated to decomposition it emits acrid smoke and irritating fumes.

**AMYL SALICILATE** • Derived from salicylic acid. A pleasant-smelling liquid used as a flavoring and in sunscreen lotions and perfumes. Insoluble in water. *See* Salicylates. NIL

**AMYLASE (Bacterial)** • *Aspergillus flavus, A. niger,* or *A. oryzae,* or *Bacillus subtilis.* Enzymes from various fungi used as antibacterial additives.

**AMYLASE FROM *ASPERGILLUS FLAVUS*** • An enzyme from aspergillus *(see)* used in starch modification. ASP

**AMYLASE FROM *ASPERGILLUS NIGER*** • An enzyme used in starch modification and in syrup, ethanol, and animal feed. *See* Aspergillus. ASP

**AMYLASE FROM *ASPERGILLUS ORYZAE*** • Enzyme from a mold. Used in starch, syrup, ethanol, and animal feed. ASP

**AMYLASE FROM *BACILLUS SUBTILIS*** • Enzyme preparation used in modifying starch. Produced by the controlled fermentation of *Bacillus subtilis* containing the gene for amylase from *Bacillus stearothermophilus.* The strain of *Bacillus subtilis* is nonpathogenic and nontoxicogenic. ASP

**AMYLASE (Swine)** • An enzyme prepared from the hog pancreas used in flour to break down starch into smaller sugar molecules. Then, in turn, the enzymes produced by yeast in the dough again split these sugar molecules to form carbon dioxide gas, which causes the dough to rise. It improves crumb softness and shelf life. It is also used medically to combat inflammation.

***a*-AMYLCINNAMALDEHYDE** • A synthetic additive, yellow, with a strong floral odor of jasmine, used in strawberry, apple, apricot, peach, and walnut flavorings for beverages, ice cream, ices, candy, baked goods, gelatin desserts, and chewing gum. Moderately toxic by ingestion. A mild skin irritant. Susceptible to oxidation by air. ASP

***a*-AMYLCINNAMALDEHYDE DIMETHYL ACETAL** • A synthetic fruit flavoring additive for beverages, ice cream, candy, and baked goods. ASP

**AMYLCINNAMATE** • Colorless to pale yellow liquid with a cocoa odor. Used as a flavoring additive.

***a*-AMYLCINNAMYL ACETATE** • A synthetic chocolate, fruit, and honey flavoring additive for beverages, ice cream, ices, candy, baked goods, and chewing gum.

***a*-AMYLCINNAMYL ALCOHOL** • A synthetic chocolate, fruit, and honey flavoring additive for beverages, ice cream, ices, candy, baked goods, and chewing gum.

***a*-AMYLCINNAMYL FORMATE** • A synthetic chocolate, fruit, nut, and maple flavoring additive for beverages, ice cream, ices, candy, baked goods, and chewing gum.

***a*-AMYLCINNAMYL ISOVALERATE** • A synthetic chocolate, fruit, grape, and nut flavoring additive for beverages, ice cream, ices, candy, baked goods, and chewing gum.

**AMYLOGLUCOSIDASE** • A sweet enzyme derived from *Rhizopus niveus* with a growth-encouraging potential. Used in the production of gelatinized starch into sugars and in the production of distilled spirits and vinegar. ASP

**AMYLOPECTIN** • Amioca. Derived from starch, it is the almost insoluble outer portion of the starch granule. The gel constituent of starch. Forms a paste with water. Used as a texturizer in foods and cosmetics. Obtained from corn. Gives a red color when mixed with iodine and does not gel when mixed with water.

**AMYLOSE** • Starches commonly processed from plants contain 18 to 27 percent amylose. It is the inner, relatively soluble portion of starch granules. Cornstarch solutions often form opaque gels after cooking and cooling; this is because of the presence of amylose. It is used as a dispersing and mixing additive for oleoresins.

**AMYRIS OIL** • Sandalwood Oil. The volatile oil obtained from a gummy wood and used as a flavoring additive in chewing gum and candy. It is a clear, pale yellow, viscous liquid with a distinct odor of sandalwood. EAF

**ANAPHYLAXIS** • Severe hypersensitivity reaction to an allergen. Symptoms may include rash, swelling, breathing difficulty, and collapse. A severe form is anaphylactic shock, which can be fatal.

**ANCHUSIN EXTRACT** • *See* Alkanet Root.

**ANETHOLE** • A flavoring additive used in fruit, honey, licorice, anise, liquor, nut, root beer, sarsaparilla, spice, vanilla, wintergreen, and birch beer flavorings for beverages, ice cream, ices, candy, baked goods, chewing gum (1,500 ppm), and liquors (1,400 ppm). Obtained from anise *(see)* oil, fennel, and other sources. Colorless or faintly yellow liquid with a sweet taste and a characteristic aniselike odor. Chief constituent of anise. Anethole is affected by light and caused irritation of the gums and throat when used in a denture cream. When applied to the skin, anethole may produce hives, scaling, and blisters. GRAS

**ANETHUM CRAVEOLENS** • *See* Dill.

**ANGELIC ACID** • *See* Angelica.

**ANGELICA** • Used in inexpensive fragrances, toothpastes, and mouthwashes. Grown in Europe and Asia, the aromatic seeds, leaves, stems, and roots have been used in medicine for flatus (gas), to increase sweating, and reduce body water. When perfume is applied, skin may break out with a rash and swell when exposed to sunlight. The bark is used medicinally as a purgative and emetic. The root oil is used in fruit, gin, and rum flavorings for beverages, ice cream, ices, candy, baked goods, gelatin desserts, chewing gum, and liquors. The root extract is used in berry, liquor, wine, maple, nut, walnut, and root beer flavorings for the same foods, up to baked goods, plus syrups. The seed extract is used in berry, fruit, walnut, maple, and spice flavorings for beverages, candy, baked goods, syrups, and condiments. The seed oil is used for fruit and gin flavoring for beverages, ice cream, ices, candy, baked goods, gelatin desserts, and liquors. The stem oil is used for fruit flavoring for the same foods as seed oil, excepting liquors. Angelica can induce sensitivity to light. GRAS. EAF

**ANGOLA WEED** • A weed from West Africa used as a flavoring additive in alcoholic beverages only. NUL

**ANGOSTURA** • Cusparia Bark. Flavoring additive from the bark of trees, grown in Venezuela and Brazil. Unpleasant musty odor and bitter aromatic taste. The light yellow liquid extract is used in bitters, liquor, root beer, and spice flavorings for beverages and liquors (1,700 ppm). Formerly used to lessen fever. GRAS. EAF

**ANHYDRIDE** • A residue resulting from water being removed from a compound. An oxide—combination of oxygen and an element—that can combine with water to form an acid, or that is derived from an acid by the abstraction of water. Acetic acid *(see)* is an example.

**ANHYDROUS** • Describes a substance that contains no water.

**ANHYDROUS AMMONIA** • Source of crude fiber and nonprotein nitrogen in animal feed. *See* Anhydrous and Ammonia.

**ANILINE** • A colorless to brown liquid that darkens with age. Slightly soluble in water, it is one of the most commonly used of the organic bases, the parent substance for many dyes and drugs. It is derived from nitrobenzene or chlorobenzene and is among the top five organic chemicals produced each year in the United States. It is used as a rubber accelerator to speed vulcanization, as an antioxidant to retard aging, and as an intermediate *(see);* it is also used in dyes, photographic chemicals, the manufacture of urethane foams, pharmaceuticals, explosives, petroleum refining, resins and adhesive products, paint removers, herbicides, and fungicides. Also used in crayons and shoe polishes. It is toxic when ingested, inhaled, or absorbed through the skin. It causes allergic reactions. It is a potential human cancer-causing ingredient. It caused cancer in mice when injected under the skin or administered orally. It can also cause contact dermatitis. In a 1991 report of a study of 1,749 workers at the Goodyear Tire & Rubber Company plant in Niagara Falls, New York, it was revealed that workers exposed directly to aniline had 6.5 times the rate of bladder cancer of the average state resident.

**ANIMAL COLLAGEN AMINO ACIDS** • The major protein of the white fibers of connective tissue, cartilage, and bone that is insoluble in water, but easily altered to gelatins by boiling in water, dilute acids, or alkalies. *See* Hydrolyzed Protein.

**ANIMAL KERATIN AMINO ACIDS** • A mixture of amino acids from the hydrolysis of keratin *(see)*. *See also* Hydrolyzed Keratin.

**ANIMAL PROTEIN HYDROLYSATE** • A source of animal protein.

**ANIMAL LIPASE** • *See* Lipase from Animals.

***p*-ANISALDEHYDE** • A colorless oil with a hawthorn odor, it is used as a flavoring additive in various foods. Moderately toxic by ingestion. A skin irritant.

**ANISE** • Anise Seed. Dried ripe fruit of Asia, Europe, and the United States. Used in licorice, anise, pepperoni sausage, spice, and vanilla flavorings for beverages, ice cream, ices, candy, baked goods, condiments (5,000 ppm), and meats (1,200 ppm). The oil is used for butter, caramel, licorice, anise, rum, sausage, nut, root beer, sarsaparilla, spice, vanilla, wintergreen, and birch beer flavorings for the same foods as above excepting condiments but including chewing gum (3,200 ppm) and liquors. Sometimes used to break up intestinal gas. Used in masculine-type perfumes, cleaners, and shampoos. Can cause contact dermatitis. *See* Star Anise. GRAS. ASP

**ANISOLE** • A synthetic additive with a pleasant odor used in licorice, root beer, sarsaparilla, wintergreen, and birch beer flavorings for beverages, ice cream, ices, candy, and baked goods. Also used in perfumery.

**ANISYL ACETATE** • Colorless liquid with a lilac odor used in perfumery and flavorings. *See* Anise and Anisyl Alcohol. ASP

**ANISYL ALCOHOL** • A synthetic berry, chocolate, cocoa, fruit, and vanilla flavoring additive for beverages, ice cream, ices, candy, baked goods, gelatin desserts, and chewing gum. ASP

**ANISYL BUTYRATE** • A synthetic fruit and licorice flavoring additive for beverages, ice cream, ices, candy, and baked goods. ASP

**ANISYL FORMATE** • Formic Acid. A synthetic raspberry, fruit, licorice, and vanilla flavoring additive for beverages, ice cream, ices, baked goods, and gelatin desserts. Also used in perfumery. Found naturally in currant and vanilla. *See* Formic Acid for toxicity. ASP

**ANISYL PHENYLACETATE** • A synthetic honey flavoring additive for beverages, ice cream, ices, candy, and baked goods. ASP

**ANISYL PROPIONATE** • Occurs naturally in quince, apple, banana, cherry, peach, and pineapple. A raspberry, cherry, and licorice flavoring additive for beverages, ice cream, ices, candy, baked goods, and gelatin desserts. ASP

**ANNATTO** • *Bixa orellana.* Extract and Seed. A vegetable dye from a tropical tree, yellow to pink, it is used in dairy products, baked goods, margarine, and breakfast cereals. It is also used to color such meat-product casings as bologna and frankfurters. A spice flavoring for beverages, ice cream, baked goods (2,000 ppm), margarine, and breakfast cereals (2,000 ppm). The government says that because of widespread consumer exposure to annatto, one of the most widely used colorings in the U.S. food supply, and because there is a lack of toxicity data for bixin and norbixin *(see both)* which are concentrated in annatto extract and oils, it is now undergoing testing by industry and FDA-sponsored testing has been deferred. Permanently listed in 1963 but certification not necessary for use *(see* Certified). ASP. E

**ANOXOMER** • An antioxidant used up to 5,000 ppm. EAF

**ANTHOCYANINS** • Intensely colored, water-soluble pigments responsible for nearly all the reds and blues of flowers and other plant parts. Such color, which is dissolved in plant sap, is markedly affected by the acidity and alkalinity of substances: red at low pH *(see)* and blue at higher pH values. There are about two hundred known anthocyanins, including those obtained from grapes, cranberries, cherries, and plums. They can be used to color acid compounds, such as wines and cranberry juice cocktail. The twenty anthocyanins in grapes are the major source of anthocyanin pigment for food color. E

**ANTHRACITE COAL, SULFONATED** • A resin for miscellaneous uses, according to the FDA. NUL

**ANTHRANILIC ACID** • *o*-Aminobenzoic Acid. Yellowish crystals with a sweet taste used in flavorings, dyes, and perfumes. *See* Benzoic Acid.

**ANTHRANILIC ACID, CINNAMYL ESTER** • Reddish yellow powder with the odor of balsam used in baked goods, beverages, and candy as a flavoring additive. May be a cancer-causing additive.

**ANTHRANILIC ACID, METHYL ESTER** • A flavoring additive used in various foods. May cause tumors. Moderately toxic by ingestion. A skin irritant.

**ANTIBIOTICS** • For growth promotion and feed efficiency. *See* Bacitracin, Bambermycin, Chlortetracycline, Erythromycin, Lincomycin, Monensin, Oleandomycin Hydrochloride, Oxytetracycline, Tylosin, Salinomycin, Flavophospholipol, and Virginiamycin. The EU has recommended phasing out of all such antibiotic growth promoters.

**ANTIBODY** • Protein in blood formed in response to invasion by a germ, virus, or other foreign body. In sensitive individuals, a special antibody, IgE *(see)*, is responsible for the allergic reaction.

**ANTICAKING ADDITIVES** • These keep powders and salt free-flowing, such as with calcium phosphates *(see)* in instant breakfast drinks and other soft-drink mixes.

**ANTIFOAMING ADDITIVE** • Defoaming Additive. A substance used to reduce foaming due to proteins, gases, or nitrogenous materials that may interfere with processing.

**ANTIGEN** • Any substance that provokes an immune response when introduced into the body.

**ANTIMYCOTICS** • Substances that migrate from food-packaging material such as calcium propionate, sodium benzoate, and sorbic acid *(see all)*.

**ANTIOXIDANTS** • Substances added to food to keep oxygen from changing the food's color or flavor. Apples, for instance, will turn brown when exposed to air, and fats will become rancid after exposure. Among the most widely used antioxidants are butylated hydroxyanisole (BHA) and butylated hydroxytoluene (BHT) *(see both)*. Vitamin E and vitamin C are natural antioxidants.

**ANTIPROTOZOAL** • A medication that combats single-celled parasites that are slightly bigger than bacteria. Many live in human and animal intestines and are harmless, but some cause a variety of ills including dysentery.
**AOX** • Abbreviation for Antioxidant.
**APPLE ACID** • *See* Malic Acid.
**APPLE ESSENCE, NATURAL** • A flavoring. ASP
*b*-**APO-8′-CAROTENAL** • A fine crystalline powder used as a color additive in orange beverages, cheese, desserts, and ice cream. *See* Carotene. ASP
**APRAMYCIN** • Ambylan. An animal drug used in pork. FDA tolerance: 0.1–0.4 ppm in swine.
**APRICOT** • Fruit and Oil. Persic Oil. The tart orange-colored fruit is used as a natural cherry flavoring additive for beverages, ice cream, ices, candy, baked goods, and soups. GRAS. ASP
**APRICOT KERNEL OIL** • The oil from the kernel of *Prunus armeniaca*. There is reported use of the chemical; it has not yet been assigned for toxicology literature.
**ARABIC GUM** • *See* Acacia.
**ARABINOGALACTAN** • A polysaccharide extracted with water from larch wood used in the minimum quantity required to be effective as an emulsifier, stabilizer, binder, or bodying additive in essential oils. Used in nonnutritive sweeteners, flavor bases, nonstandardized dressings, and pudding mixes.
**L-ARABINOSE** • A common vegetable gum, especially from gum arabic. Used as a culture medium. ASP
**ARACHIDIC ACID** • A fatty acid, also called eicosanoic acid, that is widely distributed in peanut oil fats and related compounds. It is used in lubricants, greases, waxes, and plastics.
**ARACHIDONIC ACID** • A liquid unsaturated fatty acid that occurs in liver, brain, glands, and fat of animals and humans. The acid is generally isolated from animal liver. Used essentially for nutrition and to soothe eczema and rashes in skin creams and lotions.
**ARACHIDYL PROPIONATE** • The ester of arachidyl alcohol and *n*-propionic acid used as a wax. *See* Arachidic Acid.
**ARBUTIN** • A diuretic and antiinfective derived from the dried leaves of the berry family, including blueberries, cranberries, bearberries, and most pear plants. This may explain why cranberry juice is reputed to ward off and/or treat urinary tract infections.
**L-ARGININE** • An essential amino acid *(see)*, strongly alkaline. It plays an important part in urea excretion. It has been used for the treatment of liver disease. Banned as not safe by the FDA, February 10, 1992, for use in over-the-counter diet pills but as of this writing there are a number of dietary supplement producers asking the FDA to allow the claim for it as a precursor of nitric oxide which plays a role in female sexual response. ASP

**ARGON** • A colorless and odorless gas. Argon is very inert and is not known to form true chemical compounds. E

**ARHEOL** • *See* Sandalwood Oil, Yellow.

**ARNICA** • Wolfsbane. The dried flower head has long been used as an astringent to treat skin disorders. It is used as a flavoring in alcohol beverages only. Ingestion can lead to severe intestinal upset, nervous disturbances, irregular heartbeat, and collapse. Ingestion of one ounce has caused severe illness but no death. It should not be used on broken skin. EAF

**ARNOTTA EXTRACT and SEED** • *See* Annatto.

**AROMA** • This is the term Europeans use instead of listing individual components of a flavor. In the United States labels say "flavor."

**AROMATIC** • In the context of flavorings, a chemical that has an aroma.

**AROMATIC BITTERS** • Usually made from the maceration of bitter herbs and used to intensify the aroma of perfume. The herbs selected for aromatic bitters must have a persistent fragrant aroma. Ginger and cinnamon are examples.

**ARROWROOT STARCH** • From the rhizome of *Maranta arundinacea,* a plant of tropical America. Used in the diet of babies and invalids because it is easy to digest. Arrowroot was used by the American Indians to heal wounds from poisoned arrows. The final report to the FDA of the Select Committee on GRAS Substances stated in 1980 that it should continue its GRAS status with no limitations other than good manufacturing practices. ASP

**ARSANILIC ACID** • Aminobenzene Arsonic Acid. Used in animal feed for stimulating growth and improving feed conversion. Poison by ingestion and injection. A human cancer-causing additive. Supposed to be at least five days before treated birds are slaughtered for use in food. Arsenic and its compounds are on the Community Right-To-Know List *(see).* Can cause blindness.

**ARSENIC** • Silvery black crystals used as an animal drug to promote growth for livestock and poultry. Tolerance set by the FDA of 0.5 ppm in muscle, 2 ppm in uncooked edible by-products, 0.5 ppm in eggs from chickens and turkeys. Limitation of 2 ppm in liver. A human carcinogen. Poison by subcutaneous, intramuscular, and intraperitoneal routes. Human systemic skin and gastrointestinal effects by ingestion. May cause birth defects.

**ARTEMISIA OIL** • Mugwort. A shrub and herb, native to north and south temperate climates, having strongly scented foliage and small rayless flower heads. Used as a flavoring in alcoholic beverages. The FDA says there is no reported use of the extract and there is no toxicology information available. As for the oil, the FDA has not yet done a toxicology search. *See* Wormwood. EAF

**ARTICHOKE LEAVES** • A tall herb that resembles a thistle. Used as a flavoring in alcoholic beverages only. EAF

**ARTIFICIAL** • In foods, the term follows the standard meaning: a substance not duplicated in nature. A flavoring, for instance, may have all natural ingredients but it must be called artificial if it has no counterpart in nature.

**ARTIFICIAL SWEETENERS** • *See* Intense Sweeteners.

**AS PACKAGED** • Refers to the state of the product as it is marked for purchase, while as prepared refers to the product after it has been made ready for consumption (e.g., ingredients added per instructions and cooked, such as a cake mix that has been prepared and baked, or a condensed or dry soup that has been reconstituted).

**ASAFETIDA EXTRACT** • Asafoetida. Devil's Dung. A gum or resin obtained from the roots or rhizome of *Ferula assafoetida,* any of several plants grown in Iran, Turkestan, and Afghanistan. The soft lumps, or "tears," have a garlicky odor and are used as a natural flavoring. The fluid extract is used in sausage, onion, and spice flavorings for beverages, ice cream, ices, candy, baked goods, meat, condiments, and soups. The gum is used in onion and spice flavorings for beverages, ice cream, ices, candy, baked goods, and seasonings. The gums have also been used medicinally as an expectorant and to break up intestinal gas. The oil is used for spice flavoring in candy, baked goods, and condiments. Asafetida has a bitter taste, an offensive charcoal odor, and is used in India and Iran as a condiment. There is reported use of the chemical; it has not yet been assigned for toxicology literature search. GRAS. EAF

**ASCORBATE** • Calcium and Sodium. Vitamin G salts. Antioxidants used in concentrated milk products, cooked, cured, or pulverized meat products, and in the brine in which pork and beef products are cured or packed.

**ASCORBIC ACID** • Vitamin C. A preservative and antioxidant used in frozen fruit, particularly sliced peaches, frozen fish dip, dry milk, beer and ale, flavoring oils, apple juices, soft drinks, fluid milk, candy, artificially sweetened jellies and preserves, canned mushrooms, cooked, cured, pulverized meat food products, brine in which beef or pork is cured or packed (75 ounces of vitamin C per 100 gallons). Vitamin C is necessary for normal teeth, bones, and blood vessels. The white or slightly yellow powder darkens upon exposure to air. Reasonably stable when it remains dry in air, but deteriorates rapidly when exposed to air while in solution. The final report to the FDA of the Select Committee on GRAS Substances stated in 1980 that it should continue its GRAS status with no limitations other than good manufacturing practices. ASP. E

**ASCORBYL PALMITATE** • A salt of ascorbic acid *(see),* it is used as a preservative and antioxidant for candy. Like ascorbic acid, prevents rancidity, browning of cut apples and other fruits, and is used in meat curing. Nontoxic. GRAS. ASP

**ASCORBYL STEARATE** • Nontoxic salt of a fatty acid. *See* Ascorbyl Palmitate. NIL

**ASEPTIC PROCESSING** • Dates back to at least the mid-1940s but has yet to realize its full potential. The most widely used of these new technologies, aseptic processing involves sterilizing a food product in a continuous process through a heat exchanger and then filling that food in an aseptic filler. The aseptic filler is a highly specialized piece of equipment designed to sterilize the packaging material, fill the sterile product into its container in a sterile environment, and then seal the package.

**ASP** • The U.S. Food and Drug Administration's designation that a food additive's fully up-to-date toxicology information has been sought.

**ASPARAGINE** • L Form. A nonessential amino acid *(see),* widely found in plants and animals both free and combined with proteins. It is used as a dietary supplement, a culture medium, and as a medicine. In cosmetics, it is used to help moisturizers penetrate the skin. ASP

**ASPARAGUS SEED and ROOT EXTRACT** • *Asparagus officinalis.* Sparrow Grass. The root is used in Chinese medicine as a tonic. In India, it is used as a hormonal tonic for women to promote fertility, relieve menstrual pains, increase breast milk, and generally nourish and strengthen the female reproductive system. It is also used as a tonic for the lungs in consumptive diseases and for AIDS wasting. Asparagus contains glycosides, asparagine, sucrose, starch, and mucilage. In 1992, the FDA proposed a ban on asparagus in oral menstrual drug products because it has not been shown to be safe and effective for its stated claims. There is reported use of the chemical; it has not yet been assigned for toxicology literature search.

**ASPARTAME** • NutraSweet. A compound prepared from aspartic acid and phenylalanine *(see both),* with about two hundred times the sweetness of sugar, discovered during routine screening of drugs for the treatment of ulcers. The G. D. Searle Company sought FDA approval in 1973, and it was approved in 1974, but objections that aspartame might cause brain damage led to a stay, or legal postponement, of that approval. Another problem arose. An FDA investigation of records of animal studies conducted for Searle drug approvals and for aspartame raised questions. The FDA arranged for an independent audit, which took more than two years and concluded that the aspartame studies and results were authentic. The agency then organized an expert board of inquiry and the members concluded that the evidence did not support the charge that aspartame might kill clusters of brain cells or cause other damage. However, persons with phenylketonuria, or PKU, must avoid protein foods such as meats that contain phenylalanine—one of two components of aspartame. The board did, however, recommend that aspartame not be approved until further long-term animal testing could be conducted to rule out a possibility that aspartame might cause brain tumors. The FDA's Bureau of Foods reviewed the study data already available and concluded that the board's concern was unfounded. Aspartame was approved for use as a tabletop sweetener in certain dry foods on October 22, 1981. It was also approved for breath mints, hard and soft; as a flavor enhancer in chewing gum, hard candy, instant coffee and tea beverages, ready-to-serve nonalcoholic beverages, fruit juice–based beverages, concentrates, or syrup, for malt beverages containing less than 3 percent alcohol, and for frosting, toppings, fillings, glazes, and icings for precooked baked goods.

In 1984 news reports fueled by the announcement that the Arizona Department of Health Services was testing soft drinks containing aspartame to see if it deteriorated into toxic levels of methyl alcohol under storage conditions created alarm. The Arizona Health Department acted after the director of the Food Sciences and Research Laboratory at Arizona State submitted a study alleging that higher than normal temperatures could lead to a dangerous breakdown in the chemical composition. The author of this dictionary checked with representatives of the Food and Drug Administration. They said that there are higher levels of methyl alcohol in regular fruit juices, and as far as the agency was concerned, the fears about decomposition products were unfounded. Aspartame lowers the acidity of urine and therefore reportedly makes the urinary tract more susceptible to infection. In 1988, the Mexican government stopped soda and food processors from using nutra in the name because it was "misleading." The Mexicans also required labeling that carries the following warning: "This product should not be used by individuals who are allergic to phenylalanine. Consumption by pregnant women and children under 7 years is not recommended. Users should follow a balanced diet. Consumption by diabetics must be authorized by a physician." E

**ASPARTIC ACID** • DL and L Forms. Aminosuccinate Acid. A nonessential amino acid *(see)* occurring in animals and plants, sugarcane, sugar beets, and molasses. It is usually synthesized for commercial purposes. ASP

**ASPERGILLUS** • A genus of fungi including molds found worldwide, especially in the autumn and winter in the Northern hemisphere. It contains many species of molds and spores that produce the antibiotic aspergillic acid. An *Aspergillus flavus-oryzae* group of molds has been cleared by the U.S. Department of Agriculture's Meat Inspection Division to soften tissues of beef cuts, to wit: "Solutions containing water, salt, monosodium glutamate, and approved proteolytic enzymes applied or injected into cuts of beef shall not result in a gain of more than 3 percent above the weight of the untreated product." It is also used in bakery products such as bread, rolls, and buns. It is increasingly being used to produce enzymes for producing food additives. It is an allergen, irritant, and can cause hypersensitivity pneumonitis and/or dermatitis. There is reported use of the chemical; it has not yet been assigned for toxicology literature. EAF

**ASTRINGENT** • A substance that causes skin or mucous membranes to pucker and shrink by reducing their ability to absorb water.

**ATOPIC DERMATITIS** • A chronic, itching inflammation of the skin also called eczema *(see)*.

**ATP** • Abbreviation for adenosine triphosphate. ATP serves as the major energy source within the cell to drive a number of biological processes such as photosynthesis, muscle contraction, and the synthesis of proteins.

**ATTAR OF ROSES** • *See* Rose Bulgarian.

**ATTENTION DEFICIT HYPERACTIVITY DISORDER (ADHD)** • Commonly called hyperactivity, attention deficit hyperactivity disorder is a clinical diagnosis based on specific criteria. These include excessive motor activity, impulsiveness, short attention span, and low tolerance to frustration and onset before seven years of age.

**AUBEPINE LIQUID** • *See* Hawthorn Berry.

**AUTOLYZED YEAST** • The concentrated, nonextracted, partially soluble digest obtained from food-grade yeasts. Solubilization *(see)* is accomplished with enzymes. Food-grade salts and enzymes may also be added. The additive is composed primarily of amino acids *(see),* peptides *(see),* proteins, carbohydrates, fats, and salts. Individual products may be in grains, powder, flake, or paste form. It is used as a flavoring additive or enhancer, a protein source, and as a binder. *See* Yeast.

**AVERMECTIN B and DELTA** • Broad-spectrum antiparasitic and antibiotics used on dried citrus pulp and cottonseeds. FDA tolerance 0.1 ppm on citrus pulp and 0.005 ppm on cottonseed. As a residue in or on tomato pomace 0.07; as residues in meat and meat by-products, 0.02 ppm; as a residue in milk, 0.005.

**AVG** • Abbreviation for average.

**AVOIDANCE** • Measures taken to avoid contact with allergy-producing substances. Since there are no cures for allergies as of yet, avoiding allergens is the best way to combat them.

**AZAPERONE** • A tranquilizer and sedative used to treat swine.

**AZINPHOS METHYL** • Crystals or brown waxy solid used as an insecticide for citrus pulp, soybean oil, and sugarcane. Poison by inhalation, ingestion, skin contact, intravenous, intraperitoneal, and possibly other routes. May cause tumors and birth defects.

**AZO DYES** • A large category of colorings used in both the food and cosmetic industries, the dyes are characterized by the way they combine with nitrogen. Made from diazonium compounds and phenol, the dyes usually contain a mild acid, such as citric or tartaric acid. Among the foods in which they are used are "penny" candies, caramels and chews, Life Savers, fruit drops, filled chocolates (but not pure chocolate); soft drinks, fruit drinks and ades; jellies, jams, marmalades, stewed fruit sauces, fruit gelatins, fruit yogurts; ice cream, pie fillings, vanilla, butterscotch, and chocolate puddings, caramel custard, whips, dessert sauces such as vanilla, and cream in powdered form; bakery goods (except plain rolls), crackers, cheese puffs, chips, cake and cookie mixes, waffle/pancake mixes, macaroni and spaghetti (certain brands); mayonnaise, salad dressings, ketchup (certain brands), mustard, ready-made salads with dressings, remoulade, béarnaise, and hollandaise sauces, as well as sauces such as curry, fish, onion, tomato, and white cream; mashed rutabagas, purees, packaged soups and some canned soups; canned anchovies, herring, sardines, fish balls, caviar, cleaned shellfish. Azo dyes can cause allergic reactions, particularly hives. People who become sensitized to permanent hair dyes containing phenylenediamine *(see)* also develop a cross sensitivity to azo dyes. That is, a person who is allergic to permanent phenylenediamine dyes will also be allergic to azo dyes. Also used in nonpermanent hair rinses and tints. There are reports that azo dyes are absorbed through the skin.

**AZODICARBONAMIDE** • A bleaching and maturing additive for flour. Yellow to orange red, a crystalline powder, practically insoluble in water. Used in amounts up to 45 ppm. The FDA wants further study of this chemical for both short-term and long-term effects. Although allowed as a food additive, there is no current reported use of the chemical, and, therefore, although toxicology information may be available, it is not being updated. NIL

**AZORUBIN, CARMOISINE** • Food Red No. 3. May be a cancer- and tumor-causing agent according to U.S. National Institute of Occupational Safety and Health (NIOSH). Not approved in the United States. *See* FD and C Red No. 3. E

# B

***BACILLUS STEAROTHERMOPHILUS*** • A harmless bacteria used to detect antibiotics in milk and to produce an enzyme used in modifying food starch.

**BACTERIA** • Microscopic single-cell organisms. Bacteria are among the most common microorganisms responsible for diseases in humans. Many are harmless. Those from lactic acid and propionic acid are harmless and used to produce cheeses and margarine.

**BACTERIAL CATALASE** • A catalase is an enzyme in plant and animal tissues. It exerts a chemical reaction that converts hydrogen peroxide into water and oxygen. Derived from bacteria by a pure culture fermentation process, bacterial catalase may be used safely, according to the FDA, in destroying and removing the hydrogen peroxide that has been used in the manufacture of cheese—providing "the organism *Micrococcus lysodeikticus* from which the bacterial catalase is to be derived is demonstrated to be nontoxic and nonpathogenic." The organism is removed from the bacterial catalase prior to the use of the catalase, the catalase to be used in an amount not in excess of the minimum required to produce its intended effect.

**BACTERIAL CATALASE FROM *MICROCOCCUS LYSODEIKTICUS***
• Enzyme from a bacteria used in making cheese. NUL

**BACTERIOCINS** • Antibodies having bactericidal activity, such as nisin preparation *(see)*.

**BACTERIOPHAGE** • A virus with a particular affinity for a bacteria. They are named after the bacterial strain, group, or species for which they are specific. The FDA put a petition for a mixture of several monoclonal bacteriophages for use as antimicrobial additives in ready-to-eat foods, fresh meat, meat products, fresh poultry and poultry products in abeyance *(see)*.

**BACITRACIN** • An antibiotic. White to pale with a slight odor. Used as an animal drug in beef, chicken, eggs, milk, pheasant, pork, and turkey. Used to increase weight gain, improve feed efficiency, and treat bacterial infections in swine. Tolerance set by the FDA is 0.5 ppm in uncooked tissue of cattle, swine, chickens, turkeys, pheasants, quail, and in milk and eggs. Moderately toxic by ingestion and injection. Possibly mutagenic.

**BACITRACIN METHYLENE DISALICYLATE and BACITRACIN ZINC** • White to brownish gray powder used as an animal feed drug that the FDA permits at a level not in excess of the amount reasonably required to accomplish the intended effect.

**BAKER'S YEAST EXTRACT** • The amino acids present add a bouillon-type brothy taste without adding any specific notes. Contributes to the overall savory aroma in soups, sauces, broths, stocks, bouillon. *See* Baker's Yeast Protein. GRAS. ASP

**BAKER'S YEAST GLYCAN** • Used as an emulsifier, thickener, and stabilizer in frozen desserts, sour cream, cheese spread, cheese flavored and flavored snack dips. *See* Baker's Yeast Protein. ASP

**BAKER'S YEAST PROTEIN** • *Saccharomyces cerevisiae.* A yeast strain yielding high growth and used in leavening bakery products and as a dietary supplement. ASP

**BAKING POWDER** • In baking, any powder used as a substitute for yeast, usually a mixture of sodium bicarbonate, starch as a filler, and harmless acid such as tartaric.

**BAKING SODA** • A common name for sodium bicarbonate *(see)*.

**BALM. *Melissa officinalis*** • A variation of the word "balsam." Usually means a soothing ointment, especially a fragrant one, or a soothing application. *See also* Melissa Oil. EAF

**BALM LEAVES EXTRACT** • Lemon Balm. A member of the mint family, has long been considered a "calming" herb. It has been used since the Middle Ages to reduce stress and anxiety, promote sleep, improve appetite, and ease pain and discomfort associated with digestion (including flatulence and bloating as well as colic). Even before the Middle Ages, balm leaves were steeped in wine to lift the spirits, help heal wounds, and treat venomous insect bites and stings. NUL

**BALM, LEMON** • *See* Balm Leaves Extract. GRAS

**BALM OIL** • *Melissa officinalis.* A natural fruit and liquor flavoring additive for beverages, ice cream, ices, candy, and baked goods. The balm leaves extract is also used in fruit flavors for beverages. The FDA has not yet done a search of the toxicology literature concerning this additive. GRAS. EAF

**BALSAM FIR, OIL** • *Abies balsamea.* One of the more important conifers in the northern United States and Canada. The buds, resin, and/or sap are used in folk remedies for cancers, corns, and warts and wounds. ASP

**BALSAM FIR, OLEORESIN** • *Abies balsamea. See* Basalm Fir Oil. ASP

**BALSAM PERU** • Obtained from Peruvian balsam in Central America near the Pacific coast. A dark brown viscous liquid with a pleasant lingering odor and a warm bitter taste extracted from a variety of evergreens. Used in strawberry, chocolate, cherry, grape, brandy, rum, maple, walnut, coconut, spice, and vanilla flavoring for beverages, ice cream, ices, candy, baked goods, gelatin desserts, chewing gum, and syrups. The oil is used in berry, coconut, fruit, rum, maple, and vanilla flavoring for beverages, ice cream, ices, candy, and baked goods. Balsam fir oil is a natural pineapple, lime, and spice flavoring for beverages, ice cream, ices, candy, baked goods, and gelatin desserts. Balsam fir oleoresin is a natural fruit and spice flavoring for beverages, ice cream, ices, candy, and baked goods. Balsam fir oil is yellowish green, thick, transparent liquid, with a pinelike smell and a bitter aftertaste. It is also used in the manufacture of chocolate, in face masks, perfumes, cream hair rinses, and astringents. Mildly antiseptic and irritating to the skin and may cause contact dermatitis and a stuffy nose. It is one of the most common sensitizers and may cross-react with benzoin, rosin, benzoic acid, benzyl alcohol, cinnamic acid, essential oils, orange peel, eugenol, cinnamon, clove, Tolu balsam, storax, benzyl benzoate, and wood tars. ASP

**BAMBERMYCINS** • Antibiotics used as antibacterials in feed for poultry, cattle, and swine. *See* Antibiotics.

**BAN** • The U.S. Food and Drug Administration's designation that a food additive formerly approved is now banned; there is usually new toxicology data available.

**BANTHIONINE** • *See* Acimeton.

**BARLEY FLOUR** • A cereal grass cultivated since prehistoric times. Used in the manufacture of malt beverages, as a breakfast food, and as a demulcent *(see)* in cosmetics.

**BASES** • Alkalies, such as ammonium hydroxide *(see),* used to control the acidity-alkalinity balance of food products. *See* pH.

**BASIL EXTRACT** • Sweet Basil. The extract of the leaves and flowers of *Ocimum basilicum,* an herb having spikes of small white flowers and aromatic leaves used as a seasoning. A natural flavoring distilled from the flowering tops of the plant has a slightly yellowish color and a spicy odor. Used in sausage and spice flavorings for beverages, candy, ice cream, baked goods, condiments, and meats. The oleoresin is used in spice flavorings for baked goods and condiments. The oil is used in loganberry, strawberry, orange, rose, violet, cherry, honey, licorice, basil, muscatel, meat, and root beer flavorings for beverages, ice cream, ices, candy, baked goods. Moderately toxic by ingestion. A skin irritant. GRAS. EAF

**BASIL, OIL** • *Ocimum basilicum.* Basil, both the wild and the sweet, furnishes an aromatic, volatile, camphoraceous oil, and on this account is much employed in France for flavoring soups, especially turtle soup. GRAS. ASP

**BASIL, OLEORESIN** • *Ocimum basilicum.* A flavoring. *See* Basil. ASP

**BASSU OIL** • A nondrying edible oil expressed from the kernels of the babassu palm, which grows in Brazil. Used in foods and soaps but is expensive.

**BAYBERRY BARK** • Myrica Oil. A yellow essential oil used in rum and other flavorings and fragrances. GRAS

**BAY LEAVES** • *Pimenta racemosa.* The West Indian extract is a natural flavoring used in vermouth and spice flavorings for beverages, ice cream, ices, candy, baked goods, meat, and soups. The oil is used in fruit, liquor, and bay flavorings for beverages, ice cream, ices, candy, baked goods, condiments, and meats. The oleoresin *(see)* is used in sausage flavoring for meats and soups. GRAS. ASP

**BAY, SWEET** • *Laurus nobilis.* A natural flavoring native to a Mediterranean plant with stiff, glossy, fragrant leaves. Used in vermouth, sausage, and spice flavorings for beverages, ice cream, ices, candy, baked goods, condiments, and meats. ASP

**BBC** • *See* Beta-Cyclodextrin.

**BEECHWOOD, CREOSOTE** • *See* Creosote. ASP

**BEEF TALLOW** • *See* Tallow Flakes. GRAS for packaging.

**BEESWAX** • From virgin bees and primarily used as an emulsifier. Practically insoluble in water. Yellow beeswax from the honeycomb is yellowish, soft to brittle, and has a honeylike odor. White beeswax is yellowish white and slightly different in taste but otherwise has the same properties as yellow beeswax. Used as a candy glaze and polish. Can cause contact dermatitis *(see).* The final report to the FDA of the Select Committee on GRAS Substances stated in 1980 that it should continue its GRAS status with no limitations other than good manufacturing practices. *See* Beeswax, Bleached. ASP. E

**BEESWAX, BLEACHED** • White Wax. Yellow wax bleached and purified from the honeycomb of the bee. Remains yellowish white, is solid, somewhat translucent, and fairly insoluble in water. Differs slightly in taste from yellow beeswax. Used in fruit and honey flavorings for beverages, ice cream, ices, baked goods, and honey. *See* Yellow Beeswax for medicinal uses. Mild allergen. The final report to the FDA of the Select Committee on GRAS Substances stated in 1980 that it should continue its GRAS status with no limitations other than good manufacturing practices. ASP

**BEET** • Juice and Powder. Vegetable dye used to color dairy products. Listed for food use in 1967. Exempt from color certification.

**BEETROOT JUICE POWDER** • The powdered stem base of the beet used for its reddish color in powders and rouges. Exempt from color certification. E

**BEHENIC ACID** • Docosanoic Acid. Colorless, water soluble constituent of seed fats, animal fats, and marine animal oils. It is a fatty acid *(see)*.

**BENOMYL** • Methyl-1-(Butyl Carbamoyl)-2-Benzimidazole-Carbamate. Tersan 1991. Bonide. White crystalline solid, a carbamate *(see)*. It is the generic name for a fungicide used on peaches, apples, and other fruits after they are picked. The residues in animal feed are: 70 ppm in dried apple pomace resulting from application to apples as a residue; 125 ppm in dried grape pomace and raisin waste resulting from application to growing grapes; 50 ppm in raisins resulting from application to growing grapes; 50 ppm in dried citrus pulp when present therein as a result of application to the raw agricultural citrus fruits; 50 ppm in concentrated tomato products resulting from application to growing crop; and 50 ppm in rice hulls resulting from application to raw agricultural rice. It is also used as an oxidizer in sewage treatment. It is extremely toxic by ingestion. It may cause birth defects. It is a mild irritant to human skin.

**BENSULFURON METHYL ESTER** • Herbicide. Tolerance for residue in or on rice, 0.02 ppm.

**BENTAZON** • Herbicide. FDA residue tolerance is 4 ppm in or on mint hay used for feed resulting from application to growing mint.

**BENTONITE** • A colloidal clay (aluminum silicate) that has a high swelling capacity in water. Used as a food additive, as a thickener, and as a colorant in wine. Poison if given by vein, causing blood clots, and may cause tumors. GRAS. ASP. E

**BENZALDEHYDE** • Artificial Almond Oil. A colorless liquid that occurs in the kernels of bitter almonds. Lime is used in its synthetic manufacture. As the artificial essential oil of almonds, it is used in berry, butter, coconut, apricot, cherry, peach, liquor, brandy, rum, almond, pecan, pistachio, spice, and vanilla flavorings. Occurs naturally in cherries, raspberries, tea, almonds, bitter oil, cajeput oil, and cassia bark. Used in beverages, ice cream, ices, candy, baked goods, chewing gum, and cordials. Also used in cosmetic creams and lotions, perfumes, soaps, and dyes. May cause allergic reactions. A skin irritant, contact may cause a rash. Highly toxic. Produces central nervous system depression and convulsions. Fatal dose is estimated to be two ounces. *See* Benzyl Acetate. GRAS. ASP

**BENZALDEHYDE DIMETHYL ACETAL** • A synthetic additive used in fruit, cherry, nut, and almond flavorings for beverages, ice cream, ices, candy, baked goods, gelatin, and puddings. *See* Benzyl Acetate. ASP

**BENZALDEHYDE GLYCERYL ACETAL** • A synthetic additive used in fruit, cherry, nut, and almond flavorings for beverages, ice cream, ices, candy, baked goods, and chewing gum. *See* Benzyl Acetate. ASP

**BENZALDEHYDE PROPYLENE GLYCOL ACETAL** • A synthetic additive used in fruit, cherry, nut, and almond flavorings for beverages, ice cream, ices, candy, baked goods, and chewing gum. *See* Benzyl Acetate. ASP

**BENZALKONIUM CHLORIDE (BAK)** • A widely used ammonium detergent. It is a germicide with an aromatic odor and a very bitter taste. Soluble in water and alcohol but incompatible with most detergents and soaps. Used medicinally as a topical antiseptic and detergent. Allergic conjunctivitis has been reported when used in eye lotions. Lethal to frogs in concentrated oral doses. Highly toxic. The FDA proposed a ban in 1992 for the use of benzalkonium chloride to treat insect bites and stings and in astringent *(see)* drugs because it has not been shown to be safe and effective for stated claims in OTC products.

**BENZATHINE CLOXACILLIN** • A veterinary antibiotic. The FDA tolerance for residues in milk is 0.02 ppm.

**BENZENE** • A solvent obtained from coal and used in modified hop extract for beer regulated by the FDA at 1 ppm. Derived from toluene or gasoline, it is used in the manufacture of nail polish remover, detergents, nylon, artificial leather, as an antiknock in gasoline, in airplane fuel, dope, varnish, lacquer, and as a solvent for waxes, resins, and oils. Highly flammable. Poisonous when ingested and irritating to the mucous membranes. Harmful amounts may be absorbed through the skin. Also can cause sensitivity to light in which the skin may break out in a rash or swell. Inhalation of the fumes may be toxic. The Consumer Product Safety Commission voted unanimously in February 1978 to ban the use of benzene in the manufacture of many household products. The commission took the action in response to a petition filed by the Consumer Health Research Group, an organization affiliated with consumer advocate Ralph Nader. Earlier in the year, OSHA and the EPA both cited benzene as a threat to public health. For more than a century, scientists have known that benzene is a powerful bone marrow poison, destroying the marrow's ability to produce blood cells, causing such conditions as aplastic anemia. In the past several decades evidence has been mounting that it also causes leukemia. Safety standards for cosmetic manufacturing workers and other workers have been set at 10 parts per million during an eight-hour day, but OSHA wants it reduced to 1 part per million. Although listed as a food additive, the FDA says there is no current reported use of the chemical in food and therefore it is not being updated in its data bank. NUL

**BENZENE ACETALDEHYDE** • Oily, colorless liquid that grows thicker on standing. Has a hyacinth odor. Used as a flavoring additive in bakery products, beverages, chewing gum, confections, gelatin desserts, ice cream, maraschino cherries, and puddings. Moderately toxic by ingestion. Human skin irritant.

**BENZENECARBONAL** • *See* Benzaldehyde.

**BENZENE CARBOXYLIC ACID** • *See* Benzoic Acid.

**BENZENE HEXACHLORIOE (BHC)** • Hexachlorane. Hexylan. A pesticide widely used. Poison by ingestion and by subcutaneous injection. Moderately toxic by skin contact. An experimental cancer-causing and tumor-causing additive by ingestion and skin contact. Human systemic effects by inhalation: headache, nausea or vomiting, and fever. Implicated in aplastic anemia. Possible reproductive effects. It is persistent in the environment and accumulates in mammalian tissue.

**BENZENE METHYLAL** • *See* Benzaldehyde.

**BENZENETHIOL** • Thiophenol. Phenyl Mercaptan. Flavoring additive. The FDA says there are no safety concerns at current levels of intake when used as a flavoring additive. ASP

**BENZIN** • Dark straw-colored to colorless liquid made from coal and oil. Used to dilute color, as a solvent, and as a protective coating for eggshells, fresh fruits, and vegetables. A human poison if injected into the vein. Chronic exposure may cause headache, lack of appetite, dizziness, and other symptoms of intoxication. The FDA permits its use at a level not in excess of the amount reasonably required to accomplish intended use.

**1,2-BENZISOTHIAZOL-3 (2H)-ONE-1,1-DIOXIDE** • Benzosulfimide. Zaharina. Saccharina. Saccharin Acid. Sucrette. Saccarinose. White crystals or powder, odorless with a sweet taste. Used as a masticatory substance in chewing-gum base. A nonnutritive sweetener used in artificial sweetener, bacon, beverage mixes, beverages, chewing gum, desserts, fruit juice drinks, and jams. The FDA limits it to 12 mg per fluid ounce in beverages, fruit juice drinks, and beverage mixes. Limitation of 20 mg per teaspoon of sugar sweetening equivalent and 230 mg per designated size in processed foods. Sufficient evidence of carcinogenicity in animals but not in humans, although it is a possible human cancer-causing additive. Mild acute toxicity by ingestion.

**BENZOATE OF SODA** • *See* Sodium Benzoate.

**BENZOATES** • The salts of benzoic acid *(see)* used primarily as preservatives. The Joint FAO/WHO Expert Committee on Food Additives concluded in June 1998: "The potential exists for high consumers of benzoate to exceed the ADI [Acceptable Daily Intake], but the available data were insufficient to estimate the number of high consumers or the magnitude and duration of intake above the ADI." The Committee is reviewing this additive's level in cheeses, vegetables in vinegar or brine, fish products, liquid eggs, and carbonated water-based soft drinks.

**1,2-BENZODIHYDROPYRONE** • *See* Dihydrocoumarin.

**BENZOE** • *See* Benzoin.

**BENZOEPIN** • Brown crystals used as an insecticide in dried tea. Residue tolerance of 25 ppm in dried tea. Poison by ingestion, inhalation, and skin contact and other routes. Causes tumors in laboratory animals and birth defects. A central nervous system stimulant producing convulsions in humans. A highly toxic organochlorine pesticide that does not accumulate in human tissue. Absorption is normally slow, but is increased by alcohol, oil, and emulsifiers.

**2-BENZOFURANCARBOXALDEHYDE** • Flavoring additive. The FAO/WHO said in 2000 that there was no safety concern at current levels of intake when used as a flavoring additive. ASP

**BENZOFUROLINE** • 5-Benzyl-3-Furyl Methyl(+)-cis, trans-Chrysanthemate. A pesticide used in various food products. Poison by inhalation, ingestion, and intravenous routes. Moderately toxic by skin contact. When heated to decomposition, it emits acrid and irritating fumes.

**BENZOIC ACID** • A preservative that occurs in nature in cherry bark, raspberries, tea, anise, and cassia bark. First described in 1608 when it was found in gum benzoin. Used in chocolate, lemon, orange, cherry, fruit, nut, and tobacco flavorings for beverages, ice cream, ices, candy, baked goods, icings, and chewing gum. Also used in margarine and pickles. Also an antifungal additive. Used as a chemical preservative and a dietary supplement up to 0.1 percent. A mild irritant to the skin. It can cause allergic reactions such as asthma, red eyes, and skin rashes, especially in people sensitive to aspirin. Listed by the FDA as GRAS in a reevaluation of safety in 1976. The final report to the FDA of the Select Committee on GRAS Substances stated in 1980 that it should continue its GRAS status with no limitations other than good manufacturing practices. ASP. E

**BENZOIC ALDEHYDE** • *See* Benzaldehyde.

**BENZOIC RESIN** • A flavor additive. *See* Benzoic Acid and Benzoic Resin.

**BENZOIN** • Gum Benjamin. Gum Benzoin. Any of several resins containing benzoic acid *(see),* obtained as a gum from various trees. The resin is used as a flavoring additive in chocolate, cherry, rum, spice, and vanilla flavorings for beverages, ice cream, ices, candy, baked goods, and chewing gum. Benzoin also is a natural flavoring additive for butterscotch, butter, fruit liquor, and rum. It was tested by the National Cancer Institute and found not to be a cancer-causing additive in rats and mice but may be mutagenic. ASP

**BENZOIN RESIN** • *Styrax* Spp. Flavoring. A natural resin from the small tree, *Styrax tonkinensis,* a native of Indochina. The balsamic latex flows from wounds in the bark and outer wood where incisions are made. The odor is pleasant, sweet, balsamic with a distinct note of vanillin. ASP

**BENZOPHENONES (1–12)** • At least a dozen different benzophenones exist. Synthetic additives used in berry, butter, fruit, apricot, peach, nut, and vanilla flavorings for beverages, ice cream, ices, candy, and baked goods. They are used as fixatives *(see)* for heavy perfumes (geranium, e.g.) and soaps (the smell of "new mown hay"). Obtained as a white flaky solid with a delicate, persistent roselike odor, and soluble in most fixed oils and in mineral oil. They help prevent deterioration of ingredients that might be affected by the ultraviolet rays found in ordinary daylight. May produce hives and contact sensitivity. Toxic when injected.

**BENZOPYRENE** • A hydrocarbon found in coal tar, cigarette smoke, and in the atmosphere as a product of incomplete combustion. Highly toxic and a cancer-causing additive.

**2,3-BENZOPYRROLE** • *See* Indole.

**BENZOTHIAZOLE** • BT. Used in organic synthesis. ASP

**BENZOYL EUGENOL** • *See* Eugenyl Benzoate.

**BENZOYL PEROXIDE** • A bleaching additive for flours, blue cheese, Gorgonzola, and milk. A catalyst for hardening certain fiberglass resins. A drying additive in cosmetics. Toxic by inhalation. A skin allergen and irritant. GRAS. ASP

**BENZYL ACETATE** • A colorless liquid with a pear- or flowerlike odor obtained from a number of plants, especially jasmine, for use in perfumery and soap. A synthetic raspberry, strawberry, butter, violet, apple, cherry, banana, and plum flavoring additive for beverages, ice cream, ices, candy, baked goods, chewing gum, and gelatin desserts. Can be irritating to the skin, eyes, and respiratory tract. Ingestion causes intestinal upset, including vomiting and diarrhea. The FAO/WHO Expert Committee on Food Additives has studied this additive a number of times. The Committee noted brain damage involving the cerebellum and/or hippocampus in rats and mice given benzyl acetate at a dose level of 5 percent in the diet for thirteen weeks. No such effect was observed in the long-term toxicity-carcinogenicity studies in mice or rats at lower doses. In the long-term study in rats, no adverse effects were observed at levels of up to 550 mg per kg of body weight per day in the diet. In long-term study, treated males and female mice showed lower body weights than controls. The committee has noted the absence of reproductive/birth defect studies for substances in this group, and has recommended that a full review of benzyl acetate, benzoic acid, the benzoate salts, benzaldehyde, and benzyl alcohol be performed to determine "whether these or other studies are required." ASP

**BENZYL ACETIC ACID** • *See* Cinnamic Acid.

**BENZYL ACETOACETATE** • A synthetic berry and fruit flavoring additive for beverages, ice cream, ices, candy, baked goods, gelatin desserts, and chewing gum. *See* Benzyl Acetate for toxicity. ASP

**BENZYL ACETONE** • *See* 4-Phenyl-3-Buten-2-One.

**BENZYL ACETYL ACETATE** • *See* Benzyl Acetoacetate. ASP

**BENZYL ALCOHOL** • A flavoring that is derived as a pure alcohol and is a constituent of jasmine, hyacinth, and other plants. It has a faint, sweet odor. Used in synthetic blueberry, loganberry, raspberry, orange, floral, rose, violet, fruit, cherry, grape, honey, liquor, muscatel, nut, walnut, root beer, and vanilla flavorings for beverages, ice cream, ices, candy, baked goods, gelatin desserts, and chewing gum. Irritating and corrosive to the skin and mucous membranes. Ingestion of large doses causes intestinal upsets. It may cross-react in the sensitive with balsam Peru *(see)*. ASP

**BENZYL BENZOATE** • Plasticizer in nail polishes, solvent and fixative for perfumes. Occurs naturally in balsams Tolu and Peru and in various flower oils. Colorless, oily liquid or white crystals with a light floral scent and sharp burning taste. ASP

**BENZYL BUTYL ETHER** • Synthetic fruit flavoring additive for beverages, ice cream, ices, candy, baked goods, gelatin desserts, and puddings. ASP

**BENZYL BUTYRATE** • Butyric Acid. A synthetic flavoring additive, colorless, liquid, with a plumlike odor. Used in loganberry, raspberry, strawberry, butter, apricot, peach, pear, liquor, muscatel, cheese, and nut flavorings for beverages, ice cream, ices, candy, baked goods, chewing gum, and gelatin desserts. ASP

**BENZYL CARBINOL** • *See* Phenethyl Alcohol.

**BENZYL CINNAMATE** • Sweet Odor of Balsam. Colorless prisms, used to give artificial fruit scents to perfumes. A synthetic flavoring additive found in balsams of Peru, Tolu, styrax, copaiba, and others. Used in raspberry, chocolate, apricot, cherry, peach, pineapple, plum, prune, honey, liquor, and rum for beverages, ice cream, ices, candy, baked goods, chewing gum, and gelatin desserts. Moderately toxic by ingestion. A mild allergen and skin irritant. *See* Balsam Peru for toxicity. ASP

**BENZYL DIMETHYL CARBINYL ACETATE** • *See* a,a-Dimethylphenethyl Acetate. ASP

**BENZYL DIMETHYL CARBINYL BUTYRATE** • *See* a,a-Dimethylphenethyl Butyrate.

**BENZYL DIMETHYL CARBINYL FORMATE** • *See* a,a-Dimethylphenethyl Formate.

**BENZYL 2,3-DIMETHYLCROTONATE** • A synthetic fruit and spice flavoring additive for beverages, ice cream, ices, candy, and baked goods. ASP

**BENZYLDIMETHYLDODECYLAMMONIUM CHLORIDE** • Benzyl Ammonium Chloride. An antimicrobial additive used in beets and sugarcane. A skin and eye irritant.

**BENZYL DI PROPYL KETONE** • *See* 3-Benzyl-4-Heptanone.

**BENZYL DISULFIDE** • A synthetic fruit flavoring additive for beverages, ice cream, ices, and candy. ASP

**BENZYL ETHYL ETHER** • Colorless, oily liquid, aromatic odor, insoluble in water, miscible in alcohol. Used in flavoring for beverages, ice cream, ices, candy, and baked goods. Narcotic in high concentrations. May be a skin irritant. ASP

**BENZYL FORMATE** • Formic Acid. A synthetic chocolate, apricot, cherry, peach, pineapple, plum, prune, honey, and liquor flavoring additive for beverages, ice cream, ices, candy, baked goods, and chewing gum. Pleasant fruity odor. Practically insoluble in water. There is no specific data for toxicity, but it is believed to be narcotic in high concentrations. ASP

**3-BENZYL-4-HEPTANONE** • Synthetic fruit flavoring for beverages, ice cream, ices, candy, and baked goods. ASP

**BENZYL HEXANOATE** • A flavoring determined GRAS by the Expert Panel of the Flavor and Extract Manufacturers Association.

**BENZYL o-HYDROXYBENZOATE** • *See* Benzyl Salicylate.

**BENZYL ISOAMYL ALCOHOL** • *See* a-Isobutylphenethyl Alcohol.

**BENZYL ISOBUTYL CARBINOL** • *See* a-Isobutylphenethyl Alcohol.

**BENZYL ISOBUTYRATE** • A synthetic strawberry and fruit flavoring for beverages, ice cream, ices, candy, and baked goods. ASP

**BENZYL ISOEUGENOL** • A synthetic spice flavoring for beverages, ice cream, ices, candy, and baked goods.

**BENZYL ISOVALERATE** • A synthetic raspberry, apple, apricot, banana, cherry, pineapple, walnut, and cheese flavoring additive for beverages, ice cream, ices, candy, baked goods, gelatin desserts, and chewing gum. ASP

**BENZYL MERCAPTAN** • A synthetic coffee flavoring additive used for beverages, ice cream, ices, candy, and baked goods. ASP

**BENZYL METHOXYETHYL ACETAL** • Synthetic fruit and cherry flavoring additive for beverages, ice cream, ices, candy, and baked goods. ASP

**BENZYL PHENYLACETATE** • A synthetic butter, caramel, fruit, and honey flavoring additive for beverages, ice cream, ices, candy, baked goods, and toppings. A colorless liquid with a sweet floral odor; occurs naturally in honey. ASP

**BENZYL B-PHENYL ACRYLATE** • *See* Benzyl Cinnamate.

**BENZYL PROPIONATE** • A synthetic flavoring substance, colorless liquid, with a sweet fruity odor. Used in berry, apple, banana, grape, pear, and pineapple flavorings for beverages, ice cream, ices, candy, baked goods, chewing gum, and icings. ASP

**BENZYL SALICYLATE** • Salicylic Acid. Used in floral and peach flavorings for beverages, ice cream, ices, candy, and baked goods. A fixative in perfumes and a solvent in sunscreen lotions. It is a thick liquid with a light, pleasant odor; it is mixed with alcohol or ether. As with other salicylates it may interact adversely with such medications as antidepressants and anticoagulants, and may cause skin to break out with a rash and swell when exposed to sunlight. *See* Salicylates. ASP

**BENZYLETHYL ALCOHOL** • *See* Benzyl Alcohol.
**1-BENZYLOXY (B-METHOXY) ETHOXY ETHANE** • *See* Benzyl Methoxyethyl Acetal.
**BENZYL PROPYL ACETATE** • *See* a,a-Dimethylphenethyl Acetate
**BENZYL PROPYL ALCOHOL** • *See* a,a-Dimethylphenethyl Acetate.
**BENZYL PROPYL CARBINOL** • *See* a-Propylphenethyl Alcohol.
**BENZYL THIOL** • *See* Benzyl Mercaptan.
**BERGAMOL** • *See* Linalyl Acetate.
**BERGAMOT** • Bergamot Orange or Red. Oswego Tea. An orange flavoring extracted from a pear-shaped fruit, whose rind yields a greenish brown oil much used in perfumery and brilliantine hair dressings. Used in strawberry, lemon, orange, tangerine, cola, floral, banana, grape, peach, pear, pineapple, liquor, spice, and vanilla flavorings for beverages, ice cream, ices, candy, baked goods, gelatin desserts, chewing gum, and icings. The oil can cause brown skin stains (berloque) when exposed to sunlight and is considered a prime photosensitizer (sensitivity to light). *See* Berloque Dermatitis. GRAS
**BERLOQUE DERMATITIS** • Some perfumes, which contain oil of bergamot *(see)* and other photosensitizers, may produce increased pigmentation (brown spots) in the area where the perfume has been applied, especially when it is immediately exposed to sunlight. There is no effective treatment and the pigmentation generally persists for some time.
**BETA-APO-8′-CAROTENAL** • Orange coloring additive for solid or semisolid foods. Limited to 15 mg per pound of solid or semisolid food. Does not require certification. E
**BETA-CAROTENE** • Provitamin A. Beta Carotene. Found in all plants and in many animal tissues. It is the chief yellow coloring matter of carrots, butter, and egg yolks. Extracted as red crystals or crystalline powder, it is used as a coloring in food and cosmetics and as a direct food additive. It is exempt from certification. Also used in the manufacture of vitamin A. Too much carotene in the blood can lead to carotenemia, a pale yellow-red pigmentation of the skin that may be mistaken for jaundice. It is a benign condition, and withdrawal of carotene from the diet cures it. Beta-carotene has less serious side effects than vitamin A and was given to 22,000 physicians as part of a five-year study to determine whether aspirin could protect against heart disease and beta-carotene against tumors. It is nontoxic. The FAO-WHO Expert Committee on Food Additives concluded that there was no objection to the use of vegetable extracts as coloring additives provided the level of use did not exceed the level normally present in vegetables. Implicit in this conclusion, the Committee notes, is that the extracts should not be made toxic by virtue of the concentrations of toxic compounds (including toxicants naturally occurring in the vegetables) or by the generation of reaction products or residues of a nature or in such amounts as to be lexicologically

significant. The past specifications for carotenes (vegetables) were revised to include material derived from carrots, alfalfa, and palm oil, which are known to be used commercially. Being considered for cancer-causing properties because it is positive as a mutagen in salmonella. GRAS

**BETA-CITRAURIN** • Excellent raw material for the extraction of carotinoids (*see* Carotene), or orange coloring. Found in tangerine and orange peels. Soluble in alcohol.

**BETA-CYCLODEXTRIN (BCD)** • A naturally occurring substance from the action of enzymes on starch. A white, odorless, fine crystalline solid or powder having a sweet taste. It is used as an encapsulating additive, processing aid, or stabilizer in foods. E

**BETA-GLUCANS** • Polysaccharides (*see*) that yield sugars (glucose) on hydrolysis when exposed to water treatment. Beta-glucan is in cellulose and is found in edibles such as oat fiber and barley.

**BETAINE** • Used as a coloring and as a dietary supplement. Occurs in common beets and in many vegetables as well as animal substances. Used in resins. Has been employed to treat muscle weakness medically.

**BETAINE, ANHYDROUS** • Betaine (*see*) with the water removed.

**BETULA** • Obtained from the European white birch and a source of asphalt and tar. Used in hair tonics; it reddens the scalp and creates a warm feeling due to an increased flow of blood to the area. Also used in moisturizing creams and astringents. Betula leaves were formerly used to treat rheumatism. *See* Salicylates.

**BHA** • *See* Butylated Hydroxyanisole.

**BHT** • *See* Butylated Hydroxytoluene.

**BIACETYL** • *See* Diacetyl.

**BICARBONATE OF SODA** • A buffer and neutralizing additive used in self-rising cornmeal. *See* Sodium Bicarbonate. GRAS

**BIFENTHRIN** • A synthetic pyrethroid pesticide. Used to combat insects and mites. FDA tolerances are 0.02 ppm in milk, 0.10 ppm in fat, meat, and meat by-products of cattle, goats, hogs, and sheep, and 0.50 ppm as a residue in cottonseed. Lower toxicity than most pesticides.

**BILBERRY EXTRACT** • The extract of *Vaccinium myrtillus,* a plant found in North America and the Alps that differs from the typical blueberries in having single flowers or very small buds.

**BILE SALTS and OX BILE EXTRACT** • *See* Ox Bile.

**BINDER** • Substances such as gum arabic, gum tragacanth, glycerin, and sorbitol (*see all*) that dispense, swell, or absorb water, increase consistency, and hold ingredients together. For example, binders are used to make powders in women's compacts retain their shape; binders in toothpaste provide for the smooth dispensing of the paste.

**BIOCHEMICAL** • A substance that is produced by a chemical reaction in a living organism. Some can also be made in the laboratory.

**BIOFLAVONOIDS** • Vitamin P Complex. Citrus-flavored compounds needed to maintain healthy blood vessel walls. Widely distributed among plants, especially citrus fruits and rose hips. Usually taken from orange and lemon rinds and used as a reducing additive *(see)*.

**BIOTECHNOLOGY** • The use of living cells or parts of cells to perform procedures and to make products.

**BIOTIN** • Vitamin H. Vitamin B Factor. A whitish crystalline powder used as a texturizer in cosmetic creams. Present in minute amounts in every living cell and in larger amounts in yeast and milk. Vital to growth, it acts as a coenzyme in the formation of certain essential fatlike substances and plays a part in reactions involving carbon dioxide. It is needed by humans for healthy circulation and red blood cells. EAF

**BIPHENYL** • Derived from benzene. Used as a fungistat in packaging of citrus fruits and in manufacturing processes. ASP. E

**BIRCH FAMILY** • *Betulaceae.* Sweet Oil and Tar Oil. A flavoring additive from the bark and wood of deciduous trees common in the Northern Hemisphere. The oils are obtained by distillation. They are clear, dark brown liquids with a strong leatherlike odor. Birch sweet oil is used in synthetic strawberry, pineapple, maple, nut, root beer, sarsaparilla, spice, wintergreen, and birch beer flavorings for beverages, ice cream, ices, candy, baked goods, gelatins, puddings (4,300 ppm), and syrups. Birch tar oil, which is refined, is used in chewing gum and has also been used for preserving leather. It is an ancient remedy. The medicinal properties of the plant tend to vary, depending upon which part of the tree is used. It has been used as a laxative, as an aid for gout, to treat rheumatism and dropsy, and to dissolve kidney stones. The oil is used in food flavorings. *See* Betula. EAF

**BIS-** • A prefix meaning twice

**BISABOLENE** • A colorless oily sesquiterpene found in many essential oils such as oil of bisabol and lime oil. Used as a flavoring. ASP

**BIS(2-CARBOXYETHYL) SULFIDE** • Thiodipropionic Acid. TDPA. An antioxidant used in packaging material. Poisonous by injection. Moderately toxic by ingestion. A skin and eye irritant.

**3,6-BIS(2-CHLORPHENYL)-1,2,4,5 TETRAZINE** • A pesticide with a tolerance of 20 ppm in apple pomace as a result of application to apples.

**1,1-BIS(p-CHLOROPHENYL)-2,2,2-TRICHLOROETHANOL** • Acarin. Decofol. An insecticide used on dried tea. Poison by ingestion and skin contact. May cause cancer and mutations in humans.

**BIS(DIMETHYL-3-FURYL) DISULFIDE** • Flavoring additive. WHO *(see)* Committee said there was no safety concern about it. ASP

**2,4-BIS(ETHYLAMINO)-6-CHLORO-s-TRIAZINE** • Aktinit S. Aquazine. Zeapur. An herbicide used in animal feed, molasses, potable water, sugarcane by-products, sugarcane syrups. The FDA's residue tolerances are 1 ppm in sugarcane by-products, molasses, and syrup, and 0.01 ppm in potable water. Limitation of 1 ppm in sugarcane by-product molasses when used for animal feed. It is in the EPA Genetic Toxicology Program *(see)*. Poison by intravenous route. Causes tumors in experimental animals. A skin and eye irritant in humans.

**BIS(2-ETHYLHEXYL)PHTHALATE** • BEHP. Witcizer312. A plasticizer used in packaging materials for foods of high water content. Suspected human cancer-causing additive and teratogen. Affects the human gastrointestinal tract. A mild skin and eye irritant. *See* Phthalates.

**N,N-BIS(2-HYDROXYETHYL)DODECAN AMIDE** • Lauryl Diethanolamide. Lauric Acid. Diethanolamide. Antistatic additive used in packaging materials and limited to 0.5 percent in polyethylene containers.

**BIS(2-METHYL-3-FURYL) DISULFIDE** • Flavoring additive. ASP

**BIS(2-METHYL-3-FURYL) TETRASULFIDE** • Flavoring additive. ASP

**BIS-(METHYLTHIO)METHANE** • Flavoring additive. EAF

**BIS(S-OXYQUINOLINE) COPPER** • Bioquin. Quinondo. Furitdo. A preservative for wood. Copper and its compounds are on the Community Right-To-Know List *(see)*.

**BIS(TRIS[BETA, BETA-DIMETHYLPHENETHYL]TIN)OXIDE** • Bendex. An insecticide used in animal feed, dried apples, dried citrus pulp, dried grapes, dried prunes, and raisins. The FDA's tolerances are 20 ppm in prunes, 20 ppm in raisins. Limitations of 75 ppm in dried apple pomace, 35 ppm in dried citrus pulp, 100 ppm in dried grape pomace, 20 ppm in raisin waste when used for animal feed. Moderately toxic by ingestion and skin contact.

**BITTER ALMOND OIL** • Almond Oil. Sweet Almond Oil. Expressed Almond Oil. A colorless to pale yellow, bland, nearly odorless, essential and expressed oil from the ripe seed of the small sweet almond grown in Italy, Spain, and France. It has a strong almond odor and a mild taste. Used as a flavoring. Can cause stuffy nose and skin rashes in the allergic. GRAS when free of prussic acid.

**BITTER ASH EXTRACT** • *See* Quassia Extract.

**BITTER ORANGE OIL** • The pale yellow volatile oil expressed from the fresh peel of a species of citrus used in flavorings and increasingly in "weight reducing products." It contains synephrine, a stimulant that can raise blood pressure. Bitter orange may cause skin irritation and allergic reactions.

**BITTER PRINCIPLES** • A group of chemicals in plants that are bitter tasting. They differ chemically but most belong to the iris or pine families. Bitter principles reputedly stimulate the secretion of digestive juices and stimulate the liver. They are being investigated scientifically today as antifungals and antibiotics as well as anticancer additives. The bitter principle in mallow plants is being investigated as a male contraceptive. Other bitter principles in herbs are used to combat coughs and as sedatives.

**BITTER WOOD EXTRACT** • *See* Quassia Extract.

**BIURET** • A nutrient in animal feed for ruminants except for those producing milk for human consumption. *See* Urea.

**BIXIN** • Norbixin. The active ingredients of annatto, both carotenoidlike compounds, but with five times the coloring power of carotene, and with better stability. They impart a yellow coloring to food. *See* Annatto. E

**BIX ORELLANA** • A solvent extraction of *Bixa orellana* seeds. A yellow carotenoid *(see)* solution or powder, it is a color additive in ink used for marking foods, and is used in oleomargarine, poultry, sausage casings, and shortening. May cause contact dermatitis.

**BL** • Abbreviation for bleaching agent or flour-maturing agent.

**BLACK COHOSH** • *Cimicifuga racemosa.* Cimicifuga. Snakeroot. Bugbane. Black Snakeroot. Rattleroot. Used in astringents, perennial herb with a flower that is supposedly distasteful to insects. Grown from Canada to North Carolina and Kansas. Has a reputation for curing snakebites. It is used in ginger ale flavoring. A tonic and antispasmodic. The root contains various glycosides *(see)* including estrogenic substances and tannins. Herbalists have used it to relieve nerve pains, menstrual pains, and the pain of childbirth; also used to speed delivery and reduce blood pressure. Black cohosh is believed to have sedative properties. In 1992, the FDA proposed a ban on black cohosh in oral menstrual drug products because it had not been shown to be safe and effective as claimed.

**BLACK CURRANT EXTRACT** • The extract of the fruit of *Ribes nigrum,* a European plant that produces hanging yellow flowers and black aromatic fruit.

**BLACK CUTCH EXTRACT** • *See* Catechu Extract.

**BLACK PEPPER OIL** • From steam distillation of dried fruit of *Piper nigrum.* An odorless to greenish liquid with the odor and taste of pepper. A flavoring additive used in meat, salads, soups, and vegetables. A moderate skin irritant.

**BLACK WALNUT EXTRACT** • Extract of the leaves or bark of the black walnut tree, *Juglans nigra,* found in eastern North America. It produces nuts with a thick oil and is used as a black coloring.

**BLACKBERRY BARK EXTRACT** • *Rubus fruticosus.* A natural flavoring additive extracted from the woody plant. Used in berry, pineapple, grenadine, root beer, sarsaparilla, wintergreen, and birch beer flavorings for beverages, ice cream, ices, candy, baked goods, and liquor. The berries, leaves, and root bark are also used to treat fevers, colds, sore throats, vaginal discharge, diarrhea, and dysentery. The berries contain isocitric and malic acids, sugars, pectin, monoglycoside of cyanidin, vitamins C and A. The leaves and bark are said to lower fever, are astringent, and stop bleeding. The leaves are used for a soothing bath. ASP

**BLACKBERRY FRUIT EXTRACT** • *Rubus fruticosus.* The berries, leaves, and root bark are used to treat fevers, colds, sore throats, vaginal discharge, diarrhea, and dysentery. The berries contain isocitric and malic acids, sugars, pectin, monoglycoside of cyanidin, and vitamins C and A. *See* Malic Acid. ASP

**BLACKTHORN BERRIES** • *See* Sloe Berries.

**BLEACHING ADDITIVES** • Used by many industries, particularly flour milling, to make dough rise faster. Certain chemical qualities, which pastry chefs call "gluten characteristics," are needed to make an elastic, stable dough. Such qualities are acquired during aging, but in the process flour oxidizes, that is, combines with oxygen, and loses its natural gold color. Although mature flour is white, it possesses the qualities bakers want. But proper aging costs money and makes the flour more susceptible to insects and rodents, according to food manufacturers. Hence, the widespread use of bleaching and maturing additives.

**BLOOM INHIBITOR** • Bloom is an "undesirable effect" caused by the migration of cocoa fat from the cocoa fibers to the chocolate's surface. Chocolate that has bloomed has a gray-white appearance. Nonbloomed chocolate has a bright, shiny surface, with a rich appearance. The bloom inhibitor—a surfactant *(see)* such as sorbitan or lecithin *(see both)*—controls the size of the chocolate crystals and reduces the tendency of the fat to mobilize.

**BLUE** • *See* FD and C Blue.

**BLUE NO. 1** • *See* FD and C Blue No. 1.

**B&N** • Buffer and neutralizing additive.

**BOILER WATER ADDITIVES** • Most are used in food processing as cleaning additives. Those regulated by the FDA include ammonium alginate, cobalt sulfate, lignosulfonic acid, monbutyl ether of polyoxyethylene glycol or potassium tripolyphosphate, sodium carboxymethyl cellulose, sodium glucoheptonate, sodium humate, sodium meta silicate, sodium metabisulfite, polyoxypropylene glycol, polyoxyethylene glycol, potassium carbonate, sodium acetate, sodium alginate, sodium aluminate, sodium carbonate, sodium hexametaphosphate, sodium hydroxide, sodium lignosulfonate, sodium nitrate, sodium phosphate (mono-, di-, and tri-), sodium poly acrylate, sodium poly methacrylate, sodium silicate, sodium sulfate, sodium sulfite, sodium tripolyphosphate, tannin, tetraodium EDTA, tetrasodium pyrophosphate, 1-hydroxy-ethylidene-11-diphosphonic acid and its sodium, and potassium salt. Hydrazine *(see)* must be zero in steam contacting food. Acrylamide-sodium acrylate resin is restricted to 0.05 percent of acrylamide monomer in steam contacting food. Cyclohexylamine or morpholine must be less than 10 ppm in steam contacting food except milk and milk products. Octadecylamine must be less than 3 ppm; diethylaminoethanol must be less than 15 ppm; trisodium nitrilotriacetate must be less than 5 ppm in feed water; polymaleic acid and/or its sodium salt must be less than 1 ppm in feed water and in steam contacting food.

**BOIS DE ROSE OIL** • A fragrance from the chipped wood of the tropical rosewood tree obtained through steam distillation. The volatile oil is colorless, pale yellow, with a light camphor odor. Used in citrus, floral, fruit, meat, and spice flavorings for beverages, ice cream, ices, candy, baked goods, and chewing gum. There is reported use of the chemical; it has not yet been assigned for toxicology literature. GRAS. EAF

**BOLDUS LEAVES** • Flavoring from a Chilean fir tree with a sweet edible fruit used in alcoholic beverages only. There is no reported use of the chemical and there is no toxicology information available. NIL

**BOLETIC ACID** • *See* Fumaric Acid.

**BONITO, DRIED** • Related to mackerel, the Japanese dry them and use them in soups. They're often shaved into thin flakes called bonito flakes or hanakatsuo. NUL

**BORAGE EXTRACT** • The extract of the herb *Borago officinalis*. Contains potassium and calcium and has emollient properties and is used in a "tea" for sore eyes.

**BORAX** • Illegal for use in foods including wax coating for fruits and vegetables. It is permitted for use in export meats. NUL. E

**BORIC ACID** • An antiseptic with bactericidal and fungicidal properties used as a fungus control on citrus fruit (FDA tolerance 8 ppm boron residues). It is still widely used despite repeated warnings from the American Medical Association of possible toxicity. Severe poisonings have followed both ingestion and topical application to abraded skin. NUL. E

**BORNEO CAMPHOR** • *See* Borneol. ASP

**BORNEOL** • A flavoring additive with a peppery odor and a burning taste. Occurs naturally in coriander, ginger oil, oil of lime, rosemary, strawberries, thyme, citronella, and nutmeg. Toxicity is similar to camphor oil *(see)*. Used as a synthetic nut or spice flavoring for beverages, syrups, ice cream, ices, candy, baked goods, chewing gum. Can cause nausea, vomiting, convulsions, confusion, and dizziness. ASP

**BORNYL ACETATE** • It may be obtained from various pine needle oils. Strong piney odor. As a yarrow herb and iva herb extract, it is used as synthetic fruit and spice flavorings for beverages, ice cream, ices, candy, baked goods, chewing gum, and syrups. Colorless liquid derived from borneol *(see)* is also used in perfumery and as a solvent. ASP

**BORNYL BUTYRATE** • Synthetic flavoring from valerian *(see)*. EAF

**BORNYL FORMATE** • Formic Acid. A synthetic fruit flavoring additive for beverages, ice cream, ices, candy, baked goods, and syrups. Used in perfumes, soaps, and as a disinfectant. *See* Borneol. ASP

**BORNYL ISOVALERATE** • A synthetic fruit flavoring additive with a camphorlike smell used for beverages, ice cream, ices, candy, baked goods, and syrups. Also used medicinally as a sedative. *See* Borneol. ASP

**BORNYL VALERATE** • A synthetic fruit flavoring additive for beverages, ice cream, ices, candy, and baked goods. *See* Borneol. NIL

**BORNYVAL** • *See* Bornyl Isovalerate.

**BORON SOURCES** • Boric Acid. Sodium Borate. Boron occurs in the earth's crust (in the form of its compounds, not the metal) and borates are widely used as antiseptics even though toxicologists warn about possible adverse reactions. Used in modified hop extract. Boric acid and sodium borate are astringents and antiseptics. Borates are absorbed by the mucous membranes and can cause symptoms such as gastrointestinal bleeding, skin rash, central nervous system stimulation. The adult lethal dose is 30 grams (1 ounce). Infants and young children are more susceptible. Boron is used as a dietary supplement up to 1 milligram per day. Cleared for use by the FDA in modified hops extract up to 310 ppm.

**BORONIA, ABSOLUTE** • *Boronia megastigma.* A synthetic violet and fruit flavoring additive extracted from a plant. Used as a flavoring for beverages, ice cream, ices, and baked goods. There is reported use of the chemical; it has not yet been assigned for toxicology literature. EAF

**BOSWELLIA SPECIES** • *See* Olibanum Extract.

**BOULLION** • Vegetable Smoke. There is reported use of the chemical; it has not yet been assigned for toxicology literature. ASP

**B-BOURBONENE** • *See* Ethyl Vanillin. NIL

**BOVINE MILK-DERIVED LACTOFERRIN** • Used as an antimicrobial spray on beef carcasses that will subsequently be washed to reduce the levels of the applied lactoferrin *(see)*. GRAS

**BOVINE SOMATOTROPIN (BST)** • Bovine growth hormone (BGH) is a natural protein produced by the pituitary gland of all cattle. It is a protein hormone and is not structurally or functionally related to steroid hormones. Biotechnology has enabled scientists to produce a recombinant form of this protein called BST. They have found that supplementing cows' natural levels of BST improves their efficiency as milk producers by 5 to 10 percent without proportionately increasing production costs. The mammary glands of such dairy cows take in more nutrients from the bloodstream and produce more milk. Introduced on the market in 1994, the producers of the hormone, the FDA, and some other experts claim that there is no difference in the milk of cows given the hormone since cow's milk naturally contains the hormone anyway. Consumer groups, some scientists, small farmers, and a number of dairy product producers are against the use of the hormone. Among the reasons: it increases inflammation of the udder in cows, has unknown potential effects on humans, and is unnecessary because the U.S. government already supports milk prices because there is an overabundance of milk on the market. Certain states have enacted laws that direct farmers who use BST or BGH to say that the cows have or have not been treated. They are Maine, Minnesota, West

Virginia, and Wisconsin. You can obtain more information about the addition of the hormone to milk by contacting the agencies listed on pages 44–47.

**BRAN** • The outer indigestible shell of cereal grain that is usually removed before the grain is ground into flour. It provides bulk and fiber.

**BRASSICA ALBA** • *See* Mustard.

**BREWER'S YEAST** • Originally used by beer brewers, it is a good source of vitamins and protein. It can cause allergic reactions.

**BRILLIANT BLACK** • Black Bn. This food color was evaluated by the 1974 and 1977 Joint FAO/WHO Expert Committee on Food Additives. Since the previous evaluation, additional data became available and was equivocal. The coloring did not cause tumors in rats and mice but caused cysts in the intestines of pigs. Used in dairy-based drinks, flavored and/or fermented (e.g., chocolate milk, cocoa, eggnog, drinking yogurt, whey-based drinks) in Europe. A violet-black synthetic coal tar and azo dye. Used in decorations and coatings, desserts, fish paste, flavored milk drinks, ice cream, mustard, red fruit jams, sauces, savory snacks, soft drinks, soups, and sweets. Not recommended for consumption by children. Banned in Denmark, Australia, Austria, Belgium, Canada, Finland, France, Germany, Japan, Norway, Switzerland, Sweden, the United States, and Norway. BANNED in U.S. foods. E

**BRILLIANT BLUE** • See FD and C Blue No. 1. E

**BROMATED** • Combined or saturated with bromine, a nonmetallic, reddish, volatile liquid element. *See* Bromates.

**BROMATES** • Calcium bromate is a maturing additive and dough conditioner in bromated flours and bromated whole-wheat flour. Potassium bromate is a bread improver. Sugar contaminated with potassium bromate caused a food poisoning outbreak in New Zealand. The lethal dose is uncertain but two to four ounces of a 2 percent solution causes serious poisoning in children. Death in animals and man apparently is due to kidney failure, but central nervous system problems have been reported. Bromates may also cause skin eruptions. Topical application to abraded skin has caused poisoning.

**BROMELAIN** • Bromelin. A protein-digesting and milk-clotting enzyme found in pineapple. Used for tenderizing meat, chill-proofing beer, and as an antiinflammatory medication. "Solutions consisting of water, salt, monosodium glutamate, and approved proteolytic enzymes applied or injected into cuts of beef shall not result in a gain of more than 3 percent of the weight of the untreated product." GRAS. ASP

**BROMIC ACID, POTASSIUM SALT** • White crystals used as a dough conditioner and maturing additive in baked goods, beverages, and confectionery products. A poison by ingestion. An experimental carcinogen. A powerful oxidizer. An irritant to skin, eyes, and mucous membranes.

**BROMIDES, INORGANIC** • Potassium and Sodium. Used as fumigants. Bromides can cause skin rashes; large doses can cause central nervous system depression, and prolonged intake may cause mental deterioration.

**BROMINATED VEGETABLE OIL** • Bromine, a heavy, volatile, corrosive, nonmetallic liquid element, added to vegetable oil or other oils. Dark brown or pale yellow, with a bland or fruity odor. These high-density oils are blended with low-density essential oils to make them easier to emulsify. Used largely in soft drinks, citrus-flavored beverages, ice cream, ices, and baked goods. The FDA has them on the "suspect list." Less than 15 ppm in fruit-flavored beverages are allowed according to the FDA. In 2003, the agency ruled that the food additive brominated vegetable oil may be safely used in accordance with the following prescribed conditions: (1) The additive as free fatty acids (such as oleic) shall not exceed 2.5 percent and iodine value shall not exceed 16; (2) The additive is used on an interim basis as a stabilizer for flavoring oils used in fruit-flavored beverages, for which any applicable standards of identity do not preclude such use, in an amount not to exceed 15 parts per million in the finished beverage, pending the outcome of additional toxicological studies on which periodic reports at six-month intervals are to be furnished and final results submitted to the FDA promptly after completion of the studies. *See* Bromates for toxicity. ASP

**0-(4-BROMO-2-CHLOROPHENYL)-0-ETHYL-S-PROPYLPHOS-PHORO-THIOATE** • Curacron. Profenofos. Selecron. An insecticide used in animal feed and cottonseed hulls. Poison by ingestion and skin contact.

**BROMOMETHANE** • A colorless, volatile liquid that is used as a fumigant in animal feed, apples, barley, cereal grains, corn, cracked rice, fava beans, fermented malt beverages, flour, grain sorghum, kiwifruit, lentils, macadamia nuts, oats, pistachio nuts, rice, rye, sweet potatoes, and wheat. FDA residue tolerances include 125 ppm in cereal grain, 25 ppm in fermented malt beverages, 400 ppm in dog food, 125 ppm in barley, corn, grain sorghum, oats, rice, rye, and wheat when used for animal feed. Extremely hazardous, especially by inhalation. Death following acute poisoning is usually caused by lung irritation. In chronic poisoning, death is due to injury to the central nervous system.

**BROOM EXTRACT** • *See* Genet, Absolute.

**BROWN ALGAE** • *See* Algae Brown.

**BROWN FK** • Coloring. A highly suspect brown mixture of six synthetic azo dyes together with other colorings and sodium chloride and/or sodium sulfate. Found mainly in kippers and smoked mackerel but also occasionally in cooked hams and potato chips. Not recommended for consumption by children. Banned throughout the EU (except in the United Kingdom where its use is still permitted!) Also prohibited in Australia, Austria, Canada, Finland, Ireland, Japan, Norway, Sweden, and the United States. E

**BROWN HT** • A brown synthetic coal tar and azo dye found mainly in chocolate-flavored cakes. It appears to cause allergic and/or intolerance reactions, particularly among those with an aspirin intolerance and asthma sufferers; also known to induce skin sensitivity. Not recommended for consumption by children. Its use is banned in Australia, Austria, Belgium, Denmark, France, Germany, Norway, Sweden, Switzerland, and the United States. E

**BRYONIA** • A small herb used for flavoring in alcoholic beverages only.

**BST** • Abbreviation for bovine somatotropin *(see)* hormone. NUL

**BUCHU LEAF OIL** • *Barosma betulina* and *B. crenulata.* A natural flavoring additive from a South African plant used in berry, fruit, chocolate, mint, and spice flavorings for beverages, ice cream, ices, candy, baked goods, liquors, and condiments. Has been used as a urinary antiseptic and mild diuretic. EAF

**BUCHA LEAVES OIL** • *See* Bucha Leaf Oil. EAF

**BUCKBEAN LEAVES** • *Menyanthes trifoliata.* Flavoring in alcoholic beverages only. NUL

**BUCKTHORN** • Frangula. A shrub or tree grown on the Mediterranean coast of Africa, it has thorny branches and often contains a purgative in the bark or sap. Its fruits are used as a source of yellow and green dyes.

**BUFFER** • Usually a solution with a relatively constant acidity-alkalinity ratio, which is unaffected by the addition of comparatively large amounts of acid or alkali. A typical buffer solution would be hydrochloric acid *(see)* and sodium hydroxide *(see).*

**BUQUINOLATE** • An animal drug used in chicken feed to combat parasites. FDA limitations are 0.4 ppm in uncooked liver, kidney, and skin of chickens and 0.1 ppm in uncooked chicken muscle. Limitation of 0.5 ppm in egg yokes and 0.2 ppm in whole eggs.

**BUTADIENE-STYRENE COPOLYMER** • A component for a chewing-gum base. Butadiene is produced largely from petroleum gases and is used in the manufacture of synthetic rubber. It may be irritating to the skin and mucous membranes and narcotic in high concentrations. University of Texas professor of environmental toxicology Johnathan Ward believes the link between butadiene and genetic mutations means butadiene may be carcinogenic. Indeed, he reported in 2003 that he found that many rubber plant workers exposed to butadiene either had leukemia or had died from it. Styrene, obtained from ethyl benzene, is an oily liquid with a penetrating odor. It has the same uses and toxicity. Under study by NTP *(see)* as a carcinogen.

**BUTADIENE-STYRENE RUBBER** • Latex. A chewing-gum base. ASP

**BUTANAL** • *See* Butyraldehyde.

**BUTANDIONE** • *See* Triacetyl.

**BUTANE** • N-butane. Methylsulfonal. Bioxiran. Dibutadiene Dioxide. A flammable, easily liquefiable gas derived from petroleum. A solvent, refrigerant, and food additive. Also used as a propellant or aerosol in cosmetics. The principal hazard is that of fire and explosion, but it may be narcotic in high doses and cause asphyxiation. It has been determined by the National Institute of Occupational Safety and Health to be an animal carcinogen. GRAS. NUL

**1,4-BUTANE DICARBOXYLIC ACID** • *See* Adipic Acid.

**1,3-BUTANEDIOL** • A thick liquid used as a flavoring additive and solvent for flavorings. Mildly toxic by ingestion. An eye irritant.

**2,3-BUTANEDIONE** • A greenish yellow liquid with a strong odor used as a flavoring additive with margarine. Moderately toxic by ingestion. A skin irritant. GRAS

**1,2 BUTANEDITHIOL** • Flavoring additive. WHO *(see)* says there is no safety concern. ASP

**1,3-BUTANEDITHIOL** • Flavoring additive. WHO *(see)* says there is no safety concern. ASP

**2,3-BUTANEDITHIOL** • Flavoring additive. WHO *(see)* says there is no safety concern. ASP

**1-BUTANETHIOL** • Flavoring additive. FAO/WHO *(see)* says there is no safety concern. ASP

**2-BUTANONE** • Flavoring additive. FAO/WHO *(see)* says there is no safety concern. ASP

**BUTAN-3-ONE-2-YL BUTANOATE** • Flavoring additive. FAO/WHO *(see)* says there is no safety concern. ASP

**BUTANOIC ACID** • *See* Butyric Acid.

**1-BUTANOL** • *See* Butyl Alcohol. ASP

**4-BUTANOLIDE** • A colorless liquid with a caramel odor, it is used as a flavoring additive in candy and soy milk. Moderately toxic by ingestion. May cause skin tumors. GRAS

**2,3-BUTANOLONE** • *See* Acetoin.

**2-BUTANONE** • Colorless liquid with an acetonelike odor used as a flavoring additive in various foods. On the Community Right-To-Know List and in the EPA Genetic Toxicology Program *(see both)*. Moderately toxic by ingestion, skin contact, and injection.

**BUTAN-3-ONE-2YL BUTYRATE** • White to yellow liquid used as a flavoring additive in various foods. GRAS

**(trans)-BUTANEDIOIC ACID** • *See* Fumaric Acid.

**1-BUTEN-1-YL METHYL SULFIDE** • Flavoring additive. WHO *(see)* says it has no safety concern at current levels of intake when used as a flavoring additive. EAF

**BUTOXYPOLYETHYLENE** • A synthetic antifoaming additive used in beet sugar manufacture.

**BUTTER ACIDS** • Butter contains a wide variety of fatty acids that contribute to its functional advantages and characteristics. *See* Butters. ASP

**BUTTER ESTERS** • Widely used fractionated fats that have been separated into solid and liquid components. Used to make flavorings. *See* Butters.

**BUTTERMILK** • The fluid remaining after butter has been formed from churned cream. It can also be made from sweet milk by the addition of certain organic cultures. Used as an astringent right from the bottle. Apply liberally and let dry about 10 minutes. Rinse off with cool water.

**BUTTERS** • Acids, Esters, and Distillate. Substances that are solid at room temperature but that melt at body temperature are called butters. Butter acids are synthetic butter and cheese flavoring additives for beverages, ice cream, ices, candy (2,800 ppm), baked goods. Butter esters are synthetic butter, caramel, and chocolate flavoring additives for beverages, ice cream, ices, baked goods, toppings, and popcorn (1,200 ppm). Butter starter distillate is a synthetic butter flavoring additive for ice cream, ices, baked goods, and shortening (12,000 ppm). Cocoa butter is one of the most frequently used in both foods and cosmetics. Newer butters are made from natural fats by hydrogenation *(see),* which increases the butter's melting point or alters its plasticity. *See* Trans fatty acids.

**BUTTER STARTER DISTILLATE** • A flavoring. GRAS. ASP

**BUTYL ACETATE** • Acetic Acid, Butyl Ester. A synthetic flavoring additive, a clear liquid with a strong fruit odor, prepared from acetic acid and butyl alcohol. Used in raspberry, strawberry, butter, banana, and pineapple flavorings for beverages, ice cream, ices, candy, baked goods, chewing gum, and gelatin desserts. It is an irritant and may cause eye irritation (conjunctivitis). It is a narcotic in high concentrations, and toxic to man when inhaled at 200 ppm. ASP

**BUTYL ACETOACETATE** • A synthetic berry and fruit flavoring additive for beverages, ice cream, candy, and baked goods. ASP

**BUTYL ACETYL RICINOLEATE** • See *Ricinoleate.*

**BUTYL ALCOHOL** • A synthetic butter, cream, fruit, liquor, rum, and whiskey flavoring additive for beverages, ice cream, ices, candy, baked goods, cordials, and cream. A colorless liquid with an unpleasant odor, it occurs naturally in apples and raspberries. A solvent for waxes, fats, resins, and shellac. It may cause irritation of the mucous membranes, headache, dizziness, and drowsiness when ingested. Inhalation of as little as 25 ppm causes pulmonary problems in humans. It can also cause contact dermatitis when applied to the skin. ASP

*t*-**BUTYL ALCOHOL** • *See* Butyl Alcohol.

**BUTYL ETHYL DISULFIDE** • A flavoring determined GRAS by the Expert Panel of the Flavor and Extract Manufacturers Association.

**BUTYL ALDEHYDE** • *See* Butyraldehyde.

**BUTYLAMINE** • Colorless, volatile liquid with an ammonia odor derived from butanol or butyl chloride with ammonia. Used as an intermediate for emulsifying additives, insecticides, and dyes. ASP

**sec-BUTYLAMINE** • Tutane. A fungicide used in animal feed, citrus molasses, and dried citrus pulp. Limitations of 90 ppm in citrus molasses and dried citrus pulp when used for cattle feed. Poisonous by ingestion. A powerful irritant. Moderately toxic by skin contact.

**BUTYL ANTHRANILATE** • A synthetic grape, mandarin, and pineapple flavoring additive for beverages, ice cream, ices, candy, and baked goods. ASP

**n-BUTYL n-BUTANOATE** • Colorless liquid with pineapple odor used as a flavoring additive in various foods. Mildly toxic by ingestion. Moderately irritating to eyes, skin, and mucous membranes by inhalation. Narcotic in high concentrations.

**BUTYL BUTYROLLACTATE** • Colorless liquid with a buttery, creamlike odor used as a flavoring additive in baked goods and candy. A skin irritant. ASP

**BUTYL BUTYRATE** • A colorless liquid used as a flavoring. It is an irritant and narcotic. ASP

**BUTYL BUTYRYLLACTATE** • A colorless, synthetic flavoring additive from butyl alcohol, with a fruity odor. Used in berry, butter, apple, banana, peach, pineapple, liquor, scotch, and nut flavoring for beverages, ice cream, ices, candy, baked goods, chewing gum, and gelatin desserts.

**BUTYL CARBOBUTOXYMETHYL PHTHALATE** • A plasticizer used in packaging material. Mildly toxic via injection. Causes birth defects in laboratory animals. An eye irritant in humans.

**a-BUTYL CINNAMALDEHYDE** • A synthetic fruit, nut, spice, and cinnamon flavoring additive for beverages, ice cream, ices, candy, and baked goods. ASP

**BUTYL CINNAMATE** • A synthetic chocolate, cocoa, and fruit flavoring for beverages, ice cream, ices, candy, baked goods, and liquor. ASP

**BUTYL 2-DECENOATE** • A synthetic apricot and peach flavoring additive for beverages, ice cream, ices, candy, baked goods, chewing gum (2,000 ppm). ASP

**BUTYL DECYLENATE** • *See* Butyl 2-Decenoate.

**BUTYL DODECANOATE** • *See* Butyl Laurate. ASP

**BUTYL ETHYL MALONATE** • A synthetic fruit and apple flavoring for beverages, ice cream, ices, candy, and baked goods. ASP

**BUTYL FORMATE** • Formic Acid. A synthetic fruit, plum, liquor, and rum flavoring for beverages, ice cream, ices, candy, and baked goods. *See* Formic Acid for toxicity. ASP

**BUTYL HEPTANOATE** • A synthetic fruit and liquor flavoring for beverages, ice cream, ices, candy, and baked goods. NIL

**BUTYL HEXANOATE** • A synthetic butter, butterscotch, pineapple, and rum flavoring additive for beverages, ice cream, ices, candy, and baked goods. ASP

**Tert-BUTYL HYDROQUINONE (TBHQ)** • White crystalline solid used as an antioxidant in beef products, dry cereals, edible fats, margarine, meat, pizza toppings, pork, potato chips, poultry, sausage, and vegetable oils. Moderately toxic by ingestion. May be mutagenic. The Joint FAO/WHO Expert Committee on Food Additives concluded in June 1998, "The potential exists for high consumers of TBHQ to exceed the ADI [Acceptable Daily Intake], but the available data were insufficient to estimate the number of high consumers or the magnitude and duration of intake above the ADI." The committee is reviewing this additive's level in edible fats and oils, fish and fish products, and carbonated water-based soft drinks. ASP

**BUTYL *p*-HYDROXYBENZOATE** • Butyl Paraben. Butyl *p*-Oxybenzoate. Almost odorless, small colorless crystals or white powder used as an antimicrobial preservative.

**ALPHA-BUTYL-OMEGA-HYDROXYPOLY(OXYETHYLENE) POLY(OXYPROPYLENE** • Inert ingredient used in pesticides. NIL

**3-BUTYLIDENEPHTHALIDE** • Flavoring found in celery, celery stalk. Used in soups, condiments, meats; cigarettes. FEMA *(see)* claims it is GRAS. ASP

**BUTYL ISOBUTYRATE** • A synthetic raspberry, strawberry, butter, banana, and cherry flavoring additive for beverages, ice cream, ices, candy, baked goods, and chewing gum (2000 ppm). ASP

**BUTYL ISOVALERATE** • A synthetic chocolate and fruit flavoring for beverages, ice cream, ices, candy, puddings, and gelatin desserts. ASP

**2-BUTYL-5 (or 6)-KETO-1, 4-DIOXANE** • A synthetic fruit and spice flavoring for beverages, ice cream, ices, candy, baked goods, and shortenings. ASP

**BUTYL LACTATE** • A synthetic butter, butterscotch, caramel, and fruit flavoring additive for beverages, ice cream, ices, candy, baked goods. ASP

**BUTYL LAURATE** • A synthetic fruit flavoring for beverages, ice cream, ices, candy, and baked goods. ASP

**BUTYL LEVULINATE** • A synthetic butter, fruit, and rum flavoring additive for beverages, ice cream, ices, candy, baked goods. ASP

**N-BUTYL 2-METHYLBUTYRATE** • *See* Methyl Butyrate. ASP

**BUTYL OLEATE SULFATE** • *See* Sulfated Butyl Oleate. EAF

**BUTYL PARASEPT** • *See* Butyl *p*-Hydroxybenzoate.

**BUTYL PHENYLACETATE** • Synthetic butter, honey, caramel, chocolate, rose, fruit, and nut flavoring additive for beverages, ice cream, ices, candy, baked goods, gelatin desserts, and puddings. ASP

**BUTYL PHOSPHOROTRITHIOATE** • Butifos. A defoliant used in animal feed and cottonseed hulls. A poison by ingestion, skin contact, and possibly other routes. Caused mutations in animals and affected nerve transmission. FDA limitations of 6 ppm in cottonseed hulls when used for animal feed.

**BUTYL PROPIONATE** • A synthetic butter, rum butter, fruit, and rum flavoring additive for beverages, ice cream, ices, candy, and baked goods. May be an irritant. ASP

**BUTYL RUBBER** • A synthetic rubber used as a chewing-gum base component.

**BUTYL SALICYLATE** • *See* Salycilates. ASP

**BUTYL SEBACATE** • *See* Dibutyl Sebacate.

**BUTYL STEARATE** • A synthetic antifoaming additive used in the production of beet sugar. Also a synthetic banana, butter, and liquor flavoring for beverages, ice cream, ices, candy, baked goods, chewing gum, and liqueurs. ASP

**BUTYL SULFIDE** • A synthetic floral, violet, and fruit flavoring for beverages, ice cream, ices, candy, and baked goods. ASP

**BUTYL 10-UNDECENOATE** • A synthetic butter, apricot, cognac, and nut flavoring additive for beverages, ice cream, ices, candy, baked goods, chewing gum, icing, and liquor. ASP

**BUTYL VALERATE** • A synthetic butter, fruit, and chocolate flavoring additive for beverages, ice cream, ices, candy, baked goods, puddings, and gelatin desserts. ASP

**BUTYL-** • Prefix for any class of synthetic rubbers.

**BUTYLATED HYDROXYANISOLE (BHA)** • A preservative, stabilizer, and antioxidant in many products, including beverages, ice cream, ices, candy, baked goods, chewing gum, gelatin desserts, soup bases, potatoes, glacéed fruits, potato flakes, sweet potato flakes, dry breakfast cereals, dry yeast, dry mixes for desserts, lard, shortening, unsmoked dry sausage, and in emulsions for stabilizers for shortenings. It is a white or slightly yellow waxy solid with a faint, characteristic odor. Insoluble in water. Total content of antioxidants is not to exceed 0.02 percent of fat or oil content of food; allowed up to 1,000 ppm in dry yeast; 200 ppm in shortenings; 50 ppm in potato flakes; and 50 ppm with BHT (butylated hydroxytoluene) in dry cereals. Can cause allergic reactions. BHA affects the liver and kidney functions (the liver detoxifies it). BHA may be more rapidly metabolized than BHT *(see)* and in experiments at Michigan State University it appeared to be less toxic to the kidneys of living animals than BHT. It is also used as a flavoring additive and to treat mastitis in dairy cattle. Can cause allergic reactions. The final report to the FDA of the Select Committee on GRAS Substances stated in 1980 that while no evidence in the available information demonstrates a hazard to the public at current use levels, uncertainties exist, requiring that additional studies be conducted. The FDA said in 1980 that GRAS status should continue while tests on BHA are being completed and evaluated. In the 1990 *Annual Review of Pharmacology and Toxicology,* scientists from the United Kingdom and the United States reviewed Japanese reports of a high incidence of cancerous and benign tumors in the forestomach of rats fed BHA. The reviewers concluded that because we humans don't have forestomachs and because the doses of BHA administered to the rats were so high, there was nothing to be alarmed about. In November 1990, Glenn Scott, M.D., a Cincinnati physician, filed a petition with the FDA asking the agency to prohibit the use of BHA in food. Before acting on Scott's petition, however, the FDA asked the Federation of American Societies for Experimental Biology (FASEB) to reexamine the scientific data on BHA and make a report by March 1992. The joint FAO/WHO Expert Committee on Food Additives concluded in June 1998, "The potential exists for high consumers of BHA to exceed the ADI [Acceptable Daily Intake], but the available data were insufficient to estimate the number of high consumers or the magnitude and duration of intake above the ADI." The committee is reviewing this additive's level in edible fats and oils, dried vegetables, cocoa products, processed meat, frozen fish, ready-to-eat soup and broth, and food supplements—now thirteen years after the report in the scientific journal that cited it as a potential cancer-causing agent. Petroleum derivative. Retards spoilage due to oxidation. Not permitted in infant foods. Can provoke an allergic reaction in some people. Used in edible oils, chewing gum, polyethylene food wraps. May trigger hyperactivity and other intolerances; serious concerns over carcinogenicity and estrogenic effects. BHA is banned in Japan. In 1958 and in 1963 official committees of experts recommended that BHT be banned in the UK; however reportedly industry objections killed the ban. ASP. E

**BUTYLATED HYDROXYMETHYLPHENOL** • A new antioxidant, a nearly white crystalline solid with a faint characteristic odor. Contains phenol, which is toxic.

**BUTYLATED HYDROXYTOLUENE (BHT)** • A preservative, stabilizer, and antioxidant employed in many foods. Used as a chewing-gum base, added to potato and sweet potato flakes and dry breakfast cereals, an emulsion stabilizer for shortenings used in enriched rice, animal fats, and shortenings containing animal fats. White crystalline solid with a faint characteristic odor. Insoluble in water. Total content of antioxidants in fat or oils not to exceed 0.02 percent. Allowed up to 200 ppm in emulsion stabilizer for shortenings, 50 ppm in dry breakfast cereals and potato flakes. Used also as an antioxidant to retard rancidity in frozen fresh pork sausage and freeze-dried meats up to 0.01 percent based on fat content. It is also used as a flavoring additive and to treat mastitis in dairy cattle. Can cause allergic reactions. Loyola University scientists reported on April 14, 1972, that pregnant mice fed a diet consisting of one-half of 1 percent of BHT (or BHA, butylated hydroxyanisole) gave birth to offspring that frequently had chemical changes in the brain and subsequently abnormal behavior patterns. BHT and BHA are chemically similar, but BHT may be more toxic to the kidney than BHA *(see)*, according to researchers at Michigan State University. The Select Committee of the American Societies for Experimental Biology, which advises the FDA on food additives, recommended further studies to determine "the effects of BHT at levels now present in foods under conditions where steroid hormones or oral contraceptives are being ingested." They said the possibility that BHT may convert other ingested substances into toxic or cancer-causing additives should be investigated. BHT is prohibited as a food additive in the United Kingdom. The FDA is pursuing further study. The joint FAO/WHO Expert Committee on Food Additives concluded in June 1998, "The potential exists for high consumers of BHT to exceed the ADI [Acceptable Daily Intake], but the available data were insufficient to estimate the number of high consumers or the magnitude and duration of intake above the ADI." The committee is reviewing this additive's levels in edible fats and oils, chewing gum, and fish and fish products. ASP. E

**1,3-BUTYLENE GLYCOL** • A clear, colorless, viscous liquid with a slight taste. A solvent and humectant most resistant to high humidity and thus valuable in foods and cosmetics. It retains scents and preserves against spoilage. It has a similar toxicity to ethylene glycol *(see),* which when ingested may cause transient stimulation of the central nervous system, then depression, vomiting, drowsiness, coma, respiratory failure, and convulsions; renal damage may proceed to uremia and death. One of the few humectants not on the GRAS list, although efforts to place it there have been made through the years. ASP

**BUTYLPARABEN** • Widely used in food and cosmetics as an antifungal preservative, it is the ester of butyl alcohol and *p*-hydroxybenzoic acid *(see both).*

**BUTYRALDEHYDE** • A synthetic flavoring additive found naturally in coffee and strawberries. Used in butter, caramel, fruit, liquor, brandy, and nut flavorings for beverages, ice cream, ices, candy, baked goods, alcoholic beverages, and icings. Used also in the manufacture of rubber, gas accelerators, synthetic resins, and plasticizers. May be an irritant and a narcotic. ASP

**BUTYRIC ACID** • *n*-Butyric Acid. Butanoic Acid. A clear, colorless liquid present in butter at 4 to 5 percent with a strong penetrating rancid-butter odor. Butter, butterscotch, caramel, fruit, and nut flavoring additive for beverages, ice cream, ices, candy, baked goods, gelatin desserts, puddings, chewing gum, and margarine. Found naturally in apples, butter acids, geranium rose oil, grapes, strawberries, and wormseed oil. It has a low toxicity but can be a mild irritant. GRAS. ASP

**BUTYRIC ALDEHYDE** • *See* Butyraldehyde.

**BUTYRIN** • *See* (tri-)Butyrin.

**(tri-)BUTYRIN** • A synthetic flavoring additive found naturally in butter. Butter flavoring for beverages, ice cream, ices, candy (1,000 ppm), baked goods, margarine, and puddings.

**BUTYROIN** • *See* 5-Hydroxy-4-Octanone.

**BUTYROLACTONE** • Butanolide. Liquid lactone used chiefly as a solvent for resins. It is also an intermediate *(see)* in the manufacture of polyvinylpyrrolidone *(see)*. Human toxicity is unknown but beta-butyrolactone is a cancer-causing agent according to the Environmental Defense Fund.

**BUTYRONE** • *See* 4-Heptanone.

**BUXINE** • *See a*-Amyl Cinnamaldehyde.

**BUXINOL** • *See a*-Amylcirmamyl Alcohol.

# C

**CA** • FDA abbreviation for about, approximately.

**CACAO SHELL** • Cacao shells of the seeds of trees grown in Brazil, Central America, and most tropical countries. Weak chocolatelike odor and taste, thin and peppery, with a reddish brown color. Used in the manufacture of caffeine *(see)* and theobromine, which occurs in chocolate products and is used as a diuretic and nerve stimulant. Occasionally causes allergic reactions from handling. GRAS

**CACHOU EXTRACT** • *See* Catechu Extract.

**CACTUS ROOT EXTRACT** • *See* Yucca Extract.

**CADINENE** • A general fixative that occurs naturally in juniper oil and pepper oil. It has a faint, pleasant smell. Used in candy, baked goods (1,200 ppm), and chewing gum (1,000 ppm). ASP

**CADMIUM** • A naturally occurring metal used to control molds and diseases that attack home lawns, golf courses, and other grasses. However, less than 0.1 percent of the annual U.S. consumption of 12 million pounds of cadmium is used in pesticides—most of it is used in industries. Cadmium in drinking water has been correlated with cancer of the pharynx, esophagus, intestines, larynx, lungs, and bladder. Cadmium is believed to cause mutations. It is poisonous when ingested and is also a potential cancer-causing additive. It has an extremely long biological clearance in humans and accumulates in body tissues, particularly in the liver and kidney. There are no available chelating additives to enhance cadmium excretion. The FAO/WHO Expert Committee on Food Additives allocated a Provisional Tolerable Weekly Intake (PTWI) of 400 to 500 nanograms of cadmium per person. The average dietary intake, according to the United Nations, is approximately 10 to 50 nanograms per day in areas of normal exposure. The committee noted there was a question about how much biologically active cadmium was available from various foods, such as rice or grains. For example, in a study in New Zealand, the blood concentration and urinary excretion of cadmium were found to be "surprisingly low" in a population with a high dietary intake of New Zealand oysters, which contain high levels of cadmium. The committee maintains the current PTWI of 7 nanograms per kilogram of body weight pending future research. The FDA, which previously allowed cadmium as a colorant in polystyrenes, no longer allows its use. Being reviewed by the NTP *(see)* as a carcinogen.

**CAFFEINE** • Guaranine. Methyltheobromine. Theine. Trimethylxanthine. An odorless white powder with a bitter taste that occurs naturally in coffee, cola, guarana paste, tea, and kola nuts. Caffeine is the number one psychoactive drug. Obtained as a by-product of producing caffeine-free coffee. Used as a flavor in root beer beverages and other foods. It is a central nervous system, heart, and respiratory system stimulant. Caffeine can alter blood sugar release and cross the placental barrier. It can cause nervousness, insomnia, irregular heartbeat, noises in ears, and, in high doses, convulsions. It has been linked to spontaneous panic attacks in persons sensitive to caffeine. It has been found to be addictive. It also causes increases in calcium excretion. Caffeine was considered GRAS because it was in use before 1958. However, the expert committee convened for the specific purpose of the GRAS review determined that uncertainties existed about caffeine that require additional studies. The FDA acknowledged that caffeine in cola-type beverages has been in use well before 1958. Because of its capability to cause birth defects in rats, the FDA proposed regulations to request new safety studies and to encourage the manufacture and sale of caffeine-free colas. One regulation would make the food industry's continued use of caffeine as an added ingredient in soft drinks and other foods conditional upon its funding of studies of caffeine's effects on children and the unborn. A University of Montreal study published in the *Journal of the American Medical Association,* December 22, 1993, said that women who consume the amount of caffeine in one and a half to three cups of coffee a day may nearly double their risk of miscarriage. Under present regulations, a soft drink, except one artificially sweetened, must contain caffeine if it is to be labeled as cola or pepper, and the FDA wants soda producers to be able to use this name when caffeine is not used. The FDA has asked for studies on the long-term effects of the additive to determine whether it may cause cancer or birth defects. The FDA and the American Medical Association have proposed quantitative labeling of caffeine content. By July 1, 2004, products sold in the Euopean Union containing more than 150 mg of caffeine per liter must include the term "high caffeine content" near the product name. Such products must also indicate the caffeine content expressed in mg/100. Australia already requires that caffeinated "energy drinks" state: "Not suitable for children and caffeine sensitive persons." In 2003, the National Soft Drink Association legally objected to the FDA's proposed new labeling rules for caffeine. ASP

**CAJEPUT OIL** • *Melaleuca leucadendra.* A spice flavoring from the cajeput tree native to Australia. The leaves yield an aromatic oil. Used for beverages, ice cream, ices, candy, and baked goods. EAF

**CAJEPUTENE** • *See* Limonene.

**CAJEPUTOL** • *See* Eucalyptol.

**CALAMUS** • Sweet Flag. Sweet Sedge. *Acorus calamus.* The rhizome contains essential oil, mucilage, glycosides, amino acid, and tannins. The oil is obtained by steam distillation of the stem or root and is used as a flavoring additive. Calamus root is an ancient Indian and Chinese herbal medicine used to treat stomach acid, irregular heart rhythm, low blood pressure, coughs, and lack of mental focus. Native Americans would chew the root to enable them to run long distances with increased stamina. Externally, it was used to induce a state of tranquillity. Banned as a food additive by the FDA.

**CALC** • FDA abbreviation for calculated.

**CALCIUM ACETATE** • Brown Acetate of Lime. A white amorphous powder that has been used medicinally as a source of calcium. It is used in the manufacture of acetic acid and acetone and in dyeing, tanning, and curing skins as well as a corrosion inhibitor in metal containers. Low oral toxicity. The final report to the FDA of the Select Committee on GRAS Substances stated in 1980 that it should continue its GRAS status with no limitations other than good manufacturing practices. ASP. E

**CALCIUM ACID PHOSPHATE** • *See* Calcium Phosphate

**CALCIUM ALGINATE** • A stabilizer, thickener, gelling additive, and texturizer. Also used as a solvent and vehicle for flavorings. Found in ice cream and Popsicles, soft and cottage cheeses, cheese snacks, dressings and spreads, fruit drinks, beverages, and instant desserts. *See* Alginates. GRAS. E

**CALCIUM ALUMINUM SILICATE** • Anticaking agent. *See* Calcium Silicate and Aluminum. E

**CALCIUM ASCORBATE** • A preservative and antioxidant prepared from ascorbic acid (vitamin C) and calcium carbonate *(see).* Used in concentrated milk products; in cooked, cured, or pulverized meat products; in pickles in which pork and beef products are cured and packed (up to 75 ounces per 100 gallons). *See* Ascorbic Acid for toxicity. The final report to the FDA of the Select Committee on GRAS Substances stated in 1980 that it should continue its GRAS status with no limitations other than good manufacturing practices. ASP. E

**CALCIUM BENZOATE** • Used as a preservative, both antibacterial and antifungal. Can be found in concentrated pineapple juice. People who suffer from asthma, aspirin sensitivity, or the skin disease urticaria may have allergic reactions and/or find their symptoms become worse following consumption of benzoic acid, particularly in combination with tartrazine. Not recommended for consumption by children. *See* Benzoic Acid. NUL. E

**CALCIUM BROMATE** • A maturing additive and dough conditioner used in bromated flours. The FDA allows 0.0075 part per 100 parts by weight of flour used. NIL *See* Bromate.

**CALCIUM CAPRATE** • Anticaking additive and emulsifier salt. *See* Caprylic Acid. NUL

**CALCIUM CAPRYLATE** • Anticaking additive and emulsifier salt. *See* Caprylic Acid. NUL

**CALCIUM CARBONATE** • Chalk. A tasteless, odorless powder that occurs naturally in limestone, marble, and coral. Used as a white food dye and alkali to reduce acidity in wine up to 2.5 percent, a neutralizer for ice cream and in cream syrups up to 0.25 percent, in confections up to 0.25 percent, and in baking powder up to 50 percent. Employed as a carrier for bleaches. Once widely used as a white coloring in foods and cosmetics, the FDA withdrew its use as a coloring in 1988. Calcium carbonate is still used as an alkali to reduce acidity, a neutralizer, and firming additive. Also used in dentifrices as a tooth polisher. It is used as an emulsifier under FDA regulations. A gastric antacid and antidiarrhea medicine, it may cause constipation. Female mice were bred after a week on diets supplemented with calcium carbonate at 220 and 880 times the human intake of this additive. At all dosage levels, the first and second litters of newly weaned mice were lower in weight and number, and mortality was increased. The highest level caused heart enlargement. Supplementing the maternal diet with iron prevents this, so the side effects were attributed to mineral imbalance due to excessive calcium intake. In humans, 500 milligrams per kilogram of body weight was fed to ulcer victims for three weeks. The amount ingested was 145 times the normal amount ingested as an additive. Some patients developed an excess of calcium in the blood and suffered nausea, weakness, and dizziness. Calcium carbonate can cause constipation. GRAS. ASP. E

**CALCIUM CARBONATE CUDEAR** • Logwood, chips, and extract. Purple coloring from lichens. It is the source of litmus. Previously commonly used as a coloring in food, the FDA no longer authorizes its use.

**CALCIUM CARRAGEENAN** • *See* Carrageenan.

**CALCIUM CASEINATE** • Used as a nutrient supplement for frozen desserts (except water ices) and in creamed cottage cheese. *See* Casein. ASP

**CALCIUM CHLORIDE** • The chloride salt of calcium. White, hard, odorless fragments, granules, powder, or as a solution. It absorbs water. Used in its anhydrous *(see)* form as a drying additive for organic liquids and gases. Used as a firming additive for sliced apples and other fruits, in apple pie mix, as a jelly ingredient, in certain cheeses to aid coagulation, in artificially sweetened fruit jelly, and in canned tomatoes. It is also used to treat mastitis in dairy animals. Employed medicinally as a diuretic and a urinary acidifier. Ingestion can cause stomach and heart disturbances. The final report to the FDA of the Select Committee on GRAS Substances stated in 1980 that it should continue its GRAS status with no limitations other than good manufacturing practices. ASP. E

**CALCIUM CITRATE** • A fine, white odorless powder prepared from citrus fruit. Used as a buffer to neutralize acids in confections, jellies, jams, and in saccharine at the rate of 3 ounces per 100 pounds of the artificial sweetener. It is also used to improve the baking properties of flour. *See* Citrate Salts for toxicity. The final report to the FDA of the Select Committee on GRAS Substances stated in 1980 that it should continue its GRAS status with no limitations other than good manufacturing practices. ASP. E

**CALCIUM CYCLAMATE** • BANNED. *See* Cyclamates.

**CALCIUM DIACETATE** • A sequestrant used in cereal. *See* Calcium Acetate. GRAS

**CALCIUM DIGLUTAMATE** • The salt of glutamic acid *(see)*. A flavor enhancer and salt substitute. Almost odorless white powder. The FDA says that it needs further study. As of this writing, nothing has been reported. NUL. E

**CALCIUM DIOXIDE** • Used in cereal flours. *See* Calcium Peroxide.

**CALCIUM DISODIUM EDTA** • Edetate Calcium Disodium. Calcium Disodium Ethylenediamine Tetraacetic Acid. A preservative and sequestrant, white, odorless powder with a faint salty taste. Used as a food additive to prevent crystal formation and to retard color loss. Used in canned and carbonated soft drinks for flavor retention; in canned white potatoes and cooked canned clams for color retention; in crabmeat to retard struvite (crystal formation); in dressings as a preservative; in cooked and canned dried lima beans for color retention; in fermented malt beverages to prevent gushing; in mayonnaise and oleomargarine as a preservative; in processed dried pinto beans for color retention; and in sandwich spreads as a preservative. Residue tolerances set by the FDA for this additive are: cereal flours, 25 ppm; fermented malt beverages, 25 ppm; spice extractives, 60 ppm; pecan pie filling, 100 ppm; clams (cooked canned) to promote color retention, 340 ppm; lima beans to promote color, 310 ppm; crabmeat (cooked canned) to retard struvite formation, 275 ppm; shrimp (cooked canned) to retard struvite and to promote color retention, 250 ppm; carbonated soft drinks to promote flavor, 33 ppm; canned white potatoes to promote color retention, 110 ppm; canned mushrooms, 200 ppm; pickled cucumbers or pickled cabbage to promote color, flavor, and texture retention, 220 ppm; artificially colored lemon and orange-flavored spreads, 100 ppm; potato salad preservative, 100 ppm; French dressing, mayonnaise, and salad dressing; nonstandardized dressings and sauces, preservative, 75 ppm; sandwich spread as a preservative, 100 ppm; by weight of egg yolk portion, 200 ppm; distilled alcoholic beverages to promote stability of color, flavor, and/or product clarity; oleomargarine as a preservative, 75 ppm. Promotes stability of color. Used medically as a chelating additive to detoxify poisoning by lead and other heavy metals. May cause intestinal upsets, muscle cramps, kidney damage, and blood in urine. On the FDA priority list of food additives to be studied for mutagenic, teratogenic, subacute, and reproductive effects. The European Parliament said in 2003, said that this synthetic antioxydant is building complexes with mineral salts, can increase the uptake of heavy metals, and can lead to metabolic problems. It is not authorized in Australia. E

**CALCIUM FERROCYANIDE** • Anticaking additive in salt and in icing for fish. E

**CALCIUM GLUCONATE** • Odorless, tasteless, white crystalline granules, stale in air. Used as a buffer, firming additive, sequestrant in jelly and preserves. Also used in animal feeds. It is soluble in water. May cause gastrointestinal and cardiac disturbances. The final report to the FDA of the Select Committee on GRAS Substances stated in 1980 that it should continue its GRAS status with no limitations other than good manufacturing practices. ASP. E

**CALCIUM GLYCEROPHOSPHATE** • A fine, white, odorless, nearly tasteless powder used in dentifrices, baking powder, and as a food stabilizer and dietary supplement. A component of many over-the-counter nervetonic foods. Administered medicinally for numbness and debility. The final report to the FDA of the Select Committee on GRAS Substances stated in 1980 that it should continue its GRAS status with no limitations other than good manufacturing practices. *See* Calcium Sources. ASP

**CALCIUM 5'-GUANYLATE** • Flavor potentiator. Odorless white crystals or powder having a characteristic taste. *See* Flavor Potentiators. E

**CALCIUM HEXAMETAPHOSPHATE** • An emulsifier, sequestering additive, and texturizer used in breakfast cereals, angel food cake, flaked fish (prevents struvite), ice cream, ices, milk, bottled beer, reconstituted lemon juice, puddings, processed cheeses, artificially sweetened jellies and preserves, potable water supplies to prevent scale formation and corrosion and in brine for curing hams. The final report to the FDA of the Select Committee on GRAS Substances stated in 1980 that it should continue but at this writing, its GRAS status is under review. NUL

**CALCIUM HYDROGEN SULFITE** • Preservative, antibrowning agent, antioxidant, a white crystalline or granular solid with an odor of sulfur dioxide. *See* Sulfites. E

**CALCIUM HYDROXIDE** • Slaked Lime. Calcium Hydrate. Limewater. Lye. An alkali, a white powder with a slightly bitter taste. Used as a firming additive for various fruit products, canned peas, as an egg preservative, in water treatment, in animal feeds, and for debarring hides. Used in pesticides. Accidental ingestion can cause burns of the throat and esophagus; also death from shock and asphyxia due to swelling of the glottis and infection. Calcium hydroxide also can cause burns on the skin and eyes. The final report to the FDA of the Select Committee on GRAS Substances stated in 1980 that it should continue its GRAS status with no limitations other than good manufacturing practices. ASP. E

**CALCIUM HYPOCHLORITE** • A germicide and sterilizing additive, the active ingredient of chlorinated lime, used in the curd washing of cottage cheese, in sugar refining, as an oxidizing and bleaching additive, and as an algae killer, bactericide, deodorant, disinfectant, and fungicide. Sterilizes fruits and vegetables by washing in a 50 percent solution. Under various names, dilute hypochlorite is found in homes as laundry bleach and household bleach. Occasionally cases of poisoning occur when people mix household hypochlorite solution with various other household chemicals, which causes the release of poisonous chlorine gas. As with other corrosive additives, calcium hypochlorite's toxicity depends upon its concentrations. It is highly corrosive to skin and mucous membranes. Ingestion may cause pain and inflammation of the mouth, pharynx, esophagus, and stomach, with erosion particularly of the mucous membranes of the stomach.

**CALCIUM HYPOPHOSPHITE** • Crystals of powder, slightly acid in solution, and practically insoluble in alcohol. It is a corrosion inhibitor and has been used as a dietary supplement in veterinary medicine. The final report to the FDA of the Select Committee on GRAS Substances stated in 1980 that it should continue its GRAS status with no limitations other than good manufacturing practices. NUL

**CALCIUM 5'-INOSINATE** • *See* Inosinate. E

**CALCIUM IODATE** • White odorless or nearly odorless powder used as a dough conditioner and oxidizing additive in bread, rolls, and buns. It is a nutritional source of iodine in foods such as table salt, and used also as a topical disinfectant and as a deodorant. Low toxicity, but may cause allergic reactions. GRAS. ASP

**CALCIUM IODOBEHENATE** • Dietary supplement used in animal feed as a source of iodine *(see)*. GRAS

**CALCIUM LACTATE** • White, almost odorless crystals or powder used as a buffer and as such is a constituent of baking powders and is employed in confections; also used in dentifrices and as a yeast food and dough conditioner. It improves crispness in canned bean sprouts. Also used in animal feeds. In medical use, given for calcium deficiency; may cause gastrointestinal and cardiac disturbances. The final report to the FDA of the Select Committee on GRAS Substances stated in 1980 that it should continue its GRAS status with no limitations other than good manufacturing practices. ASP. E

**CALCIUM LACTOBIONATE** • A firming additive in dry pudding mixes. *See* Calcium Lactate. NIL

**CALCIUM LAURATE** • Anticaking additive and emulsifier salt. *See* Laruic Acid. NUL

**CALCIUM LIGNOSULFONATE** • A brown, amorphous substance obtained from the pulp of wood mixed with calcium and sodium salts. It may contain up to 30 percent sugar. It is used as a dispersing additive and stabilizer for pesticides used on bananas. It is also employed in molasses fed to animals. *See* Calcium Sources. NUL

**CALCIUM MALATES** • Acidifiers. *See* Malic Acid. E

**CALCIUM METASILICATE** • White powder, insoluble in water, used as an absorbent, antacid, filler for paper coatings, and as a food additive. Use in food restricted to 5 percent in baking powder and 2 percent in table salt. Irritating dust.

**CALCIUM MYRISTATE** • Surfactant *(see)*. NUL

**CALCIUM OLEATE** • Dispersant. NUL

**CALCIUM ORTHOPHOSPHATE** • Buffer and neutralizer used in noncarbonated beverages. GRAS.

**CALCIUM OXIDE** • Quicklime. Burnt Lime. A hard, white or grayish white, odorless mass or powder that is used as a yeast food and dough conditioner for bread, rolls, and buns. It is also an alkali for neutralizing dairy products (including ice cream mixes) and alkalizes sour cream, butter, and confections, and is used in the processing of tripe. Industrial uses are for bricks, plaster, debarring hides, fungicides, insecticides, and for clarification of beet and cane sugar juices. A strong caustic, it may severely damage skin and mucous membranes. The final report to the FDA of the Select Committee on GRAS Substances stated in 1980 that it should continue its GRAS status with no limitations other than good manufacturing practices. *See* Calcium Sources. ASP. E

**CALCIUM PALMITATE** • Anticaking additive and emlsifier. *See* Palmitic Acid. NUL

**CALCIUM PANTOTHENATE** • Pantothenic Acid Calcium Salt. A B-complex vitamin, pantothenate is a white, odorless powder with a sweetish taste and bitter aftertaste. Pantothenic acid occurs everywhere in plant and animal tissue, and the richest common source is liver; jelly of the queen bee contains six times as much. Rice bran and molasses are other good sources. Acid derivatives sold commercially are synthesized. Biochemical defects from lack of calcium pantothenate may exist undetected for some time but eventually manifest themselves as tissue failures. The calcium chloride double salt of calcium pantothenate has been cleared for use in foods for special dietary uses. Moderately toxic by ingestion. The final report to the FDA of the Select Committee on GRAS Substances stated in 1980 that it should continue its GRAS status with no limitations other than good manufacturing practices. *See* Pantothenamide. ASP

**CALCIUM PANTOTHENATE CALCIUM CHLORIDE DOUBLE SALT** • *See* Calcium Panthothenate and EDTA. ASP

**CALCIUM PERIODATE** • A nutrient source of iodine in salt for livestock.

**CALCIUM PEROXIDE** • White or yellowish, odorless, almost tasteless powder that is derived from an interaction of a calcium salt and sodium peroxide with subsequent crystallization. Used in bakery products as a dough conditioner, for bleaching of oils, modification of starches, and as a seed disinfectant. Irritating to the skin. ASP

**CALCIUM PHOSPHATE** • Dibasic, Monobasic, and Tribasic. White, odorless powders used as yeast foods, dough conditioners, and firming additives. Tribasic is an anticaking additive used in table salt, powdered sugar, malted milk powder, condiments, puddings, meat, dry-curing mixtures, cereal flours, and vanilla powder. It is tasteless. Used as a gastric antacid mineral supplement and a clarifying additive for sugars and syrups. Dibasic is used to improve bread, rolls, buns, cereal flours; a carrier for bleaching; used as a mineral supplement in cereals, in dental products, and in fertilizers. Monobasic is used in bread, rolls, and buns, artificially sweetened fruit jelly, canned potatoes, canned sweet peppers, canned tomatoes, and as a jelling ingredient. Employed as a fertilizer, as an acidulant, in baking powders, and in wheat flours as a mineral supplement. Skin and eye irritant. The final report to the FDA of the Select Committee on GRAS Substances stated in 1980 that it should continue its GRAS status with no limitations other than good manufacturing practices. ASP. E

**CALCIUM PHYTATE** • Used as a sequestering additive *(see)*. When 300 milligrams per kilogram of body weight was fed to rats as a diet supplement, it successfully provided calcium for bone deposition, and the animals remained healthy. The final report to the FDA of the Select Committee on GRAS Substances stated in 1980 that it should continue its GRAS status with no limitations other than good manufacturing practices. NIL

**CALCIUM PROPIONATE** • Propanoic Acid. Calcium Salt. White crystals or crystalline solid with the faint odor of propionic acid. A mold and rope inhibitor in breads, rolls, and poultry stuffing, it is used in processed cheese, chocolate products, cakes, cupcakes, and artificially sweetened fruit jelly. It is used as a preservative in cosmetics and as an antifungal medication for the skin. GRAS. ASP. E

**CALCIUM PYROPHOSPHATE** • A fine, white, odorless, tasteless powder used as a nutrient, an abrasive in dentifrices, a buffer, and as a neutralizing additive in foodstuffs. The final report to the FDA of the Select Committee on GRAS Substances stated in 1980 that it should continue its GRAS status with no limitations other than good manufacturing practices. *See* Calcium Sources. ASP

**CALCIUM RESINATE** • Yellowish white powder or lumps used to dilute the color of eggshells. No residue is permitted.

**CALCIUM 5'-RIBONUCLEOTIDES** • Flavor potentiators *(see)*, in odorless white crystals or powder, with a characteristic taste. *See* Inosinates. E

**CALCIUM SACCHARIN** • *See* Saccharin.

**CALCIUM SALTS** • Acetate, Chloride, Citrate, Diacetate, Gluconate, Phosphate (monobasic), Phytate, Sulfate. Emulsifier salts used in evaporated milk and frozen desserts, also in enriched bread. Firming additive in potatoes and canned tomatoes. Green or red sweet peppers, lima beans, and carrots. May be gastric irritants, but they have little oral toxicity. *See* Calcium Sulfate and Calcium Phosphate.

**CALCIUM SALTS OF FATTY ACIDS** • Used as binders, emulsifiers, and anticaking additive in foods. ASP

**CALCIUM SALTS OF PARTIALLY DIMERIZED ROSIN** • Used as a coating on free citrus fruits. *See* Calcium Salts.

**CALCIUM SILICATE** • Okenite. An anticaking additive, white or slightly cream-colored, free-flowing powder. It is used up to 5 percent in baking powder and 2 percent of table salts. Also used in vanilla powder. Absorbs water. Also used as a coloring additive. Constituent of lime glass and cement, used in road construction. Practically nontoxic orally, except inhalation may cause irritation of the respiratory tract. ASP. E

**CALCIUM SORBATE** • A preservative and fungus preventative used in beverages, baked goods, chocolate syrups, soda-fountain syrups, fresh fruit cocktail, tangerine puree (sherbet base), salads (potato, macaroni, cole slaw, gelatin), cheesecake, pie fillings, cake, cheese in consumer-size packages, and artificially sweetened jellies and preserves. The final report to the FDA of the Select Committee on GRAS Substances stated in 1980 that it should continue its GRAS status with no limitations other than good manufacturing practices. ASP. E

**CALCIUM SOURCES** • Harmless calcium salts: Carbonate, Citrate, Glycerophosphate, Oxide, Phosphate, Pyrophosphate, Sulfate. Calcium is a mineral supplement for breakfast cereals, white cornmeal, infant dietary formula, enriched flour, enriched bromated flour (*see* Bromates), enriched macaroni, noodle products, self-rising flours, enriched farina, cornmeal and corn grits, and enriched bread and rolls. Calcium is a major mineral in the body. It is incompletely absorbed from the gastrointestinal tract when in the diet so its absorption is enhanced by calcium normally present in intestinal secretions. Vitamin D is also required for efficient absorption of calcium. Recommended daily requirements for adult females is 1.5 grams, for adult males 1.2 grams, and for children 0.8 gram. Calcium and phosphorus are the major constituents of teeth and bones. The ratio of calcium to phosphorus in cow's milk is approximately 1.2 to 1. In human milk the ratio is 2 to 1. The final report to the FDA of the Select Committee on GRAS Substances stated in 1980 that it should continue its GRAS status with no limitations other than good manufacturing practices.

**CALCIUM STEARATE** • Vanilla powder used in beet sugar and yeast. Prepared from lime water *(see)*, it is an emulsifier, a coloring additive. The final report to the FDA of the Select Committee on GRAS Substances stated in 1980 that it should continue its GRAS status with no limitations other than good manufacturing practices. ASP

**CALCIUM STEAROYL LACTYLATE** • *See* Calcium Stearyol-2-Lactylate. ASP

**CALCIUM STEAROYL-2-LACTYLATE** • The calcium salt of the stearic acid ester of lactyl lactate. A free-flowing, white powder dough conditioner in yeast-leavened bakery products and prepared mixes for yeast-leavened bakery products. Also a whipping additive in dried, liquid, and frozen egg whites. ASP. E

**CALCIUM SULFATE** • Plaster of Paris. A fine, white to slightly yellow, odorless, tasteless powder used as a firming additive and yeast food and dough conditioner. Utilized in brewing and other fermentation industries, in Spanish-type sherry, as a jelling ingredient, in cereal flours, as a carrier for bleaching additive, in bread, rolls, and buns, in blue cheese and Gorgonzola cheese, artificially sweetened fruit, jelly, canned potatoes, canned sweet peppers, and canned tomatoes. Used also in creamed cottage cheese as an alkali. Also used in toothpaste and tooth powders as an abrasive and firming additive. Also used as a coloring additive in cosmetics. Used in cement, wall plaster, and insecticides. Because it absorbs moisture and hardens quickly, its ingestion may result in intestinal obstruction. Mixed with flour, it has been used to kill rodents. GRAS. ASP. E

**CALCIUM SULFITE** • A white calcium salt prepared as a powder and used especially as a disinfectant and preservative. *See* Sulfites. E

**CALCIUM TARTRATE** • Derived from cream of tartar. Used as a food preservative and antacid. E

**CALENDULA** • Dried flowers of pot marigolds grown in gardens everywhere. Used as a natural flavoring additive. *See* Marigold, Pot, for foods in which it is used. GRAS

**CALORIE** • A unit used to express the heat output of an organism and the fuel or energy value of food. The amount of heat required to raise the temperature of 1 gram of water from 14.5 to 15.5°C at atmospheric pressure. When a caloric value for a serving of a food is less than 5 calories, the FDA allows the label to read "zero calories." If a fat calorie is less than 0.5 gram, it can also be listed as "calories from fat zero."

**CALUMBA ROOT** • Flavoring used in alcoholic beverages only. EAF

**CAMOMILE** • *See* Chamomile.

**2-CAMPHANOL** • *See* Borneol.

**CAMPHENE** • A synthetic spice and nutmeg flavoring additive for beverages, ice cream, ices, candy, and baked goods. Occurs naturally in calamus oil, citronella, ginger, lemon oil, mandarin oil, myrtle, petitgrain oil, and juniper berries. May be mutagenic. ASP

**CAMPHOLENE ACETATE** • Flavoring. FAO/WHO *(see)* says there is no safety concern. NIL

**CAMPHOR OIL** • Japanese White Oil. Camphor Tree. Distilled from trees at least fifty years old grown in China, Japan, Formosa, Brazil, and

Sumatra. Camphor tree is used in spice flavorings for beverages, baked goods, and condiments. Must be safrole *(see)*. It is also used in embalming fluid, in the manufacture of explosives, in lacquers, as a moth repellent, and topically in liniments, cold medications, and anesthetics. It can cause contact dermatitis. In 1980, the FDA banned camphorated oil as a liniment for colds and sore muscles because of reports of poisonings through skin absorption and because of accidental ingestion. A New Jersey pharmacist had collected case reports and testified before the FDA Advisory Review Panel on Over-the-Counter Drugs in 1980. Camphor is readily absorbed through all sites of administration. Ingestion of 2 grams generally produces dangerous effects in an adult. Ingestion by pregnant women has caused fetal deaths. As of this writing, nothing new to report. EAF

**CAMPHOR OIL FORMOSAN HO-SHO LEAVES** • *Cinnamomum camphora.* Flavoring. Although the natural oil of camphor has been largely replaced by the synthetic, a number of other components are used to make synthetic flavorings. NUL

**CAMPYLOBACTER JEJUNI** • The leading cause of bacterial diarrhea. *See* Edible Film.

**CANANGA OIL** • A natural flavor extract obtained by distillation from the flowers of the tree. Has a harsh, floral odor. Used in cola, fruit, spice, and ginger ale flavoring for beverages, ice cream, ices, candy, baked goods. May cause allergic reactions. GRAS. EAF

**CANDELILLA WAX** • Obtained from candelilla plants. Brownish to yellow brown, hard, brittle, easily pulverized, partially insoluble in water. Hardens other waxes. Used as a coating for foods. GRAS. ASP. E

**CANDIDIA GUILLIERMONDII** • An enzyme derived from *Candidia guilliermondii;* used as a production aid in citric acid. NUL

**CANDIDA LIPOLYTICA** • Derived from *Candida lypolytica;* used as a fermentation organism in the production of citric acid. NUL

**CANE SUGAR** • *See* Sucrose.

**CANOLA OIL** • A low erucic acid rapeseed oil *(see)* used in salad oils because it contains 50 percent less saturated oils than other popular oils. GRAS

**CANTHAXANTHIN** • A color additive derived from edible mushrooms, crustaceans, trout, and salmon, and tropical birds. It produces a pink color when used in foods. It is a synthetic non-provitamin A carotinoid that is easily absorbed by fat. The FDA says the color additive canthaxanthin may be safely used for coloring foods generally if the quantity does not exceed 30 milligrams per pound of solid or semisolid food or per pint of liquid food. Permanently listed in 1969 for human food and permanently listed in 1985 in chicken feed to enhance the yellow color of chicken skin. It is exempt from certification. The FAO/WHO Expert Committee on Food Additives said that up to 25 milligrams per kilogram of body weight is acceptable.

Canthaxanthin is also taken for the purpose of skin "tanning" and may be provided by tanning salons or by mail order. It is not approved as a prescription or an over-the-counter drug. A report from Vanderbilt University's Department of Pharmacy cited the case of a healthy young woman who ingested canthaxanthin given to her by a commercial tanning salon. She developed aplastic anemia and died (*JAMA*, Sep. 5, 1990, 264(9): 1141–12.). In the August 1993 issue of *American Pharmacy*, Darrell Hulisz, Pharm.D., and pharmacist Ginger Boles described this condition—called "canthaxanthin-induced retinopathy"—as "a common adverse effect associated with canthaxanthin use," adding: "The patient experiencing this form of retinopathy rarely is symptomatic, although decreased visual acuity has been reported." Oral intake, thus, may cause loss of night vision since there is some evidence that high intakes of the substance lead to deposition on the retina. The frequency of the adverse effects of this ingredient is unknown, Vanderbilt researchers say, because there is no current way to monitor distribution. Foods that contain canthaxanthin derived originally from animal feed do not have to be labeled. The need to declare the presence in a food of coloring agents used in the feed of food-producing animals was discussed by the EU Standing Committee for Foodstuffs at its meeting in 2002. A large majority of member states were in favor of draft legislation being prepared to deal with this issue, and the UK suggested the most appropriate legislative vehicle for this would be the food labeling directive. The EU has agreed to convene an expert group to discuss the issue. ASP. E

**CAPERS** • A natural flavoring from the spiny shrub. The pickled flower bud is used as a condiment for sauces and salads. GRAS. ASP

**CAPRALDEHYDE** • *See* Decanal.

**CAPRENIN** • A 5-calorie per gram fat substitute for cocoa butter in candy bars. Made of capric acid and caprylic acid, two fatty acids found in coconut and palm kernel oil. The other half is made of behenic acid, a poorly digested fat taken from hydrogenated rapeseed oil *(see)*. GRAS

**CAPRIC ACID** • Obtained from a large group of American plants. Solid crystalline mass with a rancid odor used in the manufacture of artificial fruit flavors. Also used to flavor lipsticks. *See* Decanoic Acid.

**CAPRIC ALDEHYDE** • *See* Decanal.

**CAPRINALDEHYDE** • *See* Decanal.

**CAPROALDEHYDE** • *See* Hexanal.

**CAPROIC ACID** • Hexanoic Acid. Occurs as glyceride in natural oils. Derived from coconut oil fatty acids, it is used in fruit flavors and as an intermediate for food-grade additives. It is also used in peeling solutions for fruits and vegetables.

**CAPRYLAMINE OXIDE** • *See* Caprylic Acid and Capric Acid.

**CAPRYL BETAINE** • *See* Caprylic Acid and Betaine.

**CAPRYLIC ACID** • An oily liquid that occurs naturally as a fatty acid in sweat, fusel oil, in the milk of cows and goats, and in palm and coconut oil. Cleared for use as a synthetic flavoring. The final report to the FDA of the Select Committee on GRAS Substances stated in 1980 that it should continue its GRAS status with no limitations other than good manufacturing practices. GRAS

**CAPRYLIC ALCOHOL** • *See* 1-Octanol.

**CAPSANTHIN** • *See* Paprika. E

**CAPSICUM** • African Chilies. Cayenne Pepper. Tabasco Pepper. The dried fruit of a tropical plant used as a natural spice and ginger ale flavoring for beverages, ice cream, ices, candy, baked goods, chewing gum, meats, and sauces. The oleoresin form is used in sausage, spice, ginger ale, and cinnamon flavorings for beverages, ice cream, ices, candy, baked goods, chewing gum, meats, and condiments. Used internally as a digestive stimulant. Irritating to the mucous membranes, it can produce severe diarrhea and gastritis. May cause a "hot" sensation and sweating. *See* Cayenne Pepper for toxicity. GRAS. ASP

**CAPSORUBIN** • Coloring from paprika *(see)*. E

**CAPTAN** • Agrosol. Merpan. Orthocide. Osocide. Vanguard. Vanicide. White to creamy-colored powder, practically insoluble in water, derived from tetrahydrophthalmide and trichloromethylmercaptan. Used to treat seeds, to preserve fruit, and as a fungicide on almonds, animal feed, apples, beans, beef, beets, broccoli, cabbage, carrots, corn, garlic, kale, lettuce, peaches, peas, pork, potatoes, raisins, spinach, and strawberries. The FDA permits residues of up to 50 ppm in raisins, 100 ppm on corn seed for cattle and hog feed. It is a fungicide of lower toxicity than most, but in large doses can cause diarrhea and weight loss. A skin and lung irritant, and a suspected cause of human birth defects. Pregnant women should avoid exposure to it. Also suspected of causing cancer. Moderately toxic to humans by ingestion.

**CARAMEL** • A chemically ill-defined group of material produced by heating carbohydrates. Burnt sugar with a pleasant, slightly bitter taste. Made by heating sugar or glucose and adding small quantities of alkali or a trace mineral acid during heating. Caramel color prepared by ammonia process has been associated with blood toxicity in rats. Because of this, the joint FAO/WHO Expert Committee on Food Additives temporarily removed the acceptable daily intake for ammonia-made caramel. It was found to inhibit the metabolism of $B_6$ in rabbits. Caramel is widely used as a brown coloring in ice cream, baked goods, soft drinks, and confections. As a flavoring, it is used in strawberry, butter, butterscotch, caramel, chocolate, cocoa, cola, fruit, cherry, grape, birch beer, liquor, rum, brandy, maple, black walnut, walnut, root beer, spice, ginger, ginger ale, vanilla, and cream soda beverages (2,200 ppm), ice cream, candy, baked goods, syrups (2,800 ppm), and meats (2,100 ppm). The FDA has given caramel priority for testing its mutagenic, teratogenic subacute, and reproductive effects as a food additive. Sulfite ammonia caramels tested on humans produced soft to liquid stools and increased bowel movements. The final report to the FDA of the Select Committee on GRAS Substances stated in 1980 that it should continue its GRAS status with no limitations other than good manufacturing practices. Permanently listed in 1963 as a coloring. Certification not required. ASP. E

**CARAMEL COLOR III** • Used as a color additive in beers and a variety of foods. Beer is the most important single source of this additive in the diet although consumption of dark beers has been decreasing in recent years. The FAO/WHO Expert Committee on Food Additives has established an ADI *(see)* of 200 per kilogram of body weight per day. The safety of caramel color III has been questioned during recent years following feeding studies in the rat that were associated with reduced white cells and lymphocyte counts. In studies at Hazelton Laboratories America, Madison, Wisconsin, rats given caramel color III had soft feces and lower food and fluid consumption. No other toxicity was noted.

**CARAWAY SEED and OIL** • The dried ripe seeds of a plant common to Europe and Asia and cultivated in England, Russia, and the United States. A volatile, colorless to pale yellow liquid, it is used in liquor flavorings for beverages, ice cream, baked goods, and condiments; also used as a spice in baking. The oil is used in grape, licorice, anisette, kümmel, liver, sausage, mint, caraway, and rye flavorings for beverages, ice cream, ices, candy, baked goods, chewing gum, meats, condiments, and liquors. Can cause contact dermatitis. A mild carminative, from one to two grams breaks up intestinal gas. Moderately toxic by ingestion and skin contact. A skin irritant. May be mutagenic. GRAS. ASP

**CARAZOLOL** • A beta-blocker that lowers blood pressure, chest pain, and irregular heartbeat. It is used for the treatment of stress in pigs.

**CARBADOX** • Mecadox. Fortigro. An antibacterial used in animal feed for swine. The FAO/WHO Expert Committee on Food Additives would not set an ADI or NOEL *(see both)* for this drug since it is a cancer-causing additive. FDA tolerance for carbadox residues in swine is zero. On January 4, 1994, the FDA was notified by a Quincy, Illinois, company that twenty-five dairy cows at a small Wisconsin farm had been accidentally fed for several months with swine feed containing carbadox. The agency was also notified that milk from these cows had been shipped to Wisconsin dairies for processing into mozzarella cheese, butter, and whey. The whey, in turn, had been further processed into lactose, which was used in infant formula and other products. Carbadox is approved for use in pig feed to treat swine dysentery. Studies have indicated that the drug can cause liver tumors in rodents when fed at high levels over their entire lifetime. Research reportedly had "found no significant adverse effects associated with short-term carbadox exposure in animals." Analyses by FDA, state, and other experts indicated that any carbadox residue in any of the suspect products would have been so "minuscule that it would not pose a risk to public health." A study of milk from a cow fed with carbadox-treated feed showed the amount of carbadox in the milk was less than 1 percent of the amount that was fed to the animals. Metabolism studies of carbadox in animal species show the drug can be converted to less toxic compounds. The FDA said it is likely that much of the carbadox fed to the cows was converted to less toxic compounds. In addition, any milk used that contained carbadox would have been mixed with milk from many other sources, and therefore diluted. Canada in 2001 moved to ban the use of carbadox in food animals.

**CARBAMATE** • A compound based on carbamic acid which is used only in the form of its numerous derivatives and salts. Carbamates are used in pesticides. Among the carbamate pesticides are aldicarb, 4-benzothienyl-N-methyl carbamate, bufencarb (BUX), carbaryl, carbofuran, isolan, 2-isopropyl phenyl-N-methyl carbamate, 3-isopropyl phenylmethyl carbamate, maneb, propoxur, thiram, Zectran, zineb, and ziram. Carbamic acid, which is colorless and odorless, causes depression of bone marrow and degeneration of the brain, nausea, vomiting. It is moderately toxic by many routes.

**CARBAMIDE** • The chief solid component of mammalian urine; synthesized from ammonia and carbon dioxide and used as fertilizer and in animal feed and in plastics. Increasingly popular in tooth whiteners. See Urea. E

**N-CARBAMOYL ARSANILIC ACID** • White, nearly odorless powder added to animal feed as a growth stimulant. It is an arsenic *(see)* compound that is on the Community Right-To-Know List *(see)*. Poison by ingestion. Has caused tumors in laboratory animals.

**CARBARSONE** • An antiamebic and antihistomonad used in turkey and chicken feed. FDA residue tolerance is 0.025 percent to 0.0375 percent in the feed, 2 ppm in residue in edible by-products of chicken and turkeys, and 0.5 ppm as residue in muscle meat of chickens and turkeys and in eggs.

**CARBARYL** • Sevin. Pesticide used on corn and other vegetables and fruits. FDA residue tolerances for pineapple bran for feed, 20 ppm; as residues in or on pineapples, 2 ppm; as residue in eggs, 0.25 ppm; as residue in fat, meat, meat by-products from layer chickens, 0.05 ppm; as residues in kidney and liver of cattle, goats, horses, sheep, and swine, 1 ppm; as residue in fat, meat, and meat by-products of cattle, swine, goats, horses, and shrimp, 0.1 ppm; as a residue in various raw agricultural conditions, 0.2–100 ppm. Causes nausea, vomiting, diarrhea, lung damage, blurred vision, excessive salivation, muscle twitching, cyanosis, convulsions, coma, and death. It is a poison via oral and skin absorption. It is an eye and skin irritant. Absorption through skin is slow. It does not accumulate in the tissues and is much less toxic than parathion *(see)*.

**CARBETHOXY MALATHION** • Malathion. Vegru Malatox. Vetiol. Zithiol. Malacide. Carbophos. A brown to yellow liquid used as an insecticide on animal feed, citrus pulp, grapes, nonmedicated cattle-feed concentrate blocks, packaging material, and safflower oil. The FDA permits a residue of up to 12 ppm in grapes, 0.6 ppm in safflower oil, 50 ppm in dehydrated citrus pulp, 10 ppm in nonmedicated cattle-feed concentrate blocks. A human poison by ingestion. May be mutagenic. Has caused allergic skin reactions. It can interfere with nerve transmission.

**CARBOFURAN** • A pesticide used in animal feed. FDA residue tolerances are in various raw agricultural commodities, 2 ppm; on dried grape pomace, 6 ppm; soybean soap stock, 6 ppm; in raisin waste, 6 ppm; peanut soap stock, 24 ppm.

**CARBOHYDRASE, ASPERGILLUS** • An enzyme from fermentation of *Aspergillus oryzae,* a fungi, used as a production aid and tenderizing additive in alcoholic beverages, ale, bakery products, beer, dairy products, meats, poultry, and starch syrups. Used in the production of dextrose. The FDA says that solutions of water and this enzyme applied or injected into raw meat cuts shall not result in a gain of more than 3 percent above the weight of the treated product. When heated to decomposition it emits acrid smoke and irritating fumes. GRAS. ASP

**CARBOHYDRASE and CELLULASE** • Derived from *Aspergillus niger,* this enzyme permits easy shucking of clams and peeling of shrimp. The FDA permits use at a level not in excess of the amount reasonably required to accomplish the intended effect. When heated to decomposition it emits acrid smoke and irritating fumes. NUL

**CARBOHYDRASE and PROTEASE** • An enzyme from the controlled fermentation of *Bacillus licheniformus,* it is a brown powder or liquid used in beer, alcoholic beverages, candy, dextrose, fish meal, nutritive sweeteners, protein hydrolysates, and starch syrups. When heated to decomposition it emits acrid smoke and irritating fumes. There is reported use of the chemical, but it has not yet been assigned for toxicology literature. GRAS. NUL

**CARBOHYDRASE from *BACILLUS AMYLOLIQUEFACIENS* and *BACILLUS SUBTILIS*** • *Bacillus amyloliquefaciens* strain FZB24 is found naturally in soil and leaf litter, and can be easily grown in large quantities. It seems to work as a growth enhancer and disease suppressor through an enzyme that it produces. *Bacillus subtilis,* a gram-positive harmless bacterium, is capable of producing endospores resistant to adverse environmental conditions such as heat and desiccation and is widely used for the production of enzymes and specialty chemicals. EAF

**CARBOHYDRASE, RHIZOPUS** • An enzyme derived from *Rhizopus oryzae* used in processing dextrose *(see).* When heated to decomposition, it emits acrid smoke and irritating fumes. NUL. GRAS

**CARBOHYDRASE from SACCHAROMYCES** • Enzyme from yeast used to break down protein in food processing and wine making. GRAS. NUL

**CARBOHYDRATES** • Starches and sugars contain a high proportion of carbohydrates. Carbohydrates are chemicals that contain carbon, hydrogen, and oxygen, and they are widely available in plants. In the body, however, carbohydrates in the blood supply are held at an almost constant level of about 0.05 to 0.1 percent. Carbohydrates are the fuel of life. Each gram of carbohydrate provides about four calories of energy—the same as protein but less than fat. Following digestion and absorption, available carbohydrates may be used to meet immediate energy needs of tissue cells, converted to glycogen, the storage form of glucose in liver and muscle for later energy needs, or converted to fat as a reserve for energy. It is possible that relatively pure carbohydrate solutions have different effects in young and elderly individuals. Carbohydrates can act as a supplemental fuel source during exercise. The ability of carbohydrate supplements to prolong endurance during exercising is related to preventing fatigue in a physiological sense in both body and mind. The effect of carbohydrate in increasing the tryptophan ratio in blood is considered to be a possible mechanism.

**CARBOMYCIN** • Deltamycin. An animal antibiotic used on chickens. It is also used in combination with oxytetracycline *(see)*. The FDA allows no residue in cooked edible tissues of chicken. Poison by subcutaneous route. Moderately toxic by vein and injection into the muscle. When heated to decomposition it emits toxic fumes.

**CARBON BLACK** • Several forms of artificially prepared carbon or charcoal, including animal charcoal, furnace black, channel (gas) black, lamp black, activated charcoal, and ferric sulfate. Animal charcoal is used as a black coloring in confectionery. Activated charcoal is used as an antidote for ingested poisons, and as an adsorbent in diarrhea. The others have industrial uses. Carbon black, which was not subject to certification *(see)* by the FDA was reevaluated and then banned in 1976. It was found in tests to contain a cancer-causing by-product that was released during dye manufacture. It can no longer be used in candies such as licorice and jelly beans or in drugs or cosmetics. Channel (gas) black has been BANNED.

**CARBON DIOXIDE** • Colorless, odorless, noncombustible gas with a faint acid taste. Used as a pressure-dispensing additive in gassed creams. Also used in the carbonation of beverages and as dry ice for refrigeration in the frozen food industry. Under pressure of about fifty-nine atmospheres it may be condensed into a liquid, a portion of which forms a white solid (dry ice). May cause shortness of breath, vomiting, high blood pressure, and disorientation if inhaled in sufficient amounts. GRAS. ASP. E

**CARBON DISULFIDE** • A clear, colorless liquid used as a fumigant for cereal grains. Extremely hazardous. A human poison by ingestion. Mildly toxic to humans by inhalation.

**CARBON TETRACHLORIDE** • Carbon Tet. Tetrachloromethane. Perchlormethane. A colorless, clear, heavy, nonflammable liquid obtained from carbon disulfide and chlorine. It is used as a fumigant on cereal grains. Poisonous by inhalation, ingestion, or skin absorption. Acute poisoning causes nausea, diarrhea, headache, stupor, kidney damage, and can be fatal. Chronic poisoning involves liver damage, but can also cause kidney damage. It has caused cancer in animals. Because it is so toxic, the FDA banned its use in products for the home in 1970.

**CARBONYL IRON** • Iron that has been processed with carbon and oxygen. Used as a coloring. The final report to the FDA of the Select Committee on GRAS Substances stated in 1980 that there is no evidence in the available information that it is a hazard to the public when used as it is now and it should continue its GRAS status with limitations on the amounts that can be added to food.

**CARBOPHENOTHION** • A pesticide used on citrus meal fed to cattle. FDA tolerance is 10 ppm. *See* Organophosphates.

**CARBOXINE** • Vitavax. Carboxin. A fungicide used on barley, beans, corn, oats, peanut hulls, rice, sorghum, and wheat for animal feeds. Poison by ingestion. Moderately toxic by skin contact.

**CARBOXYMETHYL CELLULOSE** • Sodium. *See* Cellulose Gums. GRAS. E

**CARBOXYMETHYL HYDROXYETHYL CELLULOSE** • A binder and emulsifier. *See* Cellulose and Ethylene Glycose. ASP

**CARDAMOM OIL** • Grains of Paradise. A natural flavoring and aromatic additive from the dried ripe seeds of trees common to India, Ceylon, and Guatemala. Used in butter, chocolate, liquor, spice, and vanilla flavorings for beverages, ice cream, ices, candy, baked goods (1,700 ppm), meats, and condiments. The seed oil is used in chocolate, cocoa, coffee, cherry liquor, liver, sausage, root beer, sarsaparilla, cardamom, ginger ale, vanilla, and cream soda flavorings for beverages, ice cream, ices, candy, baked goods, chewing gum, liquor, pickles, curry powder, and condiments. As a medicine, it breaks up intestinal gas. May be mutagenic. There is reported use of the chemical; it has not yet been assigned for toxicology literature. ASP. GRAS

**3-CARENE** • Antifungal terpene *(see)*. Can cause allergic reactions and has been found it can be toxic to the lungs. *See* Terpenes. EAF

**CARMINE** • Cochineal. *Coccus catil.* A crimson pigment derived from a Mexican and Central American species of a scaly female insect that feeds on various cacti. Carmine and cochineal extracts are permanently listed, but cochineal alone is not authorized for use. The colorings are used in red applesauce, confections, baked goods, meats, and spices. Cochineal was involved in an outbreak of salmonellosis (an intestinal infection) that killed one infant in a Boston hospital and made twenty-two patients seriously ill.

Carmine, used in the diagnostic solution to test the digestive organs, was found to be the infecting additive. Also used in cosmetics. University of Michigan medical researchers said this color additive extracted from dried bugs and used in candy, yogurt, fruit drinks, and other foods can cause life-threatening allergic reactions. It is often just listed as a "natural" ingredient on the label. A paper on the subject was published in 1997 in the November issue of *Annals of Allergy, Asthma & Immunology.* EAF. E

**CARMINIC ACID** • Natural Red No. 4. Used in mascaras, liquid rouge, paste rouge, and red eye shadows. It is the coloring matter from a scaly insect (*see* Carmine). Color is deep red in water and violet to yellow in acids. May cause allergic reactions. Not subject to certification by the FDA.

**CARNAUBA WAX** • *Copernicia cerifera.* The exudate from the leaves of the Brazilian wax palm tree used as a candy glaze and polish. The crude wax is yellow or dirty green, brittle, and very hard. It is used in many polishes and varnishes, and when mixed with other waxes makes them harder and gives them more luster. It rarely causes allergic reactions. GRAS. ASP. E

**L-CARNITINE** • Levocarnitine Carnitor. Vitacam. A B-vitamin factor found in muscle, liver, and meat extracts. Used for patients born with systemic carnitine deficiency. It is a thyroid inhibitor. Enables fatty acids to produce energy in persons carnitine deficient. Potential adverse reactions include nausea, vomiting, cramps, diarrhea, and body odor. ASP

**CAROB BEAN** • Essential Oil. *See* Locust Bean Gum. GRAS. ASP

**CAROPHYLLENE ALCOHOL** • A flavoring that occurs in essential oils, especially in clove oil. Colorless, oily, with a clovelike odor. Used as a synthetic mushroom flavoring for baked goods and condiments.

**CAROTENE** • Provitamin A. Beta-carotene. Found in all plants and many animal tissues, it is the chief yellow coloring matter of carrots, butter, and egg yolks. Extracted as red crystals or crystalline powder, it is used as a vegetable dye in butter, margarine, shortening, skimmed milk, buttermilk, and cottage cheese. It is also used to manufacture vitamin A and is a nutrient added to skimmed milk, vegetable shortening, and margarine at the rate of 5,000 to 13,000 I.U. per pound. Insoluble in water, acids, and alkalies. Too much carotene in the blood (exceeding 200 micrograms per 100 milliliters of blood) can lead to carotenemia—a pale yellow-red pigmentation of the skin that may be mistaken for jaundice. It is a benign condition and withdrawal of carotene from the diet cures it. The final report to the FDA of the Select Committee on GRAS Substances stated in 1980 that it should continue its GRAS status with no limitations other than good manufacturing practices. Beta-carotene has been permanently listed as a coloring since 1964. ASP. E

**CAROTENOID** • Any of several pigments that give fruits and vegetables yellow, orange, or red coloring.

**CARRAGEENAN** • Chondrus Extract. Irish Moss. A stabilizer and emulsifier, seaweedlike in odor, derived from Irish moss, used in oils in cosmetics and foods. It is used as an emulsifier in chocolate products, chocolate-flavored drinks, chocolate milk, gassed cream (pressure-dispensed whipped cream), syrups for frozen products, confections, evaporated milk, cheese spreads and cheese foods, ice cream, frozen custard, sherbets, ices, French dressing, artificially sweetened jellies and jams. Completely soluble in hot water and not coagulated by acids. Salts of carrageenan, such as calcium, ammonium, potassium, or sodium, are used as a demulcent to soothe mucous membrane irritation. With polysorbate 80 at 500 ppm in final food containing the additives, it is used for producing gels. Carrageenan stimulated the formation of fibrous tissue when subcutaneously injected into the guinea pig. When a single dose of it dissolved in saline was injected under the skin of the rat, it caused sarcomas after approximately two years. Its cancer-causing ability may be that of a foreign body irritant, because upon administration to rats and mice at high levels in their diet, it did not appear to induce tumors, although survival of the animals for this period was not good. The final report to the FDA of the Select Committee on GRAS Substances stated in 1980 that while no evidence in the available information demonstrates it is a hazard to the public at current use levels, uncertainties exist, requiring that additional studies be conducted. Carrageenan is at this writing on the FDA lists for cancer study since it is a carcinogen in animals. The FAO/WHO Expert Committee on Food Additives requested in 2003 that based on laboratory results, carrageenan should be restricted in infant formulas but that it is acceptable for use as a food additive. ASP. E

**CARRAGEENAN, AMMONIUM SALT** • *See* Carrageenan and Ammonium. ASP

**CARRAGEENAN, CALCIUM SALT WITH POLYSORBATE** • *See* Carrageenan and Polysorbate. NUL

**CARRAGEENAN, POTASSIUM SALT OF** • *See* Carrageenan and Potassium. ASP

**CARROT FIBER** • Used in baked goods as a texturizer at a maximum level of 5 percent by weight of flour, for use in meat substitutes (e.g., meatless sausages and meatless patties) at a maximum level of 5 percent, and for use in meat and poultry products as a binder/extender and to reduce water purging/gelling at a maximum level of 5 percent. GRAS

**CARROT JUICE POWDER** • *See* Carrot Oil.

**CARROT OIL** • *Daucus carota.* Either of two oils from the seeds of carrots. A light yellow essential oil that has a spicy odor and is used in liqueurs, flavorings. It is used as a violet, fruit, rum, and spice flavoring for beverages, ice cream, ices, candy, baked goods, gelatin desserts, puddings, condiments, and soups. Rich in vitamin A, it is also used as a coloring and has been permanently listed since 1964. A skin irritant. When heated to decomposition it emits acrid smoke and irritating fumes. GRAS. ASP

**CARROT SEED EXTRACT** • Extract of the seeds of *Daucus carota sativa*. *See* Carrot Oil.

**CARVACROL** • A colorless to pale yellow liquid with a pungent, spicy odor related to thymol but more toxic. It is found naturally in oil of origanum, dittany of Crete oil, oregano, lavage oil, marjoram, and savory. It is a synthetic flavoring used in citrus, fruit, mint, and spice flavorings for beverages, ice cream, ices, candy, baked goods, and condiments. It is used as a disinfectant and is corrosive; one gram by mouth can cause respiratory and circulatory depression and cardiac failure leading to death. ASP

**CARVACRYL ETHYL ETHER** • A synthetic spice flavoring additive for beverages, ice cream, ices, candy, and baked goods. Found naturally in caraway and grapefruit. ASP

**CARVEOL** • A synthetic mint, spearmint, spice, and caraway flavoring additive for beverages, ice cream, ices, candy, and baked goods. Found naturally in caraway and grapes, baked fruit. ASP

**4-CARVOMENTHENOL** • A synthetic citrus and spice flavoring for beverages, ice cream, ices, candy, and baked goods. Occurs naturally in cardamom oil, juniper berries.

**CARVOMENTHOL** • Flavoring. *See* Menthol. ASP

**CARVONE (*d*- or *l*-)** • Oil of Caraway. It is colorless to light yellow with an odor of caraway oil. Carvone occurs in several essential oils. *d*-Carvone is usually prepared by distillation from caraway seed and dill seed. *l*-carvone is usually isolated from spearmint oil or synthesized commercially from limonene. Carvol (*d*-carvone) is a synthetic liquor, mint, and spice flavoring additive for beverages, ice cream, ices, candy, and baked goods. It breaks up intestinal gas and is used as a stimulant. GRAS. ASP

**CIS-CARVONE OXIDE** • *See* Carvone. NIL

**CARVYL ACETATE** • A synthetic mint flavoring for beverages, ice cream, ices, candy, and baked goods. ASP

**CARVYLOPHYLLENE ACETATE** • A general fixative that occurs in many essential oils, especially in clove oil. Colorless, oily, with a clovelike odor. Used for beverages, ice cream, ices, candy, baked goods, and chewing gum. Practically insoluble in alcohol.

**CARVYL PROPIONATE** • A synthetic mint flavoring for beverages, ice cream, ices, candy, and baked goods. ASP

***b*-CARYOPHYLLENE** • A synthetic spice flavoring. Occurs naturally in cloves, black currant buds, yarrow herb, grapefruit, allspice, and black pepper. The liquid smells like oil of cloves and turpentine. Used in beverages, ice cream, ices, candy, baked goods, chewing gum, and condiments. A skin irritant. ASP

**b-CAROPHYLLENE OXIDE** • *See b*-Caryophyllene and Oxidizer. ASP

**CASCARA, BITTERLESS EXTRACT** • A natural flavoring derived from the dried bark of a plant grown from northern Idaho to northern California. Cathartic. Used in butter, maple, caramel, and vanilla flavorings for beverages, ice cream, ices, and baked goods. Also used as a laxative. The freshly dried bark causes vomiting, so it must be dried for a year before use, by which time the side effect has disappeared. It has a bitter taste and its laxative effect is due to its ability to irritate the mucosa of the large intestine. EAF

**CASCARILLA BARK** • A natural flavoring additive obtained from the bark of a tree grown in Haiti, the Bahamas, and Cuba. The dried extract is added to smoking tobacco for flavoring and is used in bitters and spice flavorings for beverages. The oil, obtained by distillation, is light yellow to amber, with a spicy odor. It is used in cola, fruit, root beer, and spice flavorings for beverages, ice cream, ices, candy, baked goods, and condiments. GRAS. EAF

**CASCARILLA BARK OIL** • Croton. *See* Cascarilla. EAF

**CASEIN** • Ammonium Caseinate. Calcium Caseinate. Potassium Caseinate. Sodium Caseinate. The principal protein of cow's milk. It is a white, water-absorbing powder without noticeable odor. Used as a texturizer for ice cream, frozen custard, ice milk, fruit sherbets, and in special diet preparations. Also used in protective cream and as the "protein" in hair preparations to make the hair thicker and more manageable. Nontoxic. The final report to the FDA of the Select Committee on GRAS Substances stated in 1980 that it should continue its GRAS status with no limitations other than good manufacturing practices. ASP

**CASHOO EXTRACT** • *See* Catechu Extract.

**CASSIA BUDS** • *Cinnamomum cassia.* A natural flavoring from the flowers of the acacia plant. Used in blackberry, violet, vermouth, and fruit flavorings for beverages, ice cream, ices, candy, baked goods, and gelatin desserts. *See* Cassia Absolute. GRAS. EAF

**CASSIA ABSOLUTE** • *Acacia farnesiana.* A natural flavoring extract from cultivated trees. Used in cola, root beer, and spice flavorings for beverages, ice cream, candy, and baked goods. The bark oil is used in berry, chocolate, lemon, coffee, cola, cherry, peach, rum, peppermint, pecan, root beer, cassia, ginger ale, and cinnamon flavorings for beverages, ice cream, ices, candy, baked goods, chewing gum, meats, and condiments. The buds are used in spice flavorings for beverages. Cassia bark can cause inflammation and erosion of the gastrointestinal tract. GRAS. EAF

**CASSIA OIL** • Cloves. Chinese Oil of Cinnamon. Darker, less agreeable, and heavier than true cinnamon. Obtained from a tropical Asian tree, it is used in bitters, fruit, liquor, meat, root beer, sarsaparilla, and spice flavorings for beverages, ice cream, candy, and baked goods (3,000 ppm). It is also used in perfumes, poultices, and as a laxative. It can cause irritation and allergy, such as a stuffy nose. EAF

**CASSIS** • *See* Currant Buds, Absolute.

**CASTOR OIL** • Palm Christi Oil. Tang Tang Oil. Ricinus Oil. Palm Cristi Oil. The seed of the castor oil plant. After the oil is expressed from the beans, a residual castor pomace remains, which contains a potent allergen. A flavoring, pale yellow and viscous, it has a slightly acrid, sometimes nauseating taste. Used in butter and nut flavorings for beverages, ice cream, ices, candy, and baked goods. Also an antisticking additive in hard-candy products and a component of protective coatings, drying oil, and releasing additive *(see)*. The raw material is a constituent of embalming fluid and a cathartic. More than 50 percent of the lipsticks in the United States use a substantial amount of castor oil. Ingestion of large amounts may cause pelvic congestion and induce abortions. ASP

**CASTOREUM EXTRACT and LIQUID** • A creamy, orange-brown substance with strong penetrating odor and bitter taste that consists of the dried perineal glands of the beaver and their secretion. The glands and secretions are taken from the area between the vulva and anus in the female beaver and from the scrotum and anus in the male beaver. Used as a fixative. GRAS. EAF

**CATALASE** • An enzyme from bovine liver used in milk, for making cheese, and for the elimination of peroxide. It is used also in combination with glucose oxidase for treatment of food wrappers to prevent oxidative deterioration of food. GRAS. EAF

**CATALASE FROM *ASPERGILLUS NIGER*** • *See* Catalase and Aspergillus. EAF

**CATALASE FROM *PENICILLIUM NOTATUM*** • Enzyme used as a mold inhibitor. Enzyme from this fungi is probably best known for being the source of penicillin. It destroys the bacterial cell wall making the bacterium very susceptible to damage. EAF

**CATALYST** • A substance that causes or speeds up a chemical reaction but does not itself change.

**CATECHU EXTRACT** • Black Cutch Extract. Cachou Extract. Cashoo Extract. Pegu Catechu Extract. A preparation from the heartwood of the *Acacia catechu* (*see* Acacia) grown in India, Sri Lanka, and Jamaica. Used in bitters, fruit, and rum flavorings for beverages, ice cream, ices, candy, baked goods, and chewing gum. The powder is used in fruit, rum, and spice flavorings for beverages, ice cream, candy, baked goods, and chewing gum. Incompatible with iron compounds, gelatin, limewater, and zinc. Used as an astringent in diarrhea. May cause allergic reactions. EAF

**CAYENNE PEPPER** • Red Pepper. A condiment made from the pungent fruit of the plant. Used in sausage and pepper flavorings for beverages, ice cream, ices, candy, meats (910 ppm), soups, and condiments. Reported to retard growth of Mexicans, South Americans, and Spaniards who eat a great deal of these peppers. Rats fed the ingredient of pepper, a reddish-brown liquid called capsaicin, used in flavoring and pickles, were stunted in growth. A report by F. M. Gannett of the Eppley Institute for Research, University of Nebraska Medical Center, Omaha, at the 1988 American Chemical Society meeting, Toronto, Canada, said that capsaicin, the substance that makes these peppers hot, is not a low-level mutagen as earlier believed but is actually antimutagenic. GRAS

**CEDAR** • Cedar Wood Oil. The oil from white, red, or various cedars obtained by distillation from fresh leaves and branches. A colorless to yellow liquid with a fresh woody scent, it is used in fruit and spice flavorings for beverages, ice cream, ices, candy, baked goods, chewing gum, and liquors. Used frequently as a substitute for oil of lavender. There is usually a strong camphor odor that repels insects. Cedar oil can be a photosensitizer, causing skin reactions when the skin is exposed to light. Similar toxicity to camphor oil *(see)*. Finished food should be thujone-free. Thujone is a toxic substance found in oils such as cedar, tansy, thuja, wormwood, and sage. EAF

**CEDAR WOOD OIL ALCOHOLS and TERPENES** • *See* Cedar and Terpenes. ASP

**CEDRO OIL** • *See* Lemon Oil.

**CEDRYL ACETATE** • Colorless liquid having a light cedar odor. Used in fragrances. ASP

**CEFTIOFUR** • An animal drug used in beef. The FDA limits residues to 3 ppm in muscle, 9 ppm in kidney, 6 ppm in liver, and 12 ppm in fat of cattle. When heated to decomposition it emits acrid smoke and irritating fumes.

**CELERY SEED** • A yellowish to greenish brown liquid, having a pleasant aromatic odor, distilled from the dried ripe fruit of the plant grown in southern Europe. Celery seed is used in sausage and celery flavorings for beverages (1,000 ppm), baked goods, condiments (2,500 ppm), soups, meats, and pickles. Celery seed solid extract is used in celery, meat, and spice flavorings for beverages, ice cream, ices, candy, baked goods, condiments, and maple syrup. Celery seed oil is used in fruit, honey, maple, sausage, nut, root beer, spice, vanilla, and cream soda flavorings for beverages, ice cream, ices, candy, baked goods, chewing gum, meats, soup, pickles, and condiments. Celery seed may cause a sensitivity to light. GRAS. ASP

**CELLULASE ENZYME** • Derived from the fungi *Aspergillus niger* or *Trichoderma longibrachiatum.* An enzyme for removal of visceral mass in clam processing and shells from shrimp. EAF

**CELLULOSE** • Chief constituent of the fiber of plants. Cotton contains about 90 percent. It is the basic material for cellulose gums *(see)*. EAF. E

**CELLULOSE GUMS** • Sodium Carboxymethylcellulose. CMC. Modified Cellulose. Occurs as a white to cream-colored powder or granules. It absorbs water. Fibrous substances consisting of the chief part of the cell walls of plants. Made from cotton by-products, it occurs as a white powder or in granules. A synthetic gum, it is used as a stabilizer in ice cream, beverages, and other foods. Cellulose acetate is obtained by treating cellulose with a food starch modifier. It has been shown to cause cancer in animals when ingested. The final report to the FDA of the Select Committee on GRAS Substances stated in 1980 that it should continue its GRAS status for packaging only with no limitations other than good manufacturing practices. Some are ASP and some are EAF.

**CELLULOSE TRIACETATE** • Used to reduce the lactose *(see)* content of milk. EAF

**CENTAURY (CENTAURIUM) HERB** • Flavoring in alcoholic beverages only. EAF

**CEPHARPIRIN** • An animal drug used in beef and milk. The FDA limits residue to 0.02 ppm in milk and 0.1 ppm in uncooked edible tissues of dairy cattle. Moderately toxic by injection into the vein. When heated to decomposition it emits toxic fumes. ASP

**CEREAL SOLIDS, HYDROLYZED** • From grains such as rice or wheat, dried and then hydrolyzed *(see)* used as an anticaking agent.

**CERESIN** • Ceresine. Earth Wax. Used in protective creams. It is a white or yellow, hard, brittle wax made by purifying ozokerite *(see),* found in Ukraine, Utah, and Texas. It is used as a substitute for beeswax and paraffin wax *(see both);* also used to wax paper and cloth, as a polish, and in dentistry for taking wax impressions. May cause allergic reactions.

**CERTIFIED** • All color additives permitted for use in foods are classified as "certifiable" or "exempt from certification." Certifiable color additives are man-made, with each batch being tested by manufacturer and FDA. This "approval" process, known as color additive certification, is aimed at assuring the safety, quality, consistency, and strength of the color additive prior to its use in foods. The manufacturer must submit samples of every batch for testing, and the lot test number accompanies the colors through all subsequent packaging.

**CETONE D** • *See* Methyl 6-Naphthyl Ketone.

**CETONE V** • *See* Allyl *a*-Ionone.

**CETYL** • Means derived from cetyl alcohol *(see).*

**CETYL ALCOHOL** • An emollient and emulsion stabilizer used in many foods and cosmetics. Cetyl alcohol is waxy, crystalline, and solid, and found in spermaceti *(see).* It has a low toxicity for both skin and ingestion and is sometimes used as a laxative. Can cause hives. *See* Fatty Alcohols. ASP

**CETYL ARACHIDATE** • An ester produced by the reaction of cetyl alcohol and arachidic acid. The acid is found in fish oils and vegetables, particularly peanut oil. A fatty compound used as an emulsifier. Nontoxic.

**CETYL ESTERS** • Synthetic spermaceti *(see)*.

**CETYLIC ACID** • *See* Palmitic Acid.

**CEYLON CINNAMON** • *See* Cinnamon.

**CEYLON CINNAMON LEAF OIL** • *See* Cinnamon Leaf Oil.

**CF-3** • Preempt. A blend of twenty-nine beneficial microbes found in the gastrointestinal tracts of mature, healthy chickens that can reduce salmonella *(see)* colonization. A single spray of bacterial suspension is administered to newly hatched chicks at a dose of approximately 0.25 milliliter per chick. The bacteria on the chick's feathers are subsequently ingested through normal grooming (preening) behavior. It is essentially replacing the mother hen. Before the advent of large modern poultry farms, hens would pass on the good microbes—and disease resistance—to their chicks. On March 13, 1998, the FDA approved this first competitive exclusion (CE) product for animals in the United States. CE products are made up of live bacteria that can be given to animals to establish normal gut microflora, thereby helping to reduce or prevent the colonization of undesirable bacteria. By populating the gut with normal microflora, thereby excluding undesirable bacteria, CE products may help reduce carcass contamination and the incidence of food-borne illness in humans. Reduction of salmonella colonization in chickens is an important step in reducing salmonella contamination in processed poultry products. While salmonella colonization is generally not a problem for the chickens, it is a problem for humans who may develop salmonellosis through the ingestion of improperly cooked or handled salmonella-contaminated chicken. While the use of Preempt will help reduce one type of contamination, poultry must be properly handled and cooked to be safe. This CE culture product was originally developed and tested by a USDA–Agricultural Research Service team at College Station, Texas. This specific culture is produced as Preempt under an exclusive licensing agreement between the USDA and MS BioScience. During clinical studies, no adverse effects were observed in the chicks following Preempt administration. In addition since Preempt is a suspension of bacteria, there are no concerns regarding chemical residues in edible tissue from treated chickens. However, since this product consists of live bacteria, using antimicrobials in feed or drinking water along with Preempt would inhibit the survival and ultimate establishment of these organisms in the gut.

**CFSAN** • Abbreviation for the FDA's Center for Food Safety and Applied Nutrition.

**CFR** • Code of Federal Regulations.

**CHACONINE** • An alkaloid in plants of the *Solanaceae* family such as potatoes and tomatoes. In laboratory animals, it causes birth defects but the World Health Organization said that the amount in potatoes is not significant.

**CHAMOMILE** • Roman, English, and Hungarian Chamomile. The daisylike white and yellow heads of these flowers provide a coloring additive known as apigenin. The essential oil distilled from the flower heads is pale blue. Roman chamomile is used in berry, fruit, vermouth, maple, spice, and vanilla flavorings. English chamomile is used as a flavoring in chocolate, fruit, and liquor flavorings for beverages, ice cream, ices, candy, and baked goods. Roman chamomile oil is used in chocolate, fruit, vermouth, and spice flavorings for beverages, ice cream, ices, candy, baked goods, gelatin desserts, and liquors. Hungarian chamomile oil is used in chocolate, fruit, and liquor flavorings for beverages, ice cream, ices, candy, baked goods, chewing gum, and liquors. Chamomile contains sesquiterpene lactones that may cause allergic contact dermatitis and stomach upsets. GRAS. The Hungarian and Roman flowers are EAF. *Anthemis nobils* is EAF while *Matricaria chamomilla* is NIL.

**CHARCOAL** • Formerly widely used as a black coloring. The FDA no longer authorizes its use.

**CHAR SMOKE FLAVOR** • A flavoring. ASP

**CHECKERBERRY EXTRACT** • *See* Wintergreen Oil.

**CHECKERBERRY OIL** • *See* Wintergreen Oil.

**CHELATING ADDITIVE** • Any compound, usually one that binds and precipitates metals, such as ethylenediamine tetraacetic acid (EDTA), which removes trace metals. *See* Sequestering Additive.

**CHEMICALS USED IN WASHING FRUITS and VEGETABLES** • Polyacrylamide, potassium bromide, sodium dodecylbenzenesulfonate, sodium hypochlorite, sodium 2-ethyl-l-hexylsulfate, sodium *n*-alkylbenzene sulfonate, sodium mono- and dimethyl-naphthalene sulfonates; alkylene oxide adducts of alkyl alcohols, and phosphate esters of alkylene oxides. Adducts of alkyl alcohols mixtures. Uses of such chemicals followed by rinsing to remove residues. Some individual chemicals remain in limited amounts in wash water, according to the FDA.

**CHERRY BARK** • ASP *See* Cherry Wild Bark.

**CHERRY LAUREL LEAVES** • *Prunus laurocerasus.* A flavoring. NUL

**CHERRY LAUREL WATER** • Flavoring. ASP

**CHERRY PIT OIL** • A natural flavoring and fragrance extracted from the pits of sweet and sour cherries. Also a cherry flavoring for beverages, ice cream, and condiments. ASP

**CHERRY PLUM** • Source of purplish red color. *See* Anthocyanins.

**CHERRY WILD BARK** • Virginian prune, black cherry, black choke, chokecherry, rum cherry dried bark. Used in cherry flavorings for food. Collected from young plants in the autumn when it has its highest prussic acid *(see)* content. Also contains cyanogenic glycosides including prunasin; volatile oil, benzaldehyde, coumarins, benzoic acid, gallitannins, resin, an enzyme (prunase). Prunus is an important cough remedy. Due to its powerful sedative action, it is used primarily in the treatment of irritating and persistent coughs. Prunus may be used as a bitter where digestion is sluggish. The cold infusion of the bark may be used as a wash in eye inflammation and as an astringent in diarrhea. Prunus causes drowsiness. Cyanogenic glycosides are moderately toxic, producing cyanic acid on hydrolysis, and should not be taken to excess. The leaves have poisoned cattle. GRAS. ASP

**CHERVIL** • *Anthriscus cereifolium.* A natural flavoring extracted from an aromatic Eurasian plant and used in spice flavorings for beverages, ice cream, ices, candy, baked goods, and condiments. A chewing-gum base. GRAS. ASP

**CHESTNUT** • *Castanea dentata.* Nuts from a European tree used as a remedy for piles, backaches, and for coughs. The bark of Spanish chestnut contains tannins *(see).* NUL

**CHESTNUT LEAVES EXTRACT** • Contains natural herbicides that the tree uses to inhibit the growth of neighboring plants. Horse chestnut leaves have been used by herbalists as a cough remedy and to reduce fevers. The leaves were also believed to reduce pain and inflammation of arthritis and rheumatism. Extract contains minerals, tannins, free amino acids, and vitamins $B_1$, $B_2$, and PP. It reportedly has antimicrobial, antiinflammatory, and healing properties. EAF

**CHEWING-GUM BASE** • Chicle, chiquibal, crown gum, guttahang kang, massaranduba balata, massaranduba chocolate, nispero lechi caspi, pendare, perillo, rosidinha, Venezuelan chicle, liche devaca, Niger gutta, tuno, chilte, natural rubber, glycerol ester of tall oil resin.

**CHICLE** • The gummy milky resin obtained from trees grown in Mexico and Central America. Rubberlike and soft at moderate temperatures. Used in the manufacture of chewing gum. ASP

**CHICORY EXTRACT** • Coffee. *Cichorium intybus.* Wild Succory. A natural flavor extract from a plant, usually with blue flowers and leaves. Related to dandelion, in ancient times it was used as a narcotic, sometimes administered before operations. Used in butter, caramel, chocolate, coffee, maple, nut, root beer, sarsaparilla, vanilla, wintergreen, and birch beer flavorings for beverages, ice cream, ices, candy, and baked goods. The root of the plant is dried, roasted, and ground for mixing. On the Continent, chicory is much cultivated, not only as a salad and vegetable, but also for fodder and more especially for the sake of its root, which though woody in the wild state, under cultivation becomes large and fleshy, with a thick rind, and is employed extensively when roasted and ground, for blending with coffee. An infusion of the herb is useful for skin eruptions connected with gout. Herbalists considered that the leaves when bruised make a good poultice for swellings, inflammations, and inflamed eyes. GRAS. ASP

**CHILI** • *Capsicum fastigatum.* Chili is the dried pod of a species of capsicum *(see)* or red pepper. The small pods have been used for heartburn and dilated blood vessels arising from drunkenness.

**CHILTE** • Cnidoscolus. Jatropha. A chewing-gum base component of vegetable origin. ASP

**CHINA BARK EXTRACT** • *See* Quillaja Extract.

**CHINESE CINNAMON** • *See* Cinnamon.

**CHINESE CINNAMON LEAF OIL** • *See* Cinnamon Leaf Oil.

**CHINESE RESTAURANT SYNDROME** • Manifested by anxiety, flushed face, and pressure in the chest, has been shown to be caused by eating large amounts of the flavor enhancer MSG. Sulfite preservatives are now known to have the potential to cause a serious attack of asthma and even death.

**CHIQUIBUL** • *Manilkara zapota.* A composition in chewing-gum bases. ASP

**CHIRATA (CHIRETTA, EAST INDIAN BOLONONG) and HERB EXTRACT** • Flavoring used in alcoholic beverages only. There is reported use of the chemical; it has not yet been assigned for toxicology literature search.

**CHIVES** • *Allium schoenoprasum.* A member of the amaryllis family, it's closely related to the onion. Some research has found it may have anticancer potential. GRAS. ASP

**CHLORAMPHENICOL** • Drug in any form may no longer be used in food-producing animals (meat, milk, and egg). Once widely used in animals. In the EPA Genetic Toxicology Program *(see)*. Poison by intraperitoneal, intravenous, and subcutaneous routes. Moderately toxic by ingestion. A human carcinogen that causes leukemia, aplastic anemia, and other bone marrow changes by ingestion.

**CHLORDANE** • An organochlorine pesticide introduced in 1945 that was among the first to be developed for insect control. Because of its persistence in the environment, most of its uses were suspended by order of the EPA in 1975. Several specified uses are still permitted, including pest control on pineapple, strawberries, and Florida citrus crops. It also can be used to remedy a number of other pest-control problems that plague certain areas of the United States. Chlordane causes cancer of the liver in mice. It is less toxic than other similar pesticides, but acute exposure has the effect of stimulating the central nervous system. It has also been implicated in acute blood abnormalities such as aplastic anemia. Can be absorbed through the skin.

**CHLORDIMEFORM** • Colorless crystals derived from ethyl formate and ammonia; it is a fumigant, an insecticide, and miticide. It also kills insect eggs. It is sold for use on cotton and vegetable crops. It is less toxic than organophosphates and is biodegradable. It is used in dried apple pomace, cottonseed hulls, and in dried prunes as a residue resulting from application to growing plums. In animal feed the tolerance is up to 25 ppm. In prunes it is 15 ppm.

**CHLORETHEPHON** • Water-absorbing needles from benzene used as a plant-growth regulator, used in animal feed, barley, raisin waste, sugarcane molasses, and wheat-milling fractions (except flour). The FDA permits a residue of 5 ppm in barley and wheat-milling fractions (except flour), 1.5 ppm in sugarcane molasses, and 65 ppm in raisin waste when used for animal feed. Moderately toxic by ingestion. Mildly toxic by skin contact. May be irritating to exposed skin and eyes or if inhaled.

**CHLORHEXIDINE DIHYDROCHLORIDE** • A veterinary drug used for cattle. The FDA tolerance residue in edible tissue of calves is zero.

**CHLORIMURON** • A pesticide and herbicide used in soybeans, peanuts, peanut hulls. FDA tolerance residues are from 0.02 to 0.05 ppm.

**CHLORINE** • A nonmetallic element, a diatomic gas that is heavy, noncombustible, and greenish yellow, it is found in the earth's crust and has a pungent suffocating odor. In liquid form it is a clear amber color with an irritating odor. It does not occur in a free state but as a component of the mineral halite (rock salt). Toxic and irritating to the skin and lungs, it has a tolerance level of one part per million in air. It is used in the manufacture of carbon tetrachloride and in flame-retardant compounds; and in processing fish, vegetables, and fruit. The chlorine used to kill bacteria in drinking water may contain carcinogenic carbon tetrachloride, a contaminant formed during the production process. Chlorination has also been found to sometimes form undesirable "ring" compounds in water, such as toluene, xylene, and the suspected carcinogen styrene—they have been observed in both the drinking water and waste water plants in the Midwest. Chlorine is a powerful irritant, and can be fatal upon inhalation. In fact it is in military arsenals as a poison gas. A National Cancer Institute study published in 1987 linked bladder cancer to people who had been drinking chlorinated surface water for forty or more years. ASP

**CHLORINE DIOXIDE** • Flour bleacher and oxidizing additive. Also used as an antimicrobial additive in poultry process water at a concentration not to exceed 3 ppm residual chlorine dioxide. Also used to wash fruits and vegetables that are not raw agricultural commodities at a level not to exceed 3 ppm residual chlorine dioxide. It is also used for a rinse for food processing equipment. A yellow to reddish yellow gas, with an unpleasant odor, highly irritating and corrosive to the skin and mucous membranes of respiratory tract. Reacts violently with organic materials. It can kill. ASP

**CHLORINE GAS** • Flour-bleaching and aging and oxidizing additive. Also used in water purification. Found in the earth's crust, it is a greenish yellow gas with a suffocating odor. A powerful irritant, dangerous to inhale, and lethal. Thirty ppm will cause coughing. The chlorine used in drinking water often contains carcinogenic carbon tetrachloride, a contaminant formed during the production process. Chlorination has also been found to sometimes form undesirable "ring" compounds in water, such as toluene, xylene, and the suspected carcinogen styrene—they have been observed in both the drinking water and waste water plants in the Midwest.

**CHLORITE** • *See* Calcium Hypochlorite.

**CHLORINE SOLUTION, AQUEOUS** • *See* Chlorine. ASP

**CHLORO-** • Signifies a substance contains chlorine *(see)*.

**CHLOROACETIC ACID** • Used in packaging adhesives and as a preservative. Not permitted in alcoholic beverages or foods. In EPA Genetic Toxicology Program *(see)* and considered an extremely hazardous substance.

**CHLOROBUTANOL** • Tetramethylene Chlorohydrin. An animal drug used to treat mastitis in cows. The FDA does not permit any residue in milk. Moderately toxic by ingestion and may be mutagenic.

**CHLOROFLUOROCARBONS (CFC)** • Any of several compounds comprised of carbon, fluorine, chlorine, and hydrogen, the best known of which are trichloromethane and dichlorodifluoromethane. Chlorofluorocarbons trap heat at the earth's surface, decreasing the amount radiated back into space and affecting the ozone layer. The ozone layer blocks ultraviolet radiation from the sun that can cause skin cancer and harm ecosystems. It has deteriorated for decades, especially in Antarctica, under an assault from synthetic chemicals. Phasing out CFCs began in 1989 with enactment of the Montreal Protocol, an international treaty. But the destructive substances take decades to decay, resulting in the long lag before beneficial effects could be measured. The use was prohibited in 1979 except for a few specialized items because of their depleting effect on stratospheric ozone. It is banned for most foods but the FDA permits it for use in cooling or freezing chickens.

**CHLOROFORM** • Used as a solvent for fats, oils, waxes, resins, and as a cleaning ingredient. It has many serious side effects and is considered a carcinogen. Exposure to it may also cause respiratory and skin allergies. The National Cancer Institute made public in June 1976 the finding that chloroform was found to cause liver and kidney cancers in test animals. It is no longer permitted in cosmetics. NUL

**CHLORMETHYLATED 2002 LAMINATED STYRENE DI-VINYL-BENZENE RESIN** • Used to clarify *(see)* sugar liquor up to 500 ppm.

**CHLOROMETHYL METHYL** • Used in the synthesis of chloromethylated compounds and as an alkylating agent and solvent used in the manufacture of water repellents, ion-exchange resins, and industrial polymers. Highly irritating to the skin and lungs. NUL

**2-CHLORO-4-NITROENZMIDE** • A feed additive. *See* Aklomide.

**CHLOROPENTAFLUOROETHANE** • Colorless gas with a slight, ethereal odor. ASP

**CHLOROPHENAMIDINE** • Acaron. Fundex. A pesticide used in animal feed, apple pomace (dried) cottonseed hulls, prunes (dried). FDA residue tolerance of 15 ppm on dried prunes, 25 ppm in dried apple pomace, 10 ppm in cottonseed hulls when used for animal feed. Poison by ingestion, skin contact, and injection. Possible cancer-causing additive and mutagen. Eye and skin irritant.

**1-(4-CHLOROPHENOXY)-3,3-DIMETHYL-1-(1,2,3-TRIAZOL-1-YL)-2-BUTAN-2-ONE** • Amiral. MEB 6447. Triadimefon. A fungicide used on barley (except flour) and wheat (except flour). FDA residue tolerance is 4 ppm in barley and wheat, milled fractions (except flour). Poisonous by ingestion.

**1-(4-CHLOROPHENYL)-3-(2,6-DIFLUOROBENZOYL) UREA** • Difluon. Dimilin. An insecticide used in animal feed, soybean hulls, and soybean soap stock when used for animal feed. In EPA Genetic Toxicology Program (see). Moderately toxic by skin contact. Mildly toxic by ingestion. May be mutagenic.

**1-(4-CHLOROPHENOXY)-3-3-DIMETHYL-1-(IH-1,2,4-TRIAZOL-1-YL)-2-BUTANONE** • A fungicide used in animal feed. FDA residue tolerances on grape pomace, 3 ppm; on apple pomace, 4 ppm; on raisin waste, 7 ppm.

**p-CHLOROPHENYL-2,4,5-TRICHLOROPHENYL SULFONE** • Tetradifon. Akaritox. A pesticide used on dried figs, dried hops, and dried tea. FDA residue tolerance is 120 ppm in dried hops, 10 ppm in dried figs, and 8 ppm in dried tea. Moderately toxic by ingestion. Mildly toxic by skin contact. May cause birth defects.

**CHLOROPHYLL** • The green coloring matter of plants, which plays an essential part in the plant's photosynthesis process. Used in antiperspirants, dentrifices, deodorants, and mouthwashes as a deodorizing additive. It imparts a greenish color to certain fats and oils, notably olive oil and soybean. Can cause a sensitivity to light. ASP. E

**CHLOROPROPANOLS** • Certain chlorinated propanols used as insecticides and herbicides contaminate hydrolyzed vegetable proteins (see). The two substances considered by the FAO/WHO Expert Committee on Food Additives were 3-chloro-1,2-propanediol and 1,30 dichloro-2-propanol, neither of which had been previously evaluated. During traditional processing of vegetable proteins with hydrochloric acid, "significant amounts" of these two contaminants have been found. With newer methods, the level of propanediol compound has been reduced to less than 2 mg per kg and the propanol compound to less than 0.02 mg per kg in hydrolyzed vegetable protein. In monkeys, the propanediol compound induced anemia, increased white blood cell count, and other blood changes following ingestion of 30 mg per kg of body weight a day for six weeks. It also reduced fertility in male rats and caused malignant and gene-damaging effects in cells in laboratory dishes. The propanediol also did the same in mouse cells in laboratory dishes. In more recent experiments in which rats were fed 1.1 to 28 mg per kg of body weight per day of either one of the compounds, the animals developed cancers of the testes, breast, and tongue among others. The committee concluded that these substances are "undesirable contaminants in food" and expressed the opinion that then levels in hydrolyzed vegetable proteins should be reduced as far as "technically possible."

**CHLORPENTAFLUOROETHANE** • Alone or with carbon dioxide. Used as propellant and aerating additive in foods. *See* Chlorofluorocarbons.

**2(m-CHLOROPHENOXY) PROPIONIC ACID** • A growth regulator used in pineapple bran. FDA residue tolerance is 3 ppm.

**CHLORPROMAZINE** • Ormazine. Thorazine. Thor-Pram. An antipsychotic and antinausea medication introduced in the 1950s, it is also used for intractable hiccups and mild alcohol withdrawal. It is used to tranquilize pigs on their way to market. Potential adverse reactions to the medication in humans include a drop in white blood cells, sedation, uncontrolled movements, Parkinsonism-like symptoms, dizziness, a drop in blood pressure when rising from a seated or prone position, vision changes, dry mouth, constipation, urine retention, male breast enlargement, inhibited ejaculation, liver dysfunction, weight gain, increased appetite, fever, photosensitivity, irregular heartbeat, and sweating. Tardive dyskinesia *(see)* may occur after prolonged use. Alcohol and other central nervous system depressants may increase central nervous system depression. Drugs used to treat Parkinsonism and antidepressants may increase chlorpromazine's nerve-suppressing activity. Blood pressure medications that act on the brain may be less effective. Oral blood thinners may be less effective and propranolol can increase the levels of both propranolol and chlorpromazine. Contraindicated in central nervous system depression, bone marrow suppression, brain damage, Reye's syndrome, and coma. Also should not be used in cardiovascular disease, or respiratory disorders, glaucoma, and enlarged prostate, and in acutely ill or dehydrated children. The ingested drug may take effect in thirty to sixty minutes and may last up to three weeks after stopping the drug.

**CHLORPYRIFOS** • O,O-Dimethyl-0-(3,5,6-Trichloro-2-Pyridyl) Phosphorothioate. Dursban. Lorsban. Used as an insecticide and acaricide on corn and other vegetables. Poison by ingestion. A skin irritant. FDA residue tolerance is 90 ppm in barley milling fractions (except flour), 130 ppm in oats milling fractions (except flour), 90 ppm in sorghum milling fractions (except flour), 30 ppm in rice-milling fractions (except flour), 30 ppm in wheat-milling fractions (except flour). The FDA tolerance as residues in milk fat is 1.25 ppm and 0.5 ppm as residues in fat, meat, and meat by-products of cattle, goats, hogs, poultry, and sheep. As a residue in barley, oat, rice, and wheat grain, the tolerance is 6 ppm.

**CHLORSULON** • Curatrem. An animal drug used to treat worms. The FDA tolerance is 1 ppm in uncooked edible muscle tissue of cattle; 2 ppm as residue in uncooked liver; 3 ppm as residue in kidney; 4 ppm as residue in uncooked cattle fat.

**CHLORTETRACYCLINE** • Aureomycin. Biomycin. Biomitsin. PfiClor. A preservative, an antibiotic, used in dip and feed to improve feed efficiency and increase weight gain. The FDA permits 4 ppm residue in uncooked kidneys of chickens and turkeys; 1 ppm in uncooked muscle, liver, fat, and skin of chickens and turkeys, and zero residue in eggs. The residues permitted in uncooked swine liver is 2 ppm, 0.2 ppm in uncooked fat of calves, 4 ppm in uncooked liver and kidneys of calves, 0.1 ppm in uncooked muscle and fat of calves, uncooked liver, and kidneys of beef cattle and nonlactating dairy cows. Residue in milk is supposed to be zero. One of the reasons for increased resistance to antibiotics in patients is believed to be the widespread use of antibiotics in food animals. In 1969, the British restricted the veterinary use of antibiotics. In 1972, the FDA-appointed committee to study the use of antibiotics in animals recommended curbs on use. Many strains of bacteria are known to be resistant to tetracycline. Use of this antibiotic has caused discoloration of permanent teeth in children given the drug prior to the eruption of the second teeth. It can also cause skin rash, gastrointestinal upsets, and inflammations in the anogenital area.

**CHOLECALCIFEROL** • Vitamin $D_3$. Used as a dietary supplement and nutrient in breakfast cereals, grain products, margarine, milk, milk products, and pasta. GRAS

**CHOLEST** • Listing on labels for cholesterol *(see)*.

**CHOLESTEROL (DIETARY)** • Cholesterol is not fat, but rather a fatlike substance classified as a lipid. Cholesterol is vital to life and is found in all cell membranes. It is necessary for the production of bile acids and steroid hormones. Dietary cholesterol is found only in animal foods. Abundant in organ meats and egg yolks, cholesterol is also contained in meats, chicken, and shellfish. Vegetable oils and shortenings are cholesterol-free.

**CHOLESTEROL (SERUM or BLOOD)** • High blood cholesterol is a risk factor in the development of coronary heart disease. Most of the cholesterol that is found in the blood is manufactured by the body at a rate of about 800 to 1,500 milligrams a day. By comparison, the average American consumes 300 to 450 milligrams daily in foods. Cholesterol travels through the blood via particles called lipoproteins—combinations of lipids and proteins. Too much cholesterol can build up in the blood and accumulate in the walls of the blood vessels, a condition known as atherosclerosis. This can ultimately reduce the flow of blood in major arteries, leading to heart attack. Blood cholesterol reflects the amount of three major classes of lipoproteins: very low-density lipoprotein (VLDL); low-density lipoprotein (LDL), which contains most of the cholesterol found in the blood; and high-density lipoprotein (HDL). LDL seems to be the culprit in coronary heart disease and is popularly known as the "bad cholesterol." By contrast, HDL is increasingly considered desirable and known as the "good cholesterol." Diet is just one factor influencing blood cholesterol levels. For some people at risk, heredity is a stronger predictor of cholesterol levels than diet. Age, race, and gender are other risk factors for high cholesterol levels.

**CHOLIC ACID** • Occurs in the bile of most vertebrates and is used as an emulsifying additive in dried egg whites and as a choleretic to regulate the secretion of bile. Bitter taste; sweetish aftertaste. The final report to the FDA of the Select Committee on GRAS Substances stated in 1980 that it should continue its GRAS status with no limitations other than good manufacturing practices. NUL

**CHOLINE** • Found in most animal tissues, either free or in combinations such as lecithin or acetylcholine. Choline is being actively studied for its effects on brain neurotransmission and memory.

**CHOLINE BITARTRATE** • A dietary supplement included in the B complex and found in the form of a thick syrupy liquid in most animal tissue. It is necessary to nerve function and fat metabolism and can be manufactured in the body but not at a sufficient rate to meet health requirements. Dietary choline protects against poor growth, fatty liver, and renal damage in many animals. Choline deficiency has not been demonstrated in man but the National Academy of Sciences lists 500 to 900 milligrams per day as sufficient for the average man. The final report to the FDA of the Select Committee on GRAS Substances stated in 1980 that it should continue its GRAS status with no limitations other than good manufacturing practices.

**CHOLINE CHLORIDE** • Ferric Choline Citrate. A dietary supplement with the same function as choline bitartrate *(see)*. The final report to the FDA of the Select Committee on GRAS Substances stated in 1980 that it should continue its GRAS status with no limitations other than good manufacturing practices. ASP

**CHOLINE HYDROCHLORIDE** • Colorless to white, water-absorbing crystals used as a fungicide on various feeds. It is listed in the Community Right-to-Know List *(see)*. Moderately toxic to humans by ingestion. May be mutagenic.

**CHOLINE XANTHATE** • A feed additive for poultry, swine, and ruminants.

**CHONDRUS** • *See* Carrageenan.

**CHROMIUM** • Occurs in the earth's crust and plays a vital role in the activities of some human enzymes. It is involved in the breakdown of sugar for conversion into energy and in the manufacture of certain fats. It works together with insulin and is essential to the body's ability to use sugar. Traces of chromium are widely available in food. However, chromium deficiency may frequently occur because the soil in the United States contains low levels. Those who are deficient may show symptoms similar to diabetes such as tiredness, mental confusion, and numbness or tingling of the hands and feet. Deficiency may worsen preexisting diabetes, depress growth in children, or contribute to the development of narrowing of the arteries.

Chromium-rich diet may prevent Type II diabetes, the non-insulin dependent form of the disease that starts in adulthood. Richard A. Anderson, a
biochemist at the USDA Human Nutrition Research Center in Beltsville,
Maryland, has shown that diets high in simple sugars such as glucose and
fructose rob the body of chromium, while those high in complex carbohydrates such as pasta preserve it. The new research builds on data from
Anderson's lab showing that chromium supplementation in rats improves
glucose tolerance—the ability to transport blood glucose into cells.
Chromium is poisonous in large amounts. Ingestion can result in violent
gastrointestinal irritation. Foods that contain chromium include fruit,
beer, oysters, liver, egg yolk, potatoes with skin, mushrooms, brewer's
yeast, and wines. Not always absorbed—for example, much of the
chromium in potatoes never gets incorporated into body cells. Simple
sugars, furthermore, cause the body to excrete large amounts of the mineral. An attempt was made to permit chromium to be listed on a food label
as reducing the risk of high blood sugar in adults. The FDA denied the
claim because it said the statements submitted as the basis for it were not
"authoritative." Chromium can be carcinogenic according to Environmental Defense.

**CHROMOSOME** • One or more small rod-shaped elements in a cell that
contains genetic information.

**CHYMOSIN** • Enzyme prepared from calf stomach. Used as a stabilizer
and thickener. GRAS. EAF

**CINCHONA EXTRACT** • The extract of the bark of various species of cinchona cultivated in Java, India, and South America. A natural flavoring, red
cinchona bark is used in bitters, fruit, rum, vermouth, and spice flavorings
for beverages, ice cream, ices, candy, liquors, and bitters (1,000 ppm).
Yellow cinchona bark is a natural flavoring from the bark of a species of
South American tree used in bitters, fruit, and vermouth flavorings for
liquors. The yellow extract is used as a bitters flavoring for beverages.
Quinine is derived from it. Cinchona stimulates digestion. May rarely cause
allergies and stomach upsets. ASP

**CINENE** • *See* Limonene.

**CINEOLE** • *See* Eucalyptol. ASP

**CINNAMAL** • *See* Cinnamaldehyde.

**CINNAMALDEHYDE** • Cinnamic Aldehyde. A synthetic yellowish oily
liquid with a strong odor of cinnamon isolated from a wood-rotting fungus.
Occurs naturally in cassia bark extract, cinnamon bark, and root oils. Used
in cola, apple, cherry, liquor, rum, nut, pecan, spice, cinnamon, vanilla, and
cream soda flavorings for beverages, ice cream, ices, candy (700 ppm),
baked goods, chewing gum (4,900 ppm), condiments, and meats. It is estimated that eaters' only exposure is 0.099 mg/kg per person per day. Also
used in perfume industry, to flavor mouthwash and toothpaste, and to scent

powder and hair tonic. It is irritating to the skin and mucous membranes, especially if undiluted. University of Illinois researchers reported in 2004 that chewing gum containing it reduced bacteria in the mouth and bad breath. Can cause inflammation and erosion of the gastrointestinal tract. One of the most common allergens. It cross-reacts with balsam Peru and benzoin. May cause depigmentation and hives. GRAS. ASP

**CINNAMALDEHYDE ETHYLENE GLYCOL ACETAL** • Cinncloval. Spice, cassia, cinnamon, and clove flavorings for beverages, ice cream, ices, candy, baked goods, chewing gum, and condiments. *See* Cinnamaldehyde for toxicity. ASP

**CINNAMEIN** • *See* Benzyl Cinnamate.

**CINNAMIC ACID** • A cherry, honey, spice, cassia, and cinnamon flavoring additive for beverages, ice cream, ices, candy, baked goods, and chewing gum. Also used in suntan lotions and perfumes. Occurs in storax, balsam Peru, cinnamon leaves, and coca leaves. Usually isolated from wood-rotting fungus. Used mainly in the perfume industry. It may cause allergic skin rashes. ASP

**CINNAMIC ALCOHOL** • Fragrance ingredient. One of the most common allergens in fragrances and flavorings. *See* Cinnamaldehyde.

**CINNAMIC ALDEHYDE** • *See* Cinnamaldehyde. Found in cinnamon oil, cassia oil, cinnamon, and patchouli oil. Used as a flavoring.

**CINNAMON (CEYLON, CHINESE, SAIGON)** • Obtained from the dried bark of cultivated trees. Used in bitters, cola, apple, plum, vermouth, sausage, eggnog, cinnamon, and vanilla flavorings for beverages, ice cream, ices, candy (4,000 ppm), baked goods (1,900 ppm), condiments, meats, and apple butter. Extracts have been used to break up intestinal gas and to treat diarrhea, but can be irritating to the gastrointestinal system. GRAS

**CINNAMON BARK** • Extract and Oil. From the dried bark of cultivated trees, the extract is used in cola, eggnog, root beer, cinnamon, and ginger ale flavorings for beverages, ice cream, baked goods, condiments, and meats. The oil is used in berry, cola, cherry, rum, root beer, cinnamon, and ginger ale flavorings for beverages, condiments, arid meats. Can be a skin sensitizer in humans and cause mild sensitivity to light. GRAS. ASP

**CINNAMON LEAF OIL** • Oil of Cassia. Chinese Cinnamon. Yellowish to brown volatile oil from the leaves and twigs of cultivated trees. About 80 to 90 percent cinnamal. It has the characteristic odor and taste of cassia cinnamon and darkens and thickens upon aging or exposure to air. Used in cola, apricot, rum, root beer, cinnamon, and ginger ale flavorings for beverages, ice cream, ices, candy, baked goods, chewing gum, gelatin desserts, condiments, pickles, and sliced fruits. Can cause contact dermatitis. EAF

**CINNAMYL ACETATE** • A synthetic flavoring, colorless to yellow liquid with a sweet floral odor. Occurs naturally in cassia bark. Used in apricot, cherry, grape, peach, pineapple, cinnamon, and vanilla flavorings for beverages, ice cream, ices, candy, baked goods, chewing gum, and condiments. Can cause allergic reactions. ASP

**CINNAMYL ALCOHOL** • A synthetic flavoring, white to slightly yellow liquid with a balsamic odor. Occurs in storax, balsam Peru, cinnamon leaves, and hyacinth oil. Used in raspberry, strawberry, apricot, peach, plum, prune, grape, liquor, brandy, nut, black walnut, spice, and cinnamon flavorings for beverages, ice cream, ices, candy, baked goods, chewing gum, gelatin desserts, and brandy. Can cause allergic reactions. ASP

**CINNAMYL ANTHRANILATE** • A synthetic flavoring additive that has been banned by the FDA. The National Cancer Institute reported on December 20, 1980, that it caused liver cancer in male and female mice and caused both kidney and pancreatic cancers in male rats in feeding studies. Earlier studies showed it increased lung tumors in mice. The FDA banned the use of it in food in 1982. Most companies voluntarily stopped using it in cosmetics after publication of the NCI information. BANNED.

**CINNAMYL BENZOATE** • A synthetic butter, caramel, and fruit flavoring additive for beverages, ice cream, ices, candy, baked goods, condiments, and chewing gum. ASP

**CINNAMYL BUTYRATE** • A synthetic citrus orange and fruit flavoring for beverages, ice cream, ices, candy, baked goods, and chewing gum.

**CINNAMYL CINNAMATE** • A synthetic fruit flavoring additive for beverages, ice cream, ices, candy, and baked goods. ASP

**CINNAMYL FORMATE** • Formic Acid. A synthetic flavoring, colorless to yellow liquid with a faint cinnamon odor. Used in banana, cherry, pear, and spice flavorings for beverages, ice cream, ices, candy, baked goods, and chewing gum. *See* Formic Acid for toxicity. ASP

**CINNAMYL ISOBUTYRATE** • A synthetic strawberry, citrus, apple, banana, grape, peach, pear, and pineapple flavoring additive for beverages, ice cream, ices, candy, baked goods, gelatin desserts, chewing gum, and toppings. ASP

**CINNAMYL ISOVALERATE** • A synthetic flavoring, colorless to yellow liquid with a spicy, fruity, floral odor. Used in strawberry, chocolate, apple, apricot, cherry, grape, maple nut, nut, spice, peach, pineapple, and plum flavorings for beverages, ice cream, ices, candy, baked goods, chewing gum, and gelatin desserts. ASP

**CINNAMYL PHENYLACETATE** • A synthetic flavoring with a fruity floral odor. Used in berry, apple, chocolate, currant, grape, peach, pear, and pineapple flavorings for beverages, ice cream, ices, candy, and baked goods. ASP

**CINNAMYL PROPIONATE** • A synthetic flavoring, colorless to yellow liquid with a fruity floral odor. Used in berry, apple, chocolate, currant, grape, peach, pear, and pineapple flavorings for beverages, ice cream, ices, candy, baked goods, chewing gum, and gelatin desserts. ASP

**CINNCLOVAL** • *See* Cinnamaldehyde Ethylene Glycol Acetal.

**CINOXATE** • *See* Cinnamic Acid.

**CIRE D'ABEILLE ABSOLUTE** • *See* Beeswax, Bleached.

**CITRAL** • A light, oily liquid that occurs naturally in grapefruit, orange, peach, ginger, grapefruit oil, oil of lemon, and oil of lime. Either isolated from citral oils or made synthetically. Used in strawberry, lemon, lime, orange, apple, cherry, grape, spice, ginger, and vanilla flavorings for beverages, ice cream, ices, candy, baked goods, and chewing gum. Also used in the synthesis of vitamin A. The compound has been reported to inhibit wound healing and tumor rejection in animals. Vitamin A counteracts its toxicity, but in commercial products to which pure citral has been added vitamin A may not be present. GRAS. ASP

**CITRAL DIMETHYL ACETAL** • A synthetic citrus, lemon, and fruit flavoring for beverages, ices, candy, and condiments. ASP

**CITRATE, CALCIUM** • *See* Calcium Citrate.

**CITRATE, ISOPROPYL** • *See* Isopropyl Citrate.

**CITRATE, MONOGLYCERIDE** • *See* Monoglyceride Citrate.

**CITRATE, SODIUM** • *See* Sodium Citrate.

**CITRATE, STEARYL** • *See* Stearyl Citrate.

**CITRATE SALTS** • Softening additive for cheese spreads; emulsifier salts to blend pasteurized processed cheeses and cheese foods. Citrates may interfere with the results of laboratory tests including tests for pancreatic function, abnormal liver function, and blood alkalinity-acidity.

**CITRIC ACID** • One of the most widely used acids in the cosmetics industry, it is derived from citrus fruit by fermentation of crude sugars. It is also extracted from citrus fruits and occurs naturally in coffee and peaches. It is a flavoring for beverages (2,500 ppm), ice cream, ices, candy (4,300 ppm), baked goods, and chewing gum (3,600 ppm). Citric acid is used to neutralize lye employed in peeling vegetables, as an adjuster of acidity-alkalinity in fruit juices, wines, jams, jellies, jelly candies, canned fruit, carbonated beverages, frozen fruit, canned vegetables, frozen dairy products, cheese spreads, sherbet, confections, canned figs, dried egg whites, mayonnaise, salad dressing, fruit butter, preserves, and fresh beef blood. Employed in curing meats, for firming peppers, potatoes, tomatoes, and lima beans and to prevent off-flavors in fried potatoes. Removes trace metals and brightens color in various commercial products. It has been used to dissolve urinary bladder stones. The final report to the FDA of the Select Committee on GRAS Substances stated in 1980 that it should continue its GRAS status with no limitations other than good manufacturing practices. ASP. E

**CITRIDIC ACID** • *See* Aconitic Acid.

**CITROFLEX A-4** • *See* Tributyl Acetylcitrate.

**CITRONELLA OIL** • A natural food flavoring extract from fresh grass grown in Asia. It consists of about 60 percent geraniol *(see)*, 15 percent citronellol *(see)*, and 10 to 15 percent camphene *(see)*. Used in citrus, fruit, and ginger ale flavorings for beverages, ice cream, ices, candy, and baked goods. Used as an insect repellent. May cause allergic reactions such as stuffy nose, hay fever, asthma, and skin rash when used in cosmetics. Can cause vomiting when ingested, cyanosis, convulsions, damage to intestinal mucosa, and when taken in sufficient amounts, death. GRAS. EAF

**CITRONELLAL** • A synthetic flavoring additive. The chief constituent of citronella oil *(see)*. Also found in lemon and lemongrass oils. Colorless liquid with an intense lemon-rose odor. Used in citrus, lemon, cherry, and spice flavorings for beverages, ice cream, ices, candy, baked goods, chewing gum, and gelatin desserts. A milk irritant. *See* Citronella Oil for toxicity. ASP

**CITRONELLOL** • A synthetic flavoring. Obtained from citronellal or geraniol, geranium rose oil, or citronella oil *(see all)*. Colorless liquid with a roselike odor. The *d* form is oilier and is the major ingredient of rhodinol *(see)*. Used in berry, citrus, cola, fruit, rose, and floral flavorings for beverages, ice cream, ices, candy, baked goods, chewing gum, and gelatin desserts. A mild irritant. *See* Citronella Oil. ASP

**CITRONELLOXY ACETALDEHYDE** • A synthetic floral, rose, and fruit flavoring additive for beverages, ice cream, ices, candy, and baked goods. *See* Citronella Oil for toxicity. ASP

**CITRONELLYL ACETATE** • A synthetic flavoring additive, colorless liquid with a fruity odor. Used in lemon, rose, apricot, banana, grape, pear, and raisin flavorings for beverages, ice cream, ices, candy, baked goods, chewing gum, and gelatin desserts. A major ingredient of rhodinyl acetate *(see)*. ASP

**CITRONELLYL BUTYRATE** • A synthetic flavoring additive, colorless liquid, with a strong rose-fruit odor. Used in cola, floral, rose, apple, pineapple, plum, prune, and honey flavorings for beverages, ice cream, ices, candy, baked goods, chewing gum, and gelatin desserts. A major ingredient of rhodinyl acetate *(see)*. ASP

**CITRONELLYL FORMATE** • Formic Acid. A synthetic flavoring additive, colorless liquid, with a strong fruity odor. Used in orange, apple, apricot, peach, plum, and honey flavorings for beverages, ice cream, ices, candy, baked goods. A major ingredient of rhodinyl acetate *(see)*. *See* Formic Acid for toxicity. ASP

**CITRONELLYL ISOBUTYRATE** • A synthetic flavoring additive, colorless liquid, with a fruit-rose odor. Used in raspberry, strawberry, floral, rose, and grape flavorings for beverages, ice cream, ices, candy, baked goods, and gelatin desserts. A major ingredient of rhodinyl acetate *(see)*. ASP

**CITRONELLYL PHENYLACETATE** • A synthetic butter, caramel, rose, fruit, and honey flavoring additive for beverages, ice cream, ices, candy, and baked goods. A major ingredient of rhodinyl acetate *(see)*. ASP

**CITRONELLYL PROPIONATE** • A synthetic flavoring additive, colorless liquid, with a rose-fruit odor. Used in lemon and fruit flavorings for beverages, ice cream, ices, candy, baked goods, and chewing gum. A major ingredient of rhodinyl acetate *(see)*. ASP

**CITRONELLYL VALERATE** • A synthetic flavoring additive for beverages, ice cream, ices, candy, and baked goods. NIL

**CITRUS BIOFLAVONOIDS** • Vitamin P complex nutrient supplement up to one gram per day. Occurs naturally in plant coloring and in the tonka bean; also in lemon juice. High concentrates can be obtained from all citrus fruits, rose hips, and black currants. Commercial methods extract rinds of oranges, tangerines, lemons, limes, kumquats, and grapefruit. P vitamin is related to healthy blood vessels and skin. Any claim for bioflavonoids renders the product illegal, according to FDA rules.

**CITRUS OILS** • Eugenol. Eucalyptol. Anethole, *a*-irone, orris, and menthol *(see all)*. Used in flavoring food products and cosmetics and as odorants in special soaps.

**CITRUS PEEL EXTRACT** • A natural flavor extract from the peel or rind of grapefruit, lemon, lime, orange, and tangerine. Color, odor, and taste characteristic of source. Used as flavoring additives in bitters, lemon, lime, orange, vermouth, beer, and ginger ale flavorings for beverages, ice cream, ices, candy, and baked goods. GRAS. ASP

**CITRUS RED NO. 2** • Monoazo. Used only for coloring orange skins that are not intended for processing and that meet minimum maturity standards established by or under laws of the states in which the oranges are grown. Used to color Florida but not California oranges. Oranges colored with Citrus Red No. 2 are not supposed to bear more than 2 ppm of the color additive calculated on the weight of the whole fruit. Citrus Red No. 2 toxicity is far from determined even though, theoretically, consumers would not ingest the dye because they peel the orange before eating. The 2-naphthol constituent of the dye if ingested in quantity can cause eye lens clouding, kidney damage, vomiting, and circulatory collapse. May cause allergic reactions and cross-react with clothing, hair dyes, and with sulfanilimides. Application to the skin can cause peeling and deaths have been reported after application to the skin. Also may cause cancer. *See* FD and C Colors. ASP

**CIVET, ABSOLUTE** • Zibeth. Zibet. Zibetum. Essential oil used as a flavoring. Derived from the unctuous secretions from the receptacles between the anus and genitalia of both the male and female civet cat. Semisolid, yellowish to brown mass, with an unpleasant odor. Used in raspberry, butter, caramel, grape, and rum flavorings for beverages, ice cream, ices, candy, baked goods, gelatin desserts, and chewing gum. A fixative in perfumery. GRAS. There is reported use of the chemical; it has not yet been assigned for toxicology literature. EAF

**CLARIFICATION** • Removal from liquid of small amounts of suspended matter; for example, the removal of particles and traces of copper and iron from vinegar and certain beverages.

**CLARIFYING ADDITIVE** • A substance that removes from liquids small amounts of suspended matter. Butyl alcohol, for instance, is a clarifying additive for clear shampoos.

**CLARY** • Clary Sage. A well-known spice in food and beverages. A fixative *(see)* for perfumes. A natural extract of an aromatic herb grown in southern Europe and cultivated widely in England. The herb is a vermouth and spice flavoring additive in vermouth (500 ppm). Clary oil is used in butter, black cherry, grape, licorice, vermouth, wine, root beer, birch beer, spice, vanilla, and cream soda flavorings for beverages, ice cream, ices, candy, baked goods, condiments, and vermouth. GRAS. EAF

**CLAYS** • Kaolin. China Clay. Used to clarify liquids *(see* Clarification) and as a filler for paper. The final report to the FDA of the Select Committee on GRAS Substances stated in 1980 that it should continue its GRAS status with no limitations other than good manufacturing practices.

**CLOPIDOL** • Additive used in chicken and turkey feeds to combat parasites. The FDA tolerance for residues in milk is 0.02 ppm; for cereal, grains, vegetables, fruits, meat of cattle, sheep, and goats, and in edible tissue of swine, it is 0.2 ppm. The tolerance is 1.5 ppm in liver of cattle, sheep, and goats; 5 ppm in muscle of chicken and turkeys; 5 ppm in liver and kidneys of chickens and turkeys.

**CLOPROSTENOL** • Estrumate. An animal drug used to treat infertility in sows and to synchronize estrus in cows.

**CLOPYRALID** • An herbicide used in animal feed, barley (milled, except flour), oats (except flour), and wheat (milled, except flour). FDA residue limits are 12 ppm in barley, oats, and wheat (except in their flours) when used for animal feed. The tolerance for residues in fat, meat, by-products of sheep is 2 ppm and 0.2 ppm for the fat, kidneys, and meat of hogs and poultry.

**CLOVE BUD EXTRACT** • A natural flavor extract from the pungent, fragrant, reddish brown dried flower buds of a tropical tree. Used in berry, fruit, meat, root beer, and spice flavorings for beverages, ice cream, candy, baked goods, condiments, and meats. Cloves are used also as a dental analgesic and germicide. They may cause intestinal upsets. Rats poisoned with clove oil have shown paralysis of hind legs and jaws, with prostration and eventually death. The FDA gave toxicity studies of clove additives top priority in 1980. GRAS. ASP

**CLOVE BUD OIL** • The volatile, colorless or pale yellow oil obtained by steam distillation from the dried flower buds of a tropical tree. A characteristic clove odor and taste. Used in raspberry, coffee, cola, banana, cherry, peach, plum, rum, sausage, eggnog, pecan, root beer flavorings for beverages, ice cream, ices, candy, baked goods, chewing gum (1,800 ppm), gelatin desserts, meats, liquors, spiced fruit (830 ppm), jelly, condiments. Used as an antiseptic and flavoring in tooth powders and as a scent in hair tonics and to flavor postage stamp glue, as a toothache treatment, as a condiment, and as a flavoring in chewing gum. It is 82 to 87 percent eugenol *(see)* and has the characteristic clove oil odor and taste. It is strongly irritating to the skin and can cause allergic skin rashes. Its use in perfumes and cosmetics is frowned upon, although in very diluted forms it is innocuous. The final report to the FDA of the Select Committee on GRAS Substances stated in 1980 that it should continue its GRAS status with no limitations other than good manufacturing practices. ASP

**CLOVE BUD OLEORESIN** • A natural resinous, viscous flavoring extract from the tree that produces clove buds. Used in fruit, meat, and spice flavorings for meat.

**CLOVE LEAF OIL** • The volatile pale yellow oil obtained by steam distillation of the leaves of the tropical tree that produces clove buds. Used in loganberry, cherry, root beer, sarsaparilla, and cinnamon flavorings for beverages, ice cream, ices, candy, baked goods, chewing gum, gelatin desserts, meats, pickles, apple butter, and condiments. *See* Clove Bud Extract for toxicity. The final report to the FDA of the Select Committee on GRAS Substances stated in 1980 that it should continue its GRAS status with no limitations other than good manufacturing practices. ASP

**CLOVE STEM OIL** • The volatile, yellow to light brown oil obtained by steam distillation from the dried stems of the tropical tree that produces clove buds. Characteristic odor and taste of cloves. Used in berry, cherry, root beer, ginger ale, and ginger beer flavorings for beverages, ice cream, ices, candy, baked goods, and condiments. *See* Clove Bud Extract for toxicity. The final report to the FDA of the Select Committee on GRAS Substances stated in 1980 that it should continue its GRAS status with no limitations other than good manufacturing practices.

**CLOVER** • An herb, a natural flavoring extract from a plant characterized by three leaves and flowers in dense heads. Used in fruit flavorings for beverages, ice cream, ices, candy, and baked goods. May cause sensitivity to light. GRAS. EAF

**CLOVER BLOSSOM EXTRACT** • Trifolium Extract. The extract of the flowers of *Trifolium pratense.* Used in fruit flavorings. May cause sensitivity to light. NUL

**CLOVERLEAF OIL** • Eugenia Caryophyllus Leaf Oil. The volatile oil obtained by steam distillation of the leaves of *Eugenia caryophyllata.* It consists mostly of eugenol *(see).* NUL

**CLOVES** • *Eugenia caryophyllata.* An evergreen tree, the clove is native to the Spice Islands and the Philippines and is cultivated in India, South America, the West Indies, and other tropical areas. The oldest medical use was in China, where it was taken for various ailments as early as 240 B.C. Medicinally, herbalists use cloves to treat flatulence, diarrhea, and for liver, stomach, and bowel ailments. It is also used as a stimulant for nerves. Clove oil is still sold in modern drugstores as a treatment for toothaches. Clove tea with mace is used for nausea. In 1992, the FDA proposed a ban on clove oil in astringent *(see)* drug products because it has not been shown to be safe and effective for its stated claims. ASP

**CLOXACILLIN** • Alcloxa. Apo-Cloxi. Austrastaph. Bactopen. Cloxapen. Novocloxin. Orbenin. Orbenin Injection. Tegopen. A penicillin antibiotic introduced in 1962 for systemic infections caused by penicillinase-producing staphylococci *(see* Staphybiotic). It is used in cattle. The FDA says residues in cattle meat should not exceed 0.1 ppm. In humans, it may cause lung problems (eosinophilia), nausea, vomiting, gastric distress, diarrhea, hypersensitivity including potentially fatal allergic reaction, liver problems, and overgrowth of nonsusceptible organisms.

**CMC** • *See* Cellulose Gums.

**CND** • FDA abbreviation for canned.

**COAL TAR** • Used in adhesives, creosotes, insecticides, phenols, wood-working, preservation of food, synthetic flavors, and dyes to make colors used in cosmetics, including hair dyes. Thick liquid or semisolid tar obtained from bituminous coal, it contains many constituents including benzene, xylenes, naphthalene, pyridine, quinolineoline, phenol, and cresol. The main concern about coal-tar derivatives is that they cause cancer in animals, but they are also frequent sources of allergic reactions, particularly skin rashes and hives.

**COBALT SALTS** • Acetate, Chloride, and Sulfate. Illegal for use. In 1960, it was discovered that cobalt salts added to beer to maintain the head caused serious heart problems in beer drinkers. Cobalt sulfate has been banned.

**COBALT SOURCES** • Acetate, Carbonate, Chloride, Oxide, and Sulfate. Cobalt is a metal occurring in the earth's crust; gray, hard, and magnetic. All here are used as a mineral supplement at the rate of 1 milligram per day. Used as a nutrient in animal feed. Excess administration can result in an overproduction of red blood cells and gastrointestinal upset. GRAS

**COCA LEAF EXTRACT (DECOCAINIZED)** • Flavoring from the dried leaves of cocaine-containing plants grown in Bolivia, Brazil, Peru, and Java. Used in bitters and cola flavoring for beverages, ice cream, ices, and candy. Once a central nervous system stimulant. GRAS. EAF

**COCCIDIOSIS** • Diseases due to coccidia, one-celled animals that cause serious infections in many species of animals. It is rare in humans except in persons suffering from AIDS.

**COCCIDIOSTAT** • A drug generally added to animal feed to partially inhibit or delay the development of coccidiosis *(see)*.

**COCHINEAL** • *See* Carmine.

**COCOA** • A powder prepared from the roasted and cured kernels of ripe seeds of *Theobroma cacao* and other species of *Theobroma*. A brownish powder with a chocolate odor, it is used as a flavoring. May cause wheezing, rash, and other symptoms of allergy, particularly in children. EAF

**COCOA BUTTER SUBSTITUTE FROM PALM KERNEL OIL** • Coating material for vitamins, citric acid, succinic acid, and spices. In lieu of cocoa butter in sweets. There is reported use of the chemical; it has not yet been assigned for toxicology literature. GRAS. ASP

**COCOA BUTTER SUBSTITUTE FROM COCONUT OIL** • GRAS. NUL

**COCOA BUTTER SUBSTITUTE FROM HIGH OLEIC SAFFLOWER** • Good substitute for olive oil and shea butter *(see both)*. EAF

**COCOA EXTRACT** • Extract of *Theobroma cacao*. *See* Cocoa Butter. ASP. EAF

**COCOA WITH DIOCTYL SODIUM SULFOSUCCINATE** • Adjuvant, emulsifier, humectant, stabilizer, and thickener. Dioctyl sodium sulfosuccinate is derived from maleic anhydride, a tissue irritant. Used in dairy-based drinks, flavored and/or fermented, for example, chocolate milk, cocoa, eggnog, drinking yogurt, whey-based drinks, condensed milk (plain) unripened cheese (5,000 mg/kg), processed cheese (5,000 mg/kg), fruit-based desserts, including fruit-flavored water-based desserts (15 mg/kg), cocoa mixes (powders and syrups; 4,000 mg/kg), edible casings (e.g., sausage casings; 200 mg/kg; white and semiwhite sugar (sucrose or saccharose), fructose, glucose (dextrose), xylose; sugar solutions and syrups, also (partially) inverted sugars, including molasses, treacle, and sugar toppings (25 mg/kg); emulsified sauces (e.g., mayonnaise, salad dressing; 5,000 mg/kg); water-based flavored drinks, including "sport" or "electrolyte" drinks and particulated drinks; alcoholic beverages, including alcohol-free and low-alcoholic counterparts (10 mg/kg). NIL

**COCOAMPHODIPRIOPIONATE** • *See* Coconut Oil.

**COCONUT ACIDS** • *See* Coconut Oil.

**COCONUT ALCOHOLS** • *See* Coconut Oil.

**COCONUT OIL** • The white, semisolid, highly saturated fat expressed from the meat of the coconut. Used in chocolate, candies, in baking, instead of lard, and in self-basting turkeys. A saturated fat that is not recommended for those worried about fat-clogged arteries. May cause allergic skin rashes. The final report to the FDA of the Select Committee on GRAS Substances stated in 1980 that it should continue its GRAS status with no limitations other than good manufacturing practices. ASP

**COFFEE** • Coffee Beans. Dry, unroasted seeds of *Coffea arabica*. Contains caffeine *(see)*. An essential oil used as a flavoring. GRAS. ASP

**COGNAC OIL** • Wine Yeast Oil. The volatile oil obtained from distillation of wine, with the characteristic aroma of cognac. Green cognac oil is used as a flavoring for beverages, ice cream, ices, candy, baked goods, chewing gum, liquors, and condiments. White cognac oil, which has the same constituents as green oil, is used in berry, cherry, grape, brandy, and rum flavorings for beverages, ice cream, ices, candy, baked goods, and gelatin desserts. GRAS. EAF

**COLA NUT** • Essential oil used for flavoring. GRAS

**COLISTIMETHATE SODIUM** • First Guard Sterile Powder. Used on one-to three-day-old chickens for control of early mortality due to *Escherichia coli* organisms. It is injected into the necks of chicks.

**COLLAGEN** • Protein substance found in connective tissue. It is usually derived from animal tissue. Collagen from hides and skins is used as an emulsifier in meat products because it can bind large quantities of fat. This makes it a useful additive or filler for meat products. Collagen can also be extracted from cattle hides to make the collagen sausage used in the meat industry. Collagen casing products were developed in Germany in the 1920s, but only gained popularity in the United States in the 1960s. The processing does not convert the collagen into a soluble product, as in the case of gelatin. Instead, it results in a product which retains a relatively high degree of the native collagen fiber and is strong enough to be used as a casing for sausages and other products. The extracted collagen is mixed with water and converted into a dough, which is extruded by either a wet or a dry process. The tube of extruded collagen is then passed through a concentrated salt solution and a chamber of ammonia to precipitate the collagen. The swollen gel contracts to produce a film of reasonable strength. It can be improved by the addition of glycerin *(see),* to make it more flexible. Allergic reactions to collagen are not infrequent. ASP

**COLLOIDAL SILICON DIOXIDE SOL** • Silica Sol. Practically insoluble in water. A free-flowing additive in salt, seasoned salt, and sodium bicarbonate. Also included in vitamin products, dietary products, spices, meat-curing compounds, flavoring powders, dehydrated honey, dehydrated molasses, and dehydrated nondiastatic malt. Chemically and biologically inert when ingested. *See* Silicon Dioxide.

**COLORING** • More than 90 percent of the food colorings now in use are manufactured, frequently from coal-tar colors. The coal-tar derivatives need to be certified, which means that batches of the dyes are chemically tested and approved by the FDA. As more and more food colors are banned, interest has grown in colors derived from natural sources such as carotene *(see)* from carrots, which is used to color margarine, and beet juice, which provides a red color for some foods. For information on the synthetics now in use, *see* FD and C Colors.

**COLORS** • *See* FD and C Colors.

**COMMUNITY RIGHT-TO-KNOW LIST** • Manufacturers that employ toxic chemicals while making products must respond, under the law, to inquiries from employees and citizens in the area. Cyanide, which is used in the manufacture of pesticides and some food additives is an example of a chemical on this list compiled by the U.S. Environmental Protection Agency.

**COMPETITIVE MICROBIAL INHIBITION** • Relies on the fact that many harmless bacteria, notably lactic acid bacteria, can inhibit the growth of both spoilage bacteria and pathogens. Inhibitory strains of lactic acid bacteria can be selected for use in dairy cultures or added to refrigerated foods to extend shelf life and enhance safety.

**CONCRETE** • A semisolid mixture of essential oil and fatty, waxy material that is obtained by the solvent extraction of flowers or plants followed by solvent removal.

**CONDENSED ANIMAL PROTEIN HYDROLYSATE** • A feed used for poultry and cattle.

**CONTACT DERMATITIS** • *See* Allergic Contact Dermatitis.

**COPAIBA OIL** • Jesuit's Balsam. From steam distillation of South American balsam, *Copaifera officinalis*. It is a yellow liquid with an aromatic odor and slightly bitter taste. It is used as a flavoring additive in various foods. EAF

**COPALS, MANILA** • A resin obtained as a fossil or as an exudate from various species of tropical plants. Must be heated in alcohol or other solvents. May cause allergic reactions, particularly skin rashes. NUL

**COPOLYMER** • Result of polymerization (*see* Polymer), which includes at least two different molecules, each of which is capable of polymerizing alone. Together they form a new, distinct molecule. They are used in the manufacture of nail enamels and face masks.

**COPOLYMER CONDENSATES OF ETHYLENE OXIDE and PROPYLENE OXIDE** • Stabilizers in flavor concentrates, processing and wetting additives in yeast-leavened bakery products, dough conditioners, surfactants, defoaming additives, and nutrient supplements in animal feed. Ethylene oxide has been found to cause cancer in animals.

**COPPER** • One of the earliest known metals. An essential nutrient for all mammals. Naturally occurring or experimentally produced copper deficiency in animals leads to a variety of abnormalities including anemia, skeletal defects, and muscle degeneration. Copper deficiency is extremely rare in man. The body of an adult contains from 75 to 150 milligrams of copper. Concentrations are highest in the brain and liver and heart. A copper intake of 2 milligrams per day appears to maintain a balance in adults. An ordinary diet provides 2 to 5 milligrams daily. Copper compounds are used as a pesticide.

**COPPER DISODIUM EDTA** • Used as an injection for cattle. *See* Copper and Copper Salts.

**COPPER GLUCONATE** • An essential nutrient. Used as a feed additive, dietary supplement, and mouth deodorant. GRAS. ASP

**COPPER SULFATE** • *See* Copper Salts. GRAS. ASP

**COPPER SALTS** • Used as nutrient supplements in animal feed. Copper itself is nontoxic, but soluble copper salts, notably copper sulfate, are highly irritating to the skin and mucous membranes, and when ingested cause serious vomiting. Copper salts include copper carbonate, chloride, gluconate, hydroxide, orthophosphate oxide, pyrophosphate, and sulfate. The final report to the FDA of the Select Committee on GRAS Substances stated in 1980 that it should continue its GRAS status with no limitations other than good manufacturing practices.

**COPRA OIL** • From the kernel of the fruit of the coconut palm *Cocos nucifera.* Fatty solid or liquid with a sweet, nutty taste. Used as a coating additive, emulsifying additive, and as a texturizer in baked goods, candy, desserts, and margarine. Nontoxic. GRAS

**CORIANDER LEAF OIL** • *Coriandrum sativum.* Coriander leaf oil is also available. It smells similar to the seed oil but is stronger, greener, and not as sweet. Coriander oil is a natural deodorant and is frequently used in perfumery. EAF

**CORIANDER OIL** • The colorless or pale yellow volatile oil from the dried ripe fruit of a plant grown in Asia and Europe. Used as a flavoring additive in raspberry, bitters, fruit, meat, spice, ginger ale, and vanilla flavorings for beverages, ice cream, ices, candy, baked goods (880 ppm), chewing gum, meats (1,300 ppm), liquors (1,000 ppm), and condiments. Used to flavor dentrifices. The oil is used in blackberry, raspberry, chocolate, coffee, cola, fruit, liquor, sausage, root beer, spice, ginger ale, and vanilla flavorings for beverages, ice cream, ices, candy, baked goods, chewing gum, condiments, meats, and liquors. Can cause allergic reactions, particularly of the skin. Coriander is used as a weak medication (up to 1 gram) to break up intestinal gas. GRAS. ASP

**CORK, OAK** • Flavoring in alcoholic beverages only. ASP

**CORN** • Corn Sugar. Dextrose. Used in maple, nut, and root beer flavorings for beverages, ice cream, ices, candy, and baked goods. The oil is used in emollient creams and toothpastes. The syrup is used as a texturizer and carrying additive in cosmetics. It is also used for envelopes, paper, stamps, sticker tapes, ale, aspirin, bacon, baking mixes, powders, beers, bourbon, breads, cheeses, cereals, chop suey, chow mein, confectioners' sugar, cream puffs, fish products, ginger ale, hams, jellies, processed meats, peanut butters, canned peas, plastic food wrappers, sherbets, whiskeys, and American wines. It may also be found in capsule vitamins, fritters, Fritos, frostings, canned or frozen fruit, graham crackers, gravies, grits, gum, monosodium glutamate, Nescafé, oleomargarine, bologna, pablum, tortillas, vinegar, yeasts, frying fats, fruit juices, laxatives. May cause allergic reactions including skin rashes and asthma. ASP

**CORN ACID** • *See* Corn Oil.

**CORN COB MEAL** • The milled powder prepared from the cobs of *Zea mays.*

**CORN DEXTRIN** • Dextri-Maltose. A white or yellow powder obtained by enzymatic action of barley malt on corn flours and used as a modifier or thickening additive in milk and milk products. Nontoxic. The final report to the FDA of the Select Committee on GRAS Substances stated in 1980 that it should continue its GRAS status with no limitations other than good manufacturing practices.

**CORN ENDOSPERM OIL** • For use in chicken feed to enhance yellow color of chicken skin and eggs. Permanently listed since 1967. NIL

**CORN FLOUR** • A finely ground powder. Used in face and bath powder. *See* Corn Oil.

**CORN GERM EXTRACT** • The extract of the germ of *Zea mays*.

**CORN GLUTEN** • A nutrient supplement for various foods. ASP

**CORN OIL** • Light yellow, clear, oily liquid used as a coating additive, emulsifying additive, and texturizer in bakery products, margarine, mayonnaise, and salad oil. Obtained as a by-product by wet-milling the grain for use in the manufacture of cornstarch, dextrins, and yellow oil. It has a faint characteristic odor and taste and thickens upon exposure to air. Human skin irritant and allergen. Has caused birth defects in experimental animals. GRAS

**CORN POPPY EXTRACT** • The extract obtained from the petals of the *Papaver rhoeas*.

**CORN SILK** • Used as a natural flavoring extract in baked goods, baking mixes, beverages, soft candies, and frozen dairy desserts. The final report to the FDA of the Select Committee on GRAS Substances stated in 1980 that there were insufficient relevant biological and other studies upon which to base an evaluation of it when it is used as a food ingredient. It remains GRAS. NUL

**CORN SUGAR** • Nutrient. *See* Corn Syrup. GRAS

**CORN SYRUP** • Corn Sugar. Dextrose. A sweet syrup prepared from cornstarch. Used in maple, nut, and root beer flavorings for beverages, ice cream, ices, candy, and baked goods. Also used for envelopes, stamps, sticking tapes, aspirin, and many food products including bacon, baking mixes, powders, beer, bourbon, breads, breakfast cereals, pastries, candy, carbonated beverages, ketchups, cheeses, cereals, chop suey, chow mein, confectioners' sugar, cream puffs, fish products, ginger ale, hams, jellies, processed meats, peanut butter, canned peas, plastic food wraps, sherbet, whiskey, and American wines. May cause allergic reactions. The final report to the FDA of the Select Committee on GRAS Substances stated in 1980 that there is no evidence in the available information that it is a hazard to the public when used as it is now, and it should continue in GRAS status with no limitations on amounts that can be added to food.

**CORNSTARCH** • Many containers are powdered with cornstarch to prevent sticking. The dietetic grade is marketed as Maizena and Mondamin. It is a demulcent for irritated colons. May cause allergic reactions, including skin rashes and asthma. The final report to the FDA of the Select Committee on GRAS Substances stated in 1980 that it should continue its

GRAS status with no limitations other than good manufacturing practices. ASP

**CORN STEEP LIQUOR** • Well defined and consistent amino acid profile and a high level of complex sugars that produce an attractive smell and taste. Used in animal feed and as a growth and fermentation medium for the production of some food additives. ASP

**CORPS PRALINE** • *See* Maltol.

**COSTMARY** • Virgin Mary. A natural flavoring derived from an herb native to Asia. Its yellow aromatic flowers are shaped like buttons. Infrequently used today as a flavoring in beer and ale. Regarded as sacred to the Virgin Mary. NUL

**COSTUS ROOT OIL** • The volatile oil is obtained by steam distillation from dried roots of an herb. Light yellow to brown viscous liquid, with a persistent violetlike odor. A natural fruit and vanilla flavoring for beverages, ice cream, ices, candy, baked goods, chewing gum, and gelatin desserts. EAF

**COTTONSEED FLOUR** • Cooked, partly defatted, and toasted flour used for pale yellow coloring. Sometimes used to make gin. It is permanently listed as a coloring. It is known to cause allergies, and because it is used in a wide variety of products without notice, it may be hard to avoid. More often, exposures to the allergens arise from the use of cottonseed meal, which may be found in fertilizers and as a constituent of feed for cattle, hogs, poultry, and dogs. Symptoms usually result from inhalation but allergic reactions also can occur from ingesting cottonseed meal used in pangreasing compounds and in foods such as some fried cakes, fig bars, and cookies. ASP

**COTTONSEED OIL** • The fixed oil from the seeds of the cultivated varieties of the plant. Pale yellow, oily, odorless liquid used in the manufacture of soaps, creams, baby creams, nail polish removers, and lubricants. The oil is used in most salad oils, oleomargarines, mayonnaises, and salad dressings. Lard compounds and lard substitutes are made with cottonseed oil. Sardines may be packed in it. Most commercial fried products such as potato chips and doughnuts are fried in cottonseed oil, and restaurants use it for cooking. Candies, particularly chocolates, often contain this oil and it is used to polish fruits at stands. It is used in baby creams, soaps, creams, nail polish removers, and lubricants. It is also used in cotton wadding or batting in cushions, comforters, mattresses, and upholstery, varnishes, fertilizers, and in animal feeds. Known to cause many allergic reactions, but because of its wide use in cosmetics, foods, and other products, it is hard to avoid.

**COTTONSEED and SOYBEAN FATTY ACIDS** • Used as a lubricant, binder, defoaming additive, and component in manufacture of other food-grade additives.

**COUCHGRASS** • *See* Dog Grass Extract.

**COUMAPHOS** • Agridip. Asunthol. Baymix 50. Used in cattle and chicken feed as an insecticide and to counteract worms. Poison by ingestion, skin contact, inhalation, and injection. May be a mutagen. The FDA tolerance in meat and meat by-products of cattle, goats, hogs, horses, poultry, and sheep is 1 ppm. In eggs and milk it is zero.

**COUMARIN** • Tonka Bean. Cumarin. A fragrant ingredient of tonka beans, sweet woodruff, cramp bark, and many other plants. It is made synthetically as well. Coumarin is prohibited in foods because it is toxic by ingestion and carcinogenic. Coumarin in Mexican vanilla has been a recurring problem for quite some time according to the FDA. Coumarin has been prohibited in food in the United States since 1940. Food containing any added coumarin as such or as a constituent of tonka beans or tonka extract is deemed to be adulterated. BANNED

**COUMARONE-IDENE RESIN** • Coating for fruit. The FDA limits it to 200 ppm on fresh-weight basis. ASP

**CRANBERRY JUICE CONCENTRATE** • Bright red coloring from the juice of the red acid berry, produced by any of several plants of the genus *Vaccinium,* grown in the United States and Europe. Food manufacturers may substitute this natural coloring for the synthetic reds that were banned.

**CRANBERRY POMACE** • Source of natural red coloring. *See* Anthocyanins.

**CREAM OF TARTAR** • A white crystalline salt in tartars from wine making, prepared especially from argols and also synthetically from tartaric acid *(see)*. Has a pleasant acid taste. Used as a thickening additive.

**CREOSOL** • *See* 2-Methoxy-4-Methylphenol. ASP

*p*-**CRESOL** • A synthetic nut and vanilla flavoring additive. Obtained from coal tar. It occurs naturally in tea and is used for beverages, ice cream, ices, candy, and baked goods. It is more powerful than phenol and less toxic. Phenol is an extremely toxic acid obtained from coal tar that has many industrial uses, including as a disinfectant for toilets and as an anesthetic. ASP

**O-CRESYL ACETATE** • *See o*-Tolyl Acetate.

*p*-**CRESYL ACETATE** • *See p*-Tolyl Acetate.

**CRETAN DITTANY** • *See* Dittany of Crete.

**CROCETIN** • Yellow coloring from saffron *(see)*.

**CROCUS EXTRACT** • *See* Saffron.

**CROSS-REACTIVITY** • When the body mistakes one compound for another of similar chemical composition.

**CROWN GUM** • Catalyst. EAF

**CRUCIFEROUS VEGETABLES** • A family of plants characterized by flowers and fruits that bear a cross in the center. The genus being studied intensively for health properties are the *Brassica,* which include brussels sprouts, cauliflower, and broccoli. These vegetables contain large quantities of some substances that have been shown to inhibit chemically induced cancers in animals.

**CRUFOMATE** • An antiworm insecticide from petroleum used on cattle, goats, and sheep. FDA residue tolerance is 1 ppm in meat, fat, and by-products.

**CRYOLITE (SODIUM ALUMINUM FLUORIDE)** • A mineral used as an insecticide. FDA tolerance on fruits and vegetables is 0.7 ppm.

**CRYPTOXANTHIN** • A natural yellow coloring from corn and marigolds. *See* Xanthophyll.

**CRYSTALLINE FRUCTOSE** • Used in baked goods, frozen foods, beverages, tabletop sweeteners. It has about one to two times the sweetness of sugar and has calories. *See* Fructose.

**CTG** • Coating for fruits and vegetables.

**CUBEBS** • *Piper cubeba.* Tailed Pepper. Java Pepper. The mature, unripe, sun-dried fruit of a perennial vine grown in South Asia, Java, Sumatra, the Indies, and Sri Lanka. It has a strong, spicy odor and is used in fruit flavoring for beverages (800 ppm). The volatile oil is obtained by steam distillation from the fruit and is colorless to light green with a characteristic spicy odor and a slightly acrid taste. It is used in berry, fruit, and ginger flavorings for beverages, ice cream, ices, candy, baked goods, meats, and condiments. Java pepper was formerly used to stimulate healing of mucous membranes. The fruit has been used as a stimulant and diuretic and sometimes is smoked in cigarettes. EAF

**CUCUMBER JUICE** • From the succulent fruit of the vine. It has a pleasant aroma and imparts a cool feeling to the skin.

**CUMALDEHYDE** • *See* Cuminaldehyde.

**CUMENEALDEHYDE** • Colorless liquid with a floral odor used as a flavoring additive in various foods. Moderately toxic by ingestion. Narcotic in high doses. ASP

**CUMIN** • Cummin. A natural flavoring obtained from the seeds of an Old World plant. Used in spice and sausage flavorings for baked goods (2,500 ppm), condiments (3,900 ppm), and meats. Volatile oil, light yellow to brown, with a strong, disagreeable odor, is distilled from the plant. Used in berry, fruit, sausage, and spice flavorings for beverages, ice cream, ices, candy, chewing gum, baked goods, meats, pickles, and condiments. Moderately toxic by ingestion and skin contact. May be mutagenic. GRAS. ASP

**CUMIN OIL** • *See* Cumin. ASP

**CUMINAL** • *See* Cuminaldehyde.

**CUMINALDEHYDE** • A constituent of eucalyptus, myrrh, cassia, cumin, and other essential oils, but often made synthetically. Colorless to yellowish, oily, with a strong, lasting odor. It is used as a synthetic flavoring in berry, fruit, and spice flavorings for beverages, ice cream, ices, candy, baked goods, chewing gum, and condiments. Used in perfumery.

**CUMINIC ALDEHYDE** • *See* Cuminaldehyde.

**CUPRIC ACETATE** • The copper salts of acetic acid and copper *(see both)*.

**CUPRIC CHLORIDE** • Copper Chloride. A copper salt used in hair dye. A yellow to brown water-absorbing powder that is soluble in diluted acids. Irritating to the skin and mucous membranes. Irritating when ingested. *See* Copper.

**CUPRIC OXIDE** • *See* Copper.

**CUPRIC SULFATE** • Copper sulfate occurs in nature as hydrocyanite. Grayish white to greenish white crystals. Used as agricultural fungicide, herbicide, and in the preparation of azo dyes *(see)*. Very irritating if ingested. Nontoxic on the skin and is used medicinally as a skin fungicide. *See* Copper.

**CUPROUS IODIDE** • A source of dietary iodide. The final report to the FDA of the Select Committee on GRAS Substances stated in 1980 that it should continue its GRAS status with no limitations other than good manufacturing practices. *See* Iodine Sources. NIL

**CURACAO PEEL EXTRACT** • A natural flavoring extracted from a plant native to the Caribbean islands. Used in orange and liquor flavorings for beverages (1,700 ppm). GRAS

**CURACAO PEEL OIL** • A natural flavoring extracted from a plant native to the Caribbean islands. Used in berry, lime, and liquor flavorings for beverages, ice cream, ices, candy, and baked goods.

**CURCUMIN** • Orange-yellow colorant derived from turmeric *(see)* and used as a natural food coloring. It does not require certification because it is a natural product, but the Expert Committee on Food Additives of the FDA recommended that the acceptable daily intake of curcumin (and turmeric) be limited to 0 to 0.5 milligrams per kilogram of body weight. Moderately toxic by injection. A skin irritant. The FAO/WHO Expert Committee on Food Additives, however, concluded in June 1998 that reproductive toxicity studies and more information concerning the solvents used in the manufacturing processes of this additive are needed. E

**CURDLAN** • Pureglucan. Received approval from the FDA. It is the first direct food additive completely developed and petitioned by a Japanese company. An enzyme that processes starch. EAF

**CURING ADDITIVES** • These include salt, nitrites *(see)*, and other compounds used to stabilize color, give flavor, and/or preserve.

**CURRANT, BLACK, BUDS and LEAVES** • *See* Currant Buds, Absolute. ASP

**CURRANT BUDS, ABSOLUTE** • A natural flavoring from a variety of small raisins grown principally in Greece. Used in fruit, berry, and raspberry flavorings for beverages, ice cream, ices, candy, and baked goods. ASP

**CUSPARIA BARK** • Essential oil from the bark of angostura used as a flavoring. *See* Angostura. GRAS

**CYANAMIDE** • Water-absorbing crystals used as fumigant for uncooked bacon, cereal flours, cereals that are cooked before being eaten, cocoa, uncooked ham, and uncooked sausage. FDA residue tolerances are 125 ppm in cereal flours, 90 ppm in cereals that are cooked before being eaten, and 50 ppm in uncooked bacon, ham, and sausage, and 200 ppm in cocoa. Cyanide and its compounds are on the Community Right-To-Know List *(see)*. Poison by ingestion, inhalation, and intraperitoneal route. Moderately toxic by skin contact. Listed as a cancer-causing agent. A severe eye irritant.

**CYANIDE** • Prussic Acid. Hydrocyanic Acid. An inorganic salt, it is one of the most rapid poisons known. Poisoning may occur when any compound releases cyanide. Cyanide is used as a fungistat, insecticide, and rodenticide. It has been reported to reduce oxygen availability in the blood even in low doses.

**CYANIDIN** • Usually isolated from bananas or cherries, it is used as a coloring in foods. It has also been used to treat night blindness.

**CYANO-, CYAN-** • From the Greek *kaynos,* meaning a dark blue. The prefix is commonly used to signify compounds containing the cyanide group CN. If the cyanide is not released from the compound, its presence is presumed not harmful.

**CYANO(4-FLURO-3-PHENOXYPHENYL)METHYL-3-(2,2-DICHLO-ROETHENYL)-2,2-DIMETHYL-PROPANECARBOXYLATE** • An insecticide used in animal feed. *See* Cyanamide.

**CYANO(3-PHENOXYPHENYL)-METHYL-4-CHLORO-ALPHA-(1-METHYL ETHYL)BENZENEACETATE** • A pesticide used in apple pomace to be used in animal feeds up to 20 ppm. The tolerance is 10 ppm in tomato pomace in animal feed and 1 ppm in peanut hulls to be used in animal feeds.

**CYANOCOBALAMIN** • *See* Vitamin $B_{12}$.

**CYANODITHIOIMIDOCARBONATE, DISODIUM** • Bacteria-killing component in the processing of sugarcane. Many organic cyano compounds are decomposed in the body to yield highly toxic cyanide.

**CYANOGENS** • Substances in almonds, and peach and apricot pits that can cause headache and heart palpitations.

**CYCLAMATES** • Sodium and Calcium. Artificial sweetening additives about thirty times as sweet as refined sugar, removed from the food market on September 1, 1969, because they were found to cause bladder cancer in rats. At that time 175 million Americans were swallowing cyclamates in significant doses in many products ranging from chewing gum to soft drinks. There has been a concerted effort to bring cyclamates back to the market, but as of this writing, they have not been approved. The FDA's Cancer Assessment Committee's review of all the evidence reportedly indicates that neither cyclamate nor its major metabolic end product, cyclohexylamine, cause cancer. However, in 2003, the FDA put in abeyance *(see)* a petition by Abbott Laboratories to allow cyclamates on the market. BANNED

**CYCLAMEN ALDEHYDE** • Colorless liquid with a strong floral odor used as a flavoring additive in various food products. Moderately toxic by ingestion. A human skin irritant. GRAS.

**CYCLAMIC ACID** • Fairly strong acid with a sweet taste. It is the acid from which cyclamates were derived *(see)*. E

**CYCLOBUTANONES** • Substances formed in fatty foods after irriadiation including beef, chicken, eggs, cheese, and certain fruits such as avocado, mango, and pawpaw. FAO/WHO has called for more studies of these compounds to determine their effect on health, if any.

**CYCLODEXTRINS** • Enzymatically modified starches shaped like doughnuts. The cavity of the molecule repels water and organic compounds can fill the cavity. As a result, caffeine can be removed from tea and coffee, bitter components can be removed from citrus fruits, flavor oils can be extracted from onion, garlic, and other plants, and cyclodextrins can be recovered and reused. The FAO/WHO Expert Committee on Food Additives *(see)* evaluated the data on β-cyclodextrin. The members found that it is poorly absorbed in the upper gastrointestinal tract in humans and is largely utilized following breakdown by the microflora in the lower gut. A small proportion may be absorbed intact. A number of acute and short-term toxicity studies were reviewed that indicated low toxicity by the oral route. Despite its low toxicity, the committee was concerned about its possible effect on fat-absorbed nutrients and drugs. The experts set a temporary ADI *(see)* of 0 to 6 mg per kg of body weight and recommended further study of its effects on fat-absorbed nutrients. They also asked for more information on production methods. The FAO/WHO Expert Committee on Food Additives requested in June 1998 that a study of human tolerance be revived in 1999 "in order to confirm the absence of adverse gastrointestinal symptoms at normal levels of intake of gamma-cyclodextrin." In 2003, a flavoring, beta Cyclodextrin, was determined GRAS by the Expert Panel of the Flavor and Extract Manufacturers Association.

**CYCLOHEPTADECA-9-EN-1-ONE** • Flavoring. ASP

**CYCLOHEXANE** • Hexamethylene. A hydrocarbon *(see)* solvent widely used in industry in the manufacture of nylon, cellulose fats, oils, waxes, resins, paint and varnish removers, glass substitutes, and fungicides. Colorless liquid with a pungent odor. It is also used to dilute colors in food. Poison by intravenous route. Moderately toxic by ingestion. A systemic irritant by inhalation and ingestion. A skin irritant. May cause mutations. ASP

**CYCLOHEXANE ETHYL ACETATE** • A synthetic fruit and honey flavoring for beverages, ice cream, ices, candy, and baked goods. *See* Cyclohexaneacetic Acid for toxicity. ASP

**CYCLOHEXANEACETIC ACID** • A synthetic butter and fruit flavoring for beverages, ice cream, ices, candy, and baked goods. Cyclohexane in high concentrations may act as a narcotic and skin irritant. ASP

**CYCLOHEXYL ANTHRANILATE** • A synthetic apple, banana, and grape flavoring for beverages, ice cream, ices, candy, baked goods, and gelatin desserts. Some cyclohexyl compounds are irritating to the skin. ASP

**CYCLOHEXYL CINNAMATE** • A synthetic apple, apricot, peach, and prune flavoring for beverages, ice cream, ices, candy, and baked goods. Some cyclohexyl compounds are irritating to the skin. ASP

**CYCLOHEXYL FORMATE** • Formic Acid. A synthetic cherry flavoring for beverages, ice cream, ices, candy, and baked goods. Some cyclohexyl compounds are irritating to the skin. ASP

**CYCLOHEXYL ISOVALERATE** • A synthetic strawberry and apple flavoring for beverages, ice cream, ices, candy, and baked goods. Some cyclohexyl compounds are irritating to the skin. ASP

**CYCLOHEXYL PROPIONATE** • A synthetic fruit flavoring for beverages, ice cream, ices, candy, and baked goods. Some cyclohexyl compounds are irritating to the skin. ASP

**CYCLOPENADECANOLIDE** • *See* Pentadecalactone.

**CYCLOIONONE** • Flavoring. *See* Ionone. EAF

**CYCLOPENTANETHIOL** • Flavoring additive. FAO/WHO says there is no safety concern. ASP

**CYCLOPENTANONE** • Colorless liquid with a peppermint odor. Used as a flavoring. EAF

**CYFLUTHRIN** • An insecticide used on cattle, goats, hogs, and sheep. FDA residues in meat are 0.05 ppm. Residues in milk 0.1 ppm.

**CYHEXATIN** • An insecticide used in animal feed. FDA residue in apple pomace and citrus pulp is 8 ppm.

*o***-CYMEN-3-OL** • *See p*-Cymene.

*p***-CYMENE** • A synthetic flavoring, a volatile hydrocarbon solvent that occurs naturally in star anise, coriander, cumin, mace oil, oil of mandarin, and origanum oil. Used in fragrances, also in citrus and spice flavorings for beverages, ice cream, candies, and baked goods. Its ingestion pure may cause a burning sensation in the mouth, nausea, salivation, headache, giddiness, vertigo, confusion, and coma. Contact with the pure liquid may cause blisters of the skin and inflammation of mucous membranes. ASP

**CYMOL** • *See p*-Cymene.

**CYMOPHENOL** • *See* Carvacrol.

**CYNARON** • *See* Acimeton.

**CYROMAZINE** • A pesticide used in poultry feed. The FDA tolerance residue in fat, meat, and meat by-products of poultry are 0.05 ppm; as residue in eggs, 0.25 ppm.

**CYSTEINE** • L-Form. An essential amino acid *(see)*, it is derived from hair and used in hair products and creams. Soluble in water, it is used in bakery products as a nutrient. It has been used to promote wound healing. GRAS. ASP

**CYSTINE** • A nonessential amino acid *(see)* found in urine and in horsehair. Colorless, practically odorless, white crystals, it is used as a nutrient supplement and in emollients. May have reproductive effects. GRAS. ASP

# D

**DAIDAI PEEL OIL** • Japanese Bitter Orange Oil. The essential oil derived from the dried peel of immature fruit, The normal types of sour orange are usually too sour to be enjoyed out-of-hand. In Mexico, however, sour oranges are cut in half, salted, coated with a paste of hot chili peppers, and eaten. The greatest use of sour oranges as food is in the form of marmalade and for this purpose they have no equal. The fruits are largely exported to England and Scotland for making marmalade. Sour oranges are used primarily for marmalade in South Africa. The juice is valued for ade and as a flavoring on fish and, in Spain, on meat during cooking. In Yucatán, it is employed like vinegar. In Egypt and elsewhere, it has been fermented to make wine. EAF

**2,4-D. (2,4-DICHLOROPHENOXY) ACETIC ACID** • Prepared from phenol and chloroacetic acid, it is an herbicide that belongs to the same class as dioxin *(see)* and is widely used by home gardeners and farmers. The FDA permits it in milled fractions (except flour) derived from barley, oats, rye, and wheat to be ingested as food or converted into food or feed as a residue. FDA tolerances for residues are 2 ppm in milled fractions, 1 ppm in potable water in western United States, and 5 ppm in processed feeds using sugarcane bagasse or molasses. 2,4-D does not cause acute toxicity, but its long-term effects are a matter of controversy and it has been linked to cancer. An excess of non-Hodgkin's lymphoma among farmers has been strongly associated with its use. It does cause eye irritation and gastrointestinal upsets.

**DAILY VALUE (DV)** • Substituted for the percentage of U.S. Recommended Dietary Allowances *(see)*. It is a guideline based on the daily needs of the general population. The percentages are supposed to help you compare the nutrients in a particular food with dietary recommendations that help reduce risk for some chronic diseases.

**DAIRY-LO** • A fat replacer containing whey protein concentrate *(see)*. It can be used in other foods including reduced-fat versions of butter, sour cream, cheese, yogurt, salad dressing, margarine, mayonnaise, and baked goods, coffee creamers, soups, and sauces. GRAS

**DALAPON** • 2,2-Dichloropropanoic Acid. Used as an herbicide in citrus pulp for cattle feed. FDA tolerance is 20 ppm.

**DAMAR** • Dammar. *Shorea dipterocarpaceae.* Damar is a Malay word meaning resin or torch made from resin. It is still applied as a collective term to a great variety of hard resins. Damars of international commerce come from the dipterocarp forests of Southeast Asia, mainly from Indonesia. Damar from the sal tree is produced in India. Production is mainly by tapping living trees, although some is still collected from the ground in fossilized form. It has a bitter taste. A little is used in foods as a clouding or glazing additive. Also used for preserving animal and vegetable specimens for science laboratories. May cause allergic contact dermatitis. EAF

*a*-**DAMASCONE** • A fragrance ingredient. ASP. EAF

*d*-**DAMASCONE** • An aroma chemical.

**DAMIANA LEAVES** • The dried leaves of a California and Texas plant used as a flavoring. Formerly used as a tonic and aphrodisiac. Now used as a flavoring. There is reported use of the chemical; it has not yet been assigned for toxicology literature.

**DAMINOZIDE** • Alar. Butanedioic Acid Mono (2,2-dimethyl hydrazide). An apple growth regulator was a particular focus of alarm in 1988–89 when its residues were reported to be hazardous to children. FDA residue tolerances were 10 ppm in dried tomato pomace, 90 ppm as residues in peanut meal (both for animal feed), 0.2 ppm in fat, meat, or meat by-products of cattle, goats, hogs, poultry, and sheep, 0.02 ppm as residues in milk, 0.2 ppm as residues in eggs, 20 ppm as residues in apples, and 30 ppm as residues in cherries, nectarines, and peaches. Probable human carcinogen. Causes multiple tumors in animals. Diaminozide was removed from the market in 1989 and is now permitted for use only on flowerbeds. EAF

**DAMMAR** • See Damar.

**DANDELION LEAF and ROOT** • Lion's Tooth. Obtained from *Taraxacum* plants that grow abundantly in the United States. The Indians used the common dandelion weed, eaten as a salad green, for heartburn. Rich in vitamins A and C, it is also used as a flavoring. Health practioners today maintain it is a gentle diuretic that does not deplete the body of potassium. Dandelion coffee is made from the dried roots of the plant. The root extract is used in bitters, butter, caramel, floral, fruit, root beer, and vanilla flavorings for beverages, ice cream, ices, candy, and baked goods. The fluid extract is used in butter, caramel, fruit, maple, and vanilla flavorings for beverages, ice cream, ices, candy, and baked goods. GRAS. ASP

**DAUCUS CAROTA** • *See* Carrot Oil.

**DAVANA OIL** • *Artemesia pallens.* A plant extract used in fruit flavoring for beverages, ice cream, ices, candy, baked goods, and chewing gum. There is reported use of the chemical; it has not yet been assigned for toxicology literature. EAF

**2-TRANS-4-DECADIENAL** • An aldehyde *(see)* with the odor reminiscent of chicken fat. ASP

**DDE** • Dichlorodiphenyldichlorethylene. It is a degradation product of DDT found as an impurity in DDT residues. It is believed to be an estrogen disrupter and is being studied by an EPA expert committee.

**DDM** • Dialkyl Dihexadecyl Malonate. A fat-based substance that is not absorbed into the body and can be used for frying and baking. It is not yet on the market as of this writing.

**DDVP** • *See* Dichlorvos.

*o*-**DECALACTONE** • A synthetic flavoring additive. Occurs naturally in butter, cream, and milk. Colorless with a fruity odor. Used in coconut and fruit flavorings for beverages, ice cream, ices, candy, baked goods, oleomargarine (10 ppm), and toppings. ASP

*γ*-**DECALACTONE** • A synthetic flavoring additive, colorless, with a fruity odor, used in citrus, orange, coconut, and fruit flavorings for beverages, ice cream, ices, candy, baked goods, and gelatin desserts. ASP

**DECANAL** • A synthetic flavoring additive. Occurs naturally in sweet orange peel, sweet mandarin oil, grapefruit oil, orris, and coriander. Colorless to light yellow, with a definite fatlike odor that becomes florallike when diluted. Used in berry, citrus, lemon, orange, fruit, and honey flavorings for beverages, ice cream, ices, candy, baked goods, chewing gum, and gelatin desserts. Moderately toxic by ingestion. A severe skin irritant. GRAS. ASP

**DECANAL DIMETHYL ACETAL** • A synthetic flavoring additive. Occurs naturally in anise, butter acid, oil of lemon, and oil of lime. Used in butter, coconut, fruit, liquor, whiskey, and cheese flavorings for beverages, ice cream, ices, candy, baked goods, chewing gum, and gelatin desserts. GRAS. ASP

**DECANOIC ACID** • A synthetic flavoring additive that occurs naturally in anise, butter acids, oil of lemon, and oil of lime and is used to flavor butter, coconut, fruit, liquor, and cheese flavorings for beverages, ice cream, ices, candy, baked goods, chewing gum, gelatin desserts, puddings, and shortenings. Also used for coating fruits and vegetables and in defoaming additives and fatty acids. Poisonous by intravenous route. A skin irritant. May be mutagenic. ASP

**1-DECANOL** • A synthetic fatty acid flavoring additive. Occurs naturally in orange and ambrette seed. Used in butter, lemon, orange, coconut, and fruit flavorings for beverages, ice cream, ices, candy, baked goods, and chewing gum. ASP

**DECANYL ACETATE** • *See* Decyl Acetate.

**2-DECENAL** • A synthetic fruit flavoring for beverages, ice cream, ices, candy, and baked goods. Moderately toxic by skin contact and mildly toxic by ingestion. A severe skin irritant. ASP

**DECENALDEHYDE** • *See* 2-Decenal.

**CIS-4-DECENYL ACETATE** • Synthetic flavoring in baked goods, beverages, chewing gum, fish products, granulated sugar, and gravies.

**DECOQUINATE** • Decox. An animal antifungal drug used in beef, chicken, and goat. FDA residues are 2 ppm in uncooked edible tissues other than muscle and 1 ppm in skeletal muscle of chickens, cattle, and goats.

**DECYL ACETATE** • A synthetic berry, orange, apple, peach, plum, and honey flavoring additive for beverages, ice cream, ices, candy, baked goods, and chewing gum. ASP

**DECYL ALCOHOL** • A synthetic fatty acid. An intermediate *(see)* for surface-active additives, an antifoam additive, and a fixative in perfumes. Occurs naturally in sweet orange and ambrette seed. Derived commercially from liquid paraffin wax *(see)*. Colorless to light yellow liquid. Used also for synthetic lubricants and as a synthetic fruit flavoring. Moderately toxic by skin contact. Mildly toxic by ingestion, inhalation, and possibly other routes. Has caused tumors in animals. A severe human skin and eye irritant.

**DECYL BENZENE SODIUM SULEONATE** • Defoaming additive and dispersing aid used on fresh citrus fruit. Poison by intravenous route. Moderately toxic by ingestion. A severe eye irritant.

**DECYL BUTYRATE** • A synthetic citrus and fruit flavoring additive for beverages, ice cream, ices, candy, and baked goods. ASP

**DECYL PROPIONATE** • A synthetic citrus and fruit flavoring additive for beverages, ice cream, ices, candy, and baked goods. NIL

**DECYLIC ACID** • *See* Decanoic Acid.

**DECYLIC ALCOHOL** • *See* 1-Decanol.

**DEER'S TONGUE** • Liatris wild vanilla. Vanilla plant. The extract of *Trilisa odoratissima* found from Virginia to Florida and Louisiana. Contains the volatile oil coumarin *(see)*. Used in perfumery and to make tobacco smell better. Once was on the GRAS list but removed because of coumarin. EAF

**DEFATTED** • Meaning the fat has been partly or totally removed from a product. If partly removed there is no minimum percentage set by the FDA.

**DEFATTED COTTONSEED OIL** • From cottonseed flour *(see)* with the fat removed.

**DEFOAMING ADDITIVE** • Antifoamer. Foam Inhibitor. Any number of surface-active additives *(see)*, such as liquid glycerides *(see)*, which are used to control the amount of foam produced in the processing of baked goods, coffee, whiteners, candies, milk products, jams, jellies, and fruit juices. They remove the head from processed drinks, such as orange and pineapple juice. Among the defoamers used are dimethylpolysiloxane, polyoxyethylene (40) monostearate, polysorbate 60, propylene glycol alginate, silicon dioxide, sorbitan monostearate, aluminum stearate, butyl stearate, fatty acids, hydroxylated lecithin, isopropyl alcohol, magnesium stearate, mineral oil, petrolatum, petroleum waxes, polyethylene glycol, polysorbate 80, potassium stearate, hydrogenated tallow alcohol, sodium polyacrylate, synthetic petroleum wax, oleic acid from tall oil and fatty acids.

**DEHA** • *See* Diethylhexyl Adipate

**DEHYDRATED** • With the water removed.

**DEHYDRATED BEETS** • Used for coloring and flavoring.

**DEHYDROACETIC ACID** • DHA. Sodium Dehydroacetate. A weak acid that forms a white, odorless powder with an acrid taste. Used as a preservative in cut or peeled squash. Used as an antienzyme additive in toothpaste to prevent tooth decay and as a preservative for shampoos. Also used as a fungi and bacteria-destroying additive in cosmetics. The presence of organic matter decreases its effectiveness. Not irritating or allergy causing, but it is a kidney-blocking additive and can cause impaired kidney function. Large doses can cause vomiting, imbalance, and convulsions. ASP

**DEHYDRODIHYDROIONOL** • A flavoring from ionone (see). ASP

**DEHYDRODIHYDROIONONE** • A flavoring from ionone. ASP

**DEHYDROMENTHOFUROLACTONE** • Flavoring used in chewing gum and cigarettes. GRAS. NUL

**DELANEY AMENDMENT** • Written by Congressman James Delaney, the amendment was part of the 1958 law requested by the Food and Drug Administration. The law stated that food and chemical manufacturers had to test additives before they were put on the market and the results had to be submitted to the FDA. Delaney's amendment specifically states that no additive may be permitted in any amount if tests show that it produces cancer when fed to man or animals or by other appropriate tests. Ever since it was enacted, the food and chemical industries have tried to get it repealed. Efforts have been made to substitute a negligible-risk standard to processed food. Up until 1996, the EPA observed different safety standards for raw and processed foods. For the latter, it used the zero-risk standard established by the Delaney amendment. That standard, however, had proved to be impractical and even counterproductive, according to the EPA and manufacturers. It prohibited foods from carrying minute traces of carcinogenic compounds, while exempting many toxic chemicals that were registered before the amendment was enacted. As a result, regulators were forced to allow the use of toxic chemicals while barring safer alternatives. Congress repealed the Delaney amendment in the Food Quality Protection Act of 1996 for pesticides substituting the negligible-risk standard that had long been used to set tolerances for raw foods. This standard allows residues of potentially carcinogenic pesticides as long as there is a "reasonable certainty of no harm" to consumers. In practice, regulators will approve a pesticide application only if it will cause no more than one additional cancer case per million people who consume it over a lifetime. Congress has held hearings to examine the pros and cons of liberalizing the Delaney amendment. At this writing, debates on the issue were in progress. Some coal-tar colors, nitrites, and nitrates that are considered cancer-causing additives are permitted in foods.

**DELAYED HYPERSENSITIVITY** • Manifested primarily as contact dermatitis due to chemicals such as neomycin sulfate or to parabens (see both), a common preservative in food products. Certain multiple allergic reactions to chemicals added to food, directly or indirectly, may also cause delayed hypersensitivity, especially the antibiotics.

**DELTAMETHRIN** • A pesticide that contains cyanide used for tomato products. The FDA permits a residue of 1 ppm.

**DELTA-TOCOPHEROL** • *See* Tocopherol. E

**DEMETON-S** • An organophosphate *(see)* pesticide used in animal feed. FDA residue limits of 5 ppm in dehydrated sugar beet pulp when used for animal feed. Poison by ingestion and other routes.

**DEMULCENT** • A soothing, usually thick, oily or creamy substance used to relieve pain in inflamed or irritated mucous surfaces. The gum acacia, for instance, is used as a demulcent.

**DENATURANT** • A substance that changes another substance's natural qualities or characteristics. For example, denatonium benzoate is added to the alcoholic content in cosmetics to make it undrinkable.

**DERMATITIS** • Inflammation of the skin.

**DESOXYCHOLIC ACID** • An emulsifying additive, white, crystalline, powdered, almost insoluble in water. Used in dried egg whites up to 0.1 percent. The final report to the FDA of the Select Committee on GRAS Substances stated in 1980 that it should continue its GRAS status with no limitations other than good manufacturing practices. Moderately toxic by ingestion. Has caused tumors in animals. NUL

**DEXTRAN** • A term applied to polysaccharides produced by bacteria growing on sugar. Used as a foam stabilizer for beer, in soft-center confections, and as a substitute for barley malt. It has also been used as a plasma expander for emergency treatment of shock. Has caused cancer in rats. The final report to the FDA of the Select Committee on GRAS Substances stated in 1980 that there is no evidence in the available information that it is a hazard to the public when used as it is now and it should continue its GRAS status with limitations on amounts that can be added to food. ASP

**DEXTRIN** • British Gum. Starch Gum. White or yellow powder produced from starch and used as a foam stabilizer for beer, a diluting additive for dry extracts and pills, in polishing cereals, for preparing emulsions, and in matches, fireworks, and explosives. May cause an allergic reaction. The final report to the FDA of the Select Committee on GRAS Substances stated in 1980 that it should continue its GRAS status with no limitations other than good manufacturing practices. ASP

**DEXTROSE** • The final report to the FDA of the Select Committee on GRAS Substances stated in 1980 that there is no evidence in the available information that it is a hazard to the public when used as it is now and it should continue its GRAS status with no limitations other than good manufacturing practices. *See* Corn Syrup. ASP

**DHC** • *See* Dihydrochalcones.

**DI-(BUTAN-3-ONE-YL) SULFIDE** • Used in the manufacture of flavorings.

**1,2(DI [1'-ETHOXY] ETHOXY) PROPANE** • A gas. *See* Propane.

**DI-(2-ETHYLHEXYL)ADIPATE** • Light-colored, oily liquid used as a plasticizer, usually in processing polyvinyl and other polymers.

**DI-(2-ETHYLHEXYL)PHTHALATE** • A light-colored, odorless liquid used as a plasticizer for many resins.

**DI-(2-ETHYLHEXYL)SODIUM SULFOSUCCINATE** • White, waxy solid widely used as an emulsifier and as a processing aid. Used in beverage mixes, cocoa, eggs, fruit juice drinks, gelatin desserts, hog carcasses, milk, molasses, and poultry. FDA limits from 9 ppm in finished foods to 25 ppm in molasses.

**DI-N-ALKYL (C8-C18 FROM COCONUT OIL) DIMETHYL AMMONIUM-CHLORIDE** • Pesticide. FDA tolerance 5 percent by weight.

**DIACETIN** • A mixture of the diesters *(see)* of glycerin *(see)* and acetic acid *(see),* used as a plasticizer, softening additive, or as a solvent for cellulose derivatives, resins, and shellacs.

**DIACETYL** • Occurs naturally in cheese, cocoa, pears, coffee, raspberries, strawberries, and cooked chicken, but is usually prepared by a special fermentation of glucose. It is a yellowish green liquid. Also used as a carrier of aroma of butter, vinegar, and coffee. Also used in blueberry, raspberry, strawberry, butter, buttermilk, butterscotch, caramel, chocolate, coffee, fruit, cheese, cherry, liquor, rum, wine, nut, almond, spice, ginger ale, vanilla, and cream soda flavorings for beverages, ice cream, ices, candy, baked goods, gelatin desserts, chewing gum, and shortening. Cleared by U.S. Department of Agriculture (Meat Inspection Division) to flavor oleomargarine in "amount sufficient for the purpose." Diacetyl compounds have been associated with cancer when ingested by experimental animals. GRAS. ASP

**DIACETYL TARTARIC OF MONOGLYCERIDES and DIGLYCERIDES** • An emulsifying additive used to improve volume and uniformity in bakery products up to 20 percent by weight of the combination such as preparation and the shortening. The final report to the FDA of the Select Committee on GRAS Substances stated in 1980 that it should continue its GRAS status with no limitations other than good manufacturing practices.

**DIALKANOLAMIDE** • A combination of methyl laurate and diethanolamine *(see both)* used to wash sugar beets prior to slicing operation. *See* Diethanolamine for potential cancer hazard.

**DIALIFOR** • Torak. An insecticide used in animal feed, apple pomace, dried citrus pulp, dried grape pomace, raisin waste, and raisins. FDA allows tolerances of up to 2 ppm in raisins, 40 ppm in dried apple pomace, 20 ppm in dried grape pomace, 115 ppm in dried citrus pulp, and 10 ppm in raisin waste when used for animal feed. Poison by ingestion and skin contact. Had adverse reproductive effects in experimental animals.

**DIALLYL POLYSULFIDES** • Used in the manufacture of flavors. ASP

**DIALLYL TRISULFIDES** • Used in the manufacture of flavors. NIL

**2,4-DIAMINO-5 (6-METHYLVERATRYL) PYRIMIDINE** • A feed additive. *See* Ormetoprim.

**DIAMMONIUM PHOSPHATE** • Used in animal feed as a source of nonprotein nitrogen and phosphorous for ruminants.

**DIAMYL KETONE** • Solvent. Toxic. EAF

**1,4-DIANILINOANTHRAQUINONE** • *See* Coal Tar.

**DIASMOL** • *See* 1,3-Nonanediol Acetate (mixed esters).

**DIATASE** • A mixture of enzymes from malt. It converts at least fifty times its weight of potato starch into sugars in thirty minutes. Used to convert starch into sugar. In 1992 diastase and diastase malt aluminum hydroxide were not shown to be safe and effective as claimed in OTC digestive-aid products. EAF

**DIATOMACEOUS EARTH** • Kieselguhr. A porous and relatively pure form of silica formed from fossil remains of diatoms—one-celled algae with shells. Inert when ingested. Used in dentrifices, as a clarifying additive, and as an absorbent for liquids because it can absorb about four times its weight in water. Used as a buffer for acid-proofing food packaging and as an insecticide. Also used in nail polishes, face powders, as a clarifying additive, and as an absorbent for liquids. The dust can cause lung damage after long exposure to high concentrations. Not recommended for use on teeth or skin because of its abrasiveness. The final report to the FDA of the Select Committee on GRAS Substances stated in 1980 that it should continue its GRAS status with no limitations other than good manufacturing practices. NIL

**DIAZIDE** • Alfa-Tox. Liquid with a faint esterlike odor widely used as an insecticide in animal feed. FDA permits 1 percent to 2 percent in animal feed. Poison by ingestion, skin contact, and other routes, except for inhalation during which it is mildly toxic. Human systemic effects by ingestion include changes in movement, muscle weakness, and sweating. Caused birth defects in animals. It is a severe skin and eye irritant in humans and emits toxic fumes when heated.

**DIAZINON** • A pesticide used in feed-handling establishments for crack and spot treatment in building floors and walls.

**DIAZO-** • A compound containing two nitrogen atoms such as diazolidinyl urea *(see)*, one of the newer preservatives, or diazepam, a popular muscle relaxant.

**DIAZOLIDINYL UREA** • Oxymethurea. 1,3-Bis(hydroxymethyl) Urea. Crystals from alcohol, soluble in water. May release formaldehyde *(see)*.

**DIBENZYL ETHER** • A synthetic fruit and spice flavoring additive for beverages, ice cream, ices, candy, baked goods, and chewing gum. The Flavor and Extract Manufacturers Association evaluated the safety of this additive. High-dose female rats had increased liver weights. A no-effect level was achieved at 196 mg/kg/day. In a 60 kg human (about 132 pounds), this would be equivalent to approximately 11.8 grams a day. ASP

**a-DIBROMO-a-CYANOACETAMIDE** • DBNPA. An antimicrobial additive used in beets and sugarcane. FDA limits are up to 10 ppm and not less than 2 ppm based on weight of raw sugarcane or raw beets. Poison by ingestion. A severe skin and eye irritant. Cyanide and its compounds are on the Community Right-To-Know List.

**2,2-DIBROMO-3-NITRILOPROPIONAMIDE** • Preservative used alone for control of microorganisms in raw sugarcane and beet sugar mills (2–10 ppm). ASP

**4,4-DIBUTYL-γ-BUTYROLACTONE** • A synthetic butter, coconut, and nut flavoring additive for ice cream, ices, candy, and baked goods. ASP

**DIBUTYL SEBACATE** • Sebacic Acid. A synthetic fruit flavoring usually obtained from castor oil and used for beverages, ice cream, and baked goods. Also used for sealing food packages. Used in fruit-fragrance cosmetics. Mildly toxic by ingestion. Oral doses in rats cause reproductive effects. ASP

**DIBUTYL SULFIDE** • *See* Butyl Sulfide.

**DI-*n*-BUTYL PHTHALATE** • An insect repellent. Used for the impregnation of clothing. May cause estrogenlike effects in humans. One of the chemicals being studied by the EPA's expert committee on environmental estrogen disrupters.

**DIBUTYLENE TETRAFURFURAL** • Derived from bran, rice hulls, or corncobs, it is used in the manufacture of medicinals and as a solvent and flavoring in cosmetics and food. Toxic when absorbed by the skin. Irritating to the eye.

**DICALCIUM PHOSPHATE** • A nutrient. *See* Calcium.

**DICAMBA** • An herbicide in or on sugarcane molasses.

**DICHLORODIFLUOROMETHANE** • Colorless, odorless gas used to freeze foods by direct contact and for chilling cocktail glasses. Narcotic in high doses. In EPA Genetic Toxicology Program *(see)*. ASP

**3,4-DICHLORO-2,6-DIMETHYL-4-PYRIDINOL** • *See* Clopidol.

**DICHLOROETHANE** • Colorless, clear liquid with a pleasant odor and sweet taste. A human poison by ingestion. The FAO/WHO Committee found it causes birth defects and that it causes cancer in mice and rats when administered orally. The committee expressed the opinion that 1,2-dichloroethane should not be used in food. *See* Ethylene Dichloride.

**DICHLOROMETHANE** • *See* Methylene Chloride.

**DICHLOROPHENOXYACETIC ACID** • A widely used herbicide on milled barley, oats, rye, wheat (except their milled flour fractions), and sugarcane. FDA residue limits are up to 5 ppm in sugarcane molasses, 2 ppm in milled fractions (except flour) in barley, oats, and wheat, and 0.1 ppm in potable water. Poison by ingestion and other routes. Moderately toxic by skin contact. A suspected human cancer-causing additive. Human systemic effects by ingestion include sleepiness, convulsions, coma, and nausea or vomiting. Can cause liver and kidney injury. A skin and severe eye irritant. Human mutagenic data. Experimental reproductive effects. When heated to decomposition it emits toxic fumes.

**3-(3,4-DICHLOROPHENYL)-1,1-DIMETHYL UREA** • Manner. Telvar Diuron Weed Killer. Vonduron. A widely used herbicide employed on animal feed. FDA limitation of 4 ppm in dried citrus pulp when used for livestock feed. In EPA Genetic Toxicology Program *(see)*. Chlorophenol compounds are on the Community Right-To-Know List *(see)*. Caused tumors and birth defects in laboratory animals.

***a,a*-DICHLOROPRIONIC ACID, SODIUM SALT** • *See* Dichloropropionic Acid.

**DICHLOROPROPIONANILIDE** • Propanil. Supernox. An herbicide used on animal feed, rice, rice bran, rice hulls, and rice polishings. FDA limitations are 10 ppm in rice bran, rice hulls, and rice polishings when used for animal feed. In EPA Genetic Toxicology Program *(see)*. Poison by ingestion. Mildly toxic by skin contact.

**DICHLOROPROPIONIC ACID** • Basinex. Crisapon. Revenge. Unipon. An herbicide used in animal feed, citrus pulp, and potable water. FDA residue allowances are 0.2 ppm in potable water and 20 ppm in citrus pulp used as animal feed. Moderately toxic by ingestion. Corrosive. A skin irritant.

**DICHLORVOS** • Dimethyl Dichlorovinyl Phosphate. Apavap. Chlbrvinphos. DDVF. VPON. 2,2-Dichlorovinyl. An organophosphate *(see)* insecticide with contact and vapor action. It has been widely used for control of agricultural, industrial, and domestic pests since the 1950s. It is used in pet flea collars and flea sprays. DDVP is available in oil solutions, emulsifiable concentration, and aerosol formulations. Its topical (skin) application has been approved for beef and dairy cattle, goats, sheep, swine, and chickens to control fleas, flies, and mites. It is also used in tomato greenhouses and applied to mushrooms, lettuce, and radishes. Aerosols and strips are used domestically for control of ants, bedbugs, ticks, cockroaches, and other pests. Nerve gases used in wars include organophosphates. It is suspected of causing cancer and birth defects. Heat decomposition causes highly toxic fumes to be emitted. In the last edition of this dictionary, the EPA was moving to have the use of dichlorvos on food packaging banned because it poses "more than a negligible risk." It is in at least 350 products. As of this writing, the EPA says that currently dichlorvos is undergoing a special review "on grounds that exposure to individuals by this compound from registered uses may pose an unreasonable risk of cancer and an inadequate margin of safety for cholinesterase inhibition [central nervous system effects]. Affected persons may include the general population from consuming foods with residues of dichlorvos, applicators, agriculture workers entering treated areas, residents/occupants of treated areas, and persons exposed to pets treated with this compound. As a result of the special review, the EPA expects to issue a proposed determination to cancel its use. It may take years to get this pesticide off the market.

**3,5-DICHOLO-2,6-DIMETHYL-4-PYRIDINOL** • *See* Clopidol.

**DICYCLOHEXYL DISULFIDE** • *See* Sulfides. ASP

**DIESTER** • A compound containing two ester groupings. An ester is formed from an alcohol and an acid by eliminating water and is usually employed in fragrant liquids for artificial fruit perfumes and flavors.

**DIETARY FOOD SUPPLEMENT** • Any food product to which enough vitamins and minerals have been added to furnish more than 50 percent of the recommended daily allowance in a single serving, according to the FDA. Such foods must, of course, have ingredients identified on the label.

**DIETHANOLAMIDE CONDENSATE FROM SOYBEAN FATTY ACIDS** • Used as a surfactant *(see)*. NUL

**DIETHANOLAMINE (DEA)** • Colorless liquid or crystalline fatty acid from soybeans or coconut oils. It is used as a solvent, emulsifying additive, and detergent. Also employed in emollients for its softening properties and as a dispersing additive and humectant in other cosmetic products. It may be irritating to the skin and mucous membranes. The FDA became aware of a National Toxicology Program (NTP) study showing an association between the topical application of diethanolamine and certain DEA-related ingredients and cancer in laboratory animals. For the DBA-related ingredients, the NTP study suggests that the cancer response is linked to possible residual levels of DEA. Although DEA itself may be used in few products, DEA-related ingredients such as oleamide DEA, lauramide DEA, cocamide DEA, are widely used as emulsifiers or foaming additives, generally at levels of 1 to 5 percent. The FDA is studying the problem and is going to consider legal options at this writing. *See* Ethanolamines.

**DIETHYL ACETALDEHYDE** • Ethyl Butyraldehyde. A flavoring additive used in many foods. Moderately toxic by ingestion. A skin irritant.

**DIETHYL ACETIC ACID** • Colorless, volatile liquid with a rancid odor used as a flavoring in a variety of foods. Moderately toxic by ingestion and skin contact.

**DIETHYL ASPARTATE** • The diester of ethyl alcohol and aspartic acid *(see both)*.

**DIETHYL DICARBONATE** • Viscous liquid with a fruity odor used as a fermentation inhibitor and fungicide. Prohibited in the United States but permitted in wine in other countries. Poison by ingestion.

**DIETHYL GLUTAMATE** • *See* Glutamate.

**DIETHYL MALATE** • Malic Acid. A synthetic apple and rum flavoring additive for beverages, ice cream, ices, candy, baked goods, gelatin, and puddings. ASP

**DIETHYL MALONATE** • A synthetic berry, fruit, apple, grape, peach, and pear flavoring for beverages, ice cream, ices, candy, and baked goods. ASP

**DIETHYL METHYLPYRAZINE, 2,3 AND 3,5** • Flavorings that taste like potatoes. EAF

**DIETHYL PALMITOYL ASPARTATE** • *See* Aspartic Acid.

**DIETHYL-*o*-PHTHALATE** • Clear, colorless liquid used as a plasticizer in packaging material. Moderately toxic by ingestion. Has caused adverse effects in experimental animals.

**DIETHYL PYROCARBONATE (DEP)** • A fermentation inhibitor in still wines, beer, and orange juice added before or during bottling at a level not to exceed 200 to 500 parts per million. DEP was widely used because it supposedly did its job of preserving and then decomposed within twenty-four hours. However, instead of disappearing, it reacted with the ammonia in beverages to form urethane, according to University of Stockholm researchers. They said that DEP caused urethane concentration of 0.1 to 0.2 milligrams per liter in orange juice and approximately 1 milligram per liter in white wine and beer. Since 1943 urethane has been identified as a cancer-causing additive. The FDA had not required listing of DEP on the label and therefore did not know how many beverages were actually treated with this additive. The FDA banned the use of DEP in 1976.

**DIETHYL SEBACATE** • Sebacic Acid. A synthetic butter, coconut, apple, melon, peach, and nut flavoring for beverages, ice cream, ices, candy, baked goods, chewing gum, and gelatin desserts. Mildly toxic by ingestion. A skin irritant. ASP

**DIETHYL SUCCINATE** • A synthetic raspberry, butter, orange, and grape flavoring for beverages, ice cream, ices, candy, and baked goods. ASP

**DIETHYL SULFIDE** • Synthetic flavoring with a garliclike odor. EAF

**DIETHYL TARTRATE** • *See* Tartaric Acid. ASP

**DIETHYL TRISULFIDE** • A flavoring determined GRAS by the Expert Panel of the Flavor and Extract Manufacturers Association.

**3,5-DIETHYL 1,2,4-TRITHIOLANE, cis and trans** • A flavoring determined GRAS by the Expert Panel of the Flavor and Extract Manufacturers Association.

**DIETHYLHEXYL ADIPATE (DEHA)** • Has received a lot of media attention in recent years. DEHA is a plasticizer, a substance added to some plastics to make them flexible. DEHA exposure may occur when eating certain foods wrapped in plastics, especially fatty foods such as meat and cheese. But the levels are very low. The levels of the plasticizer that might be consumed as a result of plastic film use are well below the levels showing no toxic effect in animal studies, according to the FDA.

**DIETHYLAMINOETHANOL** • Colorless, water-absorbing liquid with the properties of ammonia and alcohol. Toxic by ingestion. Used to obtain fatty acid derivatives, as an emulsifying additive, and as a curing additive for resin. ASP

**0,0-DIETHYL S-2 (ETHYTHIO)ETHYL PHOSPHORODITHIOATE(DI-SYSTON)** • A pesticide applied to crops. FDA tolerance is 5 ppm alone or with demeton-S *(see)* in dehydrated sugar beet pulp or pineapple bran for livestock feed.

**DIETHYLENE GLYCOL DISTEARATE** • White, waxlike solid with a faint fatty odor. Used as an emulsifying additive for oils, solvents, and waxes, a lubricating additive for paper and cardboard and as a thickening agent.

**DIETHYLENETRIAMINE** • Yellow liquid with an ammonia odor, strongly alkaline. Used as a solvent. NUL

**DIETHYLPYRAZINE** • Derived from ethyl bromide or chloride, it is used as a corrosion inhibitor and insecticide.

**DIETHYLSTILBESTEROL (DES)** • Stilbestrol. A synthetic estrogen fed to cattle and poultry to fatten them. A proven carcinogen, hormonal in nature, according to the FDA, which has given top priority to the study of the safety of DES. The FDA stipulates a zero tolerance for the compound after a proper withdrawal period. In 1971, three Harvard scientists linked DES to a rare form of vaginal cancer in the daughters of women who had taken DES during pregnancy. An estimated 100,000 to 150,000 head of cattle containing residues of the hormone are apparently getting to market. The European Union has forbidden the use of DES in cattle.

**2,5-DIETHYLTETRAHYDROFURAN** • A solvent used in processing resins. ASP

**DIFLUBENZURON** • An insecticide used on soybean crops. It is limited by the FDA to 0.5 ppm as a residue on soybean hulls for use in animal feeds.

**DIFURURYL ETHER** • Used in the manufacture of food additives.

**DIGLYCERIDES** • Emulsifiers. *See* Glycerides.

**DIHYDROANETHOLE** • *See p*-Propyl Anisole.

**DIHYDROCARVEOL** • A synthetic flavoring additive occurring naturally in black pepper. Colorless oily liquid with a spearmint odor, it is used in liquor, mint, spice, and caraway flavorings for beverages, ice cream, ices, candy, baked goods, and alcoholic beverages. A moderate skin and eye irritant. ASP

**DIHYDROCARVONE** • Colorless liquid with a spearmintlike odor used as a flavoring additive in various foods. Moderately toxic when injected under the skin. NIL

**DIHYDROCARVYL ACETATE** • Occurs in celery and mint and is used as a flavoring. *See* Dihydrocarvone. ASP

**DIHYDROCHALCONES (DHC)** • A new class of intensely sweet compounds—about fifteen hundred times sweeter than sugar—obtained by a simple chemical modification of naturally occurring bioflavonoids *(see)*. Hydrogenation *(see)* of naringin and neohesperidin (the predominant bitter constituents in grapefruit and Seville orange rind) provides the intensely sweet dihydrochalcones. DHCs are seemingly safe. There have not been any reports, thus far, of side effects in either multigenerational feeding studies or in long-term feeding trials. The disadvantage is that they cannot be easily reproduced in the laboratory so supplies are dependent upon natural sources. A more serious problem is that the intense, pleasant sweetness of DHCs is slow in onset, with considerable lingering taste, which renders them unsuitable for many food uses. Approval to use DHCs in toothpaste and chewing gum is pending. Food scientists are now trying to find derivatives and analogs of DHCs to overcome the slow onset and lingering factor in the natural compounds.

**DIHYDROCHOLESTEROL** • *See* Cholesterol.

**DIHYDROCHOLESTERYL OCTYLDECANOATE** • *See* Cholesterol and Octadecanoic Acid.

**DIHYDROCOUMARIN** • A synthetic flavoring additive occurring naturally in tonka bean, oil of lavender, and sweet clovers. Used in butter, caramel, coconut, floral, fruit, cherry, liquor, rum, nut, root beer, spice, cinnamon, vanilla, cream soda, and tonka bean flavorings for beverages, ice cream, ices, candy, baked goods, chewing gum, gelatin desserts, and puddings. Prolonged feeding has revealed a possible trend toward liver injury. ASP

**6,7-DIHYDRO-2,3-DIMETHYL-5H-CYCLOPENTAPYRAZINE** • Flavoring additive declared GRAS by FEMA *(see)*. EAF

**4,5-DIHYDRO-2,5-DIMETHYL-4-OXO-3-FURANYL BUTYRATE** • Flavoring declared GRAS by FEMA *(see)*. *See also* Butanoic Acid. EAF

**DIHYDRO-BETA-IONOL** • Synthetic flavoring. *See* Ionone. ASP

**DIHYDRO-ALPHA-IONONE** • Flavoring. *See* Ionone. ASP

**DIHYDRO-BETA-IONONE** • Flavoring. *See* ionone. ASP

**3,6-DIHYDRO-4-METHYL-2(2-METHYLPROPEN-1-YL)-2H-PYRAN** • Flavoring. EAF

**5,7-DIHYDRO-2-METHYLTHIENO(3,4-D)PYRIMIDINE** • Flavoring. ASP

**DIHYDRONOOTKATONE** • Synthetic, fruity, citruslike aroma of grapefruit used in flavors and fragrances. A derivative is used to repel termites.

**4,5-DIHYDRO-3(2H)THIOPHENONE** • Synthetic flavoring. ASP

**DIHYDRO-2,4,6-TRIMETHYL-4H-1,3,5-DITHIAZINE** • Synthetic flavoring. EAF

**DIHYDRO-2,4,6-TRIS(2-METHYLPROPYL)-4H-1,3,5-DITHIAZINE** • Synthetic flavoring. EAF

**DIHYDROFARNESOL** • A flavoring determined GRAS by the Expert Panel of the Flavor and Extract Manufacturers Association.

**DIHYDROMINTLACTONE** • A flavoring determined GRAS by the Expert Panel of the Flavor and Extract Manufacturers Association.

**5,6-DIHYDROL-2-(2,6-XYLID|NO)-4H1, 3-THIAZINE** • Bay. Xylazine. An animal drug used in meat. Poison by ingestion.

**5,7-DIHYDRO-2-METHYLTHIENO(3,4-D)PYRIMIDINE** • Derived from organic matter used in the manufacture of food additives.

**2,3-DIHYDRO-3-OXO-BENZISOSULFONAZOLE** • *See* Saccharin.

**1,2-DIHYDROPYRIDAZINE-3,6-DIONE** • A pesticide used on potato chips. FDA residue tolerance is 160 ppm. Moderately toxic by ingestion. Can cause chronic liver damage and acute central nervous system effects. Being studied as a possible cancer-causing additive.

**DIHYDROSTREPTOMYCIN** • An antibiotic used in beef and milk. FDA tolerance is zero in uncooked edible tissues of calves and in milk. May cause birth defects in humans. May be a mutagen.

**DIHYDROXYACETONE** • A flavoring determined GRAS by the Expert Panel of the Flavor and Extract Manufacturers Association. *See* Acetone.

**DIHYDROXYACETOPHENONE** • Light tan crystals that absorb ultraviolet light. It is used in plastics, dyes, fungicides, and plant-growth promoters. NIL

**2,4-DIHYDROXYBENZOIC ACID** • Intermediate in food processing derived from many plants including chamomile and buckwheat. *See* Benzoic Acid. EAF

**2,5-DIHYDROXY-1,4-DITHIANE** • A flavoring imported mostly from Asia. Has not been assigned for toxicology as yet.

**DIIODOSALYCYLIC ACID** • A dietary supplement for animals. *See* Salicylic Acid. GRAS

**DIISOBUTYL ADIPATE** • Diba. Isobutyl Adipate. A plasticizer used in packaging materials. Mildly toxic by ingestion.

**DIISOBUTYL KETONE** • Colorless liquid with mild odor used as a solvent and in coating compositions. ASP

**DIISOPROPANOLAMINE (DIPA)** • White crystalline solid that is used as an emulsifying additive for polishes, textile specialties, leather compounds, insecticides, cutting oils, and water paints. *See* Propyl Alcohol.

**DIISOPROPYL DISULFIDE** • Flavoring. FAO/WHO says it has no safety concern. EAF

**DIISOPROPYL TRISULFIDE** • Flavoring used in baked goods, beverages, condiments, frozen dairy, fruit ices, gelatins, hard candy, and gum. FEMA *(see)* says it is GRAS. EAF

**2,3-DIKETOBUTANE** • *See* Diacetyl.

**DILAURYL CITRATE** • *See* Lauryl Alcohol and Citric Acid.

**DILAURYL THIODIPROPIONATE** • An antioxidant. White crystalline flakes with a sweet odor, in general food use to extend shelf life. In fat or oil up to 0.02 percent. The final report to the FDA of the Select Committee on GRAS Substances stated in 1980 that there is no evidence in the available information that it is a hazard to the public when used as it is now and it should continue its GRAS status with no limitations other than good manufacturing practices. NIL

**DILINOLEATE** • Dimer Acid. Widely used as an emulsifier, it is derived from linoleic acid *(see).*

**DILINOLEIC ACID** • *See* Linoleic Acid.

**DILL** • *Anethum graveolens.* A natural flavoring additive from a European herb bearing a seedlike fruit. Used in sausage and spice flavorings for baked goods (4,800 ppm), meats, and pickles (8,200 ppm). Also used in medicine. Can cause sensitivity to light. The final report to the FDA of the Select Committee on GRAS Substances stated in 1980 that it should continue its GRAS status with no limitations other than good manufacturing practices. ASP

**DILL OIL** • The volatile oil obtained from the crushed, dried seeds or fruits of the herb. Slightly yellow, with a caraway odor and flavor. Used in strawberry, fruit, sausage, and dill flavorings for beverages, ice cream, ices, baked goods, gelatin desserts, chewing gum, meat, liquors, pickles, and condiments. The final report to the FDA of the Select Committee on GRAS Substances stated in 1980 that it should continue its GRAS status with no limitations other than good manufacturing practices. *See* Dill for toxicity. ASP

**DILLSEED** • Indian Dill. The volatile oil from a variety of dill herbs. Obtained by steam distillation. Light yellow, with a harsh carawaylike odor. Used in rye flavorings for baked goods, condiments, and meats. The final report to the FDA of the Select Committee on GRAS Substances stated in 1980 that it should continue its GRAS status with no limitations other than good manufacturing practices. ASP

**DILUENT** • Any component of a color additive mixture that is not of itself a color additive and has been intentionally mixed in to facilitate the uses of the mixture in coloring cosmetics or in coloring the human body, food, and drugs. The diluent may service another functional purpose in cosmetics, as, for example, emulsifying or stabilizing. Ethylcellulose is an example.

**DIMETHICONE** • *See* Dimethyl Polysiloxane.

**DIMETHIPIN** • A growth regulator in animals. The FDA permits residues of 0.02 ppm as residues in meat, meat by-products, and fat of cattle, goats, hogs, and sheep. The tolerance for residue in and on cottonseed hulls used in animal feed is 0.7 ppm.

**DIMETHOATE** • A pesticide permitted at 5 ppm in dried citrus pulp for cattle feed. The tolerance for meat, fat, and meat by-products of cattle as a residue is 0.01 ppm and 0.001 ppm in milk.

*m***-DIMETHOXYBENZENE** • Resorcinol. A synthetic fruit, nut, and vanilla flavoring for beverages, ice cream, ices, candy, and baked goods. Used on the skin as a bactericidal and fungicidal ointment. Has the same toxicity as phenol (extremely toxic), but causes more severe convulsions. ASP

**p-DIMETHOXYBENZENE** • A synthetic raspberry, fruit, nut, hazelnut, root beer, and vanilla flavoring additive for beverages, ice cream, ices, candy, and baked goods. See above for toxicity. ASP

**3,4-DIMETHOXYBENZENECARBONAL** • *See* Veratraldehyde.

**1,1-DIMETHOXYETHANE** • *See* Ethylene Glycol.

**2,6-DIMETHOXYPHENOL** • ASP *See* Phenol.

**1-([2,5-DIMETHOXYPHENYL] AZO)-2-NAPHTHOL** • A coloring used on oranges with an FDA limit of 2 ppm by weight calculated on the basis of the whole fruit. Causes cancer in animals and is under International Agency for Cancer Research review.

**S-(DIMETHOXYPHOSPHINYLOXY) n-METHYL-cis-CROTONA-MIDE** • Apadrin. Bilobran. A reddish brown solid with a mild odor widely used as an insecticide in tomato products. FDA tolerance is 2 ppm in concentrated tomato products. In the EPA Genetic Toxicology Program *(see)*. The EPA considers it extremely hazardous. It is poisonous by ingestion, inhalation, and skin contact.

**1,4-DIMETHYL-4-ACETYL-1-CYCLOHEXENE** • Prepared from acetylaldehyde and methanol *(see both)*, it is used in processing food additives. ASP

**DIMETHYLAMINE** • Gas with an ammonia odor. Derived from ammonia and methanol. Used as a solvent for the manufacture of some food additives and as a dehairing additive. Irritating. EAF

**2,4-DIMETHYLANISOLE** • Flavoring. The FAO/WHO has cited as an additive to be reevaluated. *See* Anisole. EAF

**p-ALPHA-DIMETHYLBENZYL ALCOHOL** • Flavoring. *See* Benzyl Alcohol. NIL

**a-a-DIMETHYLBENZYL ISOBUTYRATE** • Flavoring. *See* Benzyl Alcohol. ASP

**DIMETHYL BENZYL CARBINOL and CARBINYL** • Flavoring additives used in various foods. Moderately toxic by ingestion. *See* a,a-Dimethylphenethyl Alcohol.

**3,4-DIMETHYL-1,2-CYCLOPENTADIONE** • Sweet, maplelike flavoring. ASP

**3,5-DIMETHYL-1,2-CYCLOPENTADIONE** • Flavoring. ASP

**DIMETHYL DIALKYL AMMONIUM CHLORIDE** • Used as a decoloring additive in the manufacture of sugar. *See* Quaternary Ammonium Compounds.

**DIMETHYL-0-(1,2-DIBROMO-2,2-DICHLOROETHYL)PHOSPHATE** • Widely used insecticide on various foods. Poison by ingestion and inhalation. Moderately toxic by skin injection. *See* Organophosphates.

**DIMETHYL DICARBONATE** • A fungicide used in wine to inhibit yeast growth. The FDA set the tolerance of residues at 200 ppm. In ready-to-drink teas, the tolerance is 250 ppm. NEW. E

**DIMETHYL DICHLOROVINYL PHOSPHATE** • *See* Dichlorvos.

**DIMETHYL ETHER RESORCINOL** • A benzene derivative originally obtained from certain resins but now usually synthesized. *See m*-Dimethoxybenzene.

**DIMETHYL ETHERPROTOCATECHUALDEHYDE** • *See* Verataldehyde.

**2,5-DIMETHYL-3-FURANTHIOL ACETATE** • A flavoring determined GRAS by the Expert Panel of the Flavor and Extract Manufacturers Association. ASP

**2,6-DIMETHYL-5-HEPTENAL** • A synthetic fruit flavoring for ice cream, ices, candy, baked goods, gelatin desserts, and chewing gum. ASP

**3,7-DIMETHYL-7-HYDROXYOCTANAL** • *See* Hydroxycitronellal.

**DIMETHYL KETONE** • *See* Diacetyl.

**0,0-DIMETHYL METHYLCARBAMOYLMETHYL PHOSPHORODI-THIOATE** • A widely used insecticide in animal feed, citrus pulp. FDA limits are 5 ppm in dried citrus pulp when used for animal feed. Poison by ingestion, skin contact, and other routes. May cause cancer and birth defects.

**N′,N′-DIMETHYL-N-([METHYL CARBAMOYL] OXY)-1-METHYL-THIOOXA-MIMIDIC ACID** • Widely used insecticide in animal feed, pineapple bran, and pineapples. Limitations of 6 ppm in pineapple bran when used for animal feed. Poison by ingestion and inhalation. Moderately toxic by skin contact. On the EPA Extremely Hazardous Substances List.

**3,7-DIMETHYL-2,6-OCTADIENAL** • Pale yellow liquid with a strong lemon odor used as a flavoring additive in baked goods, candy, and ice cream. Mildly toxic by ingestion. A human skin irritant. *See* Citral.

**3,7-DIMETHYL-(E)-2,6-OCTADIEN-1-OL** • *See* Geraniol.

**3,7-DIMETHYL-1-OCTANOL** • A synthetic flavoring, colorless, with a sweet roselike odor. Used in floral, rose, and fruit flavorings for beverages, ice cream, ices, candy, and baked goods.

**2,6-DIMETHYL-1-OCTEN-8-OL** • *See* Rhodinol.

**2,4-DIMETHYL-2-PENTENOIC ACID** • Flavoring. *See* Pentanoic Acid. ASP

**DIMETHYL PHOSPHATE OF 3-HYDROZY-N-METHYL-CISCRO-TON-AMIDE** • A pesticide. FDA tolerance is 2 ppm in concentrated tomato products when present as a result of application of the insecticide to growing tomatoes.

**DIMETHYL POLYSILOXANE** • Dimethicone. Antifoam A. An antifoaming additive for use in processing foods in "amounts reasonably required to inhibit foaming." Used as a chewing-gum base, in molasses, soft drinks, sugar distillation, skimmed milk, wine fermentation, syrups, soups, rendered fats, and curing solutions. Not to exceed 10 ppm in nonalcoholic beverages. Zero tolerance in milk; 250 ppm in salt for cooking and in other foods, 10 ppm in foods ready for consumption. Used to combat flatulence. Very low toxicity. ASP. E

**DIMETHYL PYRAZINE** • *See* Piperazine. ASP

**2,5-DIMETHYL PYRROLE** • A colorless to yellow oily liquid that was used as a flavoring additive in various foods. GRAS. Although allowed as a food additive, there is no current reported use of the chemical, and, therefore, although toxicology information may be available, it is not being updated, according to the FDA.

**DIMETHYL RESORCINOL** • *See m*-Dimethoxybenzene.

**DIMETHYL SUCCINATE** • Succinic Acid. A synthetic fruit flavoring additive for beverages, ice cream, ices, candy, baked goods, and chewing gum. ASP

**DIMETHYL SULFATE** • Sulfuric Acid. Dimethyl Ester. Colorless, oily liquid used as a methylating additive (to add methyl) in the manufacture of cosmetic dyes, perfumes, and flavorings. Methyl salicylate *(see)* is an example. Extremely hazardous, dimethyl sulfate has delayed lethal qualities. Liquid produces severe blistering, necrosis of the skin. Sufficient skin absorption can result in serious poisoning. Vapors hurt the eyes. Ingestion can cause paralysis, coma, prostration, kidney damage, and death.

**DIMETHYL SULFIDE** • *See* Methyl Sulfide.

**2,4-DIMETHYLACETOPHENONE** • Colorless liquid with the odor of mimosa, it is used as a synthetic grape, vanilla, and cream soda flavoring additive for beverages, ice cream, ices, candy, baked goods, and liquor. It is also used in perfumery.

**2,4-DIMETHYLBENZALDEHYDE** • *See* Benzyl Acetate.

**3,4-DIMETHOXY-1-VINYLBENZENE** • *See* Benzene and Vinyl.

**2,3-DIMETHYLBENZOFURAN** • *See* Furfural and Benzene.

**DIMETHYLBENZYL ALCOHOL** • A constituent of the essential oil from *Curcuma longa* and related plants. It smells like menthol. It is used as a flavoring and scent.

*a,a*-**DIMETHYLBENZYL ISOBUTYRATE** • A synthetic fruit flavoring additive for beverages, ice cream, ices, candy, and baked goods.

**0,0-DIMETHYL(0-3METHYL-4-METHYLTHIO-M-TOLYL)PHOSPHO-ROTHIONATE** • A pesticide. FDA tolerance for residue in meat of cattle is 0.05 ppm.

**DIMETHYL-3-METHYL-4-NITROPHENYLPHOSPHOROTHIONATE** • Accothion. A widely used insecticide on wheat gluten. FDA tolerance for residue is 30 ppm in wheat gluten. In the EPA Genetic Toxicology Program and on the EPA Extremely Hazardous List *(see both)*. Poisonous by ingestion, inhalation, and other routes. Moderately toxic by skin contact. Human systemic effects upon ingestion include overactivity, diarrhea, nausea or vomiting, and shortness of breath.

**2,5-DIMETHYLTHIAZOLE** • A flavoring determined GRAS by the Expert Panel of the Flavor and Extract Manufacturers Association. *See* Thiazole. ASP

**a,a-DIMETHYLPHENYETHYL ACETATE** • Acetic Acid. A colorless liquid with a floral-fruity odor. A synthetic cherry and honey flavoring additive for beverages, ice cream, ices, candy, baked goods, and chewing gum.

**0,0-DIMETHYL-0-(3,5,6-TRICHLORO-2-PYRIDYL)PHOSPHORO-THIOATE** • *See* Chlorpyrifos.

**1,1-DIMETHYL-3-(a,a,a-TRIFLUORO-m-TOLYL)UREA** • Cottonex. Herbicide used in animal feed. FDA limit of 0.2 ppm in sugarcane when used for animal feed. In EPA Genetic Toxicology Program *(see)* and under review by the IARC *(see)*. Moderately toxic by ingestion. May be mutagenic.

**DIMETHYLGLYOXAL** • *See* Diacetyl.

**DIMETHYLKETOL** • *See* Acetoin.

**DIMETHYLOCTADECYLBENZYLAMMONIUM CHLORIDE** • Quaternol 1. Varisoft SDC. An antimicrobial additive used in beets, sugarcane, and raw sugarcane juice. FDA residue limits are 1.5–6 ppm and .05 ppm based on weight of raw sugarcane or raw beets. Moderately toxic by ingestion. A human skin irritant and severe eye irritant.

**DIMETHYLOCTANOL** • Pelargol. Colorless liquid with a sweet rose odor used as a flavoring additive in bakery products, beverages, chewing gum, confections, ice cream, and pickles. Moderately toxic by skin contact.

**a,a-DIMETHYLPHENYETHYL ALCOHOL** • A synthetic fruit flavoring additive for beverages, ice cream, ices, candy, chewing gum, jellies, gelatin desserts, and baked goods.

**a,a-DIMETHYLPHENYETHYL BUTYRATE** • Butyric Acid. A synthetic fruit flavoring additive for beverages, ice cream, ices, candy, and baked goods.

**a,a-DIMETHYLPHENYETHYL FORMATE** • Formic Acid. A synthetic spice flavoring additive for beverages, ice cream, ices, and candy.

**DIMETHYLPYRAZINE** • Flavoring additive with a nutty or potatolike taste and coffee odor used in various foods. Moderately toxic by ingestion and is an experimental mutagen. GRAS. ASP

**DIMETRIDAZOLE** • A feed additive. Not legal for animal use.

**DIMETHYL TRISULFIDE** • Isolated from soybeans, it has a strong beany odor used in flavorings. ASP

**DIMETHYL TRITHIOLANE** • Fruit flavoring. ASP

**4,5-DIMETHYL-2-ETHYL-3-THIAZOLINE** • Flavoring.

**2,5-DIMETHYL-3-FURANTHIOL** • Flavoring.

**2,6-DIMETHYL-4-HEPTANOL** • Flavoring. *See* Heptanoic Acid.

**2,6-DIMETHYL-5-HEPTENAL** • Flavoring. *See* Hepatnoic Acid.

**2,6-DIMETHYL-6-HEPTEN-1-OL** • Flavoring. *See* Heptanal.

**4,5-DIMETHYL-3-HYDROXY-2,5-DIHYDROFURAN-2-ONE** • Flavoring.

**4,5-DIMETHYL-2-ISOBUTYL-3-THIAZOLINE** • Flavoring.

**2,5-DIMETHYL-3-MERCAPTOTETRAHYDROFURAN** • Flavoring.

**2,5-DIMETHYL-4-METHOXY-3(2H)-FURANONE** • Flavoring.

**2,6-DIMETHYL-10-METHYLENE-2,6,11-DODECATRIENAL** • Flavoring.

**2,6-DIMETHYL-3-((2-METHYL-3-FURYL)THIO)-4-HEPTANONE** • Flavoring. *See* Heptanal.

**2,2-DIMETHYL-5-(1-METHYLPROPEN-1-YL) TETRAHYDROFURAN** • Flavoring. NIL

**4,8-DIMETHYL-3,7-NONADIEN-2-ONE CIS and TRANS** • New flavorings used in baked goods, beverages, chewing gum, confectionery frostings, egg products, fish products, frozen dairy, fruit ices, gelatins, gravies, hard candies, instant coffee, meat products, nut products, seasonings, soft candy, and soups. *See* Nonyl Alcohol. EAF

**2-TRANS-3,7-DIMETHYLOCTA-2,6-DIENYL 2-ETHYLBUTANOATE** • Flavoring.

**2,6-DIMETHYLOCTANAL** • Flavoring.

**3,7-DIMETHYL-1-OCTANOL** • Flavoring. *See* Octanal.

**(E)-3,7-DIMETHYL-1,5,7-OCTATRIEN-3-OL** • Flavoring. *See* Octanal.

**3,7-DIMETHYL-6-OCTENOIC ACID** • Flavoring. *See* Octanoic Acid.

**2,4-DIMETHYL-2-PENTENOIC ACID** • Flavoring. *See* Pentanoic Acid.

**ALPHA,ALPHA-DIMETHYLPHENETHYL ACETATE** • Flavoring.

**ALPHA,ALPHA-DIMETHYLPHENETHYL ALCOHOL** • Flavoring. *See* Phenethyl Alcohol

**ALPHA,ALPHA-DIMETHYLPHENETHYL BUTYRATE** • Flavoring. *See* (tri-)Butyrin. ASP

**ALPHA,ALPHA-DIMETHYLPHENETHYL FORMATE** • Flavoring. *See* Formic Acid. ASP

**2,3-DIMETHYLPYRAZINE** • See Piperidine. ASP

**2,5-DIMETHYLPYRAZINE** • *See* Piperidine. ASP

**2,6-DIMETHYLPYRAZINE** • See Piperidine. ASP

**2,6-DIMETHYLPYRIDINE** • See Piperidine. ASP

**P,ALPHA-DIMETHYLSTYRENE** • *See* Styrene. ASP

**CIS and TRANS-2-5-DIMETHYLTETRAHYDROGURAN-3-THIOL** • Synthetic flavoring used in baked goods, beverages, chewing gum, condiments, relishes, frozen dairy, fruit ices, gelatins, nut products, snack foods, soft candy, and soups. Declared GRAS by FEMA *(see)*.

**4,5-DIMETHYLTHIAZOLE** • *See* Thiazole. ASP

**2,5-DIMETHYL-3-THIOISOVALERYLFURAN** • *See* Furfuryl Alcohol. ASP

**2,6-DIMETHYLTHIOPHENOL** • *See* Phenol. EAF

**DIMETHYL TRISULFIDE** • *See* Triethyl Trisulfide. ASP

**3,5-DIMETHYL-1,2,4-TRITHIOLANE** • Flavoring. ASP

**2,4-DIMETHYL-5-VINYLTHIAZOLE** • *See* Vinyl Chloride. ASP

**3,5-DINITROBENZAMIDE** • A feed additive that the FDA says is supposed to be zero in edible tissues and by-products of chickens.

**2,6-DINITRO-N,N-DIPROPYL-4-(TRIFLUOROMETHYL)BENZENEAMINE** • Agreflan. Crisalin. Widely used herbicide on barley, carrots, peppermint oil, soybeans, spearmint oil, and wheat. Residue tolerance set by FDA is 2 ppm in peppermint oil and spearmint oil. EPA Genetic Toxicology Program. Community Right-To-Know List *(see both)*. Moderately toxic by ingestion. Caused cancer, tumors, and birth defects in experimental animals.

**2,7-DINITROSOS-1-NAPHTHOL** • Used in the manufacture of dyes. *See* Coal Tar.

**2,4-DINTRO-6-OCTYLPHENYL CROTONATE+2,6-DINTRO-4-OCTYL-PHENYL CROTONATE** • Fungicide on dried apple pomace as a result of application to growing apples as residue. FDA allows residue tolerance of 0.3 ppm. Derived from crotonic acid, which is obtained from crotonaldehyde, which is used in chemical warfare.

**DINKUM OIL** • *See* Eucalyptus Oil.

**DIOCTYL** • Containing two octyl groups. Octyl is obtained from octane, a liquid paraffin found in petroleum.

**DIOCTYL ADIPATE** • *See* Adipic Acid.

**DIOCTYL DILINOLEATE** • *See* Linoleic Acid.

**DIOCTYL MALEATE** • *See* Malic Acid.

**DIOCTYL SODIUM SULFOSUCCINATE** • Docusate Sodium. A wax-like solid that is very soluble in water. It is used as a dispersing and solubilizing additive in foods, drugs, and cosmetics. In foods and beverages it is used as a dispersing and solubilizing additive for gums, cocoa, and various hard-to-wet materials. Also a wetting additive in the cleaning of fruits, vegetables, and leafy plant material. Used in nonalcoholic beverages and sherbets at a rate not to exceed 0.5 percent of the weight of such ingredients. Finished cocoa beverages can have 75 ppm in the finished products. It is a stool softener in laxatives. Eye irritation may result from use in eye preparations. ASP

**DIOXATHION** • A widely used pesticide in animal feed and dehydrated citrus pulp. Poisonous by ingestion. *See* Organophosphates.

**DIOXIN** • The commonly used name for TCDD. 2,3,7,8-tetrachloro-dibenzo-p-dioxin. It is a halogenated aromatic hydrocarbon, and it causes mutagenic and carcinogenic changes in animals. It is a by-product of additive orange (2,4-D and 2,4,5-T). It is the most toxic of chlorine-containing dioxin compounds. The long-term human consequences of exposure to this compound are controversial but it certainly would be wise to avoid exposure to it. It is a suspected cancer-causing additive. Research at the University of Maryland has shown that children exposed to dioxins and PCBs *(see)* prenatally or during infancy can suffer behavioral, memory, and learning problems. The Maryland investigators suggest that the underlying mechanism may be thyroid hormone disruption. Even moderate impairment of thyroid hormone function has been associated with various problems in behavior and intellectual development, and certain thyroid diseases are associated with attention deficit hyperactivity disorder and language disorders. Studies of adults exposed to dioxin and PCBs show no marked neurological effects. The Maryland research was funded by the university and by the American Thyroid Association. Being removed by NTP *(see)* as a human carcinogen.

**DIOXYMETHYLENE PROTOCATECHUICALDEHYDE** • *See* Piperonal.

**DIPA** • The abbreviation for Diisopropanolamine *(see)*.

**DIPENTENE** • *See* Limonene.

**DIPHENYL ETHER** • Colorless crystals with the odor of geranium. Used in perfumery. Toxic by inhalation. Also as an intermediate in processing. ASP

**DIPHENYLKETONE** • *See* Benzophenone.

**1,3-DIPHENYL-2-PROPANONE** • A synthetic fruit, honey, and nut flavoring for beverages, ice cream, ices, candy, and baked goods. ASP

**DIPHENYLAMINE** • Big Dipper. An insecticide used on various products. Poison by ingestion. Has caused birth defects in experimental animals.

**DIPHOSPHATES** • *See* Phosphate. E

**DIPOTASSIUM EDTA** • *See* Ethylenediamine Tetraacetic Acid (EDTA).

**DIPOTASSIUM GLYCYRRHIZATE** • The dipotassium salt of glycyrrhizic acid *(see)*.

**DIPOTASSIUM GUANYLATE** • Flavor Enhancer. E

**DIPOTASSIUM INOSINATE** • Flavor Enhancer. E

**DIPOTASSIUM PERSULFATE** • White, odorless crystals used as a defoaming additive and a dispersing additive *(see both)* in fresh citrus fruit and in poultry. Moderately toxic and a skin irritant.

**DIPOTASSIUM PHOSPHATE** • A sequestrant. A white grain, very soluble in water. Used as a buffering additive to control the degree of acidity in solutions. It is used in the preparation of nondairy powdered coffee creams and in cheeses up to 3 percent by weight of cheese. It is used medicinally as a saline cathartic. GRAS. ASP

**DIPROPYL DISULFIDE** • A synthetic flavoring additive. Colorless, insoluble in water. Occurs naturally in onions. Used in imitation onion flavoring for pickle products and in baked goods.

**DIPROPYL KETONE** • See 4-Heptanone.

**DIPROPYL TRISULFIDE** • *See* Sulfides. ASP

**DIQUAT DIBROMIDE** • Yellow crystals used as an herbicide in animal feed, potable water, potato chips, potato wastes, and processed potatoes.

FDA residue tolerance for it is 0.01 ppm in potable water, 0.5 ppm in processed potatoes including potato chips, and 1 ppm in dried potato wastes when used for animal feed. EPA Genetic Toxicology Program *(see)*. Poison by ingestion and other routes. Poisoning complications include vomiting, mucosal ulcers, diarrhea, and other intestinal tract problems. Heart damage and irregular heartbeats occur in severe poisonings. Causes birth defects in experimental animals. A skin and eye irritant.

**DISODIUM ADENOSINE TRIPHOSPHATE** • A preservative derived from adenylic acid. *See* Adenosine Triphosphate.

**DISODIUM CITRATE** • White granular powder or crystals used as a buffer, nutrient for cultured buttermilk, and as a sequestrant *(see)*. It is used in cured beef, carbonated beverages, nondairy creamers, cured meat products, margarine, evaporated milk, oleomargarine, and cured and fresh pork. The FDA says it is not to exceed 500 ppm or 1.8 mg/square inch of surface. Moderately toxic if injected under the skin. *See also* Sodium Citrate. ASP

**DISODIUM CYANODITHIOMIDOCARBONATE** • Bacteria-killing component in the processing of sugarcane. Any substance that releases the cyanide ion can cause poisoning. Sodium cyanide is one of the swiftest poisons known. The FDA residue tolerance is less than 2.9 ppm in raw cane or sugar beets. ASP

**DISODIUM EDTA** • White, crystalline powder, soluble in water, used as a food preservative and sequestering additive. Promotes color retention in frozen white potatoes (100 ppm), canned potatoes (110 ppm), cooked chickpeas (165 ppm), dried banana cereal (315 ppm), canned strawberry pie filling (500 ppm), gefilte fish (50 ppm), and salad dressing (75 ppm). *See* Ethylenediamine Tetraacetic Acid (EDTA).

**DISODIUM EDTA-COPPER** • Copper Versenate. Used as a sequestering additive. *See* Ethylenediamine Tetraacetic Acid for toxicity.

**DISODIUM ETHYLENE-1,2-DISODIUM ETHYLENE-1,2-BISDITHIOCARBAMATE** • Chem Bam. Spring-Bak. An antimicrobial additive used on beets and sugarcane. The FDA limits use to 3 ppm based on weight of raw sugarcane or raw beets. EPA Genetic Toxicology Program *(see)*. Poison by ingestion. Caused birth defects and mutations in experimental animals. ASP

**DISODIUM GUANYLATE** • A flavor intensifier believed to be more effective than sodium inosinate and sodium glutamate. It is the disodium salt of 5′-guanylic acid, widely distributed in nature as a precursor of RNA and DNA. Can be isolated from certain mushrooms and is used in canned vegetables. Changes in dietary purine intake over the past decade resulting from the use of guanylate and inosinate *(see)* as flavor enhancers are no greater than those due to variability in the consumption of major dietary contributors of purines. Exposure to purines is low—approximately 4 mg per person per day, according to the FAO/WHO Expert Committee on Food

Additives. The committee concluded that on the basis of available data, the combined total daily intake of disodium 5'-guanylate and disodium 5'-inosinate is not of lexicological significance. The committee decided there was no reason to recommend that foods to which these substances have been added should be labeled and withdrew its previous recommendation for labeling. Persons suffering from gout or uric acid kidney stones should limit their dietary sources of purines *(see)*. ASP. E

**DISODIUM INDIGO-5,5-DISULFONATE** • Blue No. 2. Acid Blue W. Blue-brown powder used as a color additive on various products. EPA Genetic Toxicology Program *(see)*. Moderately toxic by ingestion. Caused tumors in experimental animals. *See* FD and C Colors.

**DISODIUM 5'-INOSINATE** • Flavor potentiator *(see)*, odorless and colorless, or white crystal or powder, with a characteristic taste. Used in canned vegetables. *See* Inosinate. ASP

**DISODIUM PHOSPHATE (DIBASIC)** • A sequestrant *(see)* used in evaporated milk, up to 0.1 percent by weight of finished product; in macaroni and noodle products at not less than 0.5 percent or more than 1 percent. It is used as an emulsifier up to 3 percent by weight in specified cheeses. Cleared by the U.S. Department of Agriculture's Meat Inspection Department to prevent cooked-out juices in cured hams, pork shoulders, and loins, canned hams, chopped hams, and bacon (5 percent in the pickling and 5 percent injected into the product). Used as a buffer to adjust acidity in chocolate products, beverages, sauces, and toppings, and enriched farina. Incompatible with alkaloids. It is a mild saline cathartic and has been used in phosphorous-deficiency treatment. It may cause mild irritation to the skin and mucous membranes, and can cause purging. GRAS

**DISODIUM PYROPHOSPHATE** • Sodium Pyrophosphate. An emulsifier and texturizer used to decrease the loss of fluid from a compound. It is GRAS for use in foods as a sequestrant. *See* Sodium Pyrophosphate.

**DISODIUM 5'-RIBONUCLEOTIDES** • Flavor enchancer. Inosinates, guanylates, and ribonucleotides, according to the FAO/WHO are substances normally present in all tissues and their role in purine metabolism as well as their breakdown in the majority of mammals, but not man, to uric acid and allantoin is well known. The various products have been studied adequately in long-term, reproduction, and teratology tests. Ingestion of large amounts of these compounds by man can increase the serum uric acid level and urinary uric acid excretion and this needs to be considered in people with gouty arthritis and those taking uric-acid retaining diuretics. Hence specific mention of the addition of these substances on the label may be indicated. The changes in dietary purine intake from the use of flavor enhancers are no greater than those likely to be occasioned by changes in consumption of those dietary items which are the main contributors of purine. Acceptable daily intake not specified. E

**DISODIUM SUCCINATE** • *See* Succinic Acid and Sodium. ASP

**DISOYAMINE** • *See* Soybean Oil.

**DISPERSANT** • A dispersing additive, such as polyphosphate, for promoting the formation and stabilization of a dispersion of one substance in another. An emulsion, for instance, would consist of a dispersed substance and the medium in which it is dispersed.

**DISTARCH PHOSPHATE** • A combination of starch and sodium metaphosphate. It is a water softener, sequestering additive, and texturizer. A modified starch once commonly used in baby foods. The final report to the FDA of the Select Committee on GRAS Substances stated in 1980 that there is no evidence in the available information that it is a hazard to the public when used as it is now and it should continue its GRAS status with no limitations other than good manufacturing practices. E

**DISTARCH PROPANOL** • A modified starch. The final report to the FDA of the Select Committee on GRAS Substances stated in 1980 that while there is no evidence in the available information that it demonstrates a hazard to the public at current use levels, uncertainties exist, requiring that additional studies be conducted. The FDA allowed GRAS status to continue while tests were being completed and evaluated. Since 1980, however, nothing new has been reported.

**DISTEARYL THIODIPROPIONATE** • Antioxidant used in packaging materials. The FDA limits it to 0.005 percent migrating from food packages.

**DISTILLATE** • The volatile material recovered by condensing the vapors of an extract or fruit material that is heated to its boiling point in a still.

**DISTILLED** • The result of evaporation and subsequent condensation of a liquid, as when water is boiled and steam is condensed.

**DISTILLED ACETYLATED MONOGLYCERIDES** • Food emulsifiers and binders in nutrient capsules and tablets to make them palatable; also food-coating additives. Use is "at level not in excess of the amount reasonably required to produce the intended effect." Cleared by the USDA Meat Inspection Department as an emulsifier for shortening.

**1,4-DITHIANE** • Flavoring. The FAO/WHO stated that it is not of concern at the levels in food. However, the EPA and some scientists say it is a contaminant and possibly carcinogenic to humans. EAF

**2,2′-(DITHIODIMETHYLENE)DIFURAN** • Flavoring. ASP

**DITTANY (FRAXINELLA) ROOTS** • *Dictamnus Albus. See* Dittany of Crete. NUL

**DITTANY OF CRETE** • *Origanum dictamnus.* A natural flavoring extracted from a small herb grown in Crete. Employed in spice flavorings for beverages and baked goods. NIL

**DIURON** • A preemergent herbicide in dried citrus pulp used as animal feed as a result of application during growing. Repeated doses produce anemia in rats.

**DNA (DEOXYRIBONUCLEIC ACID)** • The complex substance that makes up genes. It contains the genetic information for all organisms.

**2-TRANS-6-CIS-DODECADIENAL** • Flavoring. ASP

**TRANS,TRANS-2,4-DODECADIENAL** • Flavoring. EAF

***d*-DODECALACTONE** • Flavoring. ASP

***o*-DODECALACTONE** • A synthetic flavoring. Occurs naturally in butter, cream, and milk. Used in butter, fruit, and pear flavorings for candy, baked goods, oleomargarine, and toppings. Not to exceed 20 ppm in oleomargarine. ASP

***γ*-DODECALACTONE** • A synthetic flavoring, colorless, with a coconut odor that becomes butterlike in low concentrations. Used in butter, butterscotch, coconut, fruit, maple, and nut flavorings for beverages, ice cream, ices, candy, baked goods, gelatin desserts, puddings, and jellies. ASP

**1-DODECANAL** • Lauryl Aldehyde. Found in pine needles, lime, orange, and other essential oils. It is colorless to light yellow with a fatty odor. It is used as a flavoring additive in various products. Mildly toxic by ingestion. ASP

**DODECANOIC ACID** • *See* Lauric Acid.

**(Z)-4-DODECENAL** • A flavoring determined GRAS by the Expert Panel of the Flavor and Extract Manufacturers Association. ASP

**2-DODECENAL** • Flavoring with the odor of coriander *(see)*. ASP

**DODECYL ALCOHOL** • *See* Lauryl Alcohol.

**DODECYL GALLATE** • An antioxidant. The FAO/WHO Expert Committee on Food Additives found that it caused a reduction in spleen weight and pathological changes in the liver, kidney, and spleen in a 150-day study in rats in which the substance was administered by gavage. In addition the study with dodecyl gallate revealed a no-observed-effect level (NOEL) that was tenfold lower than the dietary NOEL for propyl gallate *(see)*. The committee decided that this additive was "unlikely to be carcinogenic or genotoxic" and therefore recommended a temporary acceptable daily intake (ADI) for this additive at 0–0.5 mg per kg of body weight. *See* Gallates. NIL. E

**DODECYL ISOBUTYRATE** • Flavoring. *See* Butryic Acid. ASP

***a*-(P-DODECYLPHENYL)-OMEGA-HYDROXYPOLY(OXYETHYLENE)** • Flavoring. NIL

***a*-(p-DODECYL PHENYL)-1,1-DIMETHYL UREA** • A pesticide.

**N-DODECYL SARCOSINE SODIUM SALT** • Antifogging additive, antistatic additive used in packaging material. When heated to decomposition it emits toxic fumes.

**DODECYLBENZENESULFONIC ACID** • A detergent used to sanitize glass containers for holding milk. The FDA permits a residue of less than 400 ppm in solution. May cause skin irritation. If swallowed will cause vomiting.

**DOG GRASS EXTRACT** • A natural flavoring extract used in maple flavoring for beverages, ice cream, ices, candy, and baked goods. Derives its name from the fact that it is eaten by sick dogs. GRAS. EAF

**DOPAMINE** • 3-Hydroxytyramine. An intermediate in tyrosine metabolism and the precursor of norepinephrine and epinephrine. It is a brain chemical that initiates movement.

**DOWCO 179** • *See* Chlorpyrifos.

**DRACO RUBIN EXTRACT** • *See* Dragon's Blood Extract.

**DRAGON'S BLOOD EXTRACT** • *Daemonorops* spp. The resinous secretion of the fruit of trees grown in Sumatra, Borneo, and India. Almost odorless and tasteless and available in the form of red sticks, pieces, or cakes. Makes a bright crimson powder. Used in bitters flavoring for beverages. NIL

**DRIED ALGAE MEAL** • The Food and Drug Administration (FDA) amended the color additive regulations in August 2000 to provide for the safe use of haematococcus algae meal as a color additive in the feed of salmonid fish to enhance the color of their flesh. This action was in response to a petition filed by Cyanotech Corp. NUL

**DRIED SORGHUM GRAIN SYRUP** • A corn syrup substitute produced from the starch of sorghum grain. *See* Sorghum.

**DRIED YEAST** • A dietary source of folic acid. Used to enrich farina, cornmeal, corn grits, and bakery products. Dried yeast is cleared for use in food provided the total folic acid content of the yeast does not exceed 0.04 milligrams per gram of yeast. Nontoxic.

**DRIERS** • Substances that migrate from food-packaging material including cobalt caprylate, iron caprylate, and manganese caprylate *(see all)*.

**DRY ICE** • *See* Carbon Dioxide.

**DRY MILK, NONFAT** • *See* Nonfat Dry Milk.

**DRYING ADDITIVES** • *See* Rosin.

**DRYING OILS AS COMPONENTS OF FINISHED RESINS** • Oils that migrate from food packaging (as components of finished resins) include chinawood oil (tung oil), dehydrated castor oil, and linseed oil.

**DS** • Abbreviation for dietary supplement.

**D-TAGALOSE** • A sugar from fructose. The unabsorbed facration undergoes fermentation mainly in the large intestine and therefore is said to not cause dental plaque. It is used in cereals, soft drinks, dairy desserts, diet health bars, candies, frostings, and fat-free ice cream. The Food and Drug Administration (FDA) in 2003 authorized a health claim that D-tagatose as a substance was eligible for the health claim that it did not cause dental caries. GRAS

**DULCAMARA EXTRACT** • Bittersweet Nightshade. Extract of the dried stems of *Solanum dulcamara*. Belonging to the family of the nightshades, it is used as a preservative. The ripe berries are used for pies and jams. The unripened berries are deadly. It is made into an ointment by herbalists to treat skin cancers and burns. It induces sweating. *See* Horse Nettle.

**DULCIN** • A nonnutritive sweetener that as of this writing is not legal in food. BANNED

**DULSE** • A natural flavoring extract from red seaweed. Used as a food condiment. GRAS

**DV** • Abbreviation for daily value *(see)*.

**DYSPEPSIA** • Indigestion.

# E

**E** • Signifies approval by the Federation of European Food Additives and Food Enzymes Industries and the European Union.

**EAF** • The U.S. Food and Drug Administration's designation that there is use of a food additive but it has not yet beeen assigned for toxicology literature search.

**EAR** • Estimated Average Requirement (*see* page 18).

**EARTH WAX** • General name for ozocerite, ceresin, and montan waxes. *See* Waxes.

**ECHINACEA** • *Echinacea angustifolia.* Snakeroot. Stoneflower. Coneflower. The roots and leaves of this herb served as a medicine for the Plains Indians. Said by herbalists to be a natural antibiotic and immune enhancer. Contains an antiseptic volatile oil, glycosides *(see),* and phenol, which is also an antiseptic. Echinacea has been found to increase the ability of white blood cells to fight, destroy, and digest toxic organisms that invade the body. It is taken to combat colds, infections, and inflammations. The herb produces a numbing sensation when held in the mouth for a few minutes.

**E. COLI (ESCHERICHIA COLI)** • A type of bacteria normally found in the gut of most animals including humans. Much of the work scientists have done using recombinant DNA *(see)* techniques has used *E. coli* as a carrier because it is well understood. Some types of this bacteria class have been causing food poisoning, some of it fatal. Factory farming and overuse of antibiotics are believed to be contributing to the problem of resistant and dangerous types of *E. coli.*

**ECZEMA** • Inflammation of the skin.

**EDIBLE FILMS** • The most common coatings are wax coverings for fruits, lipid films to protect meat products, and chocolate coating for a range of food items. Films made from pureed fruits and vegetables can add shelf life and tantalizing new flavors to lightly processed foods such as cut produce. Edible films may be cellulose ethers, starch, hydroxypropylated starch, corn zein, wheat gluten, soy protein, and milk proteins. This could be a problem for those with a wheat gluten intolerance, milk protein allergies, or lactose intolerance A newer film—a combination of the antimicrobials zein and nisin plus EDTA *(see all)*—to control the multiplication of the pathogen

*Campylobacter jejuni* on poultry, the most common cause of bacterial diarrhea. Most edible coatings are not obvious. Edible coatings must be GRAS.

**EDTA, CALCIUM DISODIUM** • *See* Ethylenediamine Tetraacetic Acid (EDTA) and Calcium.

**EDTA, DISODIUM** • *See* Ethylenediamine Tetraacetic Acid (EDTA) and Sodium.

**EDTA, TETRASODIUM** • Wash for peeling fruit. *See* Ethylenediamine Tetraacetic Acid (EDTA) and Sodium. ASP

**EFROTOMYCIN** • An antibiotic to improve swine-feed efficiency.

**EGG** • Particularly associated with eczema in children. May also cause reactions ranging from hives to anaphylaxis. Eggs may also be found in root beer, soups, sausage, coffee, and in cosmetics.

**EGG WHITE LYSOZYME** • Antibacterial. It occurs naturally in eggs and it is isolated and used to attack the cell walls of bacteria. GRAS. EAF

**EICOSAPENTAENOIC ACID (EPA)** • Found in fish oil *(see)*, it reduces production of thromboxane, a clotting additive, in the blood, thus making the platelets less "sticky."

**(E)-2-HEPTENOIC ACID** • Flavoring declared GRAS by FEMA *(see)*. EAF

**(E)-2-HEXENYL BUTYRATE** • Flavoring declared GRAS by FEMA *(see)*. EAF

**(E)-2-HEXENYL FORMATE** • Flavoring declared GRAS by FEMA *(see)*. EAF

**(E)-2-HEXENYL ISOVALERATE** • Flavoring declared GRAS by FEMA *(see)*. EAF

**(E)-2-HEXENYL PROPIONATE** • Flavoring declared GRAS by FEMA *(see)*. EAF

**(E)-2-HEXENYL VALERATE** • Flavoring declared GRAS by FEMA *(see)*. EAF

**ELAIDIC ACID** • *See* Oleic Acid.

**ELDER FLOWERS** • *Sambucus canadensis.* A natural flavoring from the small white flowers of a shrub or small tree. Used in fruit, wine, and spice flavorings for beverages, ice cream, ices, candy, baked goods, and wine. The leaves and bark can cause nausea, vomiting, and diarrhea. GRAS. ASP

**ELDER TREE LEAVES** • *Sambucus nigra.* Flavoring for use in alcoholic beverages only. *See* Elder Flowers. NUL

**ELDERBERRY JUICE POWDER** • Dried powder from the juice of the edible berry of a North American elder tree. Used for red coloring.

**ELECAMPANE RHIZOME** • *Inula helenium.* Flavoring in alcoholic beverages only. From a large, coarse European herb having yellow ray flowers. NIL

**ELECAMPANE ROOT** • *Inula helenium. See* Elecampane Rhizome. NUL

**ELEMI** • A soft, yellowish fragrant plastic resin from several Asiatic and

Philippine trees. Slightly soluble in water but readily soluble in alcohol. An oily resin derived from the tropical trees. The gum is used in fruit flavoring for beverages, ice cream, ices, candy, and baked goods. The oil is used in citrus, fruit, vermouth, and spice flavorings for beverages, ice cream, ices, candy, baked goods, and soups. EAF

**EMUL** • Abbreviation for Emulsifier *(see).*

**EMULSIFIERS** • Widely used additives to stabilize a mixture and to ensure consistency. They make chocolate more mixable with milk and keep puddings from separating. One of the most widely used emulsifiers is lecithin *(see)* and another is polysorbate 60 *(see).* Di- and monoglycerides *(see both)* are also used in many products.

**EMULSIFYING OIL** • Soluble Oil. An oil, which when mixed with water, produces a milky emulsion. Sodium sulfonate is an example.

**EMULSIFYING WAX** • Waxes that are treated so that they mix more easily.

**EMULSION** • What is formed when two or more nonmixable liquids are shaken so thoroughly together that the mixture appears to be homogenized. Most oils form emulsions with water.

**ENANTHIC ACID** • Used in peeling solutions for fruits and vegetables. *See* Heptanoic Acid.

**ENDOSULFAN** • Thiodan. Brown crystals made from methane and benzene, related to the long banned but still environmentally present pesticide DDT. Endosulfan is used as an insecticide on fruits and vegetables and on growing tea. It is used especially on tomatoes, carrots, lettuce, and spinach. FDA residue limit on dried tea is 24 ppm. It is toxic by ingestion, inhalation, and skin absorption. Emerging evidence indicates that this insecticide and other chemicals that imitate the human reproductive hormone estrogen may be associated with instances of breast cancer, although definite proof is lacking.

**ENDOTHAL** • Aquathol. Endothall. An herbicide in potable water. FDA residue tolerance is 0.2 ppm in potable water. Poisonous by ingestion. Very irritating to skin, eyes, and mucous membranes. Causes diarrhea.

**ENTERIC NERVOUS SYSTEM** • Our digestive systems are also chemical factories. In the linings of the esophagus, stomach, small intestine, and colon are millions of nerve cells that send stop-and-go messages to our brains. The components of this digestive control center are lumped under the title "the enteric [from the Greek *entera* meaning bowels] nervous system." Current thinking among a number of scientists is that there is a "brain" in the gut, independent from the brain encased in the skull and that the enteric nervous system may be able to learn and remember independently of the central nervous system.

**ENZ** • Abbreviation for enzyme *(see).*

**ENZYMATICALLY HYDROLYZED PROTEIN** • Enzymes are used to

break down the protein in solution. The final report to the FDA of the Select Committee on GRAS Substances stated in 1980 that it should continue its GRAS status with no limitations other than good manufacturing practices.

**ENZYMATICALLY HYDROLYZED CARBOXYMETHYL CELLULOSE** • *See* Carboxymethyl Cellulose and Enzyme. E

**ENZYME** • Any of a unique class of proteins that catalyze a broad spectrum of biochemical reactions. Enzymes are formed in living cells. One enzyme can cause a chemical process that no other enzyme can do. Among the fungi used to produce enzymes in foods are *Aspergillus niger* and *Aspergillus oryzae* for bakery products and for milk clotting. Enzymes are used to remove visceral mass in clam processing, in bakery products, for making cheese, for flavorings, and many other food-processing purposes. A number are recognized as GRAS and others have not yet been evaluated by the FDA.

**ENZYME-MODIFIED FATS** • Light to medium tan liquid, paste, or powder with strong fatty acid odor and flavor. Produced by enzyme action of fats obtained from milk, refined beef fat, or steam-rendered chicken fat. Enzyme-modified milk fat may be prepared from milk, concentrated milk, dry whole milk, cream, concentrated creams, dry cream, butter, butter oil, dried butter, or dried milk fat. Enzyme-modified milk fat may also be prepared from optional dairy ingredients including skim milk, nonfat dry milk, and buttermilk as well as dried whey. Enzymes such as lipase, for example, are used to break down fats that are used in the manufacture of cheese and similar foods. This type of additive is also used as a flavoring. GRAS. NUL

**ENZYME-MODIFIED SOY PROTEIN** • A foaming additive in soda water.

**ENZYMES, CARBOHYDRASE, and CELLULASE FROM *ASPERGILLUS NIGER*** • For the removal of visceral mass in clam processing. *See* Aspergillus. ASP

**ENZYMES from *ASPERGILLUS ORYZAE*** • Used for browning in baking products. See Aspergillus. ASP

**ENZYMES (FOR MILK CLOTTING) FROM *ENDOTHIS PARASITICA* or *BACILLUS CEREUS*** • For use in preparation of standardized cheese or cheese products.

**ENZYMES FROM PLANT and ANIMAL SOURCES** • The following are considered GRAS: bromelin, catalase, ficin, lipase, malt extract, pancreatic extract, pepsin, and trypsin *(see all)*.

**ENZYME, PROTEOLYTIC** • The decomposition of protein by enzymes. *See* various Enzyme entries. ASP

**EPA EXTREMELY HAZARDOUS LIST** • A list of highly toxic chemicals cited by the Environmental Protection Agency.

**EPHEDRA** • *Ephedra gerardiana. E. trifurca. E. sinica. E. equisetina. E. helvetica.* Ma Huang. Mormon Tea. There are about forty species of this herb mentioned in ancient scriptures of India, and it was used by the

Chinese for more than five thousand years. The stems contain alkaloids *(see)* including ephedrine *(see)*. Herbalists use the herb to treat arthritis, asthma, emphysema, bronchitis, hay fever, and hives. The Food and Drug Administration proposed in 1997 to reduce risks associated with dietary supplement products containing ephedrine alkaloids by limiting the amount in products and requiring labeling and marketing measures that give adequate warning and information to consumers. Ephedrine alkaloids are amphetaminelike compounds with potentially powerful stimulant effects on the nervous system and heart. Hundreds of consumer illnesses and injuries associated with the use of these products have been reported. Pregnant women, too, should avoid the use of dietary supplements with ephedrine alkaloids. Reported adverse events range from episodes of high blood pressure, irregularities in heart rate, insomnia, nervousness, tremors, and headaches to seizures, heart attacks, strokes, and death. Most events occurred in young to middle-aged, otherwise healthy adults using the products for weight control and increased energy. Ephedrine alkaloids in dietary supplements are usually derived from one of several species of herbs of the genus *Ephedra,* sometimes called Ma Huang, Chinese ephedra, and epitonin. Other botanical sources include *Sida cordifolia.* At this writing, the FDA was attempting to control the use of ephedra in products including those that contain other stimulants such as caffeine. *See also* Ephedrine.

**EPHEDRINE** • The alkaloid ephedrine is derived from the plant *Ephedra equisetina* and others of the forty species of ephedra or produced synthetically. Ephedra has been used for more than five thousand years in Chinese medicine and has become more and more popular in Western medicine. It acts like epinephrine *(see)* and is used as a bronchodilator, nasal decongestant, to raise blood pressure, and topically to constrict blood vessels. *See also* Ephedra.

**EPICHLOROHYDRIN** • A colorless liquid with an odor resembling chloroform. A modifier for food starches that the FDA permits to be used up to level of 0.3 percent in starch. A strong skin irritant and sensitizer. Daily administration of 1 milligram per kilogram of body weight to skin killed all of a group of rats in four days, indicating a cumulative potential. Chronic exposure is known to cause kidney damage. A two-year study of workers who had been exposed to the substance for six months or more before January 1966 showed an increase in the incidence of cancer. Chronic exposure is known to cause kidney damage in humans. Germany regulates it as a known carcinogen. FDA residue tolerances are less than 0.1 percent with propylene and less than 5 ppm in modified food starch. NUL

**EPICHLORHYDRIN CROSSLINKED WITH AMMONIA** • Decolorizing additive in clarification of sugar liquors and juices. *See* Epichlorhydrin and Ammonia. NUL

**EPIGALLOCATECHIN CALLATE (EGCG)** • Compound found in green tea that reportedly provides stronger damage protection to cells and their genetic material than vitamins E and C.

**EPINEPHRINE** • Adrenaline. The major hormone of the adrenal gland which increases heart rate and contractions, vasoconstriction or vasodilation, relaxation of the muscles in the lungs and intestinal smooth muscles, and the processing of sugar and fat.

**EPOXY** • Chemical term describing an oxygen atom bound to two linked carbon atoms. They are important chemical intermediates and the basis of epoxy resins *(see)*.

**EPSILON-DODECALACTONE** • Flavoring.

**4,5-EXPOXY-(e)-2-DECENAL** • A flavoring determined GRAS by FEMA *(see)*.

**1,8-EPOXY-*p*-MENTHANE** • *See* Eucalyptol.

**EPOXY RESINS** • The versatile epoxy resins are used widely in manufacturing for adhesive purposes and as films and durable coatings. When epoxy resins are used, the resin is combined with a curing additive. As the mixture "cures" it becomes hard. Epoxies are one of the most common causes of occupational health complaints. The Hazard Evaluation System and Information Service of California, for example, cites frequent effects of overexposure to the chemicals used in epoxy resins as eye, nose, throat, and skin irritations, allergies, and asthma. Hardened epoxy products are practically nontoxic unless they are cut, sanded, or burned.

**EXPOXIDIZED SOYBEAN OIL** • Used as a stabilizer not to exceed 1 percent in brominated soybean oil.

**EQUISETIC ACID** • *See* Aconitic Acid.

**ERGOCALCIFEROL** • Vitamin D$_2$

***ERIGERON CANADENSIS*** • *See* Erigeron Oil.

**ERIGERON OIL** • *Erigeron canadensis.* Horseweed. Fleabane Oil. Derived from the leaves and tops of a plant grown in the northern and central United States. Used in fruit and spice flavorings for beverages, ice cream, ices, candy, baked goods, and sauces. NIL

**ERIODICTYON CALIFORNIUM** • *See* Yerba Santa Fluid Extract.

**ERUCIC ACID** • Docosenoic Acid. An acid found in rapeseed, mustard seed, and wallflower seeds.

**ERYTHORBIC ACID** • Isoascorbic Acid. Antioxidant. White, slightly yellow crystals that darken on exposure to light. Isoascorbic acid contains one-twentieth the vitamin capacity of ascorbic acid *(see)*. Antioxidant used in pickling brine at a rate of 7.5 ounces per 100 gallons; in meat products at the rate of 0.75 ounces per hundred pounds; in beverages; baked goods; cured cuts and cured pulverized products to accelerate color fixing in curing, to 0.75 ounce per 100 pounds. Nontoxic. The final report to the FDA of the Select Committee on GRAS Substances stated in 1980 that it should continue its GRAS status with no limitations other than good manufacturing practices. ASP. E

**ERYTHROMYCIN** • An antibacterial obtained from the strains of *Streptomyces erythraeus* found in the soil. Used to treat a wide range of bacterial infections in humans. It is used as a drug for beef, chicken eggs, pork, and turkey. FDA tolerances are 0.1 ppm in uncooked edible tissues of swine, zero in uncooked edible tissues of beef cattle and milk, 0.025 ppm in uncooked eggs, 0.125 ppm in uncooked edible residue of chickens and turkeys. EPA Genetic Toxicology Program *(see)*. Moderately toxic by ingestion. The use of antibiotics in animal feed is highly controversial because it could lead to resistance to the antibiotic in humans as well as allergic reactions.

**ERYTHROSINE** • Sodium or potassium salt of tetraiodofluorescein, a coal-tar derivative. A brown powder that becomes red in solution. FD and C Red No. 3 is an example. *See* Coal Tar for toxicity. E

**ERYTHROXYLON COCA** • *See* Coca Leaf Extract (Decocainized).

**ESCHERICHIA COLI** • *E. coli.* A gram-negative *(see)* bacteria commonly found in fecal matter and in the human intestines, certain strains may cause intestinal and urinary tract infections. *See* E. coli.

**ESO** • Essential oil and/or oleoresin (solvent free).

**ESSENCE** • An extract of a substance that retains its fundamental or most desirable properties in concentrated form, such as a fragrance or flavoring.

**ESSENTIAL OIL** • The oily liquid obtained from plants through a variety of processes. The essential oil usually has the taste and smell of the original plant. Essential oils are called volatile because most of them are easily vaporized. The only theories for calling such oils essential are (1) the oils were believed essential to life and (2) they were the "essence" of the plant. The use of essential oils as preservatives is ancient. A large number of oils have antiseptic, germicidal, and preservative action; however, they are primarily used for fragrances and flavorings. Nontoxic when used on the skin. A teaspoon may cause illness in an adult and less than an ounce may kill.

**ESTER** • A compound formed from alcohol and acid by elimination of water, as ethyl acetate *(see)*. Usually, fragrant liquids used for artificial fruit perfumes and flavors. Esterification of rosin, for example, reduces its allergy-causing properties. Toxicity depends on the ester.

**ESTERASE-LIPASE** • Derived from *Mucor miehei.* An enzyme used as a flavor enhancer in cheese, fats, oils, and milk products. There is no reported use of the chemical and there is no toxicology information available. NUL

**ESTRADIOL** • Oestradiol. Estrace. Estinyl. Estra-L. Estraderm. depGynogen. Depo-Estradiol. Dura-Estrin. E-Cypionate. Estro-Cyp. Estrofem. Estroject-LA. Estronol-LA. Delestrogen. Dioval. Duragen 10. Estraval. Menaval. Valergen. Most potent of the natural estrogenic female hormones. In animals it is implanted in steers, heifers, and lambs. It is also implanted in combination with testosterone or progesterone, two other powerful sex hormones. The FDA permits zero tolerance in meat. Estradiol is given to humans by skin patch, tablets, injection, or vaginal cream and is used to treat menopausal symptoms, the effects of a hysterectomy, primary ovarian failure, atrophic vaginitis, postpartum breast engorgement, and inoperable prostate cancer. Potential adverse reactions include nausea, vomiting, depression, high blood pressure, dizziness, migraine, libido changes, blood clots, water retention, increased risk of stroke, blood clots to the lung, and heart attack. May also worsen nearsightedness, cause intolerance of contact lenses, and lead to loss of appetite, increased appetite, excessive thirst, pancreatitis, and bloating and abdominal cramps. Women may have breakthrough bleeding, altered menstrual flow, painful or absent menstruation, enlargement of benign tumors of the uterus, cervical erosion, abnormal secretions and vaginal candidiasis. In men there may be enlargement of the breast, testicular atrophy, and impotence. In both sexes there may be jaundice, high blood sugar, high calcium in the blood, folic acid deficiency, dark spots appearing on the skin, hives, acne, oily skin, hairiness or loss of hair, leg cramps, and hemorrhages into the skin. Contraindicated in persons with blood clot disorders, cancer of the breast, reproductive organs, or genitals, and in those with undiagnosed abnormal genital bleeding and in pregnancy. Should be used with caution in high blood pressure, asthma, mental depression, bone disease, blood problems, gallbladder disease, migraines, seizures, diabetes, absence of menstruation, heart failure, liver or kidney dysfunction, and a family history of breast or genital tract cancer. Estradiol's use as implants in animals is unnecessary and should be outlawed.

**ESTRADIOL BENZOATE** • White or slightly brownish crystalline hormone powder used as a growth promoter in beef and lamb. FDA tolerances are set at 120 parts per trillion in muscle; 480 ppt in fat; 360 ppt in kidney; 240 ppt in liver of heifers, steers, and calves. Tolerance of 120 ppm in muscles, 600 ppm in fat, kidney, and liver of lambs. Has caused cancer in experimental animals as well as birth defects. It is an estrogen used in human medication for birth control and postmenopausal symptoms and does cause side effects in humans as a medication. *See* Estradiol.

**ESTRADIOL MONOPALMITATE** • An estrogen used to promote growth in chickens. It has a zero tolerance in chickens for market. *See* Estradiol.

**ESTRADIOL VALERATE** • Used as an implant in combination with progesterone. The FDA bans its use in veal calves.

**ESTRAGOLE** • A colorless to light yellow oily liquid occurring naturally in anise, star anise, basil, estragon oil, and pimento oil. Used as a synthetic fruit, licorice, anise, and spice flavoring for beverages, ice cream, ices, candy, baked goods, chewing gum, and condiments. Has induced tumors in rats, especially newborns. It is not strongly mutagenic in bacterial or yeast systems. FEMA *(see)* says that at current doses, it probably offers no danger to humans but nevertheless, it requires further study. GRAS. ASP

**ESTRAGON** • Tarragon. A flavoring additive from the oil of leaves of a plant native to Eurasia and used in fruit, licorice, liquor, root beer, and spice flavorings for beverages, ice cream, ices, candy, baked goods, meats, liquor, and condiments. GRAS

**ESTROGEN** • A hormone produced by the ovaries that is mainly responsible for female sexual characteristics. Estrogen influences bone mass by slowing or halting bone loss, improving retention of calcium by the kidney, and improving the absorption of dietary calcium by the intestine. Estrogen is given to relieve menopausal symptoms, prevent or relieve aging changes in the vagina and urethra, and to help prevent osteoporosis *(see)*. See Estradiol.

**ETHALFLURALIN** • An herbicide. FDA tolerance for residues in fat, meat, meat by-products of cattle, hogs, goats, poultry, sheep, and milk is 0.05 ppm.

**ETHANAL** • *See* Acetaldehyde and Heptanal.

**ETHANE** • Colorless, odorless gas used as a source of ethylene *(see)*.

**1,2-ETHANEDITHIOL** • Derived from ethylene glycol, it is used as a chelating additive *(see)*. The vapors cause a severe headache and nausea. NIL

**ETHANOL** • Ethyl Alcohol. Rubbing Alcohol. Ordinary Alcohol. Used as a solvent in candy, candy glaze, beverages, ice cream, ices, baked goods, liquors, sauces, and gelatin desserts. Clear, colorless, and very flammable, it is made by the fermentation of starch, sugar, and other carbohydrates. Used medicinally as a topical antiseptic, sedative, and blood vessel dilator. Ingestion of large amounts may cause nausea, vomiting, impaired perception, stupor, coma, and death. When it is deliberately denatured *(see)*, it is poisonous. GRAS

**ETHANOLAMINES** • Three compounds—monoethanolamine, diethanolamine, and triethanolamine—with low melting points and soluble in both water and alcohol. Widely used in detergents and emulsifiers. Very large quantities are required for a lethal dose. Can be irritating to the skin if very alkaline. See Diethanolamine.

**ETHANTHALDEHYDE** • *See* Heptanal.

**ETHANTHIC ALCOHOL** • *See* Heptyl Alcohol

**ETHANTHYL ALCOHOL** • *See* Heptyl Alcohol.

**ETHEPHON** • A pesticide used in raisin water waste for use in animal feed. FDA residue tolerance is 65 ppm.

**ETHER** • An organic compound. Acetic ether *(see* Ethyl Acetate). It is obtained chiefly by the distillation of alcohol with sulfuric acid and is used chiefly as a solvent. A mild skin irritant. Inhalation or ingestion causes central nervous system depression.

**ETHION** • An insecticide to kill mites. In fat of cattle it is permitted 2.5 ppm; in meat and by-products of cattle as residue, 0.75 ppm, in milk, zero, and in animal feed from 4 to 10 ppm. It inhibits nerve signals. *See* Organophosphates.

**ETHOFUMESATE** • An herbicide with an FDA tolerance of 0.5 ppm as a residue in or on sugar beet molasses.

**ETHOPABATE** • Odorless white to pink crystals used as an animal drug in chickens. The FDA limits residue to 1.5 ppm in uncooked liver and kidney, 0.5 ppm in uncooked muscles of chickens. Used to combat bacteria.

**ETHOVAN** • *See* Ethyl Vanillin.

***p*-ETHOXY BENZALDEHYDE** • A synthetic fruit and vanilla flavoring for beverages, ice cream, ices, candy, and baked goods. *See* Benzyl Acetate. ASP

**2-(1-[ETHOXY IMINO] BUTYL)-5-(2-[ETHYL THIO] PROPYD-3-HYDROXY-2-CYCLOHEXENE-1-ONE** • An herbicide used in animal feed, flaxseed meal, potato pomace, sunflower meal, tomato products (concentrated), and peanut soap stock. FDA limitations of residue: 24 ppm in tomato products, concentrated, 15 ppm in cottonseed soap stock, 7 ppm in flaxseed meal, 75 ppm in peanut soap stock, and 20 ppm in sunflower meal used for animal feed.

**ETHOXYLATE** • An ethyl *(see)* and oxygen compound is added to an additive to make it less or more soluble in water, depending upon the mixture. Ethoxylate acts as an emulsifier.

**ETHOXYLATED MONO- and DI-GLYCERIDES** • Dough conditioners in bread used to increase the volume of the loaf not to exceed 0.5 percent of flour used. Also used as an emulsifier in pan-release additives for yeast-leavened bakery products. In solid, edible fat water emulsions as coffee creamer substitute. *See* Glycerides.

**1-ETHOXY-3-METHYL-2-BUTENE** • Flavoring. An aromatic ether. ASP

**ETHOXYQUIN** • 1,2-Dihydro-6-Ethoxy-2,2,4-Trimethylquinoline. An antioxidant *(see)* to preserve color in chili powder, paprika, and ground chili at levels not to exceed 100 ppm. The residues in or on edible products of animals are restricted to 5 ppm in or on the uncooked fat of meat from animals except poultry; 3 ppm in or on the uncooked liver and fat of poultry; and 0.5 ppm in or on the uncooked muscle meat of animals. There was a significant question about this additive in the late 1980s because its use in animal feed caused dogs to have symptoms from itchy skin and lethargy to thyroid and kidney problems. Reproductive disorders and cancer were also reported. It is used in both human and animal feed as an antioxidant. In 1995, there was a report in *Biochemical Pharmacology* by Mexican researchers that ethoxyquin affected the kidneys of rats. The FDA's toxicology program reported no adverse health effects from the additive. Then in 1997, the FDA reduced the amount of ethoxyquin allowed in dog food. It is still permitted in human food. *See* Quinoline for toxicity. *See also* Santoquin. ASP

**2-ETHOXYTHIAZOLE** • Synthetic scent of nuts, burning, frozen food, roasted food, and candies. ASP

**ETHYL** • Signifies a hydrocarbon derived from natural gas.

**ETHYL ABIETATE** • Amber-colored, thick liquid made from ethyl chloride and rosin. It is used in lacquers and coatings. Skin irritant. Although allowed as a food additive, there is no current reported use of the chemical, and therefore, although toxicology information may be available, it is not being updated, according to the FDA. NIL

**ETHYL ACETATE** • A colorless liquid with a pleasant fruity odor that occurs naturally in apples, bananas, grape juice, pineapple, raspberries, and strawberries. It is employed as a synthetic flavoring additive in blackberry, raspberry, strawberry, butter, lemon, apple, banana, cherry, grape, peach, pineapple, brandy, muscatel, rum, whiskey, mint, almond, and cream soda flavoring for beverages, ice cream, ices, candy, baked goods, chewing gum, gelatins, puddings, and liquor. It is a mild local irritant and central nervous system depressant. The vapors are irritating and prolonged inhalation may cause kidney and liver damage. Irritating to the skin. Its fat-solvent action produces drying and cracking and sets the stage for secondary infections. GRAS. ASP

**ETHYL ACETOACETATE** • Acetoacetic Ester. A synthetic flavoring that occurs naturally in strawberries. Pleasant odor. Used in loganberry, strawberry, apple, apricot, cherry, peach, liquor, and muscatel flavorings for beverages, ice cream, ices, candy, baked goods, chewing gum, and gelatin desserts. Moderately irritating to skin and mucous membranes. ASP

**ETHYL ACETONE** • *See* 2-Pentanone.

**ETHYL 3-ACETOXY-2-METHYLBUTYRATE** • A flavoring determined GRAS by FEMA *(see)*. *See* Butanoic Acid.

**S-ETHYL 2-ACETYLAMINOETHANETHIOATE** • A flavoring in baked goods, breakfast cereals, cheese, condiments, gravies, milk products, poultry, reconstituted vegetables, and many other food products. Determined GRAS by FEMA *(see)*. *See* Ethane.

**ETHYL 2-ACETYL-3-PHENYLPROPIONATE** • A synthetic fruit flavoring for beverages, ice cream, ices, candy, baked goods, chewing gum, and gelatin desserts. ASP

**ETHYL ACONITATE** • Aconitic Acid. A synthetic fruit, liquor, and rum flavoring for beverages, ice cream, ices, candy, baked goods, and gelatin desserts.

**ETHYL ACRYLATE** • A synthetic flavoring additive that occurs naturally in pineapple and raspberries. Used in fruit, liquor, and rum flavorings for beverages, ice cream, ices, candy, baked goods, and chewing gum. Highly irritating to the eyes, skin, and mucous membranes and may cause lethargy and convulsions if concentrated vapor is inhaled. The final report to the FDA of the Select Committee on GRAS Substances stated in 1980 that it should continue its GRAS status with no limitations other than good manufacturing practices. Although it was found to be carcinogenic in rats in

1986, it was delisted as a carcinogen in 2000 because it was decided that the doses given to animals were in higher concentrations than those to which humans would be exposed. ASP

**ETHYL ALCOHOL** • Contains ethanol *(see),* grain alcohol, and neutral spirits and is used as a solvent in candy glaze, beverages, ices, ice cream, candy, baked goods, liquors, sauces, gelatin desserts, and pizza crusts. It is rapidly absorbed through the gastric and intestinal mucosa. For ingestion within a few minutes, the fatal dose in adults is considered to be one and one-half to two pints of whiskey (40 to 55 percent ethyl alcohol). It was approved in 1976 for use in pizza crusts to extend handling and storage life. GRAS. EAF

**ETHYL *p*-ANISATE** • A synthetic flavoring additive, colorless to light yellow liquid with a light fruity smell. Used in berry, fruit, grape, licorice, anise, liquor, rum, and vanilla flavorings for beverages, ice cream, ices, candy, and baked goods. ASP

**ETHYL ANTHRANILATE** • Colorless liquid, fruit odor, soluble in alcohol and propylene glycol. A synthetic flavoring additive, clear, colorless to amber liquid with an odor of orange blossoms. Used in berry, mandarin, orange, floral, jasmine, neroli, fruit, grape, peach, and raisin flavorings for beverages, ice cream, ices, candy, baked goods, gelatin desserts, and chewing gum. Used in perfumery. ASP

**ETHYL ASPARTATE** • The ester of ethyl alcohol and aspartic acid *(see both).*

**4-ETHYL BENZALDEHYDE** • Flavoring. *See* Benzoic Acid. NUL

**ETHYL BENZENECARBOXYLATE** • *See* Ethyl Benzoate.

**ETHYL BENZOATE** • Essence de Niobe. Ethyl Benzenecarboxylate. An artificial fruit essence almost insoluble in water, with a pleasant odor. Used in currant, strawberry, fruit, cherry, grape, liquor, nut, walnut, vanilla, and raspberry flavorings for beverages, ice cream, ices, candy, baked goods, chewing gum, gelatin desserts, and liquors. ASP

**ETHYL BENZOYLACETATE** • A synthetic fruit flavoring additive for beverages, ice cream, ices, candy, and baked goods. Pleasant odor. ASP

**ETHYL BENZYL ACETOACETATE** • *See* Ethyl-2-Acetyl-3-Phenylpropionate.

**ETHYL BENZYL BUTYRATE** • Synthetic fruit flavoring for beverages, ice cream, ices, candy, and baked goods. NIL

**ETHYL BRASSYLATE** • Artificially synthesized flavors which have not been identified in natual products. ASP

**ETHYL BUTYL ACETATE** • A synthetic fruit flavoring for beverages, ice cream, ices, and candy. ASP

**ETHYL BUTYRATE** • Butyric Acid. Pineapple Oil. Colorless, with a pineapple odor. It occurs naturally in apples and strawberries. In alcoholic solution it is known as pineapple oil. Used in blueberry, raspberry, strawberry, butter, caramel, cream, orange, banana, cherry, grape, peach, pineapple, rum, walnut, and eggnog flavorings for beverages, ice cream, ices, candy, baked goods, gelatins, puddings, and chewing gum (1,400 ppm). Mildly toxic by ingestion. A skin irritant. GRAS. ASP

**ETHYL CAPRATE** • *See* Cognac Oil.

**ETHYL CAPROATE** • Colorless to yellowish liquid, pleasant odor, soluble in alcohol and ether. Used in artificial fruit essences. *See* Cognac Oil.

**ETHYL CAPRYLATE** • *See* Cognac Oil.

**ETHYL CARBONATE** • Carbonic Acid Diethyl Ester. Pleasant odor.

**ETHYL CARVACROL** • *See* Carvacryl Ethyl Ether.

**ETHYL CELLULOSE** • Cellulose Ether. White granules prepared from wood pulp or chemical cotton and used as a binder and filler in dry vitamin preparations up to 35 percent; chewing gum up to 0.025 percent, and in confectionery up to 0.012 percent. Also used as a diluent *(see)*. Not susceptible to bacterial or fungal decomposition. GRAS. ASP

**ETHYL CINNAMATE** • Cinnamic Acid. An almost colorless oily liquid with a faint cinnamon odor. Used as a synthetic flavoring in raspberry, strawberry, cherry, grape, peach, plum, spice, cinnamon, and vanilla flavorings for beverages, ice cream, ices, candy, baked goods, chewing gum, and gelatin desserts. Moderately toxic by ingestion. ASP

**ETHYL CITRATE** • A bitter, oily sequestrant used in dried egg whites. *See* Sequestrants.

**ETHYL CROTONATE** • Flavor identical to natural flavor from aromatic raw materials or chemically identical synthesized materials. *See* Butanoic Acid. ASP

**ETHYL CYCLOHEXANECARBOXYLATE** • Flavoring. ASP

**ETHYL CYCLOHEXANEPROPIONATE** • A synthetic pineapple flavoring additive for beverages, ice cream, ices, candy, and baked goods. ASP

**ETHYL DECANOATE** • Decanoic Acid. A synthetic flavoring occurring naturally in green and white cognac oils. Used in strawberry, cherry, grape, pineapple, liquor, brandy, cognac, and rum flavorings for beverages, ice cream, ices, candy, baked goods, gelatin desserts, and liquors. ASP

**ETHYL 2,4,7-DECATRIENOATE** • Flavoring. The FAO/WHO said it has no concern about it. EAF

**ETHYL 4,4′-DICHLOROBENZILATE** • An insecticide for citrus fruits. The FDA allows a residue of 5 ppm in and on citrus fruits and 0.5 ppm as a residue in fat, meat, and meat by-products of sheep and cattle.

**ETHYL DIHYDROXYPROPYL** • PABA. The ester of ethyl alcohol and *p*-dihydroxypropyl aminobenzoic acid. *See* Ethyl Alcohol and *para*-Aminobenzoic Acid.

**ETHYL DIISOPROPYL CINNAMATE** • *See* Cinnamic Acid.

**2-ETHYL-3,5(6)-DIMETHYLPYRAZINE** • A colorless to slightly yellow liquid with the smell of roasted cocoa used as a flavoring in various products. GRAS. ASP

**ETHYL 0-P (DIMETHYLSULFO/AMOYL) PHENYL PHOSPHORO-THIOATE** • An insecticide to combat grubs in animal feed. The FDA residue tolerance is 0.1 ppm in meat, fat, and meat by-products of cattle.

**ETHYL DODECANOATE** • *See* Ethyl Laurate.

**O,O-ETHYL-S-2 (ETHYL THIO)ETHYL PHOSPHORODITHIOATE** • Widely used insecticide on animal feed, pineapples, and dehydrated sugar beet pulp. FDA limitation of 5 ppm in dehydrated sugar beet pulp and pineapple bran when used for animal feed. Poisonous by ingestion, inhalation, and skin contact. May cause mutations. EPA considers it extremely hazardous and it is on the EPA Genetic Toxicology Program *(see)*.

**ETHYL ESTER OF FATTY ACIDS** • Compound for coating raisins. *See* Fatty Acids.

**ETHYL FORMATE** • Formic Acid. A colorless, flammable liquid with a distinct odor occurring naturally in apples and coffee extract. Used as a yeast and mold inhibitor and as a fumigant for bulk and packaged raisins and dried currants; fungicide for cashew nuts, cereals, tobacco, and dried fruits. Also a synthetic flavoring additive for blueberry, raspberry, strawberry, butter, butterscotch, apple, apricot, banana, cherry, grape, peach, plum, pineapple, tutti-frutti, brandy, rum, sherry, and whiskey flavorings for beverages, ice cream, ices, candy, baked goods, liquor, gelatin, and chewing gum. Irritating to the skin and mucous membranes, and in high concentrations it is narcotic. The final report to the FDA of the Select Committee on GRAS Substances stated in 1980 that it should continue its GRAS status with no limitations other than good manufacturing practices. *See* Formic Acid for further toxicity.

**ETHYL FORMIC ACID** • *See* Propionic Acid.

**ETHYL 2-FURAN PROPIONATE** • Synthetic raspberry, apple, cherry, and pineapple flavoring additive for beverages, ice cream, ices, candy, and baked goods. ASP

**ETHYL FURYLPROPIONATE** • *See* Ethyl 2-Furan Propionate. EAF

**ETHYL GLUTAMATE** • The ester of ethyl alcohol and glutamic acid. *See* Glutamate.

**4-ETHYL GUAIACOL** • A synthetic coffee and fruit flavoring additive for beverages, ice cream, ices, and gelatin desserts. ASP

**2-ETHYL-2-HEPTANAL** • A synthetic pineapple flavoring additive for beverages and candy. ASP

**ETHYL HEPTANOATE** • A synthetic flavoring additive, colorless, with a fruity, winelike odor and taste, and a burning aftertaste. Used in blueberry, strawberry, butter, butterscotch, coconut, apple, cherry, grape, melon, peach, pineapple, plum, vanilla, cheese, nut, rum, brandy, and cognac flavorings for beverages, ice cream, ices, candy, baked goods, gelatin desserts, chewing gum, and liqueurs. ASP

**ETHYL HEXADECANOATE** • *See* Ethyl Palmitate.

**ETHYL 2,4-HEXADIENOATE** • *See* Ethyl Sorbate.

**ETHYL HEXANEDIOL** • *See* Sorbic Acid.

**ETHYL HEXANOATE** • A synthetic flavoring additive that occurs naturally in apples, pineapples, and strawberries. Used in fruit, rum, nut, and cheese flavorings for beverages, ice cream, ices, candy, baked goods, chewing gum, gelatin desserts, and jelly. ASP

**2-ETHYL-1-HEXANOL** • A flavoring additive derived from alcohol. The FAO/WHO *(see)* concluded that doses greater than about 350 mg per kg of body weight per day administered orally to rats and mice cause changes in the liver but did not result in cancer with long-term administration. In high doses it did cause birth defects in mice but at lower doses did not. On the basis of NOEL *(see)* of 50 mg per kg of body weight per day from the long-term study in rats and a safety factor of 100, the committee established an ADI *(see)* of 0–.05 mg per kg of body weight for this additive. ASP

**ETHYL 3-HYDROXYBUTYRATE** • Used as a stabilizer and antioxidant. ASP

**ETHYL HYDROXYMETHYL OLEYL OXAZOLINE** • A synthetic wax.

**ETHYL a-HYDROXY PROPIONATE** • *See* Ethyl Lactate.

**ETHYL ISOBUTYRATE** • Isobutyric Acid. A synthetic strawberry, fruit, cherry, and butter flavoring for beverages, ice cream, ices, candy, baked goods, gelatin desserts, and toppings.

**ETHYL ISOVALERATE** • Colorless, oily liquid with a fruity odor derived from ethanol and valerate. A synthetic flavoring used in alcoholic solution for pineapple flavoring for beverages, ice cream, ices, candy, baked goods, chewing gum, and gelatin desserts. Used in essential oils and perfumery. *See* Valeric Acid. ASP

**ETHYL LACTATE** • Colorless liquid with a mild odor. Derived from lactic acid with ethanol. Used as a solvent for nitrocellulose, lacquers, resins, and enamels. Used in strawberry, butter, butterscotch, coconut, grape, rum, maple, cheese, and nut flavorings for beverages, ice cream, ices, candy, baked goods, chewing gum (3,100 ppm), gelatin desserts, syrup, and brandy (1,000 ppm). *See* Lactic Acid. ASP

**ETHYL LAURATE** • The ester of ethyl alcohol and lauric acid used as a synthetic flavoring. It is a colorless oil with a light, fruity odor. Insoluble in water, very soluble in alcohol. Used in berry, coconut, fruit, grape, liquor, cognac, rum, nut, spice, nutmeg, and cheese flavorings for beverages, ice cream, ices, candy, baked goods, chewing gum, and liqueurs. It is also used as a solvent. ASP

**ETHYL LEVULINATE** • Levulinic Acid. Colorless liquid soluble in water.

Used as a solvent for cellulose acetate and starch and flavorings. A synthetic apple flavoring for beverages, ice cream, ices, candy, and baked goods. *See* Levulinic Acid. ASP

**ETHYL LINOLEATE** • Prepared from sunflower seed oil, it is used in the vitamin industry.

**ETHYL MALATE** • *See* Diethyl Malate.

**ETHYL MALONATE** • Colorless liquid, sweet ester odor. Insoluble in water. Used in certain pigments and flavoring.

**ETHYL MALTOL** • White crystalline powder with a sweet fruity taste, it is used as a flavoring and processing aid in chocolate, desserts, and wine. Moderately toxic by injection. ASP

**4-ETHYL-2-METHOXYPHENOL** • *See* 4-Ethyl Guaiacol.

**ETHYL 3-METHYL BUTYRATE** • A synthetic fruit flavoring for beverages, ice cream, ices, and candy.

**ETHYL METHYL CELLULOSE** • *See* Methyl Cellulose. E

**ETHYL METHYL DISULFIDE** • A flavoring determined GRAS by FEMA *(see)*. *See* Pentane.

**ETHYL METHYLENE PHOSPHORODITHIOATE** • A widely used insecticide in animal feed, citrus pulp, raisins, and dried tea. The FDA allows residue tolerance of up to 10 ppm in dried tea, 4 ppm in raisins, and 10 ppm in dried citrus pulp when used for animal feed. Extremely hazardous substance. Poison by ingestion and skin contact. Human systemic effects by ingestion include paralysis, motor activity changes, fever, and interference with nerve transmission.

**ETHYL-3-METHYL-4-(METHYL THIO) PHENYL(1-METHYL-ETHYL) PHOS-PHORAMIDATE** • A pesticide allowed up to 1 ppm as residue in or on grape pomace; 2.5 in or on dried citrus pulp or citrus molasses that is fed to animals.

**ETHYL METHYLPHENYLGLYCIDATE** • Strawberry Aldehyde. Colorless to yellowish liquid having a strong odor suggestive of strawberry. A synthetic berry, loganberry, raspberry, strawberry, coconut, fruit, cherry, grape, pineapple, liquor, and wine flavoring for beverages, ice cream, ices, candy, baked goods, gelatin, pudding, and chewing gum. Caused growth retardation in rats, particularly males, and testicular atrophy. Females showed paralysis of hindquarters and deterioration of muscles. GRAS

**2-ETHYL-3-METHYLPYRAZINE** • Colorless to slightly yellow liquid with a strong raw potato odor. Used as a flavoring in various foods. GRAS

**ETHYL MYRISTATE** • The ester of ethyl alcohol and myristic acid *(see both)*. Synthetic coconut, fruit, honey, and cognac flavoring for beverages, ice cream, ices, candy, baked goods, and liqueurs. ASP

**ETHYL NITRITE** • Sweet Spirit of Niter. Spirit of Nitrous Ether. A synthetic flavoring additive, colorless or yellowish liquid with a characteristic odor and a burning, sweetish taste. Used in strawberry, cherry, pineapple, liquor, brandy, and rum flavorings for beverages, ice cream, ices, candy, baked goods, chewing gum, syrups, and icings. It may cause hemoglobinemia, in which oxygen is diminished in the red blood cells, low blood pressure, and, when it is in high concentration, narcosis. ASP

**ETHYL NONANOATE** • Nonanoic Acid. A synthetic fruit and rum flavoring additive for beverages, ice cream, ices, candy, baked goods, gelatin desserts, chewing gum, icings, and liqueurs. Mildly toxic by ingestion. A skin irritant. ASP

**ETHYL 2-NONYNOATE** • A synthetic berry, fruit, and melon flavoring additive for beverages, ice cream, ices, candy, and baked goods. ASP

**ETHYL CIS-4-7-OCTADIENOATE** • Flavoring. EAF

**ETHYL OCTANOATE** • Octanoic Acid. A synthetic flavoring additive that occurs naturally in both cognac green and cognac white oils. Used in strawberry, butter, citrus, apple, pineapple, rum, nut, and cheese flavorings for beverages, ice cream, ices, candy, baked goods, gelatin desserts, and chewing gum. Mildly toxic by ingestion. A skin irritant.

**4-ETHYLOCTANOIC ACID** • Flavoring. *See* Octanoic Acid. EAF

**ETHYL CIS-4-OCTENOATE** • Flavoring. *See* Octanoic Acid. ASP

**ETHYL TRANS-2-OCTENOATE** • Flavoring *See* Octanoic Acid. NIL

**ETHYL OCTYNE CARBONATE** • *See* Ethyl 2-Nonynoate.

**ETHYL OLEATE** • Oleic Acid. Synthetic flavoring additive used in butter and fruit flavorings for beverages, ice cream, ices, candy, baked goods, gelatin desserts, and puddings. An ingredient in nail polish remover. It is made from carbon, hydrogen, oxygen, and oleic acid *(see)*.

**ETHYL 3-OXOBUTANOATE** • *See* Ethyl Acetoacetate.

**ETHYL 3-OXOHEXANOATE** • Flavoring or flavor enhancer. NIL

**ETHYL OXYHYDRATE** • *See* Rum Ether.

**ETHYL PALMITATE** • Ethyl Hexadecanoate. The ester of ethyl alcohol and palmitic acid *(see both)*. Synthetic flavoring additive used in butter, honey, apricot, and cherry flavorings for beverages, ice cream, ices, candy, and baked goods. ASP

**ETHYL-*p*-HYDROXYBENZOATE** • *See* Hydroxy and Benzoates. E

**ETHYL *p*-ETHYLPHENOL** • Flavoring FAO/WHO's *(see)* evaluation in 2000 found no safety concern at current levels of intake when used as a flavoring additive. *See* Phenol. ASP

**ETHYL PHENYLACETATE** • Flavoring. *See* Acetic Acid. ASP

**ETHYL 4-PHENYLBUTYRATE** • Flavoring. ASP

**ETHYL 3-PHENYLGLYCIDATE** • Flavoring. ASP

**ETHYL 3-PHENYLPROPIONATE** • Flavoring. ASP

**ETHYL PROPYL DISULFIDE** • A flavoring determined GRAS by FEMA *(see)*. *See* Heptanal.

**ETHYL PROPYL TRISULFIDE** • A flavoring determined GRAS by FEMA *(see)*. *See* Octanal.

**ETHYL PERSATE** • Persic Oil Acid. Ethyl Ester. The ethyl ester of the fatty acids derived from either apricot kernel oil or peach kernel oil. *See* Apricot Kernel Oil and Peach Kernel Oil.

**ETHYL PHENYLACETATE** • Phenylacetic Acid. A synthetic flavoring additive with a sweet honey rose odor. Used in honey, butter, apricot, and cherry flavorings for beverages, ice cream, ices, candy, baked goods, and syrups. Moderately toxic by ingestion.

**ETHYL PHENYL ACRYLATE** • *See* Ethyl Cinnamate.

**ETHYL 3-PHENYL BUTYRATE** • A synthetic berry, strawberry, fruit, and cherry flavoring additive for beverages, ice cream, ices, candy, baked goods, and gelatin desserts.

**ETHYL 4-PHENYL BUTYRATE** • A synthetic fruit flavoring additive for beverages and candy.

**ETHYL PHENYLGLYCIDATE** • Colorless liquid with a strong strawberry odor used as a flavoring additive. Moderately toxic by ingestion. May be mutagenic.

**ETHYL 3-PHENYLPROPIONATE** • A synthetic fruit flavoring additive for beverages, ice cream, ices, candy, and baked goods. *See* Ethyl Cinnamate.

**ETHYL 1-PROPENE-1,2,3-TRICARBOXYLATE** • *See* Ethyl Aconitate.

**ETHYL PROPIONATE** • Propionic Acid. A synthetic flavoring additive, colorless, transparent liquid, with a fruit odor. Occurs naturally in apples. Used in butter, fruit, and rum flavorings for beverages, ice cream, gelatin desserts, baked goods, and chewing gum (1,100 ppm). Moderately toxic by ingestion. A skin irritant.

**ETHYL PYRUVATE** • Pyruvic Acid. A synthetic chocolate, fruit, rum, maple, and spice flavoring additive for beverages, ice cream, ices, candy, and baked goods.

**ETHYL SALICYLATE** • Salicylic Ether. Used in the manufacture of artificial perfumes. Occurs naturally in strawberries and has a pleasant odor. Used as a synthetic flavoring additive in fruit, root beer, sassafras, and wintergreen flavorings for beverages, ice cream, ices, candy, baked goods, chewing gum, gelatins, and puddings. At one time it was given medically to rheumatics. May interact with harmful results with medications such as anticoagulants, antidepressants, and medications for cancer such as Methotrexate. May cause allergic reaction in persons allergic to salicylates *(see)*. ASP

**ETHYL SEBACATE** • *See* Diethyl Sebacate.

**O-ETHYL S (-2-FURYLMETHYL)THIOCARBONATE** • A flavoring determined GRAS by FEMA *(see)*. *See* Heptanal.

**ETHYL SORBATE** • A synthetic fruit flavoring additive for beverages, ice cream, ices, candy, and baked goods. ASP

**ETHYL STEARATE** • The ester of ethyl alcohol and stearic acid *(see both)*.

**ETHYL TETRADECANOATE** • *See* Ethyl Myristate.

**ETHYL TIGLATE** • Tiglic Acid. A synthetic raspberry, strawberry, pineapple, and rum flavoring additive for beverages, ice cream, ices, candy, and liquor. ASP

**ETHYL TRANS-2-DECENOATE** • Flavoring agent or adjuvant. Can be used in milk. ASP

**ETHYL TRANS-4-DECENOATE** • Used as a flavoring. Can be used in milk. ASP

**ETHYL TRANS-2-METHYL-2-BUTENOATE** • *See* Ethyl Tiglate.

**ETHYL 10-UNDECENOATE** • A synthetic coconut, fruit, cognac, and nut flavoring additive for beverages, ice cream, ices, candy, baked goods, and liquor. ASP

**ETHYL UROCANATE** • The ester of ethyl alcohol and urocanic acid. *See* Imidazoline.

**ETHYL VALERATE** • Valeric Acid. A synthetic butter, apple, apricot, peach, and nut flavoring additive for beverages, ice cream, ices, candy, baked goods, gelatin desserts, and chewing gum. ASP

**ETHYL VANILLIN** • An ingredient in perfumes. Colorless flakes, with an odor and flavor stronger than vanilla. Used as a synthetic flavoring additive in raspberry, strawberry, butter, butterscotch, caramel, rum, butter, chocolate, cocoa, citrus, coconut, macaroon, cola, fruit, cherry, grape, honey, liquor, muscatel, rum, maple, nut, pecan, root beer, vanilla, and cream soda flavorings for beverages, ice cream, ices, candy, baked goods, gelatin desserts, puddings, chewing gum, imitation vanilla extract (28,000 ppm), liquor, icings, and toppings. Caused mild skin irritation in humans. In rats, it produced a reduction in growth rate and heart, kidney, liver, lung, spleen, and stomach injuries. GRAS. ASP

**ETHYL VANILLIN BETA-D-GLUCOPYRANOSIDE** • Flavoring with a very slight vanilla odor. EAF

**ETHYLACETIC ACID** • *See* Butyric Acid.

**2-ETHYLBUTYRIC ACID** • A synthetic fruit, nut, and walnut flavoring additive for beverages, ice cream, ices, candy, and baked goods.

**ETHYLENE** • The sixth-highest-volume chemical produced in the United States, it is a colorless gas with a sweet odor and taste. It is derived from heat-cracking hydrocarbon gases or from fluid removal of ethanol. It is used to make chemical compounds including those used to make plastics, refrigerants, anesthetics, and orchard sprays to accelerate fruit ripening. It is highly flammable and potentially explosive. It can asphyxiate.

**ETHYLENE BRASSYLATE** • *See* Erucic Acid.

**1,2-ETHYLENE DIBROMIDE** • A colorless, nonflammable liquid with a sweetish odor derived from bromine and ethylene. Used as a scavenger for lead in gasoline, as a fumigant, general solvent, and in waterproofing products. A cancer-causing additive, toxic by inhalation, ingestion, and skin absorption; a strong irritant to eyes and skin.

**ETHYLENE DICHLORIDE (EDC)** • Dutch Liquid. 1,2-Dichlorethane. Ethylene Chloride. The halogenate aliphatic hydrocarbon derived from the action of chlorine on ethylene. It is used in the manufacture of vinyl chloride *(see)*. Colorless, heavy liquid with a sweet odor, it is widely used as a fumigant for cereal grains, corn grits, cracked rice, and fermented malt beverages; as a solvent for fats, waxes, spices, and resins; as a lead scavenger in antiknock gasolines, in paint, varnish, and finish removers; as a wetting additive; as a penetrating additive; in organic synthesis; and in the making of polyvinyl chloride (PVC) *(see)*. It is one of the highest volume chemicals produced. It can be highly toxic whether taken into the body by ingestion, inhalation, or skin absorption. It is irritating to the mucous membranes. In cancer testing, the National Cancer Institute found this compound caused stomach cancer, vascularized cancers of multiple organs, and cancers beneath the skin in male rats. Female rats exposed to EDC developed mammary cancers—in some high-dose animals as early as the twentieth week of the study. The chemical also caused breast cancers as well as uterine cancers in female mice and respiratory tract cancers in both sexes. Deaths due to liver and kidney injury following ingestion of large amounts (30 to 70 grams) have been reported. Clouding of the eyes, hemorrhages, and destruction of the adrenal cortex have been reported in humans and dogs. Annual production in the United States is now estimated at about 10 billion pounds—the sixteenth largest of all chemicals. EDC has been found in human milk and in the exhaled breath of nursing mothers who were exposed to the chemical. FDA tolerances for residues are: 125 ppm in cereal grain; 25 ppm in fermented malt beverages. A solvent used in the production of spices, it is also used in processing animal byproducts for use in animal feeds and in pesticide compounds. The FDA's residue tolerances for spices is 30 ppm and 300 ppm in extracted by-products. On the Community Right-to-Know List and under IARC Cancer Review *(see both)*. Human poison by ingestion. Skin irritant. Implicated in worker sterility. The FAO/WHO Committee found it causes birth defects and that it causes cancer in mice and rats when administered orally. The committee expressed the opinion that this solvent (1,2-dichloroethane) should not be used in food. NIL

**ETHYLENE DIOLEAMIDE** • *See* Fatty Acids.

**ETHYLENE DISTEARAMIDE** • *See* Fatty Acids.

**ETHYLENE GLYCOL** • A slightly viscous liquid with a sweet taste. Absorbs twice its weight in water. Used as an antifreeze and humectant *(see);* also as a solvent. Toxic when ingested, causing central nervous system depression, vomiting, drowsiness, coma, respiratory failure, kidney damage, and possibly death.

**ETHYLENE GLYCOL DISTEARATE** • *See* Ethylene Glycol and Stearic Acid. NUL

**ETHYLENE GLYCOL MONOBUTYL ETHER** • *See* Ethylene Glycol and Butyl Acetate. ASP

**ETHYLENE GLYCOL MONOETHYL ETHER** • *See* Ethylene Glycol. ASP

**ETHYLENE OXIDE** • A fumigant used on ground spices and other processed natural seasonings. A colorless gas, liquid at 12°C. Derived from the oxidation of ethylene in air or oxygen with silver catalyst. Irritant to the eyes and skin. A suspected human carcinogen. On the Community Right-To-Know List and under IARC Cancer Review *(see both)*.

**ETHYLENE OXIDE (EtO)** • A high-volume chemical with production exceeding 1 million pounds annually in the United States. Used in consumer products, building materials, or furnishings that contribute to indoor air pollution. Used in pesticide products. OSHA *(see)* says EtO possesses several physical and health hazards. It is both flammable and highly reactive. Acute exposures to EtO gas may result in respiratory irritation and lung injury, headache, nausea, vomiting, diarrhea, shortness of breath, and cyanosis. Chronic exposure has been associated with the occurrence of cancer, reproductive effects, mutagenic changes, neurotoxicity, and sensitization. ASP

**ETHYLENE OXIDE-METHYL FORMATE MIXTURE** • A mold and yeast control additive in dried and glacéed fruits. Ethylene oxide is highly irritating to the mucous membranes and eyes. High concentrations may cause pulmonary edema. Inhalation of methyl formate vapor produces nasal and eye irritation, retching, narcosis, and death from pulmonary irritation. Exposure to 1 percent vapor for two and a half hours or 5 percent vapor for a half hour is lethal.

**ETHYLENE OXIDE POLYMER** • Used as a stabilizer in fermented malt beer (300 ppm by weight). *See* Ethylene Oxide and Polymers.

**ETHYLENE OXIDE POLYMER, ALKYL ADDUCT, PHOSPHATE ESTER** • *See* Ehtylene Oxide. NUL

**ETHYLENE OXIDE/PROPYLENE OXIDE COPOLYMER, ALKYL ADDUCT** • *See* Ethylene Oxide and Propylene Glycol. ASP

**ETHYLENE OXIDE/PROPYLENE OXIDE COPOLYMER, ALKYL ADDUCT, PHOSPHATE ESTER** • *See* Ethylene Oxide and Propylene Glycol. NUL

**ETHYLENE OXIDE/PROPYLENE OXIDE COPOLYMER** • *See* Ethylene Oxide and Propylene Glycol. ASP

**ETHYLENE UREA** • *See* Urea.

**ETHYLENEBUTYRALDEHYDE** • A synthetic chocolate flavoring additive for beverages, ice cream, ices, candy, and baked goods.

**ETHYLENEDIAMINE** • Colorless, clear, thick, and strongly alkaline. A component of a bacteria-killing agent in processing sugarcane. Also used as a solvent for casein, albumin, and shellac. Has been used as a urinary acidifier. It can cause sensitization leading to asthma and allergic skin rashes.

**ETHYLENEDIAMINE TETRAACETIC ACID (EDTA)** • An important compound in cosmetics used primarily as a sequestering additive *(see),* in carbonated beverages. EDTA salts are used in crabmeat (cooked and canned) to retard struvite (crystal) formation, and promote color retention. It is also used in nonstandardized dressings. It may be irritating to the skin and mucous membranes and cause allergies such as asthma and skin rashes. Also used as a sequestrant in carbonated beverages. When ingested, it may cause errors in a number of laboratory tests, including those for calcium, carbon dioxide, nitrogen, and muscular activity. It is on the FDA list of food additives to be studied for toxicity. It can cause kidney damage. The trisodium salt of EDTA was fed to rats and mice for nearly two years. According to a summary of the report, "Although a variety of tumors occurred among test and control animals of both species, the test did not indicate that any of the tumors observed in the test animals were attributed to EDTA." The tests were part of the National Cancer Institute's Carcinogenesis Bioassay Program.

**trans-1,2-ETHYLENEDICARBOXYLIC ACID** • *See* Fumaric Acid.

**EUBATUS, RUBUS** • See Blackberry Bark Extract.

**EUCALYPTOL** • Eucalyptus Oil. A chief constituent of eucalyptus and cajeput oils. Occurs naturally in allspice, star anise, bay, calamus, and peppermint oil. Eucalyptus oil is 70 to 80 percent active eucalyptol. Eucalyptol is used in mint flavorings for beverages, ice cream, ices, candy, baked goods, and chewing gum. An antiseptic, antispasmodic, and expectorant. Fatalities followed ingestion of doses as small as 3 to 5 milliliters (about a teaspoon), and recovery has occurred after doses as large as 20 to 30 milliliters (about 4 to 5 teaspoons). Symptoms of poisoning are epigastric burning with nausea, weakness, water retention, and delirium. ASP

**EUCALYPTUS EXTRACT** • *See* Eucalyptus Oil.

**EUCALYPTUS GLOBULUS LEAVES** • A flavoring. *See* Eucalyptus Oil.

**EUCALYPTUS OIL** • Dinkum Oil. The colorless to pale yellow volatile liquid from the fresh leaves of the eucalyptus tree. It is 70 to 80 percent eucalyptol and has a spicy cool taste and a characteristic aromatic, somewhat camphorlike odor. Used in fruit, mint, root beer, spice, and ginger ale flavorings for beverages, ice cream, ices, candy, baked goods, chewing gum, and liquor. Used as a local antiseptic. Has been used as an expectorant, vermifuge, and local antiseptic. Doses as small as 3 to 5 milliliters (about equal to a teaspoon) and about 1 milliliter have caused coma. Fatalities have followed doses as small as 3.5 milliliters. Symptoms include epigastric burning with nausea. Symptoms have been reported to occur as long as two hours after ingestion. ASP

**EUCHEUMA COTTON EXTRACT** • A flavoring. *See* Eucheuma Seaweed.

**EUCHEUMA SEAWEED (PROCESSED)** • *Eucheuma cottonii* Extract. *Eucheuma spinosum* Extract. A stabilizing and thickening additive derived from eucheuma seaweed used in dairy products to suspend particles and for gelling in foods. In a ninety-day study in rats, processed eucheuma administered at 0.5 percent, 1.5 percent, and 5 percent in the diet produced "no effects of toxicological significance" according to the FAO/WHO *(see)*. *See* Hydrogenation and Carrageenan. E

**EUCHEUMA SPINOSUM EXTRACT** • An emulsifier and stabilizer. *See* Eucheuma Seaweed.

**EUGENOL** • A synthetic fruit, nut, and spice flavoring for beverages, ice cream, ices, candy, baked goods, chewing gum, gelatin desserts, meats (2,000 ppm), and condiments. Used as a defoamer in yeast production, in the manufacture of vanilla. Eugenol also acts as a local antiseptic. When ingested, may cause vomiting and gastric irritation. Because of its potential as an allergen, it is left out of hypoallergenic cosmetics. Toxicity is similar to phenol, which is highly toxic. Death in laboratory animals given eugenol is due to vascular collapse. Methyl Eugenol, a flavoring, has also been found to cause tumors in rats but FEMA *(see)* says that at current use, it probably offers no danger to humans but nevertheless, it requires further study. GRAS. ASP

**EUGENYL ACETATE** • Acetic Acid. A synthetic berry, fruit, mint, spice, and vanilla flavoring additive for beverages, ice cream, ices, candy, baked goods, chewing gum, and condiments. ASP

**EUGENYL BENZOATE** • Synthetic fruit and spice flavoring additive for beverages, ice cream, ices, candy, and baked goods. ASP

**EUGENYL FORMATE** • Formic Acid. Synthetic spice flavoring additive used in condiments. *See* Formic Acid for toxicity. ASP

**EUGENYL METHYL ETHER** • Synthetic raspberry, strawberry, fruit, spice, clove, and ginger flavoring additive for beverages, ice cream, ices, candy, baked goods, and jellies. ASP

**EVERNIA FURFURACEA** • *See* Oakmoss, Absolute.

**EVERNIA PRUNASTIC** • *See* Oakmoss, Absolute.

**EXATOLIDE** • *See* Pentadecalactone.

**EXCITOTOXICOLOGY** • The study of chemicals that overstimulate and damage nerves. Glutamate *(see)* is considered an excitotoxin.

**EXCITOTOXIN** • *See* Excitotoxicology.

**EXTRACT** • The solution that results from passing alcohol or an alcohol-water mixture through a substance. Examples of extracts would be the alcohol-water mixture of vanillin, orange, or lemon extracts found among the spices and flavorings on the supermarket shelf. Extracts are not as strong as essential oils *(see)*.

**EYE ALLERGY** • There are many forms of allergy of the eye. The mucous membranes of the eye may be involved in allergic rhinitis. Such allergic conjunctivitis may also occur by itself without irritation of the nose. Dust, mold spores, foods, and eye medications may all cause conjunctivitis. There is also a less severe, chronic form of allergic conjunctivitis. Symptoms include prolonged photophobia, itching, burning, and a feeling of dryness. There may be a watery discharge and finding the source of allergy is often difficult.

**(E)-3-(Z)-6-NONADIEN-1-OL** • Flavoring declared GRAS by FEMA *(see)*. EAF

**(E,Z)-3,6-NONADIEN-1-OL ACETATE** • Flavoring declared GRAS by FEMA *(see)*. EAF

**(E,Z)-2,6-NONADIEN-1-OL ACETATE** • Flavoring declared GRAS by FEMA *(see)*. EAF

# F

**FANTESK** • A fat replacer developed by the U.S. Department of Agriculture and licensed exclusively to Opta Food Ingredients. It is based on a combination of starches or gums with a small amount of oil. It has the taste and texture of regular fat but provides less than 0.5 grams of fat per serving.

**FAO/WHO EXPERT COMMITTEE ON FOOD ADDITIVES** • An international group of experts from the World Health Organization (WHO) and the Food and Agriculture Organization of the United Nations (FAO). The members meet periodically to evaluate the safety of various food additives and contaminants with a view to recommending acceptable daily intakes for humans and to prepare specifications for the identity and purity of food additives. The preparatory work for toxicological evaluations of food additives and contaminants by the Joint FAO/WHO Expert Committee on Food Additives is actively supported by certain of the member states that contribute to the work of the International Program on Chemical Safety. The Joint FAO/WHO Expert Committee on Food Additives (JECFA) is an international expert scientific committee that is administered jointly by the Food and Agriculture Organization of the United Nations and the World Health Organization. It has been meeting since 1956, initially to evaluate the safety of food additives. Its work now also includes the evaluation of contaminants, naturally occurring toxicants, and residues of veterinary drugs in food. To date, JECFA has evaluated more than fifteen hundred food additives, approximately forty contaminants and naturally occurring toxicants, and residues of approximately ninety veterinary drugs. The committee has also developed principles for the safety assessment of chemicals in food that are consistent with current thinking on risk assessment and take account of recent developments in toxicology and other relevant sciences. JECFA normally meets twice a year with individual agendas covering either (1) food additives, contaminants, and naturally occurring toxicants in food or (2) residues of veterinary drugs in food. The membership of the meetings varies accordingly, with different sets of experts being called on depending on the subject matter of the meeting.

**FARNESAL** • Flavoring. *See* Farnesol. EAF

**FARNESENE** • Flavoring. *See* Farnesol. EAF

**FARNESOL** • A flavoring with a fresh green odor that occurs naturally in ambrette seed, star anise, cassia, linden flowers, oils of muskseed, citronella, rose, and balsam. Used in berry, apricot, banana, cherry, melon, peach, citrus, fruit, raspberry, and strawberry flavorings for beverages, ice cream, ices, candy, baked goods, and gelatin desserts. Used in perfumery to emphasize the odor of sweet floral perfumes such as lilac. Mildly toxic when ingested. Caused mutations in laboratory animals. ASP

**FARNESYL ACETATE** • Synethic flavoring with a green floral, rosy odor.

**FASEB** • Abbreviation for the Federation of American Societies for Experimental Biology, members of which evaluate studies for the FDA.

**FAT** • The most concentrated source of food energy and very necessary to health. Fat deposits provide insulation and protection for body structure as well as a storehouse for energy. Fats are composed of fatty acids and glycerol. Fatty acids consist of a long chain of carbons with a carboxyl group at one end. Depending on their structure, fatty acids can be saturated or unsaturated. While fats have been denigrated to the point that many believe that fat should be eliminated from the diet, fat serves many useful purposes. Fats store energy, help to insulate the body, and cushion and protect. Food fats are carriers of fat-soluble vitamins and include certain essential unsaturated fatty acids *(see)*. Saturated fats contain only single-bond carbon linkages and are the least active chemically. They are usually solid at room temperature. Most animal fats are saturated. The common saturated fats are acetic, butyric, caproic, caprylic, capric, lauric, myristic, palmitic, stearic, arachidic, and behenic. Butterfat, coconut oil, and peanut oil are high in saturated fats. Unsaturated fats contain one or more double-bond carbon linkages and are usually liquid at room temperature. Vegetable oils and fish oils most frequently contain unsaturated fats. Among the unsaturated fats are caproleic, lauroleic, myristoleic, palmitoleic, oleic, and linoleic. *See* Saturated Fats, Phospholipids, Steroids, and Unsaturated Fats.

**FAT CAL** • Listing on labels signifying calories from fat.

**FAT FREE** • Less than 0.5 grams per serving. However, manufacturers are permitted to "round down" and claim zero fat even if a product contains 0.6 grams of fat. Very few foods are actually completely fat free.

**FATIGUE** • Everyone's nose becomes "fatigued" when smelling a certain odor. No matter how much you like an aroma, you can only smell it for a short interval. It is nature's way of protecting humans from overstimulation of the olfactory sense.

**FAT REPLACERS** • These additives are aimed at reducing a food's fat and calorie level while maintaining some of the desirable qualities of fat such as "mouth feel," texture, and flavor. Under FDA regulations, these additives usually fall into one of two categories: food additives or "generally recognized as safe" (GRAS) substances. Food additives must be evaluated for safety and approved by the FDA before they can be marketed. They include substances with no proven track record of safety or with no known amount in food that may serve the purpose of fat replacement. Examples are polydextrose, carrageenan, and olestra *(see all)*, which are used as fat replacers. GRAS substances, on the other hand, are used in foods because they are generally recognized as safe by scientists because of their long history of use in foods. Examples of such fat replacers are cellulose gel, dextrins, guar gum, and gum arabic. Fat replacers may be carbohydrate, protein, or fat-based substances.

**FATTY ACIDS** • One of any mixture of liquid and solid acids, capric, caprylic, lauric, myristic, oleic, palmitic, and stearic. In combination with glycerin they form fat. Necessary for normal growth and skin. In foods they are used as emulsifiers, binders, and lubricants, and defoamer components in the processing of beet sugar and yeast. Polyglycerol esters of fatty acids are prepared from edible fats, oils, corn, cottonseed, palm, fruit, peanut, safflower, and soybean oils, lard, and tallow. Used as emulsifiers and defoaming additives in beet sugar and yeast production, and as lubricant binders and components in the manufacture of other food additives. Fatty acid salt (one or more of the aluminum, ammonium, calcium, magnesium, potassium, and sodium salts of all the above fatty acids) are used as emulsifiers, binders, and anticaking additives. A free fatty acid (FFA) is the uncombined fatty acid present in a fat. Some raw oils may contain as much as 3 percent FFA. These are removed in the refining process and refined fats and oils ready for use as foods usually have extremely low FFA content. *See* Stearic Acid. EAF. E

**FATTY ALCOHOLS, SYNTHETIC** • Solid alcohols made from acids. In foods, synthetic fatty alcohols include hexyl, octyl, decyl, lauryl, myristyl, cetyl, and stearyl alcohols. They are used as substitutes for the corresponding naturally derived fatty alcohols. Very low toxicity.

**FDA (FOOD and DRUG ADMINISTRATION)** • The U.S. Food and Drug Administration is part of the Public Health Service of the U.S. Department of Health and Human Services. It is the regulatory agency responsible for ensuring the safety and wholesomeness of all foods sold in interstate commerce except meat, poultry, and eggs, which are under the jurisdiction of the U.S. Department of Agriculture. The FDA develops standards for the composition, quality, nutrition, safety, and labeling of foods including food and color additives. It conducts research to improve detection and prevention of contamination. It collects and interprets data on nutrition, food additives, and pesticide residues. The agency also inspects food plants, imported food products, and feed mills that make feeds containing medications or nutritional supplements that are destined for human consumption. And it regulates radiation-emitting products such as microwave ovens. The FDA also enforces pesticide tolerances established by the Environmental Protection Agency for all domestically produced and imported foods, except for foods under USDA jurisdiction.

**FD and C COLORS** • Food, Drug, and Cosmetic Colors. A color additive is a term to describe any dye, pigment, or other substance capable of coloring a food, drug, or cosmetic, on any part of the human body. In 1900, there were more than eighty dyes used to color food. There were no regulations and the same dye used to color clothes could also be used to color candy. In 1906, the first comprehensive legislation for food colors was passed. There were only seven colors, which, when tested, were shown to be composed of known ingredients which demonstrated no harmful effects. Those colors were orange, erythrosine, ponceau 3R, amaranth, indigotin, naphthol yellow, and light green. A voluntary system of certification for batches of color dyes was set up. In 1938, new legislation was passed, superseding the 1906 act. The colors were given numbers instead of chemical names and every batch had to be certified. There were fifteen food colors in use at the time. In 1950, children were made ill by certain coloring used in candy and popcorn. These incidents led to the delisting of FD and C Orange No. 1, Orange No. 2, and FD and C Red No. 32. Since that time, because of experimental evidence of possible harm, Red 1, Yellow 1, 2, 3, and 4 have also been delisted. Violet 1 was removed in 1973. In 1976, one of the most widely used of all colors, FD and C Red No. 2, was removed because it was found to cause tumors in rats. In 1976, Red No. 4 was banned for coloring maraschino cherries (its last use), and carbon black was also banned, because both contain cancer-causing additives. Earlier, in 1960, scientific investigations were required by law to determine the suitability of all colors in use for permanent listing. Citrus Red No. 2 (limited to 2 ppm) for coloring orange skins has been permanently listed; Blue No. 1, Red No. 3, Yellow No. 5, and Red No. 40 are permanently listed but without any restrictions. In 1959, the Food and Drug Administration approved the use of "lakes," in which the dyes are mixed with alumina hydrate to make them insoluble. *See* FD and C Lakes. The other food coloring additives remained on the "temporary list." The provisional list permitted colors then in use to continue on a provisional, or interim, basis pending completion of studies to determine whether the colors should be permanently approved or terminated. FD and C Red No. 3 (erythrosin) is permanently listed for use in food and ingested drugs and provisionally listed for cosmetics and externally applied drugs. It is used in foods such as gelatins, cake mixes, ice cream, fruit cocktail cherries, bakery goods, and sausage casings. The FDA postponed the closing date for the provisionally listed color additives—FD and C Red No. 3, D and C Red No. 33, and D and C Red No. 36—to May 2, 1988, to allow additional time to study "complex scientific and legal questions about the colors before deciding to approve or terminate their use in food, drugs, and cosmetics." The agency asked for sixty days to consider the impact of the October 1987 U.S. Court of Appeals ruling that there is no exception to the Delaney Amendment *(see),* which says that cancer-causing additives may not be added to food. On July 13, 1988, the Public Citizens Health Research Group announced that the FDA agreed to revoke by July 15, 1988, the permanent listing of four color additives used in drugs and cosmetics—D and C Red No. 8, D and C Red No. 9, D and C Red No. 19, and D and C Orange No. 17. In a unanimous decision in October 1987, the U.S. Court of Appeals for the District of Columbia said the FDA lacked legal authority to approve two of the colors, D and C Orange No. 17 and D and C Red No. 19, since they had been found to induce cancer in laboratory animals. The Supreme Court ruled against an appeal on April 18, 1988. Meanwhile, Public Citizen also brought a similar suit, challenging the use of D and C Red No. 8 and D and C Red 9, which was before the U.S. Circuit Court of Appeals in Philadelphia. Under an agreement between FDA and Public Citizen, the case was sent back to the FDA, and the agency delisted these colors as well as D and C Orange No. 17 and D and C Red No. 19. Other countries as well as the World Health Organization maintain there are inconsistencies in safety data and in the banning of some colors, which in turn affects international commerce. As of this writing, there is still a great deal of confusion about the colors, with the FDA maintaining that the cancer risk is minimal—as low as one in a billion—while groups such as Ralph Nader's Public Citizen maintain that any cancer risk for a food additive is unacceptable. In 1990, the lakes of Red. No. 3 were removed for all uses from the approved list. The color itself was also removed in 1990 for cosmetic and external drug use. It is still, as of this writing, approved for food and ingested drugs.

**FD and C BLUE NO. 1** • Brilliant Blue FD and C. A bright blue, coal-tar derivative, triphenylmethane, it is used as a coloring in bottled soft drinks, gelatin desserts, ice cream, ices, dry drink powders, candy, confections, bakery products, cereals, and puddings. It is also used for hair colorings, face powders, and other cosmetics. May cause allergic reactions. On the FDA permanent list of color additives. Rated 1A—that is, completely acceptable for nonfood use by the World Health Organization. However, it produces malignant tumors at the site of injection and by ingestion in rats. Manganese dioxide is now permitted in the manufacturing process. The Food and Drug Administration (FDA) warned in 2003 of several reports of toxicity, including death, temporally associated with the use of FD and C Blue No. 1 (Blue 1) in enteral feeding solutions. In these reports, Blue 1 was intended to help in the detection and/or monitoring of pulmonary aspiration in patients being fed by an enteral feeding tube. Reported episodes were manifested by blue discoloration of the skin, urine, feces, or serum and some were associated with serious complications such as refractory low blood pressure, metabolic acidosis, and death. Case reports indicate that seriously ill patients, particularly those with a likely increase in gut permeability (e.g., patients with sepsis), may be at greater risk for these complications. Because these events were reported voluntarily from a population of unknown size, it is not possible to establish the incidence of these episodes. A causal relationship between systemic absorption of Blue 1 and the reported serious and life-threatening patient outcomes (including death) has not been definitively established. *See* Colors. ASP

**FD and C BRILLIANT BLUE NO. 1 ALUMINUM LAKE** • Aluminum salt of certified of FD and C Brilliant Blue No. 1 *(see)*. Can be used around the eye in cosmetics. Also permitted for drug use. *See* FD and C Colors, Lakes. ASP

**FD and C BLUE NO. 1, CALCIUM LAKE** • *See* FD&C Lakes. NUL

**FD and C BLUE NO. 2** • Indigotin. Indigo Carmine. A royal blue powder, a coal-tar derivative, triphenylmethane, almost always contains sodium chloride or sulfate. Easily faded by light. Used in bottled soft drinks, bakery products, cereals, candy, confections, and dry drink powders. Is also in mint-flavored jelly, frozen desserts, candy, confections, and rinses and as a dye in kidney tests and for testing milk. It is a sensitizer in the allergic. Produces malignant tumors at the site of injection when introduced under the skin of rats. The World Health Organization gives it a toxicology rating of B—available data not entirely sufficient to meet requirements acceptable for food use. Permanently listed for foods and drugs in 1987. See FD and C Colors. ASP

**FD and C BLUE NO. 2 ALUMINUM LAKE** • *See* FD&C Lakes. ASP

**FD and C BLUE NO. 2 CALCIUM LAKE** • *See* FD&C Lakes. NUL

**FD and C CITRUS RED No. 2** • Found in 1960 to damage internal organs and to be a weak cancer-causing additive. Permitted for use only to color orange skins. The World Health Organization said the color has been shown to cause cancer and that toxicological data available were inadequate to allow the determination of a safe limit; they recommended that it not be used as a food color. The FDA ruled on October 28, 1971, that the results of several rodent studies and one dog study using both oral and injected Citrus Red No. 2 showed either no adverse effect or no adverse effect levels. No abnormalities in urinary bladders were reported. The FDA noted that a paper presented in 1965 by the University of Otega Medical School reported a significant level of urinary bladder cancers in rodents fed the dye for up to twenty-four months. The FDA said that since slides of the tissues in photographs were not yet available for examination, and since there has been no confirmation of the studies, the listing of Citrus Red No. 2 should remain unchanged until the Otega results can be confirmed by examination. *See* FD and C Colors.

**FD and C GREEN NO. 1** • Guinea Green B. A dull, dark green powder used as a coloring in bottled soft drinks. The certified color industry did not apply for the extension of this color because of the small demand for its use, so it was automatically deleted from the list of color additives in 1966. Rated E by the World Health Organization, meaning it was found to be harmful and not to be used in food. No longer authorized for use by the FDA. BANNED. *See* FD and C Colors.

**FD and C GREEN NO. 2** • Light Green S.F. Yellow. Coloring used in bottled soft drinks. Because of lack of demand for this color, the certified color industry did not petition for extension and it was automatically deleted in 1966. It produces tumors at the site of injection under the skin of rats. No longer authorized for use by the FDA. BANNED. *See* FD and C Colors.

**FD and C GREEN NO. 3** • Fast Green. A sea green color permanently listed for use in food, drugs, and cosmetics, except in the area of the eye, by the FDA in 1983. Used as a coloring in mint-flavored jelly, frozen desserts, gelatin desserts, candy, confections, baking products, and cereals. Has been suspected of being a sensitizer in the allergic. On the FDA permanent list of approved color additives. Produces malignant tumors at the site of injection when introduced under the skin of rats. The World Health Organization gives it a toxicology rating of 1A, meaning that it is completely acceptable. *See* FD and C Colors. ASP

**FD and C GREEN NO. 3 ALUMINUM LAKE** • *See* FD&C Lakes. ASP
**FD and C GREEN NO. 3, CALCIUM LAKE** • *See* FD&C Lakes. NUL
**FD and C LAKES** • Aluminum or Calcium Lakes. Lakes are pigments prepared by combining FD and C colors with a form of aluminum or calcium, which makes the colors insoluble. Aluminum and calcium lakes are used in confection and candy products and for dyeing eggshells and other products that are adversely affected by water. *See* FD and C Colors for toxicity.
**FD and C RED NO. 1** • BANNED
**FD and C RED NO. 2** • Amaranth. Formerly one of the most widely used cosmetic and food colorings. A dark, reddish brown powder that turns bright red when mixed with fluid. A monoazo color, it was used in lipsticks, rouges, and other cosmetics as well as in cereals, maraschino cherries, and desserts. The safety of this dye was questioned by American scientists for more than twenty years. Two Russian scientists found that FD and C Red No. 2 prevented some pregnancies and caused some stillbirths in rats. The FDA ordered manufacturers using the color to submit data on all food, drug, and cosmetic products containing it. Controversial tests at the FDA's National Center for Toxicological Research in Arkansas showed that in

high doses Red No. 2 caused a statistically significant increase in a variety of cancers in female rats. The dye was banned by the FDA in January 1976. BANNED. Red No. 2 is still permitted in Canada and Europe.

**FD and C RED NO. 3** • Erythrosin. Bluish Pink. A cherry red coal-tar derivative, a xanthene color, used in toothpaste, canned fruit cocktail, ice cream, hot dogs, barbecue potato chips, cereals, puddings, fruit salad, sherbets, gelatin desserts, cherry pie mix (up to 0.01 percent), candy, confections, and mixes as maraschino cherries. Has been determined a carcinogen. It was reported in 1981 by NIH researchers that Red No. 3 may interfere with transmission of nerve impulses in the brain. It contains iodine and has been shown to affect the thyroid glands of laboratory animals but not of humans. Children who eat large amounts of artificially colored cherries, gelatin desserts, and other FD and C Red No. 3 colored products could be at risk. *See* FD and C Colors. The FDA was supposed to permanently list this color in 1988 but postponed the ruling "to allow the agency additional time to study complex scientific and legal questions about the color before deciding to approve or terminate its use in food." Now permanently listed for food and ingested drugs, its lake use was terminated February 1, 1990. All cosmetic uses were terminated February 1, 1990. In 1996, Red No. 3 was found to be a cancer-causing additive and may contribute to breast cancer. Scientists at Oak Ridge National Laboratory and Northeastern Illinois University reported Red No. 3 causes breast cancer in the laboratory. When the dye was added to a human cell culture, genetic damage and rapid cell growth occurred even when the concentration of the dye was quite low. The cells responded as if they had been exposed to estrogen, which damaged genetic material and caused rapid reproduction. It is still permitted in food but its lake *(see)* was removed from all uses while Red No. 3 itself was removed from the list for use in cosmetics and external drugs. The FDA has said that it intends "to propose rescinding" its use in food and internal drugs. That was in 1990. Though FDA viewed Red No. 3 cancer risks as small—about 1 in 100,000 over a seventy-year lifetime—the agency banned provisional listings because of Delaney directives. At the same time, Red No. 3 has "permanent" listings for food and drug uses that are still allowed although the agency has announced plans to propose revoking these uses as well. For now, Red No. 3 can be used in foods and oral medications. Products such as maraschino cherries, bubble gum, baked goods, and all sorts of snack foods and candy may contain Red No. 3. ASP

**FD and C RED NO. 3 ALUMINUM LAKE** • The aluminum salt of certified FD and C Red No. 3 *(see)*. Was terminated February 1, 1990. *See* FD and C Colors, Lakes. BANNED

**FD and C RED NO. 4** • A monoazo color and coal tar. Used in mouthwashes, bath salts, and hair rinses. The FDA banned it in food in 1964 when it was shown to damage the adrenal glands and bladders of dogs. The agency relented and gave it provisional license for use in maraschino cherries. It was banned in all food in 1976 because it was shown to cause urinary bladder polyps and atrophy of the adrenal glands in animals. It was also banned in orally taken drugs but is still permitted in cosmetics for external use only. *See also* FD and C Colors. BANNED

**FD and C RED NO. 20** • Permanently listed by the FDA in 1983 for general use in drugs and cosmetics (except in areas around the eyes).

**FD and C RED NO. 22** • Permanently listed by the FDA in 1983 for general use in drugs and cosmetics (except in areas around the eyes).

**FD and C RED NO. 40** • Allura Red AC. Newest color. Used widely in the cosmetic industry. Approved in 1971, Allied Chemical has an exclusive patent on it. It is substituted for FD and C Red No. 4 in many cosmetics, food, and drug products. Permanently listed because unlike the producers of "temporary" colors, this producer supplied reproductive data. However, many American scientists feel that the safety of Red No. 40 is far from established particularly because all the tests were conducted by the manufacturer. Therefore, the dye should not have received a permanent safety rating. The National Cancer Institute reported that *p*-credine, a chemical used in preparation of Red No. 40 was carcinogenic in animals. In rats, a high (3,800–8,350 mg/kg) oral dose of the coloring caused adverse reproductive effects. The FDA permanently listed Red No. 40 for use in foods and ingested drugs and cosmetics, including use around the eye area. Its lake *(see)* is permitted only for drug and cosmetic use. *See also* Azo Dyes and FD and C Colors. ASP E

**FD and C RED NO. 40 ALUMINUM LAKE** • *See* FD&C Lakes. ASP

**FD and C RED NO. 40 CALCIUM LAKE** • *See* FD&C Lakes. EAF

**FD and C VIOLET NO. 1** • Used as a coloring matter in gelatin desserts, ices, carbonated beverages, dry drink powders, candy, confections, bakery products, cereals, puddings, and as the dye used for the Department of Agriculture's meat stamp. A Canadian study in 1962 showed the dye caused cancer in 50 percent of the rats fed the dye in food. The FDA did not consider this valid evidence since the exact nature of the dye used could not be determined and all records and specimens were lost and not available for study. Furthermore, previous and subsequent studies have not confirmed evidence of Violet 1 causing cancer in rats. However, a two-year study with dogs did show noncancerous lesions on the dog's ears after being fed Violet 1. The FDA again felt the study was not adequate but that the ear lesions did appear to be dye-related and that perhaps two years may be too short a period to determine the eventual outcome. The FDA ruled on October 28, 1971, that Violet 1 should remain provisionally listed pending the outcome of a new dog study to be started as soon as possible and to last seven years. The FDA finally banned the use of Violet 1 in 1973. In 1976, however, the U.S. Department of Agriculture found that Violet 1 was still being used as a "denaturant" on carcasses, meats, and food products. The USDA ruled that any such use of mixing Violet 1 with any substance intended for food use would cause the final product to be "adulterated." *See* FD and C Colors. BANNED

**FD and C YELLOW NO. 5** • Tartrazine. A lemon yellow coal-tar derivative, is a pyrazole color used in prepared breakfast cereals, imitation strawberry, jelly, bottled soft drinks, gelatin desserts, ice cream, sherbets, dry drink powders, candy, confections, bakery products, spaghetti, and puddings. Also used as a coloring in hair rinses, hair-waving fluids, and in bath salts. Causes allergic reactions in persons sensitive to aspirin. The certified color industry petitioned for permanent listing of this color in February 1966, with no limitations other than good manufacturing practice. However, in February 1966, the FDA proposed the listing of this color with a maximum rate of use of 300 ppm in food. The color industry had objected to the limitations. Yellow No. 5 was thereafter permanently listed as a color additive without restrictions. Rated 1A by the World Health Organization—acceptable in food. It is estimated that half the aspirin-sensitive people plus 47,000 to 94,000 others in the nation are sensitive to this dye. It is used in about 60 percent of both over-the-counter and prescription drugs. Efforts were made to ban this color in over-the-counter pain relievers, antihistamines, oral decongestants, and prescription antiinflammatory drugs. Aspirin-sensitive patients have been reported to develop life-threatening asthmatic symptoms when ingesting Yellow No. 5. Since 1981, it is supposed to be listed on the label if it is used. Its lake *(see)* is for drug and cosmetic use only. *See* FD and C Colors. There is reported use of the chemical; it has not yet been assigned for toxicology literature. ASP

**FD and C YELLOW NO. 5 ALUMINUM LAKE** • For drug and cosmetic use only. *See* FD and C Yellow No. 5, Colors, Lakes. ASP

**FD and C YELLOW NO. 5 CALCIUM LAKE** • *See* FD and C Lakes. EAF

**FD and C YELLOW NO. 6** • Monoazo. Sunset Yellow FCF. A coal-tar, monoazo color, used in carbonated beverages, bakery products, candy, confectionery products, gelatin desserts, and dry drink powders. It is also used in hair rinses as well as other cosmetics. It is not used in products that contain fats and oils. Since there is evidence that this causes allergic reactions, alcoholic beverages that contain it must list it on the label according to the Bureau of Alcohol. Rated 1A by the World Health Organization—acceptable in foods. Permanently listed December 22, 1986. In 1989, a ruling went into effect that it had to be listed on the labels because of its ability to induce allergic reactions. *See* FD and C Colors. ASP. E

**FD and C YELLOW NO. 6 ALUMINUM LAKE** • *See* FD and C Yellow No. 6, Colors, Lakes. ASP

**FD and C YELLOW NO. 6 CALCIUM LAKE** • *See* FD and C Lakes. EAF

**FECULOSE STARCH ACETATE** • *See* Modified Starch.

**FEED** • Substance under the Food Additives Ammendment added directly to feed.

**FEMA** • Stands for the Expert Panel of the Flavor and Extract Manufacturers Association. In 1960, it created the FEMA GRAS program in which "the safety of flavor ingredients would be evaluated for potential GRAS *(see)* status by an independent panel of experts in the fields of chemistry, toxicology, pharmacology, medicine, pathology, and flavor assessment." The FDA has acknowledged the validity of the FEMA GRAS program and has recognized the FEMA GRAS publications as "reliable industry GRAS lists."

**FENAMIPHOS** • A worm killer used in animal feeds, pineapples, and raisins. The FDA's residue tolerance is 25 ppm in citrus oil, 0.3 ppm in raisins, 5 ppm in dried apple pomace, 2.5 ppm in citrus molasses, 10 ppm in pineapple bran, and 3 ppm in raisin waste when used for animal feed. The EPA considers it extremely hazardous. Poison by ingestion, inhalation, and skin contact.

**FENARIMOL** • White odorless crystals used as a fungicide in animal feed and apples. Limited to 0.2 ppm in wet and dry apple pomace when used for animal feed. The FDA residue tolerance for meat and meat by-products of cattle, goats, hogs, or sheep is 0.01 ppm; as a residue in fat, kidney, and livers of cattle, sheep, hogs, goats, and poultry, it is 0.1; in eggs, 0.01; in milk 0.003. Moderately toxic by ingestion. Caused mutations in experimental animals.

**FENBENDAZOLE** • Panacur. Animal drug used to combat worms in animal feed and in beef and pork. FDA tolerance of residues in liver of cattle is 0.8 ppm, 5 ppm in swine muscle, and 20 ppm in swine kidney and skin. Can cause mutations.

**FENCHOL** • *See* Fenchyl Alcohol.

***d*-FENCHONE** • A synthetic flavoring occurring naturally in common fennel *(see)*. It is an oily liquid with a camphor smell and practically insoluble in water. Used in berry, liquor, and spice flavorings for beverages, ice cream, ices, candy, baked goods, and liquors. ASP

**FENCHYL ALCOHOL** • A synthetic berry, lime, and spice flavoring additive for beverages, ice cream, ices, candy, and baked goods.

**FENNEL** • Common. Sweet. One of the earliest known herbs from the tall beautiful shrub. The fennel flowers appear in June and are bright yellow, with a characteristic fennel taste. Common fennel is used as a sausage and spice flavoring for beverages, baked goods, meats, and condiments. Sweet fennel has the same function but includes ice cream, ices, and candy. Sweet fennel oil is used in raspberry, fruit, licorice, anise, rye, sausage, root beer, sarsaparilla, spice, wintergreen, and birch beer flavorings for beverages, ice cream, ices, candy, baked goods, gelatin desserts, condiments, meats, and liquors. Organic cosmeticians use compresses of fennel tea to soothe inflamed eyelids and watery eyes. May cause allergic reactions. GRAS. ASP

**FENOXAPROP-ETHYL** • Acclaim. Furore. Puma. Whip. A selective postemergent herbicide to control grassy weeds in broad-leaved crops and turf grass. The FDA limits residue to 0.05 ppm on cottonseed, peanuts, peanut hulls, rice grain, and soybeans. The tolerance limits in meat, meat by-products, and fat of cattle, goats, hogs, and sheep is also 0.05 ppm, and in milk, 0.02 ppm.

**FENPROSTALENE** • Bovilene. An animal drug used to treat beef. FDA residue limits 20 ppb in liver; from 10 to 30 ppm in uncooked edible parts, and 100 ppb at injection site in cattle. A prostaglandin used to induce abortion in feedlot heifers and for estrus control in beef and nonlactating dairy cattle.

**FENRIDAZON** • A pesticide. The residues allowed by the FDA in fat, meat, and meat by-products of cattle, goats, hogs, and sheep is 0.5 ppm. Residues in kidney and liver of cattle, goats, hogs, and sheep is 1 ppm. Residues in eggs and milk is 0.05 ppm and in poultry, fat, meat, and meat by-products, 0.3 ppm.

**FENTHION** • Mercaptophos. Widely used insecticide in fish, meat, and sauces. The FDA limits residues in grass, alfalfa, and rice as well as in fat, meat, and meat by-products of hogs, poultry, and in milk to 1 ppm. EPA Genetic Toxicology Program *(see)*. A human poison by any route. Caused tumors and birth defects in experimental animals. *See* Organophosphates.

**FENUBTATIN OXIDE** • A spider and mite-killing compound. The FDA now has a project under way to develop a method to evaluate residues on apples, oranges, and cucumbers as to toxicity. At this writing, the agency does not have a method to identify this pesticide.

**FENUGREEK SEED** • Greek Hay. An annual herb grown in southern Europe, North Africa, and India. The seeds are used in making curry. Fenugreek is a butter, butterscotch, maple, black walnut, and spice flavoring for beverages, ice cream, ices, candy, baked goods, syrups, meats, and condiments. The extract *(see)* is a butter, butterscotch, caramel, chocolate, coffee, fruit, maple, meat, black walnut, walnut, root beer, spice, and vanilla flavoring additive for beverages, ice cream, ices, pickles, liquors, and icings. The oleoresin *(see)* is a fruit, maple, and nut flavoring additive for beverages, ice cream, ices, candy, baked goods, puddings, and syrups. GRAS. ASP

**FENVALERATE** • Sumifly. An insecticide used in animal feed, sunflower seeds, and tomatoes. Insecticide residue tolerance of 0.05 ppm on all food items. Limitation of 20 ppm in animal feed. Cyanide and its compounds are on the Community Right-To-Know List. Poison by ingestion. Moderately toxic by skin contact. Highly toxic to fish and bees. Corrosive and causes eye damage. A skin irritant.

**FERMENTED AMMONIATED CONDENSED WHEY** • *See* Whey.

**FERMENTATION DERIVED MILK-CLOTTING ENZYME** • Used in the production of cheese as permitted by Standards of Identity *(see)*.

**FERRIC AMMONIUM CHLORIDE** • A nutrient. *See* Ferric Chloride. GRAS

**FERRIC AMMONIUM CITRATE** • Food and water purification. Green powder very soluble in water and having a mild iron-metallic taste. It is odorless and its solutions are acid to litmus. GRAS. EAF

**FERRIC CHLORIDE** • Flavoring additive for various foods. EPA Genetic Toxicology Program *(see)*. Withdrawn as a coloring additive. Moderately toxic by ingestion. Corrosive. Causes adverse reproductive effects in experimental animals. GRAS as a nutrient. ASP

**FERRIC CHOLINE CITRATE** • *See* Iron Salts.

**FERRIC CITRATE** • White crystals odorless with a metallic taste. Used as a nutrient supplement in various foods. *See* Ferric Chloride. GRAS. NUL

**FERRIC ORTHOPHOSPHATE** • *See* Iron Salts.

**FERRIC OXIDE** • Occurs naturally as hematite ore and rust and is used in pigments and metal polishes and on magnetic tapes. Underground hematite miners have a higher incidence of lung cancer. No conclusive carcinogenic effect was observed in mice, hamsters, or guinea pigs given ferric oxide intratracheally or by inhalation. Ferric oxide is not classifiable as to its carcinogenicity to humans, according to IARC *(see)*. NEW

**FERRIC PEPTONATE** • Nutrient. GRAS. NUL

**FERRIC PHOSPHATE** • A nutrient supplement. The final report to the FDA of the Select Committee on GRAS Substances stated in 1980 that there is no evidence in the available information that it is a hazard to the public when used as it is now and should continue its GRAS status with limitations on the amounts that can be added to food. *See* Iron Salts. GRAS. ASP

**FERRIC PYROPHOSPHATE and FERRIC SODIUM PYROPHOS-PHATE** • Nutrients. There is reported use of the chemical; it has not yet been assigned for toxicology literature by the FDA. *See* Iron Salts. GRAS. ASP

**FERRIC SULFATE** • A flavoring additive. GRAS. There is reported use of the chemical; it has not yet been assigned for toxicology literature. *See* Iron Salts. NEW

**FERROCYANIDE SALTS** • Salts of ferrocyanic acid obtained by the reaction of cyanide with an iron sulfate. Used as a coloring. ASP

**FERROCHOLINATE** • Greenish brown solid used as a nutrient supplement. *See* Iron Salts.

**FERROUS ASCORBATE** • Blue-violet solid used as a nutrient supplement. *See* Iron Salts. GRAS. NUL

**FERROUS CARBONATE** • A nutrient supplement. *See* Iron Salts. GRAS. NIL

**FERROUS CITRATE** • A nutrient supplement. *See* Iron Salts. GRAS. NUL

**FERROUS FUMARATE** • Dietary supplement. *See* Iron Salts. GRAS. ASP

**FERROUS GLUCONATE** • Gluconic Acid. Iron Salt. Iron Gluconate.

Used as a food coloring for ripe olives only. It is also used to treat iron-deficiency anemia. It may cause gastrointestinal disturbances. When painted on mouse skin in 2,600 milligram doses per kilogram of body weight, it caused tumors. GRAS. ASP. E

**FERROUS LACTATE** • Lactic Acid. Iron Salt. Iron Lactate. Greenish white crystals that have a slightly peculiar odor. It is derived from the interaction of calcium lactate with ferrous sulfate or the direct action of the lactic acid on iron fillings. It is used as a food additive and dietary supplement. Used to color black olives. Causes tumors when injected under the skin of mice. GRAS. ASP. E

**FERROUS SULFATE** • Green or Iron Vitriol. A source of iron used medicinally. *See* Iron Salts. GRAS. ASP

**FERROUS SULFATE HEPTAHYDRATE** • Pale green crystals or granules used as clarifying additive, dietary supplement, nutrient supplement, processing aid, or stabilizer in baking mixes, cereals, infant foods, pasta products, and wine. Moderately toxic by ingestion. Caused mutations in rats. Withdrawn by the FDA as a coloring additive for food. *See* Iron Salts. BANNED

**FERULA ASAFOETIDA** • *See* Asafoetida Extract.

**FIBER** • Commonly termed "bulk"—the indigestible carbohydrates, including cellulose, hemicellulose, and gums. Fiber is added to food to reduce calorie content, as a thickening additive, and a stabilizer. If an apple a day keeps the doctor away, it may be because of the fiber content. Scientists have suspected that the high intestinal cancer rate in the United States may be linked to the 80 percent decrease of consumption of fiber in the average diet during the past century. Essentially, there are three classes of fiber found in the fruit, leaves, stems, seeds, flowers, and roots of different plants. The first class is the insoluble cellulose found in the plant-cell wall. Some of the other polysaccharides constitute a second class and are also found in the cell wall (hemicellulose and pectic polyerms), in the endosperm of seeds (mucilages), or in the plant's surface (gums). The third class, the lignins, are noncarbohydrates that infiltrate and contribute to the death of the plant cell, which then becomes part of the woody reinforcing plant structure. Enzymes from a number of the more than four hundred kinds of bacteria in the human colon are capable of digesting many components of plant fiber. Doctors have found that the water-holding capacity of some fibers may be helpful in treating colon disease. The fiber's bile absorption properties might be used in modifying cholesterol metabolism. Plant fibers are also capable of binding trace metals and bile acids. These properties modify the action of the gut contents. Fibers pass through the gut somewhat like a sponge, probably altering metabolism in the intestine. The fibers appear to protect intestinal cells by removing foreign substances, such as carcinogens produced by charbroiling. Increased fiber consumption has been recommended for relief of some symptoms of diverticular disease, irritable bowel syndrome, and constipation.

**FICIN** • An enzyme occurring in the latex of tropical trees. A buff-colored powder with an acrid odor. Absorbs water. Concentrated and used as a meat tenderizer. Ten to twenty times more powerful than papain tenderizers. Used to clot milk, as a protein digestant in the brewing industry, and as a chill-proofing additive in beer. Also in cheese as a substitute for rennet in the coagulation of milk, and used for removing casings from sausages. Can cause irritation to the skin, eyes, and mucous membranes, and in large doses can cause purging. GRAS. EAF

**FIELD POPPY EXTRACT** • Extract of the petals of *Papaver rhoeas* used in coloring and as an odorant.

**FILLED MILK** • A combination of skim milk and vegetable oil to replace milk fat. Usually has the same amount of protein and calories as whole milk. Used as a milk substitute. It often contains the high cholesterol fatty acids *(see)* of coconut oil.

**FINOCCHIO** • *See* Fennel.

**FIR NEEDLE OIL** • Fir Oil. Pine. Balsam. An essential oil obtained by the steam distillation of needles and twigs of several varieties of pine trees native to both Canada and Siberia. Used as a flavoring. ASP

**FIR NEEDLES AND TWIGS** • *Abies sibirica.* Flavoring. See Fir Needle Oil. EAF

**FISH GLYCERIDES** • *See* Fish Oil and Glycerin.

**FISH OIL** • A fatty oil from fish or marine mammals used in soap manufacturing. Rich in Omega-3 fatty acids that were reported in the 1980s to reduce fats in the blood and are believed to reduce the risk of coronary artery disease. The final report to the FDA of the Select Committee on GRAS Substances stated in 1980 that it should continue its GRAS status for food packaging with no limitations other than good manufacturing practices. There is reported use of the chemical; it has not yet been assigned for toxicology literature. NEW

**FISH PROTEIN CONCENTRATE WHOLE AND ISOLATE** • Dietary supplement. ASP

**5-A-DAY** • Refers to the dietary recommendation to consume five servings of fruits and vegetables every day. The tagline 5-a-day became a promotional message in campaigns to increase fruit and vegetable consumption.

**FIXATIVE** • A chemical that reduces the tendency of an odor or flavor to vaporize by making the odor or flavor last longer. An example is musk *(see),* which is used in perfume and undecylaldehyde as a fixative for citrus flavors.

**FLAV** • Natural flavoring agent.

**FK/AD** • Substance used in conjunction with flavors.

**FLAVONOIDS** • A large group of compounds widely distributed throughout nature. They include quercetin, present in onion skins, and anthocyanins, the major commercially used group. *See* Bioflavonoids.

**FLAVOPHOSPHOLIPOL** • An antibiotic used as an antimicrobial growth promoter (AMGP) in animal feeds, although some studies show that this substance does not cause as much antibiotic-resistant bacteria as some other antibiotics used in feed. EU and U.S. agencies believe that it might cause resistance in humans because it is used in human medicine.

**FLAVOR ENHANCERS** • *See* Flavor Potentiators.

**FLAVOR POTENTIATORS** • One of the newest and fastest-growing categories of additives, potentiators enhance the total seasoning effect, generally without contributing any taste or odor of their own. They are effective in minute doses—in parts per million or even less. A potentiator produces no identifiable effect itself but exaggerates one's response. They alter the response of the sensory nerve endings on the tongue and in the nose. The first true potentiators in the United States were the 5′-nucleotides, which are derived from a natural seasoning long in use in Japan: small flakes of dry bonito (a tunalike fish) are often added to modify and improve the flavor of soups, and from bonito a 5′-nucleotide, disodium inosinate *(see),* has been isolated and identified as a flavor potentiator. Another 5′-nucleotide is disodium guanylate *(see),* one of the newer additives on the market, which gives one a sensation of "fullness" and "increased viscosity" when eating. The product is advertised as being able to give diners a sense of "full-bodied flavor" when ingesting a food containing it.

**FLAVORING COMPOUND** • A flavoring composed of two or more substances. The substances may be natural or synthetic, and they are usually closely guarded secrets. Normally, a flavoring compound is complete; that is, it is added to a food without any additional flavorings being necessary. A strawberry flavoring compound, for example, may contain twenty-eight separate ingredients before it is complete.

**FLAVORINGS** • There are more than two thousand flavorings added to foods, of which approximately five hundred are natural and the rest synthetic. This is the largest category of additive. Lemon and orange are examples of natural flavorings, while benzaldehyde and methyl salicylate *(see both)* are examples from the laboratory.

**FLAXSEED** • The seed of the flax plant may be "hidden" in cereals and milk of cows fed flaxseed. It is also in flaxseed tea and the laxative Flaxolyn. It is a frequent allergen when ingested, inhaled, or in direct contact. Flaxseeds are the source of linseed oil. Among other hidden sources are: dog food, Roman meal, and muffins.

**FLEABANE OIL** • Oil of Canada Fleabane. Erigeron Oil. The pale yellow volatile oil from a fresh flowering herb. It takes its name from its supposed ability to drive away fleas. Used in fruit and spice flavorings for beverages, ice cream, ices, candy, baked goods, and sauces.

**FLUAZIFOP-BUTYL** • An herbicide used on animal feed. The FDA permits a residue of from 0.2 to 1 ppm on various feeds.

**FLUCYTHRINATE** • An herbicide used on animal feed. FDA tolerance is 10 ppm for apple pomace; 0.2 on cottonseed oil; 0.1 ppm in cottonseed, and corn grain, 2 on cabbage, 3 on corn forage, and 0.2 on sugar bagasse.

**FLUORIDE** • An acid salt used in toothpaste to prevent tooth decay. *See* Sodium Fluoride.

**FLUORIDONE** • An herbicide. The FDA residue tolerance in fish and crayfish is 0.05 ppm; as a residue in milk and eggs, 0.05 ppm; as a residue in fat, meat, and meat by-products of cattle, goats, or hogs, 0.05 ppm. As a residue in kidney and liver of cattle, hogs, or goats, 0.1 ppm, and 0.1 to 1 ppm as a residue on various fruits and vegetables.

**FLUORINE COMPOUNDS** • Calcium Fluoride. Hydrofluorsillic Acid. Potassium Fluoride. Sodium Fluoride. Sodium Silicofluoride. All have been used in the fluoridation of water. Fluorides cross the placental barrier and the effects on the fetus are unknown. New clinical evidence shows that kidney disturbance sometimes is due to the amount of fluoride it contributes to the blood. Fluorine-containing compounds (sodium, potassium, or calcium fluoride) are illegal. A petition for extension in dietary supplements was terminated in 1973. Addition of fluorine compounds to food is limited to that from fluoridation of public water supplies and to that resulting from the fluoridation of bottled water within limits set by the FDA. The Commissioner of Food and Drugs has concluded that it is in the interest of the public health to limit the addition of fluorine compounds to foods to that resulting from the fluoridation of public water supplies and to that resulting from the fluoridation of bottled water.

**4′-FLUORO-4-(4-[2-PYRIDYL]-1*p* IPERAZINYL)BUTYROPHENONE** • Azaperone. Suicahn. A sedative and tranquilizer used on animals. Poison by ingestion.

**FOAM INHIBITOR** • An antifoaming additive such as dimethyl polysiloxane *(see)* used in chewing-gum bases, soft drinks, and fruit juices to keep them from foaming. *See* Defoaming Additive.

**FOAM STABILIZERS** • Used in soft drinks and brewing. See Vegetable Gums.

**FOAMING ADDITIVE** • Used to help whipped topping peak when it is being whipped with cold milk. A commonly added foaming additive is sodium caseinate *(see)*.

**FOLIC ACID** • A yellowish orange compound and member of the vitamin B complex, used as a nutrient. Occurs naturally in liver, kidney, mushrooms, and green leaves. Aids in cell formation, especially red blood cells.

As of January 1, 1998, manufacturers of enriched breads, flours, cornmeals, pastas, rice, and other grain products were required to add the nutrient folic acid to their products—a move to reduce the risk of neural tube birth defects in newborns. Folic acid, when consumed in adequate amounts by women before and during early pregnancy, reduces the risk of such birth defects as spina bifida. It is estimated that folic acid supplementation will reduce by about two thousand per year the number of American babies born with birth defects. It took ten years for U.S. government agencies to recommend that "all women of child-bearing age in the United States who are capable of becoming pregnant should consume 0.4 mg. of folic acid per day for the purpose of reducing their risk of having a pregnancy affected by spina bifida or other neural tube defects." ASP

**FOOD-BORNE DISEASE** • Disease, usually gastrointestinal, caused by organisms or their toxins carried in ingested food. Also commonly known as "food poisoning."

**FOOD GUIDE PYRAMID** • The Food Guide Pyramid is a graphic design used to communicate the recommended daily food choices contained in the 1995 Dietary Guidelines for Americans. The information provided is developed and promoted by the U.S. Department of Agriculture and the U.S. Department of Health and Human Services. The Food Guide Pyramid shows at its wide base what should form the foundation of a healthful diet— six to eleven servings daily from the bread, cereal, rice, and pasta group. The next level up the tapered pyramid is divided between the vegetable group, three to five servings daily, and the fruit group, two to four servings daily. The next level up the narrowing pyramid is divided between the milk, yogurt, and cheese group, two to three servings daily, and the meat, poultry, fish, dry beans, eggs, and nuts group, two to three servings daily. The smallest part of the pyramid at the top shows the fats, oils, and sweets in the diet that should be used sparingly. The Food Guide Pyramid's guide to daily food choices are:

- Eat a variety of foods.
- Balance the food you eat with physical activity—maintain or improve your weight.
- Choose a diet with plenty of grain products, vegetables, and fruits.
- Choose a diet low in fat, saturated fat, and cholesterol.
- Choose a diet moderate in sugars.
- Choose a diet moderate in salt and sodium.
- If you drink alcoholic beverages, do so in moderation.

**FOOD RED 6** • Formerly Ext. FD and C Red No. 15, FD and C Red No. 1, and Ponceau 3R. One of the first approved certified coal-tar colors. Food

Red 6 was delisted as a food additive as possibly harmful. Dark red powder, it changes to cherry red in solution. *See* FD and C Colors.

**FOOD STANDARDS** • Standards of Identity. The FDA and USDA previously established a "recipe" for about three hundred foods, such as peanut butter and mayonnaise, fixing the ingredients by law. Many of these foods were exempted from the need for ingredient listing. The new labeling law, effective in 1994, requires manufacturers to give full ingredient listings for all foods.

**FOOD STARCH ESTERFIED WITH *n*-OCTENYL SUCCINIC ANHYDRIDE TREATED WITH BETA-AMYLASE** • Esters *(see)* and enzymes such as beta-amylase change the properties of a compound, often making it more soluble or reducing its allergenic potential. *See* Modified Starch.

**FOOD STARCH MODIFIED** • Various chemicals are permitted in modifying food starch and are listed under individual chemical names. *See* Modified Starch.

**FORMALDEHYDE** • Paraformaldehyde. Preservative in defoaming additives and in animal feeds. A colorless gas obtained by the oxidation of methyl alcohol and generally used in watery solution. Formaldehyde generally is known as a disinfectant, germicide, fungicide, defoamer, and preservative, and is used in animal feed, in defoaming additives, and embalming fluid. One ounce taken by mouth causes death within two hours. Skin reaction after exposure. It is a highly reactive chemical that is damaging to the hereditary substances in the cells of several species. It causes lung cancer in rats and has a number of other harmful biological consequences. Researchers from the Division of Cancer Cause and Prevention of the National Cancer Institute recommended in April 1983 that since formaldehyde is involved in DNA damage and inhibits its repair, and potentiates the toxicity of x-rays in human lung cells, and since it may act in concert with other chemical additives to produce mutagenic and carcinogenic effects, it should be "further investigated." The question is whether we ingest any formaldehyde when we ingest the animals that ate the feed and the products that had undergone "defoaming" by formaldehyde. The ADI *(see)* set for formaldehyde is 3 mg/kg of body weight. Researchers at Italy's University of Milan studied the health risk from consumption of cheese made using formaldehyde (grana padano) and concluded there was no appreciable health risk. ASP

**FORMALIN** • Fungicide in water of salmon, trout, largemouth bass, catfish, and bluegills. *See* Formaldehyde.

**FORMESAFEN SODIUM** • A pesticide used on soybeans. FDA tolerance is 0.05 ppm on soybeans.

**FORMETANATE HYDROCHLORIDE** • A pesticide in citrus molasses resulting from application to growing fruit. The FDA tolerance is 10 ppm in citrus and 8 ppm on growing fruit.

**FORMIC ACID** • Colorless, pungent, highly corrosive, it occurs naturally in apples and other fruit. Used as a decalcifier and for dehairing hides. Chronic absorption is known to cause albuminuria—protein in the urine. It caused cancer when administered orally in rats, mice, and hamsters in doses from 31 to 49 milligrams per kilogram of body weight. Used as a preservative for silage. Silage is not supposed to be fed to livestock within four weeks of treatment. FDA residue tolerance is 2.25 percent of silage on a dry basis and 0.45 percent when direct cut. ASP

**FORMIC ETHER** • *See* Ethyl Formate.

**FORTIFIED** • Fortification of food refers to the addition of nutrients such as vitamin C to breakfast drinks and vitamin D to milk. It actually increases the nutritional values of the original food.

**FOS** • Abbreviation for fructooligosaccyarides *(see)*.

**FRANKINCENSE** • Aromatic gum resin obtained from African and Asian trees and used chiefly as incense. For food use, *see* Olibanum Extract.

**FREE** • Product contains none or only insignificant amounts of a substance.

**FREE RADICALS** • Certain oxygen molecules that are underlying factors in aging and degenerative diseases because they damage DNA, the blueprint for life, within the cells. They also adversely affect enzymes, the workhorses of the cells, and damage cell membranes. Free radicals are formed during the course of normal metabolism, as well as from exposure to cigarette smoke and other environmental influences. Fat-soluble antioxidants, beta-carotene and other carotenoids, as well as vitamins C and E and pycnogenol *(see),* are believed to fight the damage from free radicals.

**FRESH** • A food that has not been heat processed or frozen and supposedly contains no preservatives.

**FRUCTOOLIGOSACCHARIDES (FOS)** • Sugars that occur naturally in plants such as tomatoes, onions, and bananas. They are not digestible in the stomach and travel unabsorbed to the intestine. In the intestines they promote the growth of beneficial bacteria such as those used to culture yogurt. They are now used in poultry feed to enhance growth and reduce intestinal pathogens. Applications have been made to use them as a food additive for human foods.

**FRUCTOSE** • A sugar occurring naturally in large numbers of fruits and honey. It is the sweetest of the foodstuffs. It is also used as a medicine, preservative, common sugar, and to prevent sandiness in ice cream. Researchers at the General Clinical Research Center at the University of Colorado School of Medicine in Denver report that fructose is absorbed in the gastrointestinal tract more slowly than sugars like sucrose, which contain glucose. As a result, even though the body converts some fructose to glucose, 80 to 90 percent of the sugar is absorbed intact, and there is only a slight increase in blood glucose levels immediately after consumption. Fructose can be up to two times sweeter than sucrose. However, in 2004, a Louisiana state biomedical researcher linked high-fructose corn syrup to the increase in obesity since the

1980s. Recent advances in enzyme technology have made it possible to produce fructose on a commercial scale. It caused tumors in mice when injected under the skin in 5,000-milligram doses per kilogram of body weight.

**FRUIT JUICE** • Used to color foods consistent with good manufacturing practices. Permanently listed. ASP

**FSIS** • Abbreviation for Food Safety and Inspection Service of the United States Department of Agriculture. Personnel are responsible for inspecting meat and poultry facilities.

**FULLER'S EARTH** • A white or brown naturally occurring earthy substance. A nonplastic variety of kaolin *(see)* containing an aluminum magnesium silicate. Used as an absorbent and to decolorize fats and oils. No longer permitted as a coloring in food. It is used to keep fish eggs from sticking together in hatcheries. ASP

**FUM** • Fumigant.

**FUMARIC ACID** • White, odorless, derived from many plants and essential to vegetable and animal tissue respiration; prepared industrially. An acidulant used as a leavening additive and a dry acid for dessert powders and confections (up to 3 percent). Also as apple, peach, and vanilla flavoring additive for beverages, baked goods (1,300 ppm), and gelatin desserts (3,600 ppm). Used in baked goods as an antioxidant and as a substitute for tartaric acid *(see).* ASP. E

**FUMARIC ACID FERROUS SALT** • A dietary supplement. *See* Ferrous Fumarate.

**FUMICANTS** • Chemicals and gases used to kill pests on crops. Among those approved for use by the FDA are carbon tetrachloride with either carbon disulfide or ethylene chloride, with or without pentane; or methyl bromide. Also carbon disulfide, carbon tetrachloride, ethylene dichloride, and ethyl bromide. All are highly toxic and should be applied only by experts. Ethyl bromide is a cancer-causing agent.

**FUNCTIONAL FOODS** • Foods that may provide health benefits beyond basic nutrition.

**FUNG** • Fungicide.

**FUNGAFLOR** • Imazalil. Fungicide used in animal feed. Poison by ingestion and causes adverse reproductive effects in experimental animals.

**FUNGAL HEMICELLUASE** • Enzyme used in food processing. NUL

**FUNGAL PECTINASE** • Enzyme used in fruit juice and wine processing. *See* Pectins. ASP

**FUNGI** • A group of simple plantlike organisms that don't have the green coloring known as chlorophyll. Fungi include mushrooms, yeasts, rusts, molds, and smuts.

**FURADAN** • White crystalline solid widely used as an insecticide in animal feed. Limitation in animal feed is from 2 ppm in grape pomace to 24 ppm in peanut soap-stock fatty acids. Insecticide residue tolerance of 2 ppm in raisins. Extremely hazardous substance, it is on the EPA Genetic Toxicology Program *(see)*. Poisonous by inhalation, ingestion, and skin contact. Causes birth defects in experimental animals.

**2-FURALDEHYDE** • *See* Furfural.

**FURANS** • Furans are extremely toxic and are also found with dioxins. They are created in two major ways: 1) by the processes used to manufacture some products, for example, certain pesticides, preservatives, disinfectants, flavorings, and paper products; 2) when materials are burned at low temperatures, for example, certain chemical products, leaded gasoline, plastic, paper, and wood. Furan resins are made by the polymerization or poly condensation of furfural, furfural alcohol *(see both)*, or other compounds containing a furan ring, or by the reaction of these furan compounds with other compounds. Furans are persistent, bioaccumulative, and result predominantly from human activity. They are also carcinogenic.

**2-FURAN ACROLEIN** • *See* Furyl Acrolein.

**2-FURANMETHANETHIOL FORMATE** • Furfuryl Mercaptan. Flavoring. Colorless oily liquid; extremely powerful and diffusive odor which on dilution becomes agreeable, coffeelike, caramellic-burnt, and sweet. NUL

**4-((FURANMETHYL)THIO)-2-PENTANONE** • Flavoring. Clear yellow liquid; meaty aroma. NUL

**FURCELLERAN** • Sodium, Calcium, Potassium, and Ammonium. Extracted from red seaweed grown in northern European waters. It is a natural colloid and gelling additive. The processed gum is used as an emulsifier, stabilizer, and thickener in foods. Also used in puddings, ice cream, and jams, in products for diabetics, as a carrier for food preservatives, and in bactericides. It is also used in over-the-counter drugs for weight reduction and toothpastes. On the FDA list of additives to be studied for mutagenic, teratogenic, subacute, and reproductive effects since 1980. It is reportedly more stable than vegetable gums. EAF

**FURFURAL** • Artificial Ant Oil. 2-Furaldehyde, Furfuraldehyde,I, Fural, 2-Furancarboxaldehyde, Pyromucic Aldehyde, 2-Formylfuran, 2-Furylmethanal. A colorless liquid with a peculiar odor. Occurs naturally in angelica root, apples, coffee, peaches, and skim milk. Used as a solvent, insecticide, fungicide, to decolor resins, and as a synthetic flavoring in butterscotch, butter, caramel, coffee, fruit, brandy, rum, rye, molasses, nut, and cassia flavorings for beverages, ice cream, ices, candy, gelatin desserts, syrups (the biggest user; up to 30 ppm), and spirits. It irritates mucous membranes and acts on the central nervous system. Causes tearing and inflammation of the eyes and throat. Ingestion or absorption of 0.06 grams produces persistent headache. Used continually, it leads to nervous disturbances and eye disorders (including photosensitivity). The FAO/WHO Expert Committee on Food Additives in June 1998 requested animal studies to investigate whether this additive interacts with DNA in mice and a ninety-day study in rats to identify a no-observed-effect level (NOEL) for liver damage. Other studies, however, have demonstrated different results: Exposure of rats to furfural by ingestion or subcutaneous injection caused unsteadiness, paralysis, seizures, coma, and changes in liver, kidneys, blood, and bone marrow. Cats exposed to 2,800 ppm for thirty minutes developed fatal pulmonary edema. Solutions to 10 percent and 100 percent furfural instilled in rabbits' eyes caused pain in addition to transient swelling and redness of the lids and conjunctivitis. Chronic dietary exposure to furfural caused liver cirrhosis in rats. Dogs exposed at 130 ppm for six hours a day for four weeks developed liver damage, but dogs exposed at 63 ppm did not. Rabbits exposed to furfural vapors for several hours daily developed liver and kidney lesions as well as changes in their blood. Furfural is mutagenic in at least one bacterial species. Furfural is an irritant of the skin, eyes, mucous membranes, and respiratory tract. Concentrations of 1.9 to 14 ppm produced headache, itching of the throat, and redness and tearing of the eyes in some exposed workers. Workers exposed to furfural vapors in a plant with inadequate ventilation reported numbness of the tongue and mucous membranes of the mouth, loss of taste sensation, and difficulty in breathing. Exposure to high concentrations has produced pulmonary edema. Damage to the eyesight of some individuals has also been reported. Chronic skin exposure may produce eczema, allergic skin sensitization, and photosensitization. A worker exposed to furfural who has consumed alcohol may experience warmth and redness of the face, a throbbing sensation and pain in the head and neck, difficulty in breathing, nausea, vomiting, sweating, thirst, chest pain, uneasiness, weakness, dizziness, blurred vision, and confusion. This effect may last from thirty minutes to several hours but does not appear to have residual side effects. By analogy with effects seen in animals—liver lesions, death from respiratory effects, toxicity by ingestion—furfural may affect the central nervous system, liver, kidneys, blood, and bone marrow of humans; however, these effects have not been reported in exposed workers. Listed as a cancer-causing agent by Environmental Defense. ASP

**FURFURAL ACETONE** • A flavoring with a sweet balsamic, vanilla odor, woody odor and taste. Used in nut flavors. *See* Furfural.

**FURFURYL ACETATE** • Acetic Acid. A synthetic raspberry, fruit, and ginger ale flavoring for beverages, ice cream, ices, candy, baked goods, and chewing gum. *See* Furfuryl Alcohol for toxicity. ASP

**FURFURYL ALCOHOL** • A synthetic flavoring obtained mainly from corncobs and roasted coffee beans. Derived from furfural. Has a faint burning odor and a bitter taste. Used in butter, butterscotch, caramel, coffee, fruit, and brandy flavorings for beverages, ice cream, ices, candy, baked goods, gelatin desserts, and icings. Toxicity: Workers warned inhalation, ingestion, or skin contact may cause severe injury or death. Contact with molten substance may cause severe burns to skin and eyes. Any skin contact should be avoided. Effects of contact or inhalation may be delayed. ASP

**FURFURYL BUTYRATE** • Flavoring. *See* Furfural. ASP

**FURFURYL HEXANOATE** • Flavoring with a green, fatty, musty, waxy taste. *See* Furfural.

**FURFURYL MERCAPTAN** • A synthetic fruit, liquor, rum, nut, chocolate, and spice flavoring additive that occurs naturally in coffee and is used in beverages, ice cream, ices, candy, and baked goods. *See* Furfural. ASP

**FURFURYL MERCAPTAN (2-FURANMETHANETHIOL)** • Flavoring that occurs in coffee, cooked beef, and chicken. *See* Furfural.

**2-FURFURYLIDENE BUTYRALDEHYDE** • A synthetic fruit, liquor, rum, nut, and spice flavoring additive for beverages, ice cream, ices, candy, and baked goods. *See* Furfural. ASP

**FURFURYL ISOPROPYL SULFIDE** • Flavoring. *See* Furfural. ASP

**FURFURYL 3-METHYLBUTANOATE** • Flavoring. *See* Furfural. ASP

**FURFURYL METHYL ETHER** • Flavoring. *See* Furfural. ASP

**FURFURYL METHYL DISULFIDE** • Flavoring with a bread or roast beef–like taste. It is a roast note for pork, liver, chicken, salami, chocolate, coffee, toffee, bread. See Furfural. ASP

**FURFURYL METHYL SULFIDE** • Synthetic flavoring with a pungent onion and garlic odor and taste. *See* Furfural.

**ALPHA-FURFURYL OCTANOATE** • Flavoring. *See* Furfural. ASP

**ALPHA-FURFURYL PENTANOATE** • Flavoring with a woody, fruity pineapple odor and fruity taste, used in pineapple. *See* Furfural. ASP

**FURFURYL PROPIONATE** • Flavoring. *See* Furfural. ASP

**FURFURYL PROPYL DISULFIDE** • Flavoring. *See* Furfural. EAF

**N-FURFURYLPYRROLE** • Flavoring with a vegetable, green, earthy, pungent horseradish taste. Used in garnish flavors for soup. *See* Furfural. ASP

**FURFURYL THIOACETATE** • Flavoring. *See* Furfural. ASP

**FURFURYL THIOPROPIONATE** • Flavoring used in tuna fish at 5ppm; in onion at 3ppm; coffee at 1 ppm and in seafood and mocha. *See* Furfural. ASP

**FURYL ACETONE** • *See* (2-Furyl)-2-Propanone.

**FURYL ACROLEIN** • A synthetic coffee, fruit, cassia, and cinnamon flavoring additive for beverages, ice cream, ices, candy, baked goods, gelatin desserts, and puddings. ASP

**4-(2-FURYL)-3-BUTEN-2-ONE** • A synthetic nut, almond, and spice flavoring additive for beverages, ice cream, ices, candy, baked goods, and gelatin desserts. ASP

**(2-FURYL)-2-PROPANONE** • A synthetic fruit flavoring additive for ice cream, ices, candy, and baked goods. ASP

**FUSEL OIL (REFINED)** • A synthetic flavoring that occurs naturally in cognac oil. It is also a product of carbohydrate fermentation to produce ethyl alcohol *(see)* and varies widely in composition. Used in grape, brandy, cordial, rum, rye, scotch, whiskey, and wine flavorings for beverages, ice cream, ices, candy, baked goods, chewing gum, gelatin desserts, puddings, and liquor. Commercial amyl alcohol *(see),* its major ingredient, is more toxic than ethyl alcohol and as little as 30 milligrams has caused death. Smaller amounts cause methemoglobinuria (blood cells in the urine) and kidney damage. ASP

# G

**G** • Abbreviation for gram *(see).*

**a-GALACTOSIDASE** • Derived from *Mortierella vinaceae,* it is an enzyme used in sugar beet production. NUL

**GALANGAL GREATER** • *Alpinia galanga.* Very popular spice in all Southeast Asia and especially typical of the cuisine of Thailand. The rhizome contains up to 1.5 percent essential oil (1,8 cineol, α-pinene, eugenol, camphor, methyl cinnamate, and sesquiterpenes). May be used fresh or dried, which makes a great difference in flavor. Fresh galangal has a pure and refreshing odor and a mildly spicy gingerlike flavor. NUL

**GALANGAL ROOT** • East Indian Root. Chinese Ginger. The pungent aromatic oil of the galangal root is a bitters, vermouth, spice, and ginger ale flavoring additive for beverages. The extract is a bitters, fruit, liquor, spice, and ginger ale flavoring additive for beverages, ice cream, ices, candy, baked goods, and liquors. Related to true ginger, it was formerly used in cooking and in medicine to treat colic. GRAS. EAF

**GALANGAL ROOT OIL** • Natural flavor isolated by physical method. *See* Galangal Root. GRAS. NIL

**GALBANUM OIL** • A yellowish to green or brown aromatic bitter gum resin from an Asiatic plant used as incense. The oil is a fruit, nut, and spice flavoring for beverages, ice cream, ices, candy, baked goods, and condiments. Has been used medicinally to break up intestinal gas and as an expectorant. EAF

**GALLATES (DODECYL, OCTYL and PROPYL)** • These antioxidants are derived from gallic acid, obtained from tannins and molds. The FAO/WHO *(see)* has held many meetings about these additives. Although the committee noted there are similarities in the metabolism of the different gallates, it concluded that there was not enough evidence to allocate a group ADI for the gallates. In addition, a 150-day gavage study with dodecyl gallate revealed a no-observed-effect level (NOEL) that was tenfold lower than the dietary NOEL for propyl gallate. In the ninety-day toxicity study in rats, propyl gallate administered in the diet at 7,450 mg per kg caused changes in blood, spleen, and liver. The committee allocated an ADI *(see)* of 0–1.4 mg per kg of body weight for propyl gallate. The committee concluded that neither octyl or dodecyl gallate were likely to be cancer-causing or gene-toxic. Therefore, the committee allocated temporary ADIs for these substances. With octyl gallate, a slight anemia was observed at 100 mg per kg of body weight per day in rats when it was administered for two generations. A temporary ADI of 0–.01 mg per kg of body weight was allocated for octyl gallate. With dodecyl gallate, reduction in spleen weight and pathological changes in the liver, kidney, and spleen were observed in a 150-day study in rats in which the substance was administered by gavage. A temporary ADI of 0.05 mg per kg of body weight was allocated for dodecyl gallate based on a NOEL of 10 mg per kg of body weight per day in this study and a safety factor of 200. The committee concluded that additional studies on dodecyl, octyl, and propyl gallate may help to explain the differences in toxicological potency of these compounds. If these studies do not resolve the issue, then the committee said long-term toxicity and cancer studies and gene toxicity studies "might be required."

**GALLIC ACID** • *See* Propyl Gallate.

**GALLOTANNIC ACID** • *See* Tannic Acid.

**GAMBIR CATECHU** • A flavoring. *See* Catechu Extract.

**GAMBIR GUM** • *See* Catechu Extract. EAF

**GAMMA-TOCOPHEROL** • *See* Tochoperol. E

**GARDEN ROSEMARY OIL** • *See* Rosemary Extract.

**GARDENOL** • *See* a-Methylbenzyl Acetate.

**GARLIC EXTRACT** • An extract from *Allium sativum,* a yellowish liquid with a strong odor used in fruit and garlic flavorings. Garlic is a member of the onion family and was cultivated in Egypt from earliest times and known in China more than two thousand years ago. Garlic contains lots of potassium, fluorine, sulfur, phosphorus, vitamins A and C, as well as seventy-five different sulfur compounds. In addition it contains quercetin, cyanidin, and bioflavonoids *(see all).* Garlic also contains selenium, which has been found to have anticancer potential. Garlic has been used since ancient times to treat all sorts of ailments, including the Great Plague in Europe and dysentery during World War I. The herb has recently been found to contain antibiotic, antiviral, and antifungal ingredients. It has also been reported in the scientific literature that garlic may decrease nitrosamines, modulate cancer cell multiplication, increase immunity, and protect the body against ionizing radiation. Three Rutgers University researchers in 1992 reported at the American Chemical Society meeting in Washington, D.C., that chemicals in garlic may protect the liver from damage caused by large doses of the popular nonaspirin painkiller acetaminophen (in Tylenol and dozens of other painkillers and cold medications) and may prevent growth of lung tumors associated with tobacco smoke. Garlic also reportedly inhibits the production of prostaglandins *(see),* which may explain why allium oils have antitumor activity. Phytochemicals in garlic are under intensive study for cholesterol-lowering, immune-enhancing, and cancer-preventive activity. GRAS. ASP

**GARLIC OIL** • Yellow liquid with a strong odor, obtained from the crushed bulbs or cloves of the plant. Used in fruit and garlic flavorings for beverages, ice cream, ices, candy, baked goods, chewing gum, and condiments. Has been used medicinally to combat intestinal worms. Reevaluated and found to be GRAS by the FDA in 1976. *See* Garlic Extract.

**GAS** • A product from the controlled combustion in air of butane, propane, or natural gas. It is used for removing or displacing oxygen in the processing, storage, or packaging of citrus products, vegetable fats, vegetable oils, coffee, and wine. No known toxicity when used in packaging. ASP

**GASTRONOMY** • The study and appreciation of good food and good eating, and a culture's culinary customs, style, and lore. Any interest or study of culinary pursuits relates essentially to the kitchen and cookery, and to the higher levels of education, training, and achievement of the professional chef and the chef apprentice.

**GEL** • A semisolid, apparently homogenous substance that may be elastic and jellylike (gelatin) or more or less rigid (silica gel) and that is formed in various ways such as by coagulation or evaporation.

**GELATINS** • Gelatin is a protein obtained by boiling skin, tendons, ligaments, or bones with water. It is colorless or slightly yellow, tasteless, and absorbs five to ten times its weight of cold water. Used as a food thickener and stabilizer and a base for fruit gelatins and puddings and sausage casings. The raw material can also be rendered into lard. In the United States and some Asian countries, pork skin is immersed, boiled, dried, and then fried to make a snack food (pork rinds). Employed medicinally to treat malnutrition and brittle fingernails. ASP

**GELLAN GUM** • Used as a stabilizer and thickener in various foods. ASP. E

**GENE** • The smallest genetic unit of a chromosome. It is a piece of DNA which contains the hereditary information for the production of a protein.

**GENET, ABSOLUTE** • A natural flavoring from flowers used in fruit and honey flavorings for beverages, ice cream, ices, candy, baked goods, and chewing gum. The extract is a raspberry and fruit flavoring for beverages. There is reported use of the chemical; it has not yet been assigned for toxicology literature. EAF

**GENETIC TOXICOLOGY PROGRAM** • The U.S. Environmental Protection Agency has certain chemicals under study to determine their effects on genes, the parts of the cell that carry inherited characteristics. Damage to the mechanisms of genes can lead to birth defects and cancer, as well as other illnesses.

**GENTAMYCIN SULFATE** • Garamycin Sulfate. An antibiotic used to treat pork and turkey. FDA residue limitations are 0.1 ppm in turkey and in swine muscle. This drug is also used to treat serious infections in humans and theoretically, resistance to the drug could build up by eating treated pork or turkey. Allergic reactions to the drug in the meat could also occur.

**GENTIAN ROOT EXTRACT** • The yellow or pale bitter root of central and southern European plants used in angostura, chocolate, cola, fruit, vermouth, maple, root beer, and vanilla flavorings for beverages, ice cream, ices, candy, and liquors. It has been used as a bitter tonic. ASP

**GERANIAL** • *See* Citral.

**GERANIALDEHYDE** • *See* Citral.

**GERANIOL** • Oily sweet, with a rose odor, it occurs naturally in apples, bay leaves, cherries, grapefruit, ginger, lavender, and a number of other essential oils. A synthetic flavoring additive that occurs naturally in apples, bay leaves, cherries, coriander, grapefruit, oranges, tea, ginger, mace oil, and the oils of lavender, lavandin, lemon, lime, mandarin, and petitgrain. A berry, lemon, rose, apple, cherry, peach, honey, root beer, cassia, cinnamon, ginger ale, and nutmeg flavoring for beverages, ice cream, ices, candy, baked goods, chewing gum, and toppings. Geraniol is omitted from hypoallergenic cosmetics. Can cause allergic reactions. Whereas no specific toxicity information is available, deaths have been reported from ingestion of unknown amounts of citronella oil *(see)* which is 93 percent geraniol; gastric mucosa was found to be severely damaged. GRAS. ASP

**GERANIUM** • An essential oil used as flavoring. See Geranium Rose Oil. GRAS. NUL

**GERANIUM ROSE OIL** • A synthetic flavoring additive that occurs naturally in geranium herbs and rose petals. Used in strawberry, lemon, cola, geranium, rose, violet, cherry, honey, rum, brandy, cognac, nut, vanilla, spice, and ginger ale flavorings for beverages, ice cream, ices, candy, baked goods, gelatin desserts, chewing gum, and jelly. A teaspoon may cause illness in an adult and less than an ounce may kill. May affect those allergic to geraniums. EAF

**GERANYL ACETATE** • Geraniol Acetate. Clear colorless liquid with the odor of lavender, it is a constituent of several essential oils. Used in berry, lemon, orange, floral, apple, grape, peach, pear, honey, spice, and ginger ale flavorings for beverages, ice cream, ices, candy, baked goods, gelatin desserts, chewing gum, and syrup. It is obtained from geraniol *(see)*. GRAS. ASP

**GERANYL ACETOACETATE** • A synthetic fruit flavoring additive for beverages, ice cream, ices, candy, and baked goods. ASP

**GERYANYL ACETONE** • Flavoring with a rosy, leafy, fruity taste. *See* Gerianol. ASP

**GERANYL BENZOATE** • A synthetic flavoring additive, slightly yellowish liquid, with a floral odor. Used in floral and fruit flavorings for beverages, ice cream, ices, candy, baked goods, and candy. *See* Benzoate. ASP

**GERANYL BUTYRATE** • Geraniol Butyrate. Colorless liquid that occurs in several essential oils, it is used as a synthetic attar of roses in berry, citrus, fruit, apple, cherry, pear, and pineapple flavorings for beverages, ice cream, ices, candy, baked goods, chewing gum, and gelatin desserts. *See* Geraniol. ASP

**GERANYL FORMATE** • Geraniol Formate. Colorless liquid with a roselike odor, insoluble in alcohol, it occurs in several essential oils. Used in perfumes and soaps as a synthetic neroli bigarade oil *(see)*. A fresh, leafy, rose odor, it is used in berry, citrus, apple, apricot, and peach flavorings for beverages, ice cream, ices, candy, baked goods, gelatins, chewing gum, and puddings. *See* Geraniol. ASP

**GERANYL HEXANOATE** • A synthetic citrus and pineapple flavoring additive for beverages, ice cream, ices, candy, and baked goods. *See* Hexanoic Acid. ASP

**GERANYL ISOBUTRATE** • Salt of Isobutyric Acid *(see)*. A synthetic floral, rose, apple, pear, and pineapple flavoring additive for beverages, ice cream, ices, candy, baked goods, chewing gum, gelatin desserts, and puddings. ASP

**GERANYL ISOVALERATE** • A synthetic berry, lime, apple, peach, and pineapple flavoring additive for beverages, ice cream, ices, candy, and baked goods. ASP

**GERANYL PHENYLACETATE** • A synthetic flavoring, yellow liquid with a honey-rose odor. Used in fruit flavorings for beverages, ice cream, ices, candy, baked goods, and chewing gum. *See* Phenylacetic Acid. ASP

**GERANYL PROPIONATE** • Geraniol Propionate. Colorless liquid with a roselike odor, it is used as a synthetic flavoring in berry, geranium, apple, pear, pineapple, and honey flavorings for beverages, ice cream, ices, candy, baked goods, chewing gum, and gelatin desserts. ASP

**GERANYL TIGLATE** • A flavoring determined GRAS by FEMA *(see)*. *See* Allyl Tiglate.

**GERMANDER** • *Teucrium chamaedrys* or *Teucrium scorodonia.* Flavoring from an American plant used in alcoholic beverages only. *See* Sage. NUL

**GHATTI GUM** • Indian Gum. The gummy exudate from the stems of a plant abundant in India and Ceylon. Used as an emulsifier and in butter, butterscotch, and fruit flavorings for beverages. Limited to 0.1 to 0.2 percent of foods in which it is used. Has caused an occasional allergy but when ingested in large amounts has not caused obvious distress. The FDA's reevaluation in 1976 found the gum was GRAS if used at the rate of 0.2 percent for alcoholic beverages and 0.1 percent for all other food categories.

In pharmaceutical preparations one part ghatti usually replaces two parts acacia *(see)*. The final report to the FDA of the Select Committee on GRAS Substances stated in 1980 that there is no evidence in the available information that it is a hazard to the public when used as it is now and it should continue its GRAS status with limitations on the amount that can be added to food. ASP

**GIBBERELLIC ACID and ITS SALTS** • Used for malt beverages and distilled spirits. A plant growth–promoting hormone synthesized in 1978. Mildly toxic by ingestion. It is limited to less than 2 ppm in malt and 0.5 ppm in finished malt beverages. Its tolerance is zero in distilled spirits. Caused tumors in experimental animals. ASP

**GIGARTINA EXTRACTS** • A stabilizer from red algae of the sea. *See* Algae.

**GINGER** • *Zingiber officinale.* Derived from the rootlike stem of plants cultivated in all tropical countries, it is used in apple, plum, sausage, eggnog, pumpkin, ginger, ginger ale, and ginger beer flavorings for beverages, ice cream, ices, baked goods (2,500 ppm), and meats. The extract is used for cola, sausage, root beer, ginger, ginger ale, and ginger beer flavorings for beverages, ice cream, ices, candy, baked goods, chewing gum, meats, and condiments. Ginger has been used to break up intestinal gas and colic. GRAS. ASP

**GINGER OIL** • Obtained from the dried rhizomes of *Zingiber officinale,* it is used in flavorings for beverages, ice cream, ices, candy, baked goods, chewing gum, meats, and condiments. It is also used in perfumes. Employed medicinally to break up intestinal gas. A skin irritant. Has been shown to be mutagenic in rabbits. GRAS. ASP

**GINGER OLEORESIN** • Produced by extraction of the dried and unpeeled rhizome of *Zingiber officinale,* ground to a moderately coarse powder. The removal of the last few percentages of solvent is a problem which has yet to be solved satisfactorily. Certain solvents can be removed almost quantitatively through the use of small amounts of ethyl alcohol as a chaser during the last stages of evaporation. Ginger oleoresin is extracted from various types of ginger, but the majority of all ginger oleoresins are derived from Nigerian and Jamaican ginger, the former being the most inexpensive material, the latter having the most refined aroma. From the southwest coast of India comes a highly appreciated quality of ginger which is preferred for the production of oleoresin for use in carbonated beverages. It is used in root beer and ginger ale for the same products. ASP

**GINSENG** • *Panax ginseng* (Asia). *Panax quinquefolius* (North America). *Eleutherococcus senticosus* (Siberia). Root of the ginseng plant, grown in China, Korea, and the United States. The Chinese esteem ginseng as an herb of many uses and have been using it in medicine for more than five thousand years. The Chinese and Koreans also use it in combination with chicken soup. The word *panax* in its botanical name comes from the Greek *panakos,* a panacea. Among its active ingredients are amino acids, essential oils, carbohydrates, peptides, vitamins, minerals, enzymes, and sterols. In Asia, it is esteemed for its abilities to preserve health, invigorate the system, and prolong life. It is taken in an herbal tea as a daily tonic. North American Indians used ginseng as a love potion. It has been found to normalize high or low blood sugar. It produces a resin, a sugar starch, glue, and volatile oil. Ginseng is used as a flavoring additive in the United States and has a sweetish, licoricelike taste but is widely used in Asian medicines as an aromatic bitter.

**GLUCAMINE** • An organic compound that is prepared from glucose *(see).*

**GLUCITOL** • Sorbitol. Sorbol. White crystalline powder with a sweet taste used as an anticaking additive, curing additive, drying additive, emulsifier, firming additive, flavoring additive, formulation aid, free-flowing additive, humectant, lubricant, nutritive sweetener, pickling additive, releasing additive, sequestrant, stabilizer, surface-finishing additive, texturizing additive, and thickener. Used in baked goods, baking mixes, low-calorie beverages, hard and soft candy, chewing gum, chocolate, cough drops, frankfurters, frozen dairy desserts, jams, jellies, sausage, and shredded coconut. Limitation of 99 percent in hard candy and cough drops, 75 percent in chewing gum, 98 percent in soft candy, 30 percent in nonstandardized jams and jellies, 30 percent in baked goods, 17 percent in frozen dairy desserts, 12 percent in all other foods. Mildly toxic by ingestion and may cause diarrhea. *See also* Sorbitol. GRAS

**GLUCOAMYLASE** • An enzyme used to break down sugars in food processing.

**GLUCODELTA LACTONE** • White crystalline powder used as an acidifier, binder, curing additive, leavening additive, pH control additive, pickling additive, and sequestrant *(see).* Used in meat mixes, dessert mixes, frankfurters, Genoa salami, and sausages. GRAS

**GLUCOMANNAN** • A powder extracted from the roots of the konjac plant. The promoters claim that the powder, taken in a capsule before meals, absorbs liquid and swells in the stomach to form a gel and reduces hunger. The FDA was asked to approve it as GRAS but refused to do so unless scientific data were submitted. *See* Konjac Flour.

**GLUCONATE** • Calcium and Sodium. Sequestrants *(see)* derived from glucose, a sugar. Odorless, tasteless. Buffer *(see)* for confections and a firming additive for tomatoes and apple slices. Sodium gluconate is also used as a nutrient and dietary supplement. Final report to the FDA of the Select Committee on GRAS Substances in 1980 said it should continue its GRAS status with no limitations other than good manufacturing practices.

***d*-GLUCONIC ACID** • A light, amber liquid with the faint odor of vinegar, produced from corn. Used as a dietary supplement and as a sequestrant *(see)*. The magnesium salt of gluconic acid has been used as an antispasmodic. GRAS. NUL. E

**GLUCONO-DELTA-LACTONE** • An acid with a sweet taste; fine, white, odorless. It is used as a leavening additive in jelly powders and soft drink powders where dry food acid is desired. Used in the dairy industry to prevent milk stone, by breweries to prevent beer stone, and is also a component of many cleaning compounds. Also used as a pickling additive. Cleared by the USDA *(see)* for use at 8 ounces for each 100 pounds of cured, pulverized meat, or meat food product to speed up the color-fixing process and to reduce the time required for smoking. GRAS. ASP. E

**GLUCOSE** • Occurs naturally in animal blood, grape, and corn sugars. A source of energy for plants and animals. Sweeter than sucrose *(see),* glucose syrup is used to flavor sausage, hamburger, meat loaf, luncheon meat, chopped or pressed ham. It is also used as an extender in maple syrup. It is used medicinally for nutritional purposes and in the treatment of diabetic coma. Candymakers who work with it sometimes lose their nails.

*d***-GLUCOSE** • Corn sugar. *See* Glucose.

**GLUCOSE GLUTAMATE** • Used as a humectant in hand creams and lotions, it occurs naturally in animal blood, grape, and corn sugars, and is a source of energy for plants and animals. It is sweeter than sucrose. Glucose syrup is used to flavor sausage, hamburger, and other processed meats. Also used as an extender in maple syrup and medicinally as a nutrient. Glutamate is the salt of glutamic acid and is used to enhance natural food flavors. The FDA asked for further studies as to its potential mutagenic, teratogenic, subacute, and reproductive effects in 1980. Since then, the FDA has not reported any action.

**GLUCOSE ISOMERASE FROM *BACILLUS COAGULANS* or FROM IMMOBILIZED *ARTHROBACTER GLOBIFORMS* or FROM *STREPTOMYCES OLIVOCHROMOGENES* or FROM *STREPTOMYCES RUBIGINOSUS*** • Immobilized glucose isomerase is used on a massive scale throughout the world in the production of high-fructose syrups for the confectionery and soft-drink industries. Made from harmless bacteria and sugar. Yet, the FDA says it is NUL.

**GLUCOSE OXIDASE PREPARATION** • From *Aspergillis niger* or *Penicillium notatum.* Used to make sweetners. *See* Glucose Isomerase. NUL

**GLUCOSE PENTAACETATE** • Sugar substitute used for diabetics. ASP

**GLUCURONIC ACID** • A carbohydrate that is widely distributed in the animal kingdom.

**GLUTAMATE** • Ammonium and monopotassium salt of glutamic acid *(see)*. Used to enhance natural flavors and to improve the taste of tobacco. Used to impart meat flavor to foods, to enhance other natural food flavors, and to improve the taste of tobacco. It is used as an antioxidant in cosmetics to prevent spoilage. It is being studied by the FDA for mutagenic, ter-atogenic, subacute, and reproductive effects. The final report to the FDA of the Select Committee on GRAS Substances stated in 1980 that there is no evidence in the available information that it is a hazard to the public when used as it is now and it should continue its GRAS status with limitations on the amount that can be added to food. The European Parliament stated in 2003 that these taste enhancers can provoke in certain cases nervous symp-toms (decreased sensibility in neck, arms, and back) and irregular heartbeat. In animal testing, they provoked reproductive disorders in rats. They also are reported to cause problems for asthmatic persons.

**GLUTAMIC ACID** • L-Glutamic Acid. A white, practically odorless, free-flowing crystalline powder, a nonessential amino acid *(see)* usually manu-factured from vegetable protein. A salt substitute, it has been used to treat epilepsy and to correct stomach acids. It is used to enhance food flavors and to add meat flavor to foods. Glutamic acid with hydrochloride (*see* Hydro-chloric Acid) is used to improve the taste of beer. The final report to the FDA of the Select Committee on GRAS Substances stated in 1980 that there is no evidence in the available information that it is a hazard to the public when used as it is now and it should continue its GRAS status with limitations on the amount that can be added to food. ASP. E

**GLUTAMINE** • L-Glutamine. A nonessential amino acid *(see)* used as a medicine, dietary supplement, and as a culture medium. Mildly toxic by ingestion. Caused adverse reproductive effects in experimental animals.

**GLUTARAL** • *See* Glutaraldehyde and Glutaric Acid.

**GLUTARALDEHYDE** • A food flavoring. An amino acid *(see)* that occurs in green sugar beets. It has a faint agreeable odor and is used as a fixing additive for enzymes added to foods. It is also used as a flavor enhancer in foods. A petition to use glutaraldehyde-crosslinking additive in the manu-facture of edible collagen sausage casings was put in abeyance *(see)* by the FDA in 2003. Glutaraldehyde has caused birth defects in experimental ani-mals. A severe human skin irritant. *See* Glutaric Acid. ASP

**GLUTARIC ACID** • Pentanedioic Acid. A crystalline fatty acid that occurs in green sugar beets, meat, and in crude wood. Very soluble in alcohol and ether. Widely used in Asian medicine as an aromatic bitter.

**GLUTEN** • A mixture of proteins from wheat flour, obtained as an extremely sticky, yellowish gray mass by making a dough and then wash-ing out the starch. It consists almost entirely of two proteins, gliadin and glutelin, the exact proportions of which depend upon the variety of wheat. Contributes to the porous and spongy structure of bread. NUL

**GLY-** • The abbreviation for glycine *(see)*.

**(MONO)GLYCERIDE CITRATE** • Aids the action of and helps dissolve antioxidant formulations for oils and fats, such as shortenings for cooking.

**GLYCERIDES** • Monoglycerides, Diglycerides, and Monosodium Glycerides of Edible Fats and Oils. Any of a large class of compounds that are esters *(see)* of the sweet alcohol glycerin. They are also made synthetically. Emulsifying and defoaming additives. Used in bakery products to maintain "softness," in beverages, ice cream, ices, ice milk, milk, chewing-gum base, shortening, lard, oleomargarine, confections, sweet chocolate, chocolate, rendered animal fat, and whipped toppings. The diglycerides are on the FDA list of food additives to be studied for possible mutagenic, teratogenic, subacute, and reproductive effects. The glycerides are also used in cosmetic creams as texturizers, emulsifiers, and emollients. The final report to the FDA of the Select Committee on GRAS Substances stated in 1980 that it should continue its GRAS status with no limitations other than good manufacturing practices.

**GLYCERIN** • Glycerol. Any by-product of soap manufacture obtained by adding alkalies *(see)* to fats and fixed oils. A sweet (about 0.6 times that of cane sugar), warm-tasting substance. Used as a humectant in tobacco and in marshmallows, pastilles, and jellylike candies; as a solvent for colors and flavors; as a bodying additive in combination with gelatins and edible gums; as a plasticizer in edible coatings for meat and cheese. It is also used in beverages, confectionery, baked goods, chewing gum, gelatin desserts, meat products, soda-fountain fudge. In concentrated solutions it is irritating to the mucous membranes, but as used, nontoxic, nonirritating, nonallergenic. Contact with a strong oxidizing additive such as chromium trioxide, potassium chlorate, or potassium permanganate *(see)* may produce an explosion. The final report to the FDA of the Select Committee on GRAS Substances stated in 1980 that it should continue its GRAS status with no limitations other than good manufacturing practices. ASP

**GLYCERIN, SYNTHETIC** • Made from petroleum. ASP

**GLYCEROL** • *See* Glycerin. E

**GLYCEROL ESTER OF GUM ROSIN** • Turned down for GRAS because of insufficient information. *See* Rosin and Glycerol.

**GLYCEROL TRIBUTYRATE** • A synthetic flavoring. There is reported use of the chemical; it has not yet been assigned for toxicology literature. EAF

**GLYCERYL ABIETATE** • A density adjuster for citrus oil used in the preparation of alcoholic beverages and still and carbonated fruit drinks. Also cleared as a plasticizing material in chewing-gum base. No known toxicity.

**GLYCERYL BEHENATE** • Used to form tablets. There is no reported use of the chemical and there is no toxicology information available. *See* Behenic Acid. GRAS. NUL

**GLYCERYL CAPRATE** • The monoester of glycerin and caprylic acid *(see both)*.

**GLYCERYL CAPRYLATE** • *See* Glycerin and Caprylic Acid.

**GLYCERYL CAPRYLATE/CAPRATE** • A mixture of caprylic acid and capric acid (see both).

**GLYCERYL DILAURATE** • See Glycerin and Lauric Acid.

**GLYCERYL DIOLEATE** • The diester of glyceric and oleic acid *(see both)*.

**GLYCERYL DISTEARATE** • The diester of glycerin and stearic acid *(see both)*.

**GLYCEROL ESTER OF PARTIALLY DIMERIZED ROSIN** • A hard, pale, amber-colored resin produced by combining rosin *(see)* with food-grade glycerin. It is used in chewing-gum bases.

**GLYCEROL ESTER OF POLYMERIZED ROSIN** • Softener for chewing-gum base.

**GLYCEROL ESTERS OF WOOD ROSIN** • There are three general methods of producing rosins commercially, these methods (and their products) being: solvent extraction of pure stump wood (wood rosin); tapping of gum from the living tree (gum rosin); separation from tall oil (tall oil rosin). The three rosins, freed of extraneous impurities and refined, differ somewhat quantitatively and in color but all three may be glycinerated to produce the glycerol ester. It is used as a chewing-gum base and as a beverage stabilizer. The FDA turned down its GRAS designation in 2002 on the basis of insufficient data.

**GLYCEROL ESTER OF TALL OIL ROSIN** • A softener for chewing-gum base.

**GLYCEROL TRIBUTYRATE** • A synthetic flavoring. GRAS. EAF

**GLYCERYL ABIETATE** • A density adjuster for citrus oil used in the preparation of alcoholic beverages and still and carbonated fruit drinks. Also cleared as a plasticizing material in chewing-gum base.

**GLYCERYL BEHENATE** • Used to form tablets. *See* Behenic Acid. GRAS. NUL

**GLYCERYL CAPRATE** • The monoester of glycerin and caprylic acid *(see both)*.

**GLYCERYL CAPRYLATE** • *See* Glycerin and Caprylic Acid.

**GLYCERYL CAPRYLATE/CAPRATE** • A mixture of caprylic acid and capric acid *(see both)*.

**GLYCERYL DILAURATE** • *See* Glycerin and Lauric Acid.

**GLYCERYL DIOLEATE** • The diester of glycerin and oleic acid *(see both)*.

**GLYCERYL DISTEARATE** • The diester of glycerin and stearic acid *(see both)*.

**GLYCERYL HYDROSTEARATE** • *See* Glyceryl Monostearate.

**GLYCERYL 5-HYDROXYDECANOATE** • Artificially synthesized flavor. NIL

**GLYCERYL 5-HYDROXYDODECANOATE** • Artificially synthesized flavor. NIL

**GLYCERYL HYDROXYSTEARATE** • The monoester of glycerin and hydroxystearic acid. *See* Glycerin and Stearic Acid.

**GLYCERYL ISOSTEARATE** • *See* Glyceryl Monostearate.

**GLYCERYL-LACTO ESTERS OF FATTY ACIDS** • Emulsifiers. *See* Glycerol and Fatty Acids. ASP

**GLYCERYL LACTOOLEATE and LACTOPALMITATE OF FATTY ACIDS** • Food emulsifiers used in shortening where free and combined lactic acid does not exceed 1.75 percent of shortening plus additive. They add calories but are considered nontoxic. The final report to the FDA of the Select Committee on GRAS Substances stated in 1980 that it should continue its GRAS status with no limitations other than good manufacturing practices. NIL

**GLYCERYL LANOLATE** • The monoester of glycerin and lanolin *(see both)*.

**GLYCERYL LINOLEATE** • The monoester of glycerin and linoleic acid *(see both)*.

**GLYCERYL MONO- and DIESTERS** • Manufactured by reacting edible glycerides with ethylene oxide. These are used as defoamers in yeast production. The final report to the FDA of the Select Committee on GRAS Substances stated in 1980 that it should continue its GRAS status with no limitations other than good manufacturing practices.

**GLYCERYL MONOOLEATE** • A flavoring additive. *See* Glyceryl and Oleic Acid. GRAS. ASP

**GLYCERYL MONOSTEARATE** • An emulsifying and dispersing additive used in oleomargarine, shortenings, and other food products including noodles. Restricted to less than 2 percent of macaroni and less than 3 percent of noodle products. It is a mixture of two glyceryls. GRAS. ASP

**GLYCERYL MYRISTATE** • *See* Glycerin and Myristic Acid.

**GLYCERYL OLEATE** • *See* Glycerin and Oleic Acid.

**GLYCERYL-PABA** • The ester of glycine and para-aminobenzoic acid *(see both)*.

**GLYCERYL PALMITOSTEARATE** • A mixture of fatty acid glycerides, it is a fine powder or waxy solid. It is used in food processing. *See* Glycerides and Fatty Acids. GRAS. ASP

**GLYCERYL RICINOLEATE** • *See* Glycerin.

**GLYCERYL SESQUIOLEATE** • *See* Glycerin.

**GLYCERYL STARCH** • *See* Starch and various Glycerols.

**GLYCERYL STEARATE** • An emulsifier. *See* Glycerin.

**GLYCERYL TRIACETATE** • *See* Triacetin. GRAS. E

**GLYCERYL TRIBENZOATE** • Flavoring and flavor enhancer. *See* Glyceryl and Benzoic Acid. ASP

**GLYCERYL TRIBUTYRATE** • *See* Tributyrin.

**GLYCERYL TRIMYRISTATE** • *See* Glycerin and Myristic Acid.

**GLYCERYL TRIPROPANOATE** • Flavoring. *See* Glycerin and Proponoic Acid. ASP

**GLYCERYL TRISTEARATE** • Surface-finishing additive, formulation aid, lubricant, or release *(see)* additive. *See* Stearic Acid and Glycerin. ASP

**GLYCERYL TRIUNDECANOATE** • The triester of glycerin and unde-
cenoic acid *(see both)*.

**GLYCINE** • Aminoacetic Acid. Gly. Glycocoll. L-Glycine. An amino acid
*(see)* classified as nonessential. Found in beans, brewer's yeast, brown rice
bran, caseinate, dairy products, eggs, fish, gelatin, lactalbumin, legumes,
meat, nuts, seafood, seeds, soy, sugarcane, whey, whole grains. Reaction of
ammonia with chloroacetic acid. Made up of sweet-tasting crystals, it is
used as a dietary supplement and as a gastric antacid. Used with saccharin
to mask its aftertaste. Mildly toxic by ingestion. Restricted to less than 0.2
percent of the finished beverage or beverage base. The Food and Drug
Administration has expressed the opinion in trade correspondence that
glycine is GRAS for certain technical effects in human food when used in
accordance with good manufacturing practice; however, reports in scientific literature indicate that adverse effects were found in cases where high
levels of glycine were administered in diets of experimental animals and
current usage information indicates that the daily dietary intake of glycine
by humans may be substantially increasing due to changing use patterns in
food technology. Therefore, the Food and Drug Administration on April 1,
2003, said that it no longer regards glycine and its salts as GRAS for use in
human food and all outstanding letters expressing sanction for such use are
rescinded. The FDA said producers must reformulate food products for
human use to eliminate added glycine and its salts; or must bring such products into compliance with an authorizing food additive regulation. A food
additive petition supported by toxicity data is required to show that any proposed level of glycine or its salts added to foods for human consumption
will be safe. The additive is considered an essential nutrient in certain animal feeds and the FDA believes it is safe for such use under conditions of
good feeding practice. ASP. E

**GLYCOCHOLIC ACID** • A product of mixing cholic acid and glycine, it
is the chief ingredient of bile in vegetarian animals. It is used as an emulsifying additive for dried egg whites up to 0.1 percent. The final report to the
FDA of the Select Committee on GRAS Substances stated in 1980 that it
should continue its GRAS status with no limitations other than good manufacturing practices. There is no reported use of the chemical and there is
no toxicology information available. NUL

**GLYCOFUROL** • *See* Furfural.

**GLYCOGEN** • Distributed throughout cell protoplasm, it is an animal
starch found especially in liver and muscle. Used as a violet dye.

**GLYCOLIC ACID** • Contained in sugarcane juice, it is an odorless, slightly
water-absorbing acid used to control the acid-alkali balance in cosmetics and
whenever a cheap organic acid is needed. It is also used in copper brighten-
ing, decontamination procedures, and in dyeing. It is a mild irritant to the skin
and mucous membranes. The final report to the FDA of the Select Committee

on GRAS Substances stated in 1980 that it should continue its GRAS status with no limitations other than good manufacturing methods.

**GLYCOL DISTEARATE** • Alcohol from glycol. *See* Glycols.

**GLYCOLS** • Propylene Glycol. Glycerin. Ethylene Glycol. Carbitol. Diethylene Glycol. Glycol literally means "glycerin" plus "alcohol." A group of syrupy alcohols derived from hydrocarbons *(see)* and used in foods as emulsifiers and in chewing-gum bases and in cosmetics as humectants. The FDA cautions manufacturers that glycols may cause adverse reactions in users. Propylene glycol and glycerin *(see both)* are considered safe. Other glycols in low concentrations may be harmless for external application but ethylene glycol, carbitol, and diethylene glycol are hazardous in concentrations exceeding 5 percent even in preparations for use on small areas of the body. Wetting additives *(see)* increase the absorption of glycols and therefore their toxicity.

**GLYCOL STEARATE** • An emulsifier. *See* Glycols and Stearates.

**GLYCOPHEN** • Promidione. Rovral. A fungicide used in animal feed, ginseng (dried), grape pomace (dried), raisin waste, raisins, and soap stock. FDA residue tolerance of 300 ppm in raisins, 4 ppm in dried ginseng, and 225 ppm in dried grape pomace and raisin waste for animal feed. Moderately toxic by ingestion.

**GLYCOSIDES** • Many flowering plants contain cardiac glycosides. The most well known are foxglove, lily of the valley, and squill. The cardiac glycosides have the ability to increase the force and power of the heartbeat without increasing the amount of oxygen needed by the heart muscle. Among the glycosides are cyanogens, goitrogens, estrogens, and saponins. They are found in lima beans, cassava, flax, broccoli and other brassicas, most legumes, and grasses.

**GLYCYRRHETINIC ACID** • Used as a flavoring. Prepared from licorice root, it has been used medicinally to treat a disease of the adrenal gland.

**GLYCYRRHETINYL STEARATE** • The stearic acid ester of glycyrrhetinic acid *(see)*.

**GLYCYRRHIZA and GLYCYRRHIZA EXTRACT** • *See* Glycyrrhizin, Ammoniated. GRAS

**GLYCYRRHIZIC ACID** • Used as a flavoring, coloring. Extracted from licorice. *See* Glycyrrhetinic Acid.

**GLYCYRRHIZIN, AMMONIATED** • Glycyrrhiza. Licorice. Product of dried root from the Mediterranean region used in licorice, anise, root beer, wintergreen, and birch beer flavorings for beverages, ice cream, ices, candy, and baked goods. It is used as a sugar substitute. It is one hundred times as sweet as sugar. It is also used to flavor tobacco and pharmaceuticals, as a demulcent and expectorant, and as a drug vehicle. It doesn't have calories. The final report to the FDA of the Select Committee on GRAS Substances stated in 1980 that it should continue its GRAS status with limitations on amounts that can be added to food. Cases have been reported of avid licorice eaters who develop high blood pressure. *See* Licorice. ASP

**GLYOXYLIC ACID** • Used as a coloring. Syrup or crystals that occur in unripe fruit, young leaves, and baby sugar beets. Forms a thick, malodorous syrup. It absorbs water from the air and condenses with urea to form allantoin *(see)* and gives a nice blue color with sulfuric acid. It is a skin irritant and corrosive.

**GLYPHOSATE** • A broad spectrum, postemergent herbicide used in animal feed. FDA residues allowed are 0.4 ppm in dried citrus pulp, 20 ppm in soybean hulls, and 30 ppm in sugarcane molasses.

**GOLD** • As a food additive it is used solely for external decoration where it can be found on chocolate confectionery, in the covering of dragées, and the decoration of sugar-coated flour confectionery. E

**GONADORELIN** • A hormone used as an injection for cattle to increase growth. In humans it can cause such side effects as nausea, headache, and flushing.

**GONADOTROPIN (SERUM)** • A hormone capable of promoting growth and function of testes and ovaries when injected into cattle. It is also used in human medicine.

**GRADE** • Grading and inspection assure purity, wholesomeness, and appearance. The USDA has established grades for more than three hundred food products. Grading for most products is done voluntarily at the manufacturers' request (and expense) by a USDA inspector, and a USDA grade symbol may then appear on the package; lack of a symbol does not mean substandard product. Unfortunately, these grades lack continuity among product categories (Grade AA is the highest grade for eggs; Grade A is the highest for milk). Meat and poultry, however, whether fresh or processed and packaged must be inspected and carry an inspection stamp.

**GRAINS OF PARADISE** • *Aframomum melegueta.* Pungent aromatic seeds of a tropical African plant of the ginger family. It is a natural flavoring used in fruit, ginger, ginger ale, and pepper flavorings for beverages, ice cream, ices, and candy. GRAS. EAF

**GRAM (g)** • A metric unit of weight—28.3 grams equals 1 ounce. There are 1,000 mgs in a gram. Food labels list fat, protein, carbohydrate, and fiber in grams (g) per serving.

**GRAMINIS** • *See* Dog Grass Extract.

**GRAM-NEGATIVE, -POSITIVE** • Classification of bacteria according to whether or not they accept a stain named after Hans Gram, a Danish bacteriologist. Different life processes and vulnerabilities of germs are reflected by their gram-positive or gram-negative characteristics. An antibiotic may be effective against certain gram-positive germs and have no effect on gram-negative ones and vice versa.

**GRAPE COLOR EXTRACT** • Enocianina. A purple-red liquid extracted from the residue of grapes pressed for use in grape juice and wine. Used for coloring in still and carbonated drinks and ales, beverage bases, and alcoholic beverages. ASP

**GRAPE ESSENCE, NATURAL** • The liquid expressed from fresh grapes used as a coloring.

**GRAPE POMACE** • Source of natural red and blue colorings. Also used as an animal feed. *See* Anthocyanins.

**GRAPE SEED EXTRACT** • A flavoring determined GRAS by FEMA *(see)*. It is being reviewed at the request of the National Cancer Institute for subchronic, reproductive, and developmental toxicity.

**GRAPE SEED OIL** • An ingredient in fragrances obtained by expression from the fresh peel of the grape. The yellow, sometimes reddish liquid is also used in fruit flavorings.

**GRAPE SKIN EXTRACT** • Enocianina. Used in still and carbonated drinks and ades, beverage bases, and alcoholic beverages. Permanently listed since 1966. Does not require certification. GRAS. ASP

**GRAPFRUIT ESSENCE, NATURAL** • *See* Grapefruit Oil. ASP

**GRAPEFRUIT EXTRACT** • *See* Grapefruit Oil. EAF

**GRAPEFRUIT, JUICE** • Flavoring. EAF

**GRAPEFRUIT OIL** • The yellow, sometimes reddish liquid is an ingredient obtained by expression from the fresh peel of the grapefruit. Used for lemon, lime, orange, and peach flavorings for beverages, ice cream, ices, candy, baked goods, gelatin desserts, chewing gum (1,500 ppm), and toppings. An experimental tumor-causing additive. Grapefruit is promoted in weight-loss diets and it has been found to interfere with the work of a liver and intestinal enzyme, CYP3A4. As a result, grapefruit can interact with a wide range of medications including those for cholesterol-lowering, heart disease, antibiotics, and antianxiety medicines. Grapefruit oil can irritate the skin. GRAS. ASP

**GRAPEFRUIT OIL, TERPENELESS (CITRUS PARADISI)** • *See* Grapfruit Oil and Terpenes. EAF

**GRAS** • The Generally Recognized As Safe List was established in 1958 by Congress. Those substances that were being added to food over a long time, which under conditions of their intended use were generally recognized as safe by qualified scientists, would be exempt from premarket clearance. Congress had acted on a very marginal response—on the basis of returns from those scientists sent questionnaires. Approximately 355 out of 900 responded, and only about 100 of those responses had substantive comments. Three items were removed from the originally published list. Since then, developments in the scientific fields and in consumer awareness have brought to light the inadequacies of the testing of food additives and, ironically, the complete lack of testing of the Generally Recognized as Safe List. President Nixon directed the FDA to reevaluate items on the GRAS list. The reevaluation was completed and a number of items were removed from the list. Although there were a number of others on the list, some of them top priority, to be studied in 1980, nothing has been reported by the FDA on their status since then.

**GREEN** • *See* FD and C Green (Nos. 1, 2, 3).

**GREEN S** • Coloring. E

**GREEN BEAN EXTRACT** • The extract of the unripe beans of domesticated species of *Phaseolus.*

**GREEN TEA EXTRACT** • A number of studies in the 1990s have suggested green tea may help prevent certain human illnesses. An ingredient, epigallocatechin gallate (EGCG), reportedly carries twice the antioxidant power of red wine and vitamins C and E. *See* Antioxidants.

**GROUND LIMESTONE** • Used as a flavoring. GRAS. EAF

**GROUNDSEL EXTRACT** • Extract of *Senecio vulgaris,* a North American maritime shrub or tree.

**GUAIAC GUM (GUAIACUM)** • *See* Gum Guaiac. Used as a flavoring in alcoholic beverages.

**GUAIAC WOOD OIL** • Guaiacum. Yellow to amber, semisolid mass with a floral odor. Derived from steam distillation of guaiac wood. A gum resin used in fruit and rum flavorings for beverages, ice cream, ices, candy, and baked goods. The oil is a raspberry, strawberry, rose, fruit, honey, ginger, and ginger ale flavoring for beverages, ice cream, candy, baked goods, gelatin desserts, and chewing gum. Formerly used to treat rheumatism. *See* Guaiac Gum.

**GUAIACYL ACETATE** • A synthetic berry flavoring for beverages, ice cream, ices, candy, gelatin, chewing gum, and baked goods. ASP

**GUAIACYL PHENYLACETATE** • A synthetic berry, coffee, honey, tobacco, and smoke flavoring additive for beverages, ice cream, ices, candy, baked goods, and toppings.

**GUAIOL** • An alcohol from guaiac wood *(see)* ASP

**GUANIDOETHYL CELLULOSE** • *See* Guaiac Wood Oil.

**GUANYLIC ACID SODIUM SALT** • Disodium Guanylate. A flavor enhancer used in canned foods, poultry, sauces, snack items, and soups. Mildly toxic by ingestion. Has caused mutations in experimental animals. E

**GUAR GUM** • *Cyamopsis tetragonolobus.* Guar Flour. From ground nutritive seed tissue of plants cultivated in India, it has five to eight times the thickening power of starch. A free-flowing powder, it is used as a stabilizer for frozen fruit, icings, glazes, and fruit drinks, and as a thickener for hot and cold drinks. Also a binder for meats, confections, baked goods, cheese spreads, cream cheese, ice cream, ices, French dressing, and salad dressing. Keeps tablet formulations from disintegrating, and is used in cosmetic emulsions, toothpastes, lotions, and creams. Employed also as a bulk laxative, appetite suppressant, and to treat peptic ulcers. The FDA's reevaluation in 1976 found guar gum to be GRAS if used as a stabilizer, thickener, and firming additive at 0.35 percent in baked goods, 1.2 percent in breakfast cereals, 2 percent in fats and oils, 1.2 percent in gravies, 1 percent in sweet sauces, toppings, and syrups, and 2 percent in processed vegetables and vegetable juices. In large amounts, it may cause nausea, flatulence, or abdominal cramps. The final report to the FDA of the Select Committee on GRAS Substances stated in 1980 that there is no evidence in the available information that it is a hazard to the public when used as it is now and it should continue its GRAS status with limitations on amounts that can be added to food. In 1997, however, the FDA banned it from use as an active ingredient in drugs because it swells when wet and had been used in weight-loss products to produce a feeling of fullness. One brand resulted in hospitalization of at least ten patients and one death from a blood clot after surgery to remove a throat blockage. GRAS. ASP. E

**GUARANA GUM** • *Paullina cupana.* The dried paste consisting mainly of crushed seed from a plant grown in Brazil. Contains about 4 percent caffeine. Used in cola flavorings for beverages and candy. *See* Caffeine for toxicity. There is reported use of the chemical; it has not yet been assigned for toxicology literature.

**GUARANINE** • *See* Caffeine.

**GUAVA** • Psidium. Extracted from the fruit of a small shrubby American tree widely cultivated in warm regions. The fruit is sweet, sometimes acid, globular, and yellow. It is used to flavor jelly. GRAS. ASP

**GUINEA GREEN B** • *See* FD and C Green No. 1.

**GUM** • True plant gums are the dried exudates from various plants obtained when the bark is cut or other injury is suffered. Gums are soluble in hot or cold water and sticky. Today the term gum, both for natural and synthetic sources, usually refers to resins. Gums are also used as emulsifiers, stabilizers, and suspending additives.

**GUM ACACIA** • *See* Gum Arabic.

**GUM ARABIC** • Acacia Gum. The exudate from acacia trees grown in the Sudan. Used in face masks, hairsprays, setting lotions, rouge, and powders for compacts. Serves as an emulsifier, stabilizer, and gelling additive. Used in ice cream and vanilla powder. It may cause allergic reactions such as hay fever, dermatitis, gastrointestinal distress, and asthma. GRAS

**GUM BENJAMIN** • *See* Benzoin.

**GUM BENZOIN** • It is the balsamic resin from benzoin grown in Thailand, Cambodia, Sumatra, and Vietnam. Used to glaze and polish confections.

**GUM DAMMAR** • *See* Damar.

**GUM GHATTI** • *See* Ghatti Gum.

**GUM GLUTEN** • Used as a stabilizer in macaroni products. *See* Gluten.

**GUM GUAIAC** • Resin from the wood of the guaiacum used widely as an antioxidant in edible fats or oils, beverages, rendered animal fat, or a combination of such fats and vegetable fats. Also used as a flavoring. According to FAO/WHO *(see)*, very little is absorbed. It is also used in cosmetic creams and lotions. Brown or greenish brown. Formerly used in treatment of rheumatism. The FDA of the Select Committee on GRAS Substances stated in 2003 that it should continue its GRAS with tolerance of 0.01 percent antioxidant activity.

**GUM KARAYA** • Sterculia Gum. It is the dried exudate of a tree native to India. Karaya came into wide use during World War I as a cheaper substitute for gum tragacanth *(see)*. Karaya swells in water and alcohol but does not dissolve. It is used as a stabilizer in cheese, dressings for foods, ice cream, and fruit jelly and jam. Because of its high viscosity at low concentrations, its ability to produce highly stable emulsions, and its resistance to acids, it is widely used in frozen food products. In 1971, however, the FDA put this additive on the list of chemicals to be studied for teratogenic, mutagenic, subacute, and reproductive effects. It can cause allergic reactions such as hay fever, dermatitis, gastrointestinal diseases, and asthma. GRAS

**GUM ROSIN** • *See* Rosins.

**GUM SUMATRA** • *See* Gum Benzoin.

**GUM TRAGACANTH** • The dried gummy exudate from plants found in Iran, Asia Minor, and Syria. A thickener and stabilizer, odorless, and with a gluelike taste. Used in fruit jelly, ornamental icings, fruit, sherbets, water ices, salad dressing, French dressing, confections, and candy. An emulsifier used in brilliantine, shaving cream, toothpaste, face packs, foundation cream, hairspray, mascara, depilatories, compact powder, rouge, dentifrice, setting lotion, eye makeup, and hand lotion. Also employed in compounding drugs and pastes. One of the oldest known natural emulsifiers, its history predates the Christian era by hundreds of years; it has been recognized in the U.S. Pharmacopoeia since 1829. It has a long shelf life and is resistant to acids. Aside from occasional allergic reactions, it can be ingested in large amounts with little harm except for diarrhea, gas, or constipation. When reevaluated it was found to be GRAS in the following percentages: 0.2 percent for baked goods; 0.7 percent in condiments and relishes; 1.3 percent in fats and oils; 0.8 percent in gravies and sauces; 0.2 percent in meat products; 0.2 percent in processed fruits; and 0.1 percent in all other categories.

**GUTTA HANG KANG** • *Palaquium leiocarpum.* A chewing-gum base. Natural masticatory substances of vegetable origin. ASP

# H

**HAEMATOCOCCUS ALGAE MEAL** • The color additive haematococcus algae meal is used to enhance the pink to orange-red color of the flesh of salmonid fish. It consists of the comminuted and dried cells of the alga

*Haematococcus.* The FDA says that the meal must have the following restrictions: Lead, not more than 5 parts per million; arsenic, not more than 2 ppm; mercury, not more than 1 ppm; heavy metals (as lead), not more than 10 ppm; astaxanthin, not less than 1.5 percent pluvials. EAF

**HALOXON** • Galloxon. An antiworm medicine for animals. FDA residue tolerance is 0.1 ppm in edible tissues of cattle, sheep, and goats.

**HALSOSALT** • Made from cornstarch that is fermented to produce lysine, a salty amino acid, it is being proposed as a salt substitute.

**HAW BARK** • Black Extract. Extract of the fruit of a hawthorn shrub or tree. Used in butter, caramel, cola, maple, and walnut flavorings for beverages, ice cream, ices, candy, and baked goods. Has been used as a uterine antispasmodic. ASP

**HAWTHORN BERRY** • *Crataegus oxyacantha.* A spring-flowering shrub or tree. A number of scientific studies in Central Europe and in the United States have found that hawthorn berries can dilate the blood vessels and lower blood pressure. The berries reportedly also can increase the enzyme metabolism of the heart and make the heart's use of oxygen during exercise more efficient. Hawthorn extracts are also believed to have some diuretic properties. In the 1800s, the berries were used to treat digestive problems and insomnia. They contain bioflavonoids, compounds that are necessary for vitamin C function and also help strengthen blood vessels. In Germany, this herb is used to treat early-stage congestive heart failure and in the United States, it is used by health practioners to lower blood pressure. *See* Haw Bark.

**HAZELNUT OIL** • The oil obtained from the various species of the hazelnut tree, genus *Corylus.*

**HCL** • The abbreviation for hydrochloride.

**HEATHER EXTRACT** • An extract of *Calluna vulgaris,* also called ling extract.

**HECTORITE** • An emulsifier and extender. A clay consisting of silicate of magnesium and lithium, it is used in the chill-proofing of beer. The dust can be irritating to the lungs.

**HEDEOMA OIL** • *See* Pennyroyal Oil.

**HELIOTROPIN** • Piperonal. Used in cherry and vanilla flavors. A purple diazo dye *(see)* with a heliotrope odor. Usually made from oxidation of piperic acid. Ingestion of large amounts may cause central nervous system depression. Applications to the skin may cause allergic reactions and skin irritations.

**HELIOTROPINE** • *See* Heliotropin.

**HELIOTROPYL ACETATE** • *See* Piperonyl Acetate.

**HELIUM** • This colorless, odorless, tasteless gas is used as propellant for foods packed in pressurized containers. The final report to the FDA of the Select Committee on GRAS Substances stated in 1980 that it should continue its GRAS status with no limitations other than good manufacturing practices. NUL. E

**HEMICELLULOSE EXTRACT** • Used in feed as a source of metabolizable energy. It is in the cell walls of all plants and some seaweeds and contains a variety of sugars. Nontoxic.

**HEMLOCK NEEDLES AND TWIGS OIL** • Tsuga. Spruce Oil. A natural flavoring extract from North American or Asian nonpoisonous hemlock. Used in fruit, root beer, and spice flavorings for beverages, ice cream, ices, candy, baked goods, gelatin desserts, puddings, and chewing gum. NUL

**HENDECANAL** • *See* Undecanal.

**HENDECEN-9-OL** • *See* 9-Undecanal.

**2,4-HEPTADIENAL** • Used as a flavoring additive in various foods. Moderately toxic by ingestion. Severe skin irritant. ASP

*g*-**HEPTALACTONE** • A synthetic coconut, nut, and vanilla flavoring for beverages, ice cream, ices, candy, and baked goods. ASP. E

**HEPTALDEHYDE** • *See* Heptanal.

**HEPTANAL** • Heptaldehyde. Oily, colorless liquid with a penetrating fruit odor made from castor oil. A synthetic flavoring additive used in citrus, apple, melon, cognac, rum, and almond flavorings for beverages, ice cream, ices, candy, baked goods, and liqueurs. Mildly toxic by ingestion. ASP

**HEPTANAL DIMETHYL ACETAL** • A synthetic fruit, melon, and mushroom flavoring additive for beverages, ice cream, ices, candy, baked goods, chewing gum, and condiments. ASP

**HEPTANAL GLYCERYL ACETAL** • A synthetic mushroom flavoring for beverages, ice cream, ices, candy, and baked goods. ASP

**2,3-HEPTANEDIONE** • A synthetic raspberry, strawberry, butter, fruit, rum, nut, and cheese flavoring additive for beverages, ice cream, ices, candy, baked goods, and chewing gum. ASP

**HEPTANOIC ACID** • Enanthic Acid. Found in various fusel oils and in rancid oils, it has the faint odor of tallow. It is made from grapes and is a fatty acid used chiefly in making esters *(see)* for flavoring materials. ASP

**2-HEPTANOL** • A synthetic flavoring additive, liquid, and miscible with alcohol and ether. *See* Heptyl Alcohol for use. ASP

**2-HEPTANONE** • A synthetic flavoring additive, liquid, with a penetrating odor, used to give a "peppery" smell to such cheeses as Roquefort. Found in oil of cloves and in cinnamon bark oil. Used in berry, butter, fruit, and cheese flavorings for beverages, ice cream, ices, candy, baked goods, chewing gum, and condiments (25 ppm). Found naturally in oil of cloves and in cinnamon bark oil. The lethal concentration in air for rats is 4,000 ppm. In high doses it is narcotic, and a suspected irritant to human mucous membranes. ASP

**3-HEPTANONE** • A synthetic melon flavoring additive for beverages, ice cream, ices, candy, and baked goods. *See* 2-Heptanone, which is a similar compound.

**4-HEPTANONE** • A synthetic strawberry and fruit flavoring additive for beverages, ice cream, ices, candy, baked goods, and gelatin desserts. *See* 2-Heptanone, which is a similar compound. ASP

**cis-4-HEPTENAL** • Synthetic mushroom flavoring. ASP

**2-HEPTENAL** • Green grassy, herbaceous, spicy, fruity esterlike synthetic flavoring. Suggested use in apple, fruit, cucumber, pear, grape flavorings; also used in fragrances for fruity top notes; also geranium and galbanum. ASP

**4 HEPTENAL DIETHYL ACETAL** • Synthetic flavoring. FAO/WHO *(see)* has no safety concern at current levels of intake. NIL

**(Z)-4-HEPTEN-1-OL** • Synthetic flavoring that is described as creamy grass or banana. EAF

**2-HEPTEN-4-ONE** • Synthetic flavoring derived from hazelnuts. ASP

**3-HEPTEN-2-ONE** • Synthetic flavoring derived from peppers. FAO/WHO *(see)* says there is no safety concern. ASP

**TRANS-3-HEPTENYL ACETATE** • Synthetic flavoring. FAO/WHO says there is no safety concern. ASP

**TRANS-3-HEPTENYL-2-METHYLPROPANOATE** • Synthetic flavoring. FAO/WHO says there is no safety concern. ASP

**HEPTYL ACETATE** • A synthetic berry, banana, melon, pear, and pineapple flavoring additive for beverages, ice cream, ices, candy, and baked goods. *See* 2-Heptanone. EAF

**3-HEPTYL ACETATE** • Synthetic flavoring. FAO/WHO says there is no safety concern. ASP

**HEPTYL ALCOHOL** • 1-Heptanol. Colorless, fragrant liquid miscible with alcohol. A synthetic flavoring additive with a fatty, citrus odor, used in fruit flavorings for beverages, ice cream, ices, candy, and baked goods. Moderately toxic by ingestion and skin contact. *See* 2-Heptanone. ASP

**HEPTYL ALDEHYDE** • *See* Heptanal.

**HEPTYL BUTYRATE** • Butyric Acid. A synthetic raspberry, floral, violet, apricot, melon, and plum flavoring additive for beverages, ice cream, ices, candy, baked goods. ASP

**2-HEPTYL BUTYRATE** • Synthetic flavoring. FAO/WHO says there is no safety concern. EAF

**HEPTYL BUTYROLACTONE** • Synthetic flavoring. *See* Undecalactone and Butyrolactone.

**HEPTYL CINNAMATE** • A synthetic cinnamon flavoring. ASP

**3-HEPTYLDIHYDRO-5-METHYL-2(3H)-FURANONE** • Synthetic flavoring. FAO/WHO *(see)* has no safety concern. ASP

**HEPTYL FORMATE** • Used in artificial fruit essences. A skin irritant. *See* 2-Heptanone. ASP

**2-HEPTYL FURAN** • Synthetic flavoring. *See* Furans. NIL

**HEPTYL HEPTANOATE** • Colorless liquid with fruity odor used in artificial fruit essences. *See* 2-Heptanone.

**HEPTYL ISOBUTYRATE** • A synthetic coconut, apricot, peach, pineapple, and plum flavoring additive for beverages, ice cream, ices, candy, and baked goods. NIL

**HEPTYL OCTANOATE** • Synthetic flavoring. NIL

**HEPTYL PELARGONATE** • Liquid with pleasant odor used in flavors and perfumes. *See* 2-Heptanone.

***n*-HEPTYLIC ACID** • *See* Heptanoic Acid.

**HEPTYLPARABEN** • A preservative used in fermented malt beverages to inhibit microbiological spoilage. It is also used in noncarbonated soft drinks and fruit-based beverages when allowed by established standards of identity. FDA tolerance is 12 ppm. *See* Parabens. ASP

**HERB** • FDA abbreviation for herbicide.

**HERB ROBERT EXTRACT** • Extract of the entire plant, *Geranium robertianum. See* Geranium Oil.

**HESPERIDIN** • A natural bioflavonoid *(see)*. Fine needles from citrus fruit peel. Used as a synthetic sweetener. EAF

**HEXACHLOROPHENE** • An antibacterial used in animal products, but the FDA restricts its use. In 1969 scientists reported microscopically visible brain damage in rats from small concentrations of this chemical. The company that had the patent on hexachlorophene, the Swiss-based Givaudan Corporation, sold the chemical only to those companies that could demonstrate a safe and effective use for it. However, when the patent ran out, it was sold for many purposes. It is still used in small amounts in some cosmetic products for humans.

**1-HEXADECANOIC ACID** • *See* Palmitic Acid.

**1-HEXADECANOL** • Cetyl Alcohol. A synthetic chocolate flavoring additive for ice cream, ices, and candy. Moderately toxic by ingestion. An eye and human skin irritant.

**OMEGA-6-HEXADECENLACTONE** • Ambrettolide. 6-Hexadecenolide. A synthetic fruit flavoring additive for beverages, ice cream, ices, candy, baked goods, gelatin desserts, and chewing gum. ASP

**6-HEXADECENOLIDE** • *See* Omega-6-Hexadecenlactone.

**HEXADECYLIC ACID** • *See* Palmitic Acid

**trans,trans-2-4-HEXADIENAL** • Hexa-2,4-Dienal; 2,4-Hexadienal; 2,4-Hexadien-1-ol; 2,4-Hx; 1,3-Pentadiene-1-Carboxaldehyde; 2-Propylene Acrolein; Sorbaldehyde; Sorbic Aldehyde 2,4-Hexadienal. A colorless to yellow liquid with a pungent "green" or citrus odor, is used as a food additive for flavor enhancement, as a fragrance agent, as a starting material or intermediate in synthetic reactions in the chemical and pharmaceutical industries, as a fumigant, and as a corrosion inhibitor for steel. 2,4-

hexadienal was nominated for study by the National Cancer Institute because of the potential for carcinogenicity based on its a,b-unsaturated aldehyde structure and the potential link between exposure to lipid peroxidation products in the diet and human malignancies. The commercial product is a mixture containing chiefly trans,trans-2,4-hexadienal in equilibrium with cis,trans-2,4-hexadienal. Male and female rats and mice received 2,4-hexadienal (89 percent trans, trans; 11 percent cis,trans) in corn oil by gavage for sixteen days, fourteen weeks, or two years. Under the conditions of these two-year gavage studies, there was clear evidence of carcinogenic activity of 2,4-hexadienal in rats and mice based on increased incidences of squamous cell neoplasms of the forestomach. The occurrence of squamous cell carcinoma of the oral cavity (tongue) in male mice may have been related to the administration of 2,4-hexadienal. The NTP Board of Scientific Counselors Technical Reports Review Subcommittee, October 18, 2001, accepted the toxicology findings. This additive, of course, should be banned. ASP

**2,4 HEXADIENAL-1-OL** • It occurs naturally in many foods including kiwi, mango, peanuts, clams, and beer. In concentrated form, it exhibits a powerful irritating odor but at concentrations used in flavorings (less than 1 ppm) it provides a sweet green aroma. Based on 1999 reports, the daily per capita intake for "eaters only" is estimated at 0.003 mg/kg body weight per day as a flavoring. After two years of gavage studies, there was clear evidence of cancer-causing activity in rats and mice. The NTP concluded that the high doses given the rodents caused chronic irritation. Gavage administrations provides a bolus dose that exerts traumatic effect on the lining of the rodents forestomach. Thus, the experts concluded, it would not be expected in the diet and concluded it was safe as a flavoring. ASP

**2,4-HEXADIENOATE** • *See* Allyl Sorbate.

**HEXAHYDROPYRIDENE** • *See* Piperidine

**HEXAHYDROTHYMOL** • *See* Menthol.

**HEXAKIS** • A pesticide to kill mites in animal feeds. The residue tolerance set by the FDA ranges from 20 ppm in raisin waste to 100 ppm in dried grape pomace. A corrosive skin and eye irritant.

**HEXALACTONE (d, g, or y)** • Synthetic butter, fruit, honey, and vanilla flavoring for beverages, ice cream, ices, candy, baked goods, chewing gum, and gelatin desserts.

**HEXALDEHYDE** • *See* Hexanal.

**HEXAMETHYLENETETRAMINE (HMT)** • Methenamine. Odorless powder or crystals used in adhesives, coatings, as a stabilizers for lubricating and insulating oils, as a urinary antibacterial, and as a urinary antiseptic for animals. It is used in production of Provolone cheese. Studies at Italy's University of Milan concluded there was no appreciable health risk from ingestion of cheese made with this additive. E

**HEXANAL** • Hexaldehyde. Hexoic Aldehyde. A synthetic flavoring additive occurring naturally in apples, coffee, cooked chicken, strawberries, tea, and tobacco leaves (oils). Used in butter, fruit, honey, and rum flavorings for beverages, ice cream, ices, candy, baked goods, chewing gum, and gelatin desserts. ASP

**1-HEXANAL** • *See* Hexyl Alcohol. ASP

**HEXANE** • Made from crude oil. Pure *n*-hexane is a colorless liquid with a slightly disagreeable odor. It is highly flammable, and its vapors can be explosive. The major use for solvents containing *n*-hexane is to extract vegetable oils from crops such as soybeans. ASP

**HEXANEDIOIC ACID** • *See* Adipic Acid.

**2,3,HEXANEDIONE** • Synthetic flavoring. ASP

**1,6-HEXANEDITHIOL** • Synthetic flavoring. *See* Hexane. EAF

**1-HEXANETHIOL** • Synthetic Flavoring. *See* Hexane. EAF

**1,2,6-HEXANETRIOL** • An alcohol used as a solvent. No known skin toxicity.

**HEXANOIC ACID** • A synthetic flavoring additive that occurs naturally in apples, butter acids, cocoa, grapes, oil of lavender, oil of lavandin, raspberries, strawberries, and tea. Used in butter, butterscotch, chocolate, berries, strawberries, and tea. Used in butter, butterscotch, chocolate, berry, fruit, rum, pecan, and cheese flavorings for beverages, ice cream, ices, candy, baked goods, chewing gum, and condiments. Moderately toxic by ingestion and skin contact. Severe eye irritant. Has caused mutations in laboratory animals. ASP

**HEXANOL** • Hexyl Alcohol. Used as an antiseptic and preservative, it occurs as the acetate *(see)* in seeds and fruits of *Hercleum sphondylium* and *Umbelliferae*. *See* Hexyl Alcohol.

**3-HEXANOL** • Hexyl Alcohol. Used as an antiseptic and preservative in cosmetics, it occurs as the acetate *(see)* in seeds and fruits of *Heracleum sphondylium* and *Umbelliferae*. Colorless liquid slightly soluble in water, it is miscible with alcohol. ASP

**3-HEXANONE** • A solvent. Toxic by ingetion. ASP

**HEXAZINONE** • A weed killer used in various plant products. Moderately toxic by ingestion and by skin contact. Has caused adverse reproductive effects in laboratory animals.

**trans-3-HEXENAL** • Synthetic flavoring. It is a spoilage protectant in potatoes and has a pineapple taste. ASP

**2-HEXENAL** • A synthetic berry and fruit flavoring additive that occurs naturally in apples and strawberries and is used for beverages, ice cream, ices, candy, and baked goods. ASP

**cis-3-HEXENAL** • A synthetic fruit flavoring additive for beverages, ice cream, ices, and candy. ASP

**trans-4-HEXANAL** • A flavoring determined GRAS by FEMA *(see)*.

**(E)-2-HEXENAL DIETHYL ACETAL** • A flavoring determined GRAS by FEMA *(see)*.

**3-HEXENOIC ACID** • *See* Methyl Hexenoate. ASP

**1-HEXEN-3-OL** • Artificial odorant with a green smell. ASP

**2-HEXEN-1-OL** • A synthetic flavoring that is a colorless liquid with a fruity odor. It occurs naturally in grapes; similar in compound to 3-Hexen-1-ol. Used in fruit and mint flavorings for beverages, ice cream, ices, candy, and baked goods. Moderately toxic by ingestion and mildly toxic by skin contact.

**2-HEXEN-1-YL ACETATE** • A synthetic fruit flavoring additive for beverages, ice cream, ices, candy, and baked goods.

**cis-3-HEXEN-1-YL ACETATE** • Green grassy, herbaceous, fruity odor. Used in pear, apple, strawberry, melon, and peach flavorings.

**trans-2-HEXEN-1-YL ACETATE** • Green grassy, spicy, fruitlike flavoring used in soft fruits, apple, pear, melon, honeydew, wintergreen, and tea. ASP

**cis-3-HEXENYL BENZOATE** • Synthetic flavor with a sweet fruity odor and a taste of grapes. ASP

**cis-3-HEXENYL BUTYRATE** • Flavoring with an intense fruity green leafy odor. ASP

**cis-3-HEXENYL CROTONATE** • Green rosy, floral odor. EAF

**cis-3-HEXENYL FORMATE** • Used to add green and vegetable notes to broccoli and asparagus flavors. ASP

**cis-3-HEXENYL HEXANOATE** • Flavoring with a taste of red fruits, peach, passionfruit. ASP

**trans-2-HEXENYL HEXANOATE** • Fruity flavoring. EAF

**3-HEXENYL ISOVALERATE** • Flavoring used in apple and butter products. ASP

**cis-3-HEXENYL LACTATE** • Flavoring with a fruity note used for berries. ASP

**cis-3-HEXENYL 2-METHYL BUTYRATE** • Colorless liquid with a strong fruity odor used as a flavoring in various foods. ASP

**3-HEXENYL PHENYLACETATE** • Honey, apricot, cherry, peach, butter, tobacco flavoring. ASP

**cis-3 and trans-2-HEXENYL PROPIONATE** • Fresh, green, fruity, slightly waxy and vegetablelike character. Used in apple, strawberry, guava and other tropical fruit flavorings. ASP

**HEXITOL OLEATE** • An emulsifier that was used in ice cream but has been banned by the FDA.

**HEXOIC ACID** • *See* Caproic Acid.

**HEXOIC ALDEHYDE** • A synthetic berry, apple, pear, and pineapple flavoring additive for beverages, ice cream, ices, candy, baked goods, and chewing gum.

**HEXONE** • Colorless liquid with a fruity odor used as a flavoring additive in various foods. Moderately toxic by ingestion. Mildly toxic by inhalation. Very irritating to the skin, eyes, and mucous membranes. A human systemic irritant by inhalation. Narcotic in high concentration.

**HEXYL ACETATE** • Acetic Acid. Hexyl Ester. A synthetic berry, apple, pear, and pineapple flavoring additive for beverages, ice cream, ices, candy, baked goods, and chewing gum. Mildly toxic by ingestion. ASP

**2-HEXYL-4-ACETOXYTETRAHYDROFURAN** • A synthetic fruit flavoring additive for beverages, ice cream, ices, candy, and baked goods. NIL

**HEXYL ALCOHOL** • 1-Hexanol. A synthetic flavoring additive that occurs naturally in apples, oil of lavender, strawberries, and tea. Used in berry, coconut, and fruit flavorings for beverages, ice cream, ices, candy, baked goods, chewing gum, and gelatin desserts *See* 3-Hexanol and also Fatty Alcohols. ASP

**HEXYL-2-BUTENOATE** • Colorless liquid with a fruity odor used as a flavoring in various foods. GRAS. ASP

**HEXYL BUTYRATE** • Fruity flavoring. ASP

**a-HEXYLCINNAMALDEHYDE** • *See* Hexyl Cinnamaldehyde. ASP

**HEXYL CINNAMALDEHYDE** • A synthetic flavoring, pale yellow liquid with a jasminelike odor. Used in berry, fruit, and honey flavorings for beverages, ice cream, ices, candy, baked goods, and gelatin desserts. Moderately toxic by ingestion. A skin irritant

**HEXYL ESTER** • *See* Hexyl Acetate.

**2-HEXYL-4,5-DIMETHYL-1,3-DIXOLANE** • A flavoring determined GRAS by FEMA *(see)*. *See* Heptanal.

**HEXYL FORMATE** • Formic Acid. A synthetic raspberry and fruit flavoring additive for beverages, ice cream, ices, candy, and baked goods. ASP

**HEXYL 2-FUROATE** • A synthetic coffee, maple, and mushroom flavoring additive for candy and condiments. ASP

**HEXYL HEXANOATE** • Hexanoic Acid. A synthetic fruit flavoring additive for beverages, ice cream, ices, candy, and baked goods. ASP

**2-HEXYLIDENE CYCLOPENTANONE** • Synthetic flavoring approved by the FDA. ASP

**HEXYL ISOBUTYRATE** • Fruity, esterlike, tropical flavoring used in tropical fruit and fresh flavors. ASP

**HEXYL ISOVALERATE** • A colorless liquid with a fruity odor used as a flavoring in various foods. ASP

**2-HEXYL-5 (or 6)-KETO-1,4-DIOXANE** • A synthetic cream flavoring additive for beverages, ice cream, ices, candy, and baked goods. NIL

**HEXYL LAURATE** • See Lauric Acid.

**HEXYL 2-METHYL BUTYRATE** • Colorless liquid; strong, fresh, green fruity odor used as a flavoring additive.

**HEXYL OCTANOATE** • Octanoic Acid. A synthetic fruit flavoring additive for beverages and puddings. ASP

**HEXYL PHENYLACETATE** • Green grassy, fruity, esterlike, tropical flavoring used in tropical fruits and fresh green flavors. ASP

**HEXYL PROPIONATE** • Propionic Acid. A synthetic fruit flavoring additive for beverages, ice cream, ices, candy, and baked goods. ASP

**HEXYLENE GLYCOL DIACETATE** • *See* 1,3-Nonanediol Acetate.

**2-HEXYLIDENE CYCLOPENTANONE** • A synthetic fruit flavoring additive for beverages, ice cream, ices, candy, and baked goods.

**4-HEXYLRESORCINOL** • It has a pungent odor and a sharp astringent taste and has been used medicinally as an antiworm medicine and antiseptic. In foods, it is used as a color stabilizer, enzyme browning inhibitor, and a processing aid. It can cause severe gastrointestinal irritation; bowel, liver, and heart damage has been reported. Concentrated solutions can cause burns of the skin and mucous membranes.

**HEXYTHIAZOX** • A white, odorless, crystalline pesticide used to kill mites on pears. FDA residue tolerance is 0.3 ppm.

**HICKORY BARK EXTRACT** • *Carya* spp. A natural flavoring extract from the hickory nut tree and used in butter, caramel, rum, maple, nut, spice, tobacco, and smoke flavorings for beverages, ice cream, ices, candy, baked goods, condiments, and liquors. GRAS. NIL

**HICKORY SMOKE COMPENSATE (HSC)** • A food flavoring popular in the United States. Available data have suggested that this additive has tumor-initiating and -promoting potential. Researchers at Japan's Nagoya City University Medical School gave rats a diet containing 5 percent HSC and the animals developed precancerous lesions. No effect was observed at lower doses. ASP

**HIGH AMYLOSE CORNSTARCH** • Cornstarch that has been treated with enzymes to make it sweeter.

**HIGH FRUCTOSE CORN SYRUP** • Corn syrup *(see)* that has been treated with enzymes to make it sweeter. It is about one and a half times sweeter than sugar. It does have calories. Used in beverages, candy, frozen desserts, dairy drinks, canned fruits, processed ham, hamburger, ice cream, luncheon meat, meat loaf, poultry, and sausage. A combination of fructose and dextrose *(see both)* it is a low-cost addition to pickles, ketchup, and syrups. There is reported use of the chemical; it has not yet been assigned for toxicology literature. GRAS. ASP

**HIGH POTENCY** • A nutrient in a food that is 100 percent or more of the RDI *(see)* established for that product. The term may also be used with multi-ingredient products if two-thirds of the nutrients are present at 100 percent of the RDI.

**HINOKITIOL** • The organic compound distilled from the leaves of arborvitae, it is a pale yellow oil with a camphor smell and is used in perfumery and flavoring. Low toxicity.

**HIP BERRY EXTRACT** • *See* Rose Hips Extract.

**HISTAMINE** • A chemical released by mast cells and considered responsible for much of the swelling and itching characteristics of hay fever and other allergies.

**HISTIDINE** • L forms only (L-histidine is the natural form). A basic essential amino acid *(see)* used as a nutrient. It is a building block of protein, used as a nutrient. Soluble in water. It is used in cosmetic creams. GRAS. ASP

**HOMOCYSTEINE** • An amino acid found in high concentrations in blood when there is a risk of a heart attack in young women. Women who have high homocysteine levels tend to have low folate levels.

**HONEY** • Used as a coloring, flavoring, and emollient in cosmetics. Formerly used in hair bleaches. The common, sweet, viscous material taken from the nectar of flowers and manufactured in the sacs of various kinds of bees. The flavor and color depend upon the plants from which it was taken. Honey has been used to cure meat for thousands of years. Researchers at Clemson University in South Carolina rediscovered that this natural preservative confers excellent protection against oxidation and boosts shelf life in popular processed meats.

**HONEYDEW MELON JUICE** • Liquid expressed from fresh honeydew.

**HONEYSUCKLE** • The common fragrant tubular flowers filled with honey, which are used in perfumes.

**HOPS** • *Humulus lupulus.* Used in beer brewing and in fruit and root beer flavorings for beverages. Derived from the carefully dried pineconelike fruit of the hop plant grown in Europe, Asia, and North America. Light yellow or greenish, it is an oily liquid with a bitter taste and aromatic odor. A solid extract is used in bitters, fruit, and root beer flavorings for beverages, ice cream, ices, candy, and baked goods. Hops oil is used in raspberry, grape, whiskey, and spice flavorings for beverages, ice cream, ices, candy, baked goods, chewing gum, and condiments. Hops at one time were thought to be a sedative. GRAS. ASP

**HOPS OIL** • *See* Hops.

**HOR** • FDA abbreviation for hormone.

**HOREHOUND EXTRACT** • *Marrubium vulgare.* Hoarhound. A flavoring extracted from a mintlike plant cultivated in Europe, Asia, and the United States, *Marrubium vulgare.* It has a very bitter taste and is used in maple, nut, and root beer flavorings for beverages, ice cream, ices, candy, and baked goods. It is also a bitter tonic and expectorant. GRAS. ASP

**HORMONES** • A hormone is a chemical produced by a gland and secreted into the bloodstream, affecting the function of distant cells or organs. U.S. beef producers have been using growth hormones, a very powerful chemical from the pituitary gland at the base of the brain, to increase the weight of cattle by from 10 to 20 percent for the same amount of feed. Diethylstilbestrol, another hormone, an estrogen, was used by beef and poultry producers to increase the weight of meat for which they are paid by the pound. The FDA has tried to ban diethylstilbestrol for that purpose because it has been shown to be carcinogenic, but spot checks have shown that it is still present in some meat and poultry products. In 1988, the twelve-nation European Community put a ban on U.S. beef because of the use of growth hormones in raising cattle for meat. The U.S. position is that the growth hormones approved for cattle by the Department of Agriculture are not harmful to humans. Environmentalists who testified in favor of the European legislators have maintained that such hormones create tumors and genetic deformities in children. Hormones are still being used in feed and by implantation in cattle, chickens, and turkeys, as you can determine by checking listings, including those for estradiol, mibolerone, testosterone propionate, and trenbolone.

**HORSE CHESTNUT** • The seeds of *Aeschulus hippocastanum.* A tonic, natural astringent for skin, and fever-reducing substance that contains tannic acid *(see).*

**HORSEMINT LEAVES EXTRACT** • *Monarda* spp. A flavoring extract from any of several coarse, aromatic plants, grown from New York to Florida and from Texas to Wisconsin. Used in fruit flavorings for beverages (600 ppm). Formerly used as an aromatic stimulant and to break up intestinal gas. GRAS. NIL

**HORSE NETTLE** • Solanum. Bull Nettle. Radical Weed. Air-dried ripe fruit of *Solanum carolinense,* a South American nightshade plant. It is also grown in Florida. It is used as a sedative and anticonvulsant.

**HORSERADISH EXTRACT** • Scurvy Grass. *Armoracia lapathifolia.* A condiment ingredient utilizing the grated root from the tall, coarse, white-flowered herb native to Europe. Often combined with vinegar or other ingredients. Contains ascorbic acid *(see)* and acts as an antiseptic in cosmetics. It contains vitamin C and is used by herbalists to treat arthritis pain by stimulating blood flow to inflamed joints. Potential adverse reactions include diarrhea and sweating if taken internally in large amounts. GRAS. ASP

**HOUSELEEK EXTRACT** • Extract of the common houseleek *Sempervivum tectorum* native to the mountains of Europe and to the Greek Islands. Its longevity led to its being named sempervivum, which means "ever alive." It has been used to treat shingles, gout, and to get rid of bugs. Its pulp was applied to the skin for rashes and inflammation, and to remove warts and calluses. The juice was used to reduce fever and to treat insect stings. Houseleek juice mixed with honey was prescribed for thrush, and an ointment made from the plant was used to treat ulcers, burns, scalds, and inflammation.

**HPP** • Hydrolyzed plant protein. *See* Hydrolyzed Vegetable Protein.

**HUMECTANT** • A substance used to preserve the moisture content of materials, used to preserve moisture in confections and tobacco. Glycerin, propylene, glycol, and sorbitol *(see all)* are widely used humectants. See individual substances for toxicity.

**HUMULUS** • A hop plant, a herbaceous vine with palmate leaves and pistillate flowers. *See* Hops.

**HVP** • *See* Hydrolyzed Vegetable Protein.

**HYACINTH, ABSOLUTE** • *Hyacinthus orientalis.* The extract of the common fragrant flower. Once used as a flavoring for chewing gum and in perfumes and soaps, it is now permitted only for alcoholic beverage flavoring. Dark green liquid with a penetrating odor, the juice of hyacinth is very irritating to the skin and can cause allergic reactions. The bulb can cause severe gastrointestinal symptoms. There is reported use of the chemical; it has not yet been assigned for toxicology literature. EAF

**HYACINTHIN** • *See* Phenylacetaldehyde.

**HYBRID SAFFLOWER OIL** • The oil derived from the seeds of a genetic strain that contains mostly oleic acid triglyceride, as distinct from safflower oil.

**HYDRATED** • Combined with water.

**HYDRATED ALUMINA** • *See* Aluminum Hydroxide.

**HYDRATED SILICA** • An anticaking additive used to keep loose powders free-flowing. *See* Silica and Hydrated.

**HYDRATROPALDEHYDE** • *See* Phenylpropionaldehyde.

**HYDRATROPIC ALDEHYDE PROPLYENE GLYCOL ACETAL** • Synthetic flavoring. ASP

**HYDRATROPALDEHYDE DIMETHYL ACETAL** • *See* Phenylpropionaldehyde Dimethyl Acetal.

**HYDRAZINE** • Colorless fuming liquid used as a solvent and catalyst for inorganic materials. Used in steam in contact with food. The FDA allows zero residue. A reducing additive *(see)* and chlorine scavenger, it is a highly toxic chemical. It is a cancer-causing additive and direct liquid contact with skin or eyes may produce severe burns. Vapors are highly irritating to the nose and throat and may cause injury to the lungs, liver, and kidneys. The FDA has zero tolerance for residue on food. NASA has requested studies because it has been shown to cause nasal cancers in animals. NUL

*a*-**HYDRO-OMEGA-HYDROXY-POLY(OXYETHYLENE)POLY(OXYPROPYLENE)(51-57 MOLES)POLY (OXYETHYLENE)BLOCK CO-POLYMERS (MOL WT. 14,000)** • Dough conditioner. FDA tolerance, 0.5 percent of flour used. *See* Copolymer Condensates of Ethylene Oxide and Propylene Oxide.

*a*-**HYDRO-OMEGA-HYDROXY-POLY(OXYETHYLENE)POLY(OXYPROPYLENE)(55-61 MOLES)POLY(OXYETHYLENE)BLOCK CO-POLYMERS (MOL WT. 9,760-13,200)** • Solubilizer and stabilizer in flavor concentrations. The FDA permits use according to general manufacturing principles. *See* Copolymer Condensates of Ethylene Oxide and Propylene Oxide.

**a-HYDRO-OMEGA-HYDROXY-POLY(OXYETHYLENE)POLY(OXY-PROPYLENE)(53-59 MOLES)POLY(OXYETHYLENE)(14-16 MOLES) BLOCK COPOLYMER (MOL WT. 3,500-4,125)** • A solubilizing and dispersing additive in combination with dioctyl sodium sulfosuccinate *(see)*. FDA tolerance is 10 ppm total in finished beverages or fruit drinks. *See* Copolymer Condensates of Ethylene Oxide and Propylene Oxide.

**HYDROBIOTIC FEED** • *See* Verxite Granule and Flakes.

**HYDROCARBONS** • A large class of organic compounds containing only carbon and hydrogen. Petroleum, natural gas, coal, and bitumens are common hydrocarbon products. Hydrocarbons also include mineral oils, paraffin wax, and ozokerite. *See all.*

**HYDROCHLORIC ACID** • An acid used as a modifier for food starch, in the manufacture of sodium glutamate *(see),* and gelatin, for the conversion of cornstarch to syrup (0.012 percent), and to adjust the pH (acidity-alkalinity balance) in the brewing industry (0.02 percent). Also used as a solvent. A clear, colorless, or slightly yellowish corrosive liquid, it is a water solution of hydrogen chloride of varying concentrations. Used in hair bleaches to speed up oxidation in rinses and to remove color. Inhalation of the fumes causes choking and inflammation of the respiratory tract. Ingestion may corrode the mucous membranes, esophagus, and stomach, and cause diarrhea. Circulatory collapse and death can occur. GRAS. ASP. E

**HYDROCHLOROFLUOROCARBON, 22,142b, 152a** • Propellants and refrigerants derived from chlorofluorocarbon, any of several compounds comprised of carbon, fluorine, chlorine, and hydrogen. Though safer than many propellant gases, their use has diminished because of suspected effects on stratospheric ozone.

**HYDROCINNAMALDEHYDE** • Colorless to slightly yellow liquid with a strong hyacinth odor used as a flavoring additive in various foods. A human skin irritant.

**HYDROCINNAMIC ALCOHOL** • Colorless, thick liquid with a sweet hyacinth odor used as a flavoring additive in various foods. Moderately toxic by ingestion. Mildly toxic by skin contact.

**HYDROCINNAMYL ACETATE** • Colorless liquid with a spicy, floral odor used as a flavoring additive in various foods. Mildly toxic by ingestion.

**HYDROCORTISONE SODIUM SUCCINATE** • A-Hydrocort. Solu-Cortef. An adrenal gland hormone used to decrease severe inflammation. Used to treat cows, and the FDA permits up to 10 ppb in milk. The drug also suppresses the immune response. Has caused adverse reproductive effects in laboratory animals.

**HYDROGEN CYANIDE** • A colorless gas or liquid with a characteristic odor. In veterinary preparations used to treat mastitis, inflammation of the udders. As a fumigant, the FDA tolerances are 200 ppm in cocoa, 125 ppm in cereal flours, 90 ppm in cereals cooked before eaten, and 50 ppm in uncooked ham, bacon, and sausage. In humans, high concentrations may cause shortness of breath, paralysis, unconsciousness, convulsions, and respiratory arrest. Chronic exposure over long periods may cause fatigue and weakness. Exposure to 150 ppm from thirty minutes to an hour may endanger life. Death may result from a few minutes' exposure to 300 ppm. Average fatal dose is 50 to 60 mg. The compressed gas is used for exterminating rodents and insects. Must be handled by specially trained experts.

**HYDROGEN PEROXIDE** • A bleaching and oxidizing additive, a detergent, and antiseptic. An unstable compound readily broken down into water and oxygen. It is made from barium peroxide and diluted phosphoric acid. Generally recognized as safe as a preservative and germ killer in milk and cheese as well as in cosmetics. Bleaches tripe and butter; used in the treatment of eggs before drying and in cheddar and Swiss cheeses. A 3 percent solution is used medicinally as an antiseptic and germicide. A strong oxidizer, undiluted it can cause burns of the skin and mucous membranes. In 1980, the Japanese notified the World Health Organization that hydrogen peroxide was a suspect as a cancer-causing additive. It was widely used in Japanese fish cakes. The noodles were dipped in diluted hydrogen peroxide for disinfection. The fish meat and raw flour were also mixed with hydrogen peroxide. In laboratory rats, it was discovered that in the sixty-fifth week, the lining of the duodenum was thickened but no cancers occurred. The Japanese Welfare Ministry decided that hydrogen peroxide is safe for food when it is entirely decomposed and that the food should not contain any residual. GRAS. ASP

**HYDROGEN SULFIDE** • Colorless gas with a terrible odor. It is derived from sulfuric acid and as a by-product of petroleum refining. Highly flammable. Toxic by inhalation. Strong irritant to the eyes. Used as a source of sulfur and hydrogen in the manufacture of food additives. ASP

**HYDROGENATED CORN SYRUP** • Used in cat and dog food as a humectant (see). See also Corn Syrup.

**HYDROGENATED HONEY** • Controlled hydrogenation (see) of honey.

**HYDROGENATED MENHADEN OIL** • Obtained along the west coast of North America from the menhaden fish, somewhat larger than herring. The oil contains myristic acid, palmitic acid, and linoleic acid (see all). Used as a substitute for linseed oil. Hydrogenated menhaden oil is used as a substitute for tallow. GRAS

**HYDROGENATED OIL** • Oil that is partially converted from naturally polyunsaturated fats to saturated. Makes liquid oils partially solid. May adversely affect the levels of fat in the blood and has been linked to colon cancer in some reports. See Hydrogenation.

**HYDROGENATED PEANUT OIL** • See Hydrogenation and Peanut Oil.

**HYDROGENATED POLY-1-DECENE** • Used as a glazing agent in products like candy. In 2003, the European Parliament said that its use must be revised especially with respect to children.

**HYDROGENATED SOYBEAN OIL** • *See* Soybean Oil and Hydrogenation.

**HYDROGENATED SOY GLYCERIDE** • *See* Soybean Oil and Hydrogenation.

**HYDROGENATED SPERM OIL** • Used to coat bakery pans so the products will not stick.

**HYDROGENATED STARCH HYDROLYSATE** • The end product of the hydrogenation of corn syrup. *See* Hydrogenation and Corn Syrup.

**HYDROGENATED TALLOW** • A component used in the production of beet sugar and yeast in amounts to inhibit foaming. *See* Hydrogenation. No known toxicity. The final report to the FDA of the Select Committee on GRAS Substances stated in 1980 that it should continue its GRAS status with no limitations other than good manufacturing practices.

**HYDROGENATED TALLOW ACID** • *See* Hydrogenated Tallow.

**HYDROGENATED TALLOW ALCOHOL** • *See* hydrogenated tallow, which has the same uses. The final report to the FDA of the Select Committee on GRAS Substances stated in 1980 that it should continue its GRAS status with no limitations other than good manufacturing practices.

**HYDROGENATED TALLOW BETAINE** • *See* Hydrogenated Tallow and Betaine.

**HYDROGENATED TALLOW GLYCERIDE** • *See* Hydrogenated Tallow and Glycerides.

**HYDROGENATED TALLOWTRIMONIUM CHLORIDE** • *See* Quaternary Ammonium Compounds.

**HYDROGENATED VEGETABLE GLYCERIDE** • An emollient to prevent the skin from losing moisture. *See* Vegetable Oils and Hydrogenation.

**HYDROGENATED VEGETABLE OIL (HVP)** • Used in instant soups, frankfurters, sauces, and beef stew. Consists of vegetable—usually soybean—protein that has been chemically broken down to its amino acids that built it. HVP is a "flavor enhancer." It contains MSG *(see)*. *See also* Partially Hydrogenated Vegetable Oil.

**HYDROGENATION** • The process of adding hydrogen gas under high pressure to liquid oils. It is the most widely used chemical process in the edible fat industry. Used in the manufacture of petrol from coal and in the manufacture of margarine and shortening. Used primarily in the cosmetic and food industries to convert liquid oils to semisolid fats (Crisco and maragarine, for example) at room temperature. Reduces the amount of acid in the compound and improves color. Usually the higher the amount of hydrogenation the lower the unsaturation in the fat and the less possibility of flavor degradation or spoilage due to oxidation. Hydrogenated oils still contain some unsaturated components that are susceptible to rancidity.

Therefore, the addition of antioxidants is still necessary. Hydrogenation leads to trans fats which have been found to contribute to fat-clogged arteries. *See* Trans Fats.

**HYDROLYSIS** • Decomposition that changes a compound into other compounds by taking up the elements of water. For example, hydrolysis of salt into an acid and a base or hydrolysis of an ester into an alcohol and an acid. *See* Hydrolyzed.

**HYDROLYZED** • Subject to hydrolysis or turned partly into water. Hydrolysis is derived from the Greek *hydro,* meaning "water," and *lysis,* meaning "a setting free." It occurs as a chemical process in which the decomposition of a compound is brought about by water, resolving into a simpler compound. Hydrolysis also occurs in the digestion of foods. The proteins in the stomach react with water in an enzyme reaction to form peptones and amino acids *(see).*

**HYDROLYZED ANIMAL PROTEIN** • Protein from animals that has been split into smaller units by acids, alkalis, or enzymes.

**HYDROLYZED CASEIN** • *See* Casein and Hydrolyzed.

**HYDROLYZED KERATIN** • The widely used hydrolysate of keratin, a protein obtained from hair, wool, horn, nails, claws, beaks, membranes of eggshells, and nerve tissues. Acid, enzyme, or other forms of hydrolysis derive the hydrolysate. The word *animal* was removed from this ingredient name. Used in dietary protein supplements.

**HYDROLYZED LEATHER MEAL** • Used in swine feed up to 1 percent of weight.

**HYDROLYZED MILK PROTEIN** • *See* Acid Hydrolyzed Proteins.

**HYDROLYZED PLANT PROTEIN** • A protein obtained from various foods such as soybeans, corn, or wheat and then broken down into amino acids by a chemical process, acid hydrolysis. Hydrolyzed plant or vegetable protein is used as a flavor enhancer in numerous processed foods like soups, chilies, sauces, and some meat products like frankfurters. *See* Hydrolyzed Vegetable Protein.

**HYDROLYZED PROTEIN** • Used as a flavoring and flavor enhancer. The word *animal* was removed from this ingredient's name. Also used in gels and in animal feed. *See* Acid Hydrolysates of Protein and Hydrolyzed.

**HYDROLYZED (SOURCE) PROTEIN EXTRACT** • *See* Acid Hydrolysates of Proteins.

**HYDROLYZED SOY PROTEIN** • *See* Soybean and Hydrolyzed.

**HYDROLYZED VEGETABLE PROTEIN (HPP, HVP)** • The hydrolysate (liquefaction) of vegetable protein derived by acid, enzyme, or other method of hydrolysis. A flavor enhancer used in soup, beef, and stew. High salt and glutamate content with low-quality protein. On the GRAS list, but the Select Committee of the Federation of American Societies for

Experimental Biology (FASEB) advised the FDA that hydrolyzed vegetable protein contains dicarboxylic amino acid (a building block of the protein that affects growth) when used at present levels in strained and junior baby foods. They said that the effects of this substance on children should be studied further. The effects on adults of vegetable and animal protein hydroxylates demonstrate "no current hazard," but the FASEB voiced uncertainties about future consumption levels for those products and recommended further studies. The source of HVP must now be listed on the label. *See* Acid Hydrolysates of Protein.

**HYDROLYZED YEAST** • The hydrolysate of yeast (liquefaction) derived from acid, enzyme, or other method of hydrolysis.

**HYDROLYZED YEAST PROTEIN** • *See* Hydrolyzed Yeast.

**HYDROQUINONE** • Used in bleach, freckle creams, and in suntan lotions. A white crystalline phenol *(see)* that occurs naturally but is usually manufactured in the laboratory. Hydroquinone combines with oxygen very rapidly and becomes brown when exposed to air. Death has occurred from the ingestion of as little as 5 grams. Ingestion of as little as one gram (one-twenty-eighth of an ounce) has caused nausea, vomiting, ringing in the ears, delirium, a sense of suffocation, and collapse. Industrial workers exposed to the chemical have suffered clouding of the eye lens. Application to the skin may cause allergic reactions. It can cause depigmentation in a 2 percent solution. When injected into the abdomen of mice in 28 milligram doses per kilogram of body weight, it caused bladder cancers, but other studies in which animals were fed the chemical did not show it to induce cancer. However, it did cause atrophy of the liver and aplastic anemia. ASP

**HYDROQUINONE MONOETHYL ETHER** • White flakes with sweet clover odor used as a fixative in foods, perfumes, dyes, cosmetics, and especially in suntan preparations. *See* Hydroquinone. ASP

**HYDROXY PROPYLMETHYL CELLULOSE CARBONATE** • Prepared from wood pulp or cotton by treatment with methyl chloride. Used as a substitute for water-soluble gums, to render paper greaseproof, and as a thickener. The final report to the FDA of the Select Committee on GRAS Substances stated in 1980 that it should continue its GRAS status with limitations on amounts that can be added to food. ASP

**2-HYDROXYACETOPHENONE** • Flavoring additive. The FAO/WHO said in 2000 that there was no safety concern at current levels of intake when used as a flavoring additive. NIL

***p*-HYDROXYANISOLE** • *See* Guaiacol

**0-HYDROXYBENZALDEHYDE** • *See* Benzyl Acetate.

**4-HYDROXYBENZALDEHYDE** • Flavoring evaluated by FAO/WHO *(see)* which in 2001 said there was no safety concern at current levels of intake when used as a flavoring additive. EAF

***p*-HYDROXYBENZOATE** • *See* Propylparaben.

***p*-HYDROXYBENZOIC ACID** • Prepared from *p*-bromophenol. Used as a preservative and fungicide. *See* Benzoic Acid for toxicity.

**4-HYDROXYBENZOIC ACID** • Flavoring additive. FAO/WHO said in 2001 that there was no safety concern at current levels of intake when used as a flavoring additive. However, other institutions say that ingestion of this chemical can be irritating. Declared GRAS by FEMA *(see)*. EAF

**4-HYDROXYBENZYL ALCOHOL** • *See* Benzylaldehyde. EAF

***p*-HYDROXYBENZYL ISOTHIOCYANATE** • A derivative of mustard oil used in flavoring. The final report to the FDA of the Select Committee on GRAS Substances stated in 1980 that it should continue its GRAS status with no limitations other than good manufacturing practices.

**4-HYDROXYBUTANOIC ACID LACTONE** • *See* Butanoic Acid and Lactic Acid. ASP

**1-HYDROXY-2-BUTANONE** • *See* Acetoin. ASP

**2-HYDROXYCAMPHANE** • *See* Borneol.

**HYDROXYCITRONELLAL** • Colorless liquid obtained by the addition of citronellol. Used as a fixative and a fragrance in perfumery for its sweet lilylike odor. It can cause allergic reactions. ASP

**HYDROXYCITRONELLAL DIETHYL ACETAL** • A synthetic citrus and fruit flavoring additive for beverages, ice cream, ices, candy, and baked goods. ASP

**HYDROXYCITRONELLAL DIMETHYL ACETAL** • A synthetic flavoring additive, colorless liquid, with a light floral odor. Used in fruit and cherry flavorings for beverages, ice cream, ices, candy, and baked goods. ASP

**HYDROXYCITRONELLOL** • A synthetic lemon, floral, and cherry flavoring additive for beverages, ice cream, ices, candy, baked goods, gelatin desserts, and chewing gum. ASP

**2-HYDROXY-2-CYCLOHEXEN-1-ONE** • Flavoring. ASP

**2-HYDROXY-*p*-CYMENE** • *See* Carvacrol.

**5-HYDROXY-2,4-DECADIENOIC ACID DELTA-LACTONE** • Flavoring. EAF

**5-HYDROXY-2-DECENOIC ACID DELTA-LACTONE** • Flavoring. EAF

**5-HYDROXY-7-DECENOIC ACID DELTA-LACTONE** • Flavoring. NIL

**4-HYDROXY-3,5-DIMETHOXYBENZALDEHYDE** • A flavoring determined GRAS by the Expert Panel of the Flavor and Extract Manufacturers Association. *See* Benzaldehyde.

**4-HYDROXY-2,5-DIMETHYL-3(2H)-FURANONE** • Flavoring. *See* Furans. ASP

**4-HYDROXY-2,3-DIMETHYL-2-4 NONADIENOIC ACID GAMMA LACTONE** • A flavoring determined GRAS by FEMA *(see)*. ASP

**6-HYDROXY-3,7-DIMETHYLOCTANOIC ACID LACTONE** • Flavoring. *See* Octanoic Acid.

**(Z)-4-HYDROXY-6-DODECENOIC ACID LACTONE** • One of the newer synthetic flavorings. *See* Dodecenoic Acid and Lactic Acid. EAF

**5-HYDROXY-6-DODECENOIC ACID LACTONE** • Flavoring. EAF

**1-HYDROXYETHYLIDENE-1,1-DIPHOSPHONIC ACID** • Flavoring. ASP

**HYDROXYLAMINE HCL** • An antioxidant for fatty acids *(see)*. May be slightly irritating to skin, eyes, and mucous membranes, and may cause a depletion of oxygen in the blood when ingested. In the body it is reported to decompose to sodium nitrite.

**HYDROXYLATE** • The process in which an atom of hydrogen and an atom of oxygen are introduced into a compound to make the compound more soluble.

**HYDROXYLATED LECITHIN** • An emulsifier and antioxidant used in baked goods, ice cream, and margarine. It is also used as a defoaming additive for processing beet sugar and yeast. According to the FAO/WHO Expert Committee on Food Additives, the safety of hydroxylated lecithin (*see* Lecithin) has not been adequately established. It has been cleared by the FDA for use as a food emulsifier. ASP

**HYDROXYLATION** • The process in which an atom of hydrogen and an atom of oxygen are introduced into a compound to make that compound more soluble.

**N-(4-HYDROXY-3-METHOXYBENZYL)-8-METHYL-6-NONENAMIDE** • Flavoring. ASP

**2-HYDROXY-4-METHYLBENZALDEHYDE** • Flavoring. EAF

**HYDROXYMETHYLCELLULOSE** • Thickener and bodying additive derived from plants. Used as a thickener. *See* Carboxymethyl Cellulose.

**4-HYDROXY-4-METHYL-7-cis-DECANOIC ACID GAMMALACTONE** • Flavoring. ASP

**4-HYDROXYMETHYL-2,6-DI-TERT-BUTYLPHENOL** • Used as an antioxidant. Shall not exceed 0.02 percent of oil in food. ASP

**2-HYDROXYMETHYL-6,6-DIMETHYLBICYCLO(3.1.1)HEPT-2-ENYL FORMATE** • Flavoring. ASP

**10-HYDROXYMETHYLENE-2-PINENE** • Flavoring. *See* Pinene. EAF

**4-HYDROXY-5-METHYL-3(2H)-FURANONE** • Flavoring. *See* Furans. ASP

**3-(HYDROXYMETHYL)-2-HEPTANONE** • Flavoring. *See* Heptanoic Acid. ASP

**2-HYDROXY-5-METHYL-3-HEXANONE** • Flavoring. *See* Hexanoic Acid. EAF

**3-HYDROXY-5-METHYL-2-HEXANONE** • Flavoring. *See* Exanoic Acid. EAF

**4-HYDROXY-4-,METHYL-5-HEXENOIC ACID GAMMA LACTONE** • Flavoring determined GRAS by FEMA *(see)*.

**4-HYDROXY-3-METHYLOCTANOIC ACID LACTONE** • Flavoring. *See* Octanoic Acid and Lactic Acid. EAF

**HYDROXYNONANOIC ACID, DELTA-LACTONE** • Flavoring. *See* Octanoic Acid and Lactic Acid. ASP

**HYDROXYOCTACOSANYL HYDROXYSTEARATE** • *See* Stearic Acid and Hydroxylation.

**5-HYDROXY-4-OCTANONE** • A synthetic butter, butterscotch, fruit, cheese, and nut flavoring additive for beverages, ice cream, ices, candy, and baked goods. ASP

**3-HYDROXY-2-OXOPROPIONIC ACID** • Flavoring. *See* Propionic Acid. EAF

**3-HYDROXY-2-PENTANONE** • Flavoring. *See* Pentanoic Acid. ASP

**4-HYDROXY-3-PENTENOIC ACID LACTONE** • Flavoring. *See* Pentenoic Acid and Lactic Acid. ASP

**3-HYDROXY-4-PHENYLBUTAN-2-ONE** • Flavoring determined GRAS by FEMA *(see)*. *See* Butanoic Acid. ASP

**4-(p-HYDROXYPHENYL)-2-BUTANONE** • Synthetic fruit flavoring for beverages, ice cream, ices, candy, baked goods, gelatin desserts, and chewing gum. ASP

**HYDROXYPHENYL GLYCINEAMIDE** • Derived from the nonessential amino acid glycine *(see)* used as a buffering additive and as a violet scent.

**HYDROXYPROLINE** • L-Proline. The hydroxylated *(see)* amino acid used to add "protein" to a compound. NUL

**L-HYDROXYPROLINE** • An amino acid analog of proline. NUL

**HYDROXYPROPYLAMINE NITRITE** • *See* Isopropanolamine and Nitrites.

**HYDROXYPROPYL CELLULOSE** • Thickener. *See* Hydroxymethylcellulose. ASP

**HYDROXYPROPYL GUAR** • Guar Gum. 2-Hydroxypropyl Ether. *See* Guar Gum.

**HYDROXYPROPYL METHYLCELLULOSE** • An emulsifier used in food except standard foods which do not provide for such use. *See* Cellulose Gums. ASP

**HYDROXYPROPYL STARCH, HYDROXYPROPYL STARCH OXI-DIZED, and HYDROXYPROPYL DISTARCHPHOSPHATE** • These are all modified starches. The final report to the FDA of the Select Committee on GRAS Substances stated in 1980 that while no evidence in the available information on these starches demonstrates a hazard to the public when they are used at levels that are now current and in the manner now practiced, uncertainties exist requiring that additional studies should be conducted. In 1980, the FDA said GRAS status would continue while tests were being completed and evaluated. The FDA has reported nothing new since then. E

**HYDROXYQUINOLINE SULFATE** • Was used as a component of a cottage cheese coagulant but has been banned by the FDA.

**HYDROXYSTEARIC ACID** • *See* Stearic Acid.

**HYDROXYSTEARMIDE MEA** • Mixture of ethanolamide of hydroxystearic acid. *See* Stearic Acid.

**HYDROXYSTEARYL METHYLGLUCAMINE** • An amino sugar. *See* Glucose.

**2-HYDROXY-3,5,5-TRIMETHYL-2-CYCLOHEXENONE** • Flavoring used in tobacco.

**5-HYDROXYUNDECANOIC ACID LACTONE** • Flavoring. *See* Decanoic Acid and Lactic Acid.

**5-HYDROXY-8-UNDECENOIC ACID DELTA-LACTONE** • Flavoring. *See* Decanoic Acid and Lactic Acid.

**HYGROMYCIN** • A broad spectrum antibiotic from *Streptomyces hygroscopicus* used in animal feed. The FDA allows zero residue in poultry eggs and in uncooked edible tissues and by-products of swine and poultry.

**HYPERACTIVITY** • *See* Attention Deficit Hyperactivity Disorder (ADHD).

**HYPERICUM** • Hypericin. Blue black needles obtained from pyridine *(see)*. The solutions are red or green with a red cast. Small amounts seem to be a tranquilizer and have been used as an antidepressant in medicine. It can produce a sensitivity to light.

**HYPERSENSITIVITY** • The condition in persons previously exposed to an antigen in which tissue damage results from an immune reaction to a further dose of the antigen. Classically, four types of hypersensitivity are recognized, but the term is often used to mean the type of allergy associated with hay fever and asthma.

**HYPERTENSION** • High Blood Pressure. Hypertension is persistently elevated arterial blood pressure. It is the most common public health problem in developed countries. Emphasis on lifestyle modifications has given diet a prominent role for both the primary prevention and management of hypertension.

**HYPO** • Prefix from the Greek, meaning "under" or "below," as in hypoacidity—acidity in a lesser degree than is usual or normal.

**HYPOGLYCEMIA** • Low blood sugar—the opposite of diabetes.

**HYPOPHOSPHORIC ACID** • Crystals used in baking powder, sodium salt.

**HYPOTHALAMUS** • Brain control area involved in emotion, movement, and eating. Less than the size of a peanut and weighing a quarter of an ounce, this small area deep within the brain also oversees appetite, blood pressure, sexual behavior, sleep, and emotions, and sends orders to the pituitary gland.

**HYSSOP EXTRACT** • Extract of *Hyssopus officinalis*. A synthetic flavoring from the aromatic herb. Used in bitters. The extract is liquor flavoring for beverages, ice cream, and ice. Native to southern Europe. It was used to calm the nerves. The oil is a liquor and spice flavoring. GRAS. NIL

**HYSSOP OIL** • *Hyssopus officinalis.* A historical and biblical herb whose name is derived from the Greek word *azob* or holy herb has a pleasant mild fragrance which is used in aromatherapy. People with high blood pressure or seizures are warned not to ingest or smell this oil. EAF

# I

**ICELAND MOSS EXTRACT** • The extract of *Lichen islandicus.* A water-soluble gum that gels on cooling. Used to flavor alcoholic beverages only.

**IgE** • Antibodies that are responsible for the majority of allergic reactions. Medical scientists feel that if their efforts succeed in suppressing IgE formation they will have a method of not only more effectively treating allergies but also of preventing many of them from occurring. *See also* Antibody.

**IGF-1** • Abbreviation for insulinlike growth factor. A natural protein required for normal growth, it is associated with the use of recombinant bovine somatotropin *(see).* Allegations have been made that milk from treated cows may cause breast cancer. The consumption of dietary IGF-1 in milk, the FDA maintains, plays no role in inducing or promoting any human disease, including breast cancer. NIL

**IMAZALIL** • An antifungal used on dried citrus pulp for animal feed. FDA residue tolerance is 25 ppm in the pulp and 0.01 to 0.50 ppm in cattle fats, swine, sheep, and milk.

**IMAZETHAPYR** • An herbicide used on soybeans. FDA residue tolerance is 0.1 ppm.

**IMIDAZOLE** • Glyoxaline. White crystalline base made by the action of ammonia and formaldehyde on glyoxal. It is used as a biological control of pests and as an antihistamine.

**IMIDAZOLIDINYL UREA** • A bactericidal preservative with a low toxicity in animals. Sensitivity reactions have been reported in humans.

**IMIDAZOLINE** • A derivative of imidazole *(see)* also called glyoxalidine.

**IMITATION** • A flavor containing any portion of nonnatural materials. For instance, unless a strawberry flavoring is made entirely from strawberries, it must be called imitation. When a processor fails to use all the standard ingredients in mayonnaise, he used to have to call it salad dressing. Imitation used to mean that the product contains fewer vitamins, minerals, or other nutrients than the food it resembles. The rules have changed.

**IMMORTELLE EXTRACT** • *Erythrina micopteryx. Helichrysum angustifolium.* A natural flavoring extract from a red-flowered tropical tree. The name derives from the French *immortel,* "immortal" or "everlasting." Used in raspberry, fruit, and liquor flavoring for beverages, ice cream, ices, baked goods, candy, gelatin desserts, and chewing gum. GRAS. EAF

**IMPERATORIA** • *Peucedanum ostruthium* A flavoring from a tropical grass used in malt beer. Used in alcoholic beverages only.

**INDIAN GUM** • *See* Ghatti Gum.

**INDIAN TRAGACANTH** • *See* Karaya Gum.

**INDIGO** • Probably the oldest known dye. Prepared from various Indigofera plants native to Bengal, Java, and Guatemala. Dark blue powder with a coppery luster. No known skin irritation.

**INDIGO CARMINE** • See FD and C Blue No. 2. E

**INDOLE** • A white, lustrous, flaky substance with an unpleasant odor, occurring naturally in jasmine oil and orange flowers and used as a synthetic flavoring additive in raspberry, strawberry, bitters, chocolate, orange, coffee, violet, fruit, nut, and cheese flavorings for beverages, ice cream, ices, candy, baked goods, and gelatin desserts. It can be extracted from coal tar and feces; in highly diluted solutions, the odor is pleasant. The lethal dose in dogs is 60 milligrams per kilogram of body weight. Moderately toxic by ingestion and skin contact. Has caused tumors and cancer in laboratory animals. ASP

**INH** • FDA abbreviation for inhibitor.

**INORGANIC BROMIDES PRESENT AS A RESULT OF FUMIGA-TION OF PROCESSED FOODS WITH ORGANIC BROMIDES and/or FROM USE ON RAW PRODUCTS** • The FDA's residue tolerances are: less than 25 ppm in malt beverages; 125 ppm on all processed food; less than 125 ppm in animal feed grain milled fractions; less than 250 ppm in concentrated tomato products and dried figs; less than 325 ppm in Parmesan or Roquefort cheeses; less than 400 ppm in dried egg, or processed herbs, spices, and dog food; less than 90 in dried citrus pulp for use as cattle feed. *See* Bromides.

**INOSINATE** • A salt of inosinic acid used to intensify flavor, as with sodium glutamate *(see)*. Inosinic acid is prepared from meat extract; also from dried sardines.

**INOSINIC ACID** • Flavor enhancer. A substance found in muscle and on hydrolysis yields inosine. E

**INOSITOL** • A dietary supplement of the vitamin B family used in emollients. Found in plant and animal tissues. Isolated commercially from corn. A fine, white crystalline powder, it is odorless with a sweet taste. Stable in air. The final report to the FDA of the Select Committee on GRAS Substances stated in 1980 that it should continue its GRAS status with no limitations other than good manufacturing practices. ASP

**INSECTICIDE** • A class of crop protection and specialty chemicals used to control insects on farms and in forests, as well as nonagricultural applications such as residential lawns, golf courses, and public tracts of land.

**INSOL. FIBER** • Label listing for insoluble fiber *(see both)*.

**INSOLUBLE** • A substance that cannot be dissolved.

**INSOLUBLE GLUCOSE ISOMERASE ENZYME PREPARATIONS** • *See* Enzymes. GRAS. EAF

**INTENSE SWEETENERS** • Intense sweeteners are nonnutritive sweeteners, also referred to as low-calorie sweeteners or artificial sweeteners. Intense sweeteners can replace nutritive sweeteners in most foods at a caloric saving of approximately 16 calories per teaspoon (the calories of a teaspoon of sugar). Examples of intense sweeteners in use in the U.S. food supply are saccharin, aspartame, and acesulfame K *(see all)*.

**INTERMEDIATE** • A chemical substance found as part of a necessary step between one organic compound and another, as in the production of dyes, pharmaceuticals, or other artificial products that develop properties only upon oxidation. Used frequently for artificial colors.

**INTERNATIONAL AGENCY FOR RESEARCH ON CANCER (IARC)** • A United Nations organization that gathers information on suspected environmental carcinogens and summarizes available data with appropriate references. Included in these reviews are synonyms, physical and chemical properties, uses and occurrence, and biological data relevant to the evaluation of the risk of cancer to humans.

**INTRINSIC FACTOR COMPLEX** • A dietary supplement of liver-stomach concentration. The FDA has deemed it illegal.

**INULIN** • Flavoring from chicory *(see)*. GRAS

**INVERT SUGAR** • Inversol. Colorose. A mixture of 50 percent glucose and 50 percent fructose. It is sweeter than sucrose. Commercially produced by "inversion" of sucrose. Honey is mostly invert sugar. Invert sugar is used in confectionery and in brewing. Like glycerin *(see)* it holds in moisture and prevents drying out. Used medicinally in intravenous solutions. The final report to the FDA of the Select Committee on GRAS Substances stated in 1980 that there is no evidence in the available information that it is a hazard to the public when used as it is now and it should continue its GRAS status with limitations on amounts that can be added to food. ASP

**INVERTASE FROM SACCHAROMYCES CEREVISIAE** • An enzyme used in processing. GRAS. ASP. E

**IODINE SOURCES** • Calcium Iodate, Cuprous Iodide, Potassium Iodate, and Potassium Iodide. Discovered in 1811 and classed among the rarer earth elements, it is found in the earth's crust as bluish black scales. Iodine is an integral part of the thyroid hormones, which have important metabolic roles, and is an essential nutrient for humans. Iodine deficiency leads to thyroid enlargement or goiter. Nutritionists have found that the most efficient way to add iodine to the diet is through the use of iodized salt. The FDA has ordered all table salts to specify whether the product contains iodide. However, many commercially prepared food items do not contain iodized salt. Iodized salt contains up to 0.01 percent; dietary supplements contain

0.16 percent. Cuprous and potassium iodides are used in table salts; potassium iodide is in some drinking water; and potassium iodate is used in animal feeds. Dietary iodine is absorbed from the intestinal tract, and the main human sources are from food and water. Seafoods are good sources, and dairy products may be good sources if the cows eat enriched grain. Adult daily iodine requirement is believed to be 110 to 150 milligrams. Growing children and pregnant or lactating women may need more. Iodine compounds can produce a diffuse red pimply rash, hives, asthma, and sometimes, anaphylactic shock.

**A-IONOL** • See BHT. ASP

**B-IONOL** • See BHT. ASP

**IONONE** • Flavoring. It occurs naturally in boronia, an Australian shrub. Colorless to pale yellow with an odor reminiscent of cedar wood or violets. It may cause allergic reactions.

**IPRODIONE** • Glycophene. A fungicide used on various commodities including cattle, goats, hogs, chickens, sheep, and eggs. FDA residue tolerance on animal feed ranges from 10 to 300 ppm.

**IPRONIDAZOLE** • A feed additive, antiprotozoal agent, it also promotes growth and feed utilization in poultry. Withdrawn for animal use January 17, 1989, in the United States and in 1997 in Europe. It was found to cause tumors, mutations, and fetal harm. It was supposed to be stopped originally six days before slaughter but residues were still a problem.

**IRIS** • Integrated Risk Information System prepared and maintained by the U.S. Environmental Protection Agency (U.S. EPA).

**IRIS FLORENTINA** • *See* Orris.

**IRISH MOSS** • Emulsifier for frozen desserts, dressings, fruits, jelly, and preserves. *See* Carrageenan.

**a-IRISONE** • *See* Ionone.

**ft-IRISONE** • *See* Ionone.

**IRON, ELEMENTAL** • An essential mineral element that occurs widely in foods, especially organ meats such as liver, red meats, poultry, and leafy vegetables. The principal foods to which iron or iron salts are added are enriched cereals, some beverages, including milk, poultry stuffing, cornmeal, corn grits, and bread. Iron ammonium citrate is an anticaking additive in salt. Iron-choline citrate is cleared for use as a source of iron in foods for special dietary use. Iron peptonate, a combination of oxide and peptone, is made soluble by the presence of sodium citrate and is used in the treatment of iron-deficiency anemia. The recommended daily allowances for children and adults is from 0.2 milligram to 1 milligram and 18 milligrams per day for pregnant women. Iron ascorbate, carbonate, chloride, citrate, fumarate, gluconate, lactate, oxide, phosphate, pyrophospate, sulfate, and reduced iron are dietary supplements. Iron is potentially toxic in all forms. GRAS. ASP

**IRON AMMONIUM CITRATE** • A salt for human or animal consumption. An anticaking additive that the FDA says should be less than 25 ppm. *See* Iron Salts. ASP

**IRON CAPRYLATE, IRON LINOLEATE, IRON NAPHTHENATE, and IRON TALLATE** • All are used in packaging. Iron naphthenate was said by the Select Committee on GRAS Substances to have so little known about it that there was nothing upon which to base an evaluation of it when it is used as a food ingredient. As for the others, the final report to the FDA of the Select Committee on GRAS Substances stated in 1980 that they should continue GRAS status with no limitations other than good manufacturing practices. No reported use of iron caprylate, iron naphthenate, or iron linoleate and there is no toxicology information available so all are NUL.

**IRON-CHOLINE CITRATE COMPLEX** • Used in animal feed. *See* Iron and Citrate Salts. ASP

**IRON (HARMLESS SALTS OF)** • Used as nutrients in flour, macaroni and noodles, and bakery products. *See* Iron Salts.

**IRON OXIDE** • Any of several natural or synthetic oxides of iron (iron combined with oxygen) varying in color from red-brown or black-orange to yellow. Used for dyeing eggshells and for pet food. There is no reported use of the chemical and there is no toxicology information available. *See* Iron for toxicity. NUL. E

**IRON, REDUCED** • Elemental iron obtained by a chemical process. It is a grayish black powder used as a nutrient and dietary supplement.

**IRON SALTS** • Iron Sources. Ferric, Choline Citrate, Ferric Orthophosphate, Iron Peptonate, Ferric Phosphate, Ferric Sodium Pyrophosphate, Ferrous Fumarate, Ferrous Gluconate, Ferrous Lactate, and Ferrous Sulfate. Widely used as enrichment for foods, ferric phosphate is used as a food supplement, particularly in bread enrichment. Ferric pyrophosphate is a grayish blue powder used in ceramics. Ferric sodium pyrophosphate is used in prepared breakfast cereals, poultry stuffing, enriched flours, self-rising flours, farina, cornmeal, corn grits, bread, and rolls. The final report to the FDA of the Select Committee on GRAS Substances stated in 1980 that there is no evidence in the available information that it is a hazard to the public when used as it is now and should continue as GRAS with limitations on amounts that can be added to food. It may cause gastrointestinal disturbances. Ferrous lactate is greenish white with a sweet iron taste. Air and light affect it. It is also used to treat anemia. The final report to the FDA of the Select Committee on GRAS Substances stated in 1980 that there is no evidence that ferrous lactate is hazardous and therefore it should continue as GRAS with limitations. Ferrous sulfate is blue-green and odorless and oxidizes in air and is used as a wood preservative, weed killer, and to treat anemia. Large quantities can cause gastrointestinal disturbances. For ferric choline citrate, *see* Choline Chloride. Among other irons used are ferrous gluconate, ferrous fumarate, sodium ferric EDTA, sodium ferric-itropyrophosphate, ferrous citrate, and ferrous ascorbate. All NUL

**IRON POLYVINYLPYRROLIDONE** • Nutrient. NUL

**a-IRONE** • A synthetic flavoring derived from the violet family and usually isolated from irises and orris oil. A light yellow, viscous liquid, it gives off the delicate fragrance of violets when put in alcohol. It is also used to flavor dentifrices and in perfumery. *See* Orris for toxicity.

**IRRADIATED ENZYMES** • Used to control insects. The FDA requires that the dose not exceed 10 kilograys.

**IRRADIATED ERGOSTEROL** • *See* Vitamin $D_2$.

**IRRADIATED FISH** • The FDA put in abeyance *(see)* the request to use cobalt-60 gamma radiation as an antimicrobial treatment for fresh seafood. The FDA also put in abeyance a petition to use low-dose radiation to sanitize shellfish.

**IRRADIATED FOOD** • Food is loaded onto a conveyor belt and passed through a radiation cell, where it is showered with beams of ionizing radiation produced by high radioactive isotopes. The radiation can inhibit ripening and kill certain bacteria and molds that induce spoilage, so that food looks and tastes fresh for up to several weeks. The process does not make food radioactive and does not change the food's color or texture in most cases. Does it destroy nutrients? Does it create radiolytic products in food after exposure that may cause genetic damage? Is irradiation less dangerous than some of the other chemicals added to foods as preservatives? These questions are being hotly debated. The FDA requires foods that have been irradiated to reveal that on the label and to display an international logo, a flower in a circle so you will be able to decide for yourself. FDA regulations say the dose cannot exceed 1 kilogray. *See* Radiation and Radiation Sources.

**IRRADIATED MEATS** • Minimum dose 10 kilogray for sterilization of frozen packaged meats.

**IRRADIATED PORK** • Control of *Trichinella spiralis*. The FDA says minimum dose is 10 kilogray.

**IRRADIATED POULTRY** • To control pathogens in fresh or frozen uncooked poultry. The FDA says minimum dose is 10 kilogray.

**IRRADIATED POULTRY FEED** • Dose ranges from 2 to 25 kilogray gamma radiation from cobalt-60 to render poultry feed salmonella *(see)* negative.

**IRRADIATED SPICES, HERBS, and SEASONINGS** • To control insects and/or microorganisms. The FDA says dose is not to exceed 30 kilograys.

**IRRADIATED YEAST** • A nutrient in enriched farina, a source of vitamin D.

**ISO** • Greek for "equal." In chemistry, it is a prefix added to the name of one compound to denote another composed of the same kinds and numbers of atoms but different from each other in structural arrangement.

**ISOAMYL ACETATE** • A synthetic flavoring additive that occurs naturally in bananas and pears. Colorless, pearlike odor and taste, it is used in raspberry, strawberry, butter, caramel, coconut, cola, apple, banana, cherry, grape, peach, pea, pineapple, rum, cream soda, and vanilla flavorings for beverages, ice cream, ices, candy, baked goods, chewing gum (2,700 ppm), and gelatin desserts. Exposure to 950 ppm for one hour has caused headache, fatigue, shoulder pain, and irritation of the mucous membranes. ASP

**ISOAMYL ACETOACETATE** • A synthetic fruit and apple flavoring for beverages, ice cream, ices, candy, and baked goods. ASP

**ISOAMYL ALCOHOL** • A synthetic flavoring additive that occurs naturally in apples, cognac, lemons, peppermint, raspberries, strawberries, and tea. Used in chocolate, apple, banana, brandy, and rum flavorings for beverages, ice cream, ices, candy, baked goods, gelatin desserts, chewing gum, and brandy. A central nervous system depressant. Vapor exposures have caused marked irritation of the eyes, nose, and throat, and headache. Amyl alcohols are highly toxic, and ingestion has caused human deaths from respiratory failure. Isoamyl alcohol may cause heart, lung, and kidney damage. ASP

**ISOAMYLASE FROM PSEUDOMONAS AMYLODERAMOSA** • Enzymes used to modify starch. GRAS

**ISOAMYL BENZOATE** • A synthetic berry, apple, cherry, plum, prune, liquor, rum, and maple flavoring additive for beverages, ice cream, ices, candy, gelatin desserts, baked goods, and chewing gum. Also used in perfumery and cosmetics. ASP

**ISOAMYL CINNAMATE** • A synthetic strawberry, butter, caramel, chocolate, cocoa, fruit, peach, pineapple, and honey flavoring additive for beverages, ice cream, candy, and baked goods. ASP

**ISOAMYL FORMATE** • Formic Acid. A synthetic flavoring additive, colorless, liquid, with a fruity smell. Used in strawberry, apple, apricot, banana, peach, and pineapple flavorings for beverages, ice cream, candy, baked goods, gelatin desserts, and chewing gum. *See* Formic Acid for toxicity. ASP

**ISOAMYL 2-FURANBUTYRATE** • A synthetic chocolate, coffee, fruit, and whiskey flavoring additive for beverages, ices, candy, baked goods, and gelatin.

**ISOAMYL 2-FURANPROPIONATE** • A synthetic chocolate, coffee, fruit, and whiskey flavoring additive for beverages, ice cream, ices, candy, and baked goods.

*a*-**ISOAMYL FURFURYLACETATE** • *See* Isoamyl 2-Furanpropionate.

**ISOAMYL 3-(2-FURAN)BUTYRATE** • Artificial flavoring. *See* Furans. ASP

*a*-**ISOAMYL FURFURYLPROPIONATE** • *See* Isoamyl 2-Furanbutyrate.

**ISOAMYL HEXANOATE** • Synthetic flavoring. *See* Hexanoic Acid. ASP

**ISOAMYL ISOBUTYRATE** • A synthetic fruit and banana flavoring additive for beverages, ice cream, ices, candy, baked goods, gelatin desserts, puddings, and chewing gum (2,000 ppm). Used in manufacture of artificial rum and fruit essences. ASP

**ISOAMYL ISOVALERATE** • A synthetic flavoring additive, clear, colorless, liquid, with an apple odor. Occurs naturally in bananas and peaches. Used in raspberry, strawberry, apple, apricot, banana, cherry, peach, pineapple, honey, rum, walnut, vanilla, and cream soda flavorings for beverages, ice cream, ices, candy, baked goods, gelatin desserts, puddings, jellies, liqueurs, and chewing gum. ASP

**ISOAMYL LAURATE** • The ester of isoamyl alcohol and lauric acid *(see both)* used as a synthetic fruit flavoring for beverages, ice cream, ices, candy, and baked goods. ASP

**ISOAMYL NONANOATE** • A synthetic chocolate, fruit, and liquor flavoring additive for beverages, ice cream, ices, candy, baked goods, and gelatin desserts. ASP

**ISOAMYL OCTANOATE** • A synthetic chocolate, fruit, and liquor flavoring additive for beverages, ice cream, ices, candy, baked goods, and gelatin desserts. ASP

**ISOAMYL PHENYLACETATE** • A synthetic butter, chocolate, cocoa, peach, honey, licorice, and anise flavoring additive for beverages, ice cream, ices, candy, baked goods, toppings, and gelatin desserts. ASP

**ISOAMYL PYRUVATE** • A synthetic flavoring additive, colorless liquid, with a pleasant odor. Used in root beer and fruit flavorings for beverages, ice cream, ices, candy, and baked goods. Also used in perfumery and soaps. *See* Salicylic Acid for toxicity. ASP

**ISOAMYL SALICYLATE** • Synthetic flavoring. *See* Salicylates. ASP

**ISOASCORBIC ACID** • Preservative. *See* Erythorbic Acid. GRAS

**ISOBORNEOL** • A synthetic fruit and spice flavoring additive for beverages, ice cream, ices, candy, and chewing gum. *See* Borneol for toxicity. ASP

**ISOBORNYL ACETATE** • Synthetic pine odor used as a fruit flavoring for beverages, ice cream, ices, candy, baked goods, and gelatin.

**ISOBORNYL FORMATE** • Synthetic flavoring. *See* Isoborneol. ASP

**ISOBORNYL ISOVALERATE** • Synthetic flavoring. *See* Isoborneol. ASP

**ISOBORNYL PROPIONATE** • Synthetic flavoring. *See* Isoborneol. ASP

**ISOBUTANE** • A propellant. *See* Butanes. GRAS. NUL

**ISOBUTYL ACETATE** • The ester of isobutyl alcohol and acetic acid used as a synthetic flavoring additive. A clear, colorless liquid with a fruity odor. Used in raspberry, strawberry, butter, banana, and grape flavorings for beverages, ice cream, ices, candy, baked goods, gelatin desserts, chewing gum, and icings. It may be mildly irritating to mucous membranes, and in high concentrations it is narcotic. ASP

**ISOBUTYL ACETOACETATE** • A synthetic berry and fruit flavoring additive for beverages, ice cream, ices, candy, and baked goods. *See* Isobutyl Acetate for toxicity. ASP

**ISOBUTYL ALCOHOL** • Present in fusel oil; also produced by fermentation of carbohydrates. Colorless liquid with an odor of amyl alcohol, it is used in the manufacture of synthetic fruit flavorings and as a solvent. It is mildly irritating to skin and mucous membranes and, in high concentrations, narcotic. ASP

**ISOBUTYL ALDEHYDE** • A synthetic flavoring additive that occurs naturally in soy sauce, tea, tobacco, and coffee. It has a pungent odor. Used in berry, butter, caramel, fruit, liquor, and wine flavorings for beverages, ice cream, ices, candy, baked goods, and liquor.

**ISOBUTYL ANTHRANILATE** • Synthetic mandarin orange, cherry, and grape flavoring additive for beverages, ice cream, ices, candy, baked goods, and chewing gum (1,700 ppm). ASP

**ISOBUTYL BENZOATE** • Synthetic berry, cherry, plum, and pineapple flavoring additive for beverages, ice cream, ices, candy, and baked goods. ASP

**ISOBUTYL BUTYRATE** • Synthetic berry, apple, banana, pineapple, liquor, and rum flavoring additive for beverages, ice cream, ices, candy, puddings, liquors, and baked goods. ASP

**ISOBUTYL CINNAMATE** • Flavor said to be identical to natural flavor from aromatic raw materials. ASP

**2(4)-ISOBUTYL-4(2),DIMETHYLDIHYDRO-4H-1,3,5-DIMETHYLDI-HYDRO-4H-1,3,5-DITHIAZINE** • A newer synthetic flavoring. EAF

**ISOBUTYL FORMATE** • Synthetic flavoring. ASP

**ISOBUTYL 2-FURANPROPIONATE** • A synthetic berry and pineapple flavoring additive for beverages, ice cream, ices, gelatin desserts, and chewing gum.

**ISOBUTYL HEPTANOATE** • Synthetic flavoring. *See* Heptanoic Acid. ASP

**ISOBUTYL HEXANOATE** • A synthetic apple and pineapple flavoring additive for beverages, ice cream, ices, chewing gum, and baked goods.

**ISOBUTYL ISOBUTYRATE** • A synthetic strawberry, butter, fruit, banana, and liquor flavoring additive for beverages, ice cream, ices, candy, gelatin desserts, puddings, liquors, and baked goods. ASP

**ISOBUTYLENE-ISOPRENE COPOLYMER** • Thickener used in chewing gum. *See* Butyl Rubber. ASP

**2-ISOBUTYL-3-METHOXYPYRAZINE** • Thickener. *See* Butyl Rubber. ASP

**ISOBUTYL N-METHYLANTHRANILATE** • Synthetic flavoring. ASP

**2-ISOBUTYL-3-METHYLPYRAZINE** • Syntheic flavoring. *See* Piperazine. ASP

**ISOBUTYL PABA** • *See* Propylparaben.

**ISOBUTYL PALMITATE** • *See* Palmitate.

**ISOBUTYL PARABEN** • *See* Parabens.

**ISOBUTYL PELARGONATE** • The ester of isobutyl alcohol and pelargonic acid *(see both)*.

**ISOBUTYL PHENYLACETATE** • A synthetic butter, caramel, chocolate, fruit, honey, and nut flavoring additive for beverages, ice cream, ices, candy, puddings, maraschino cherries, and baked goods. ASP

**ISOBUTYL PROPIONATE** • A synthetic strawberry, butter, peach, and rum flavoring additive for beverages, ice cream, candy, and baked goods. Used in the manufacture of fruit essences. ASP

**ISOBUTYL SALICYLATE** • A synthetic flavoring additive; colorless liquid with an orchid odor. Used in fruit and root beer flavorings for beverages, ice cream, ices, candy, and baked goods. *See* Salicylic Acid for toxicity. ASP

**ISOBUTYL STEARATE** • The ester of isobutyl alcohol and stearic acid. *See* Fatty Alcohols.

**ISOBUTYLENE/ISOPYRENE COPOLYMER** • A copolymer of isobutylene and isoprene monomers derived from petroleum and used as resins. A chewing-gum base. Isobutylene is used to produce antioxidants for foods, food supplements, and packaging. Vapors may cause asphyxiation.

**ISOBUTYLENE/MALEIC ANHYDRIDE COPOLYMER** • A copolymer of isobutylene and maleic anhydride monomers derived from petroleum and used as a resin. Strong irritant.

**ISOBUTYLENE RESIN, POLYISOBUTYLENE** • A component of chewing-gum base.

**a-ISOBUTYLPHENETHYL ALCOHOL** • A synthetic butter, caramel, chocolate, fruit, and spice flavoring additive for beverages, ice cream, ices, candy, baked goods, liqueurs, and chocolate. *See* Isoamyl Alcohol for toxicity.

**ISOBUTYRIC ACID** • A synthetic flavoring additive that occurs naturally in bay, bay leaves, parsley, and strawberries. It has a pungent odor. Used in butter, butterscotch, fruit, liquor, rum, cheese, nut, vanilla, and cream soda flavorings for beverages, ice cream, ices, candy, baked goods, chewing gum, and margarine. It is a mild irritant. A pungent liquid that smells like butyric acid *(see)*. ASP

**ISOCETYL ALCOHOL** • *See* Cetyl Alcohol.

**ISOCETYL ISODECANOATE** • *See* Cetyl Alcohol.

**ISOCETYL PALMITATE** • *See* Cetyl Alcohol.

**ISOCETYL STEARATE** • *See* Cetyl Alcohol and Stearic Acid.

**ISOCETYL STEAROYL STEARATE** • The ester of isocetyl alcohol, stearic alcohol, and stearic acid. *See* Fatty Acids.

**ISOCYCLOCITRAL** • Synthetic flavoring with a green, aldehydic, herbal, leafy odor. Has a sharp leafy note. It is used in hyacinth and sweet pea compositions. *See* Citral. ASP

**ISOEUGENOL** • An aromatic liquid phenol oil obtained from eugenol *(see)* by mixing with an alkali. A synthetic flavoring additive, pale yellow, viscous, with a floral odor. Occurs naturally in mace oil. Used in mint, fruit, spice, cinnamon, and clove flavorings for beverages, ice cream, ices, baked goods, chewing gum (1,000 ppm), and condiments. Used in the manufacture of vanillin *(see)*. Moderately toxic by ingestion. Has caused mutations in experimental animals. ASP

**ISOEUGENOL ACETATE** • *See* Acetylisoeugenol. ASP

**ISOEUGENYL ACETATE** • A synthetic berry, fruit, and spice flavoring additive for beverages, ice cream, ices, candy, baked goods, and chewing gum. ASP

**ISOEUGENYL ETHYL ETHER** • A synthetic flavoring additive, white, crystalline, with a spicy, clovelike odor. Used in fruit and vanilla flavorings for beverages, ice cream, ices, candy, and baked goods.

**ISOEUGENYL FORMATE** • A synthetic spice flavoring additive used in condiments. *See* Formic Acid for toxicity. ASP

**ISOEUGENYL METHYL ETHER** • A synthetic raspberry, strawberry, cherry, and clove flavoring additive for beverages, ices, ice cream, candy, baked goods, gelatin desserts, and chewing gum. ASP

**ISOEUGENYL PHENYLACETATE** • A synthetic fruit, honey, and spice flavoring additive for beverages, ice cream, ices, candy, and baked goods. ASP

**ISOJASMONE** • *See* Jasmone. ASP

**ISOLATE** • A substance that is freed from chemical contaminants.

**ISOLEUCINE** • L Form. An essential amino acid not synthesized within the human body. Isolated commercially from beet sugar, it is a building block of protein. Used as a nutrient and dietary supplement. The FDA asked for further study of this nutrient in 1980. GRAS. ASP

**ISOMALT** • A candidate for an artificial sweetener, it has 45 to 65 percent the sweetness of sugar. A component of bread obtained by the action of enzymes on starch. It contains calories and is physically similar to sugar. It has a sweet taste reportedly without any aftertaste. While it is not as sweet as sugar, it may be enhanced with an intense sweetener such as acesulfame K *(see)*. It is used in fifteen countries in candies, gums, ice cream, jams, and baked goods. E

**DL-ISOMENTHONE** • Synthetic flavoring. *See* Menthol. ASP

**ALPHA-ISOMETHYLIONONE** • Flavoring. *See* Ionone. ASP

**ALPHA-ISOMETHYLIONYL ACETATE** • Synthetic flavoring. ASP

**ISONONYL ISONONANOATE** • The ester *(see)* produced by the reaction of nonyl alcohol with nonanoic acid. Used in fruit flavorings for lipsticks and mouthwashes. Occurs in cocoa, oil of lavender.

**ISOPARAFFINIC PETROLEUM HYDROCARBONS, SYNTHETIC** • Coating additive, insecticide formulations, used on eggs, fruits, pickles, vegetables, wine, and vinegar. *See* Paraffin. NIL

**ISOPENTYLAMINE** • Used in processing. Irritating to the skin. ASP

**ISOPENTYLIDENEISOPENTYLAMINE** • Synthetic flavoring. Widely used in baked goods, beverages, breakfast cereals, chewing gum, confectionery frostings, egg products, frozen dairy, fruit ices, gelatins, hard candy, imitation dairy, instant coffee, meat products, snack foods, soups, and soft candy. Declared GRAS by FEMA *(see)*. EAF

**ISOPHORONE** • White, watery liquid that is irritating to skin and eyes. It is used in solvents for polyvinyl and nitrocellulose resins, and pesticides.

**ISOPROPANOL** • *See* Isopropyl Alcohol.

**ISOPROPANOLAMINE** • An emulsifying additive with a light ammonia odor that is soluble in water.

**cis-5-ISOPROPENYL-cis-2-METHYLCYCLOPENTAN-1-CARBOXALDEHYDE** • Synthetic flavoring. FAO/WHO has no safety concern about it. ASP

**ISOPROPENYLPYRAZINE** • Synthetic flavoring. NIL

**ISOPROPYL ACETATE** • Synthetic nutty flavoring. ASP

**P-ISOPROPYLACETOPHENONE** • Synthetic flavoring. NIL

**ISOPROPYL ALCOHOL** • Isopropanol. An antibacterial, solvent, and denaturant *(see)*. Solvent for the spice oleoresins. The FDA permits residues of 250 ppm or less in modified hop extract; 50 ppm in spice oleoresins; 6 ppm in manufacture of lemon oil; 2 percent by weight in hop extract as residue from extraction of hops in manufacture of beer. It is also used in defoaming additives for processing beet sugar and yeast, on food-processing equipment and on food-contact surfaces as well as on glass containers for holding milk. It is prepared from propylene, which is obtained in the cracking of petroleum. Also used in antifreeze compositions and as a solvent for gums, shellac, and essential oils. Ingestion or inhalation of large quantities of the vapor may cause flushing, headache, dizziness, mental depression, nausea, vomiting, narcosis, anesthesia, and coma. The fatal ingested dose is around a fluid ounce. ASP

**ISOPROPYL BENZOATE** • Preservative. *See* Benzoic Acid. NIL

**P-ISOPROPYLBENZYL ALCOHOL** • *See* Benzyl Alcohol. ASP

**ISOPROPYL BUTYRATE** • Occurs naturally in apples, cranberries, strawberries, and wine. Used as a flavoring for apple, blackberry, cherry, cranberry, ginger, and grape. ASP

**ISOPROPYL CINNAMATE** • Synthetic flavoring. ASP

**ISOPROPYL CITRATE** • A sequestrant and antioxidant additive used in oleomargarine and salad oils. The final report to the FDA of the Select Committee on GRAS Substances stated in 1980 that it should continue its GRAS status with no limitations other than good manufacturing practices. When heated to decomposition it emits acrid smoke and irritating fumes. ASP

**ISOPROPYL-2-CYCLOHEXENONE** • *See* Isopropyl Alcohol. EAF

**ISOPROPYL FORMATE** • Formic Acid. A synthetic berry and melon flavoring additive for beverages, ice cream, candy, and baked goods. ASP

**ISOPROPYL HEXANOATE** • A synthetic pineapple flavoring additive for beverages, ice cream, ices, candy, and baked goods. ASP

**ISOPROPYL ISOBUTYRATE** • A synthetic pineapple flavoring additive for beverages, ice cream, ices, candy, and baked goods. ASP

**ISOPROPYL ISOSTEARATE** • *See* Stearic Acid and Propylene Glycol.

**ISOPROPYL ISOVALERATE** • A synthetic pineapple and nut flavoring additive for beverages, ice cream, ices, candy, and baked goods. ASP

**ISOPROPYL 2-METHYLBUTYRATE** • Synthetic flavoring. EAF

**2-ISOPROPYL-5-METHYL-2-HEXENAL** • Synthetic flavoring. ASP

**2-ISOPROPYL-4-METHYLTHIAZOLE** • Synthetic flavoring. ASP

**ISOPROPYL MYRISTATE** • A widely used fatty compound derived from isopropyl alcohol and myristic acid. Used as a solvent in pesticide formulations. ASP

**ISOPROPYL PALMITATE** • Colorless and odorless, used as a lubricant. ASP

**2-ISOPROPYLPHENOL** • Synthetic flavoring. *See* Thymol. ASP

**P-ISOPROPYLPHENYLACETALDEHYDE** • Synthetic flavoring. FAO/WHO has no safety concern about it. ASP

**ISOPROPYL PHENYLACETATE** • A synthetic butter, caramel, and honey flavoring additive for beverages, ice cream, ices, candy, and baked goods. ASP

**ISOPROPYL PROPIONATE FLAVORING** • Flavoring. FAO/WHO *(see)* said in 1998 that there was no safety concern at current levels of intake when used as a flavoring additive. Toxic. ASP

**2-ISOPROPYLPYRAZINE** • Synthetic green pepper flavoring. EAF

**ISOPROPYL TIGLATE** • Synthetic sweet mint flavoring. ASP

**2-ISOPROPYL-N,2,3-TRIMETHYLBUTYRAMIDE** • Synthetic flavoring with a menthol taste. EAF

**ISOPULEGOL** • Synthetic flavoring with a menthol taste. FAO/WHO says it has no safety concern. ASP

**ISOPULEGONE** • Synthetic flavoring with a mint taste. *See* Pennyroyal oil. ASP

**ISOPULEGYL ACETATE** • Synthetic fragrance. ASP

**ISOQUINOLINE** • Synthetic flavoring. ASP

**ISOSAFROEUGENOL** • White crystalline powder with a vanilla odor used as a flavoring additive in various foods. Moderately toxic by ingestion.

**ISOSTEARIC ACID** • A saturated fatty acid that has the same uses as stearic acid and oleic acids *(see both)*.

**ISOTHIOCYANATES** • Found in mustard, horseradish, radishes, they seem to induce protective enzymes.

**ISOTHIOUREA** • Antifungal additive used on citrus fruit. Prohibited from direct addition or use in human food.

**ISOVALERIC ACID** • Occurs in valerian, hop oil, tobacco, and other plants. Colorless liquid with a disagreeable taste and odor used in flavors and perfumes. A poison by skin contact. Moderately toxic by ingestion. A corrosive skin and eye irritant. *See* Valeric Acid. ASP

**ISOVALERIC ACID, ALLYL ESTER, BENZYL ESTER, BUTYL ESTER, ETHYL ESTER** • Flavoring additives in various foods. The allyl ester is under IARC review. The allyl form is poisonous by ingestion. The others are mildly toxic by ingestion. Moderately toxic by skin contact. Skin irritants.

**ISOVINYL FORMATE** • Formic Acid. A synthetic fruit flavoring additive for beverages, ice cream, ices, candy, and baked goods. *See* Formic Acid for toxicity.

**ISOVINYL PROPIONATE** • *See* Isovinyl Formate.

**I.U.** • International Unit. A term for measurement of vitamins that are fat soluble (do not mix with water and need fat for proper absorption). Vitamins A, E, D, and K are usually measured in I.U.s.

**IVA** • *Achillea moschata.* A flavoring for alcoholic beverages only from a small American ground pine that smells like skin. There is no reported use of the chemical and there is no toxicology information available. NUL

**IVERMECTIN** • Mectizan. Hyvermectin. A drug used to treat river blindness in humans, it is used to treat worms in animals, especially beef, pork, and reindeer. The FDA limits residues to 15 ppb in cattle and reindeer liver, and 20 ppb in swine liver. Poison by injection under the skin. Potential adverse human effects include dizziness, fever, headache, tender swollen glands, rash, and fatigue. *See* Guar Gum.

# J

**JAMBUL OLEORESIN** • Java Plum. *Syzygium jambolanum.* Used as a flavoring in foods. Used medically as an antidiarrheal medication. ASP

**JAPAN WAX** • Japan Tallow. Sumac Wax. Vegetable Wax. A fat squeezed from the fruit of a tree grown in Japan and China. Pale yellow, flat cakes, disks, or squares, with a fatlike rancid odor and taste. It is related to poison ivy and may cause allergic contact dermatitis. The final report to the FDA of the Select Committee on GRAS Substances stated in 1980 that there were insufficient relevant biological and other studies upon which to base an evaluation of it when it is used as a food ingredient. It remains GRAS for packaging. NUL

**JAPONICA** • *See* Honeysuckle. GRAS

**JASMINE** • Oil and Spiritus (alcoholic solution). The oil is extracted from a tropical shrub with extremely fragrant white flowers and is used in raspberry, strawberry, floral, and cherry flavorings for ice cream, ices, candy, baked goods, gelatin desserts, chewing gum, and jelly. The spiritus is used in blackberry, strawberry, and fruit flavorings for beverages, ice cream, ices, candy, baked goods, gelatin, and cherries. Used in perfumes. May cause allergic reactions. GRAS. EAF

**JASMINE ABSOLUTE** • Oil of jasmine obtained by extraction with volatile or nonvolatile solvents. Sometimes called the "natural perfume" because the oil is not subjected to heat and distilled oils. *See* Absolute. May cause allergic reactions. EAF

**JASMINE SPIRITUS** • *Jasminum grandiflorum*. Natural flavoring. *See* Jasmine Absolute. EAF

**JASMONATES** • Derived from fragrant compounds with the odor of jasmine flowers (*see* Jasmine Absolute), these have been found to keep stored potatoes from sprouting.

**JASMONE, CIS** • Derived from the oil of jasmine flowers, it is used in flavorings and perfumery. ASP

**JASMONYL** • *See* 1,3-Nonanediol Acetate.

**JELUTONG** • Any of several trees with a milky white exudate. Resembles chicle and is used chiefly in waterproofing and in chewing gum. ASP

**JUNIPER** • *Juniperus communis*. Extract, Oil, and Berries. A flavoring from the dried ripe fruit of trees grown in northern Europe, Asia, and North America. The greenish yellow extract is used in liquor, root beer, sarsaparilla, wintergreen, and birch beer flavorings for beverages, ice cream, ices, candy, and baked goods. The oil is used in berry, cola, pineapple, gin, rum, whiskey, root beer, ginger, and meat flavorings for beverages, ice cream, ices, candy, baked goods, gelatin desserts, chewing gum, meats, and liquors. The berries are used in gin flavoring for condiments and liquors. Juniper is used also in fumigating and was formerly a diuretic for reducing body water. The oil is mildly toxic by ingestion, a human skin irritant and allergen, and if taken internally, a severe kidney irritation similar to that caused by turpentine may result. GRAS. NIL. The oil is ASP.

**JUNIPER OIL** • *See* Juniper.

# K

**KABAT** • Altosid. Methoprene. Amber liquid used as an insect growth regulator in animal feed, dried apples, apricots, barley cereal, beef, corn cereal, cornmeal, grits, hominy, macaroni, oat cereal, dried peaches, potable water, dried prunes, raisins, rice cereal, rye cereal, spices, wheat cereal, and wheat flour. The FDA's insect growth regulator residue tolerance is 10 ppm in the grains, rice, and dried fruits. Exempt from the tolerance is potable water. Moderately toxic by skin contact. Mildly toxic by ingestion. Has caused mutations in laboratory animals.

**KADAYA** • *See* Karaya Gum.

**KAOLIN** • China Clay. Used as an anticaking additive in food. Aids in the covering ability of face powder and in absorbing oil secreted by the skin. Used in baby powder, bath powder, face masks, foundation cake makeup, liquid powder, face powder, dry rouge, and emollients. Originally obtained from

Kaoling Hill in Kiangsi Province in southeast China. Essentially a hydrated aluminum silicate *(see)*. It is a white or yellowish white mass or powder, insoluble in water and absorbent. Used medicinally to treat intestinal disorders, but in large doses it may cause obstructions, perforations, or granuloma (tumor) formation. The final report to the FDA of the Select Committee on GRAS Substances stated in 1980 that it should continue its GRAS status with no limitations other than good manufacturing practices. *See also* Clays.

**KARAYA GUM** • Kaday. Katilo. Kullo. Kuterra. Sterculia. Indian Tragacanth. Mucara. The exudate of a tree found in India. The finely ground white powder is used as a stabilizer in gelatins, gumdrops, prepared ices, and ice cream, and as a filler for lemon custard. Also a citrus and spice flavoring additive for beverages, ice cream, ices (1,300 ppm), candy, meats, baked goods, toppings (3,500 ppm), and emulsions (18,000 ppm). Used instead of the more expensive gum tragacanth *(see)* and in bulk laxatives. Reevaluated by the FDA in 1976 and found to be GRAS in the following percentages: 0.3 percent for frozen dairy desserts and mixes; 0.02 percent for milk products; 0.9 percent for soft candy; and 0.002 percent for all other food categories. GRAS. ASP. E

**KATILO** • *See* Karaya Gum.

**KAUTSCHIN** • *See* Limonene.

**KELP** • Recovered from the giant Pacific marine plant *Macrocystis pyriferae.* Used as seasonings or flavoring and to provide iodine when used in dietary foods. It has many minerals that are associated with seawater and, as a result, is very high in sodium. The FDA residue tolerance is less than 0.225 mg per day without reference to age or physical state; 0.045 mg per day for infants; 0.105 mg per day for those under four years; 0.225 mg per day for adults and children. For pregnant or lactating women, 0.20 mg per day. It is a source of iodine in foods for special dietary use. The Japanese report that kelp reduced normal thyroid function, probably because of its iodine content. The FDA has also reported that high levels of arsenic have been found in people who eat a lot of kelp as a vegetable. The final report to the FDA of the Select Committee on GRAS Substances stated in 1980 that it should continue its GRAS status with no limitations other than good manufacturing practices. *See* Algae, Brown. ASP

**2-KETO-4-BUTANETHIOL** • Flavoring. ASP

**KETONAROME** • *See* Methylcyclopentenolone.

**KETONE C-7** • *See* 2-Heptanone.

**2-KETOPROPIONALDEHYDE** • *See* Pyruvaldehyde.

**KETOPROPIONALDEHYDE** • *See* Pyruvic Acid.

**KG** • Abbreviation for kilogram, which is equal to about 2.205 pounds.

**KIDNEY BEAN EXTRACT** • Extract of *Phaseolus vulgaris,* the beans were used as a nutrient and a laxative by the American Indians.

**KILOGRAM (kg)** • Equal to about 2.205 pounds.

**KOLA NUT EXTRACT** • Guru Nut. A natural extract from the brownish seed, about the size of a chestnut, produced by trees in Africa, the West Indies, and Brazil. Contains caffeine *(see)*. Used in butter, caramel, chocolate, cocoa, coffee, cola, walnut, and root beer flavorings for beverages, ice cream, ices, candy, and baked goods. Has been used to treat epilepsy. GRAS. ASP

**KONJAC FLOUR** • Konjac Mannan. Konnyaku. Yam Flour. It is derived from the tubers of *Amorphophallus konjac,* a large plant grown in Japan for its flour. A food additive that is expected to increase in use as a gelling additive, thickener, emulsifier, and stabilizer in such foods as soup, gravy, mayonnaise, and jam. There is a long history of use in traditional Japanese and Chinese foods; the average consumption of konjac flour from these uses is estimated to be between 2 and 3 grams per person per day and sometimes as high as 4 grams. The anticipated maximum consumption of konjac flour from food additive uses is about 3 grams per person per day. Human studies conducted for up to sixty-five days at dose levels of up to 8.6 grams of konjac flour per person per day. Volunteers consuming approximately 5.2 grams or more reported loose stools, flatulence, diarrhea, and abdominal pain or distension. Studies with normal and diabetic volunteers demonstrated that consumption of 7.2 to 8.6 grams of konjac flour per day for seventeen days significantly decreased mean fasting blood sugar levels; in addition, a dose of 3.9 to 5 grams consumed in a single meal or administered with glucose was reported to delay the increase in blood sugar and insulin levels for several hours following the meal, also delaying their return to baseline levels. The test meal also appeared to impair vitamin E absorption (up to 30 percent decrease) and influenced the absorption of the coadministered drug glibenclamide (a diabetes medication). On the basis of the available toxicological data and the long history of use of konjac in food, the committee allocated temporary ADI *(see)* "not specified" for konjac flour and said a review should be done of konjac's affect on vitamin E and other fat-soluble vitamins. Also, it was noted that consumption of dry konjac has been associated with obstruction of the esophagus and that it should be consumed only in hydrated form. E

**KONNYAKU** • *See* Konjac Flour.

**KOSHER** • Parve. U. Hebrew word meaning "proper" or "fit," used especially for food prepared according to Orthodox dietary and religious laws. Forbidden are pork, horseflesh, shellfish, and parts of beef and lamb. All meat and poultry must be killed by a Jew trained in the prescribed ritual, then soaked or salted to remove all blood. Milk and its products must not be eaten with meat. The notifications on packages meaning the product has been prepared under dietary laws are U or Parve.

**KRAMERIA EXTRACT** • Rhatany Extract. A synthetic flavoring derived from the dried root of either of two American shrubs. Used in raspberry, bitters, fruit, and rum flavorings. Used in cosmetics as an astringent. Low oral toxicity. Large doses may produce gastric distress. Can cause tumors and death after injection, but not after ingestion.

**KULLO** • *See* Karaya Gum.

**KUTEERA** • *See* Karaya Gum.

# L

**LABDANUM** • Absolute, Oil, and Oleoresin. A synthetic musk flavoring additive. It is a volatile oil obtained by steam distillation from gum extracted from various rockrose shrubs. Golden yellow, viscous, with a strong balsamic odor and a bitter taste. The absolute is used in raspberry, fruit, and vanilla flavorings for beverages, ice cream, ices, candy, baked goods, gelatin desserts, and chewing gum. The oil is used in fruit and spice flavorings for beverages, ice cream, ices, candy, and baked goods. The oleoresin *(see)* is used in fruit and vanilla flavorings for beverages, ice cream, ices, candy, and baked goods. Also used in perfumes, especially as a fixative. Mildly toxic by ingestion. A skin irritant. There is reported use of the chemical; it has not yet been assigned for toxicology literature. EAF

**LABRADOR TEA EXTRACT** • Hudson Bay Tea. Marsh Tea. The extract of the dried flowering plant or young shoots of *Ledum palustre* or *Ledum groenlandicum,* a tall, resinous evergreen shrub found in bogs, swamps, and moist meadows. Brewed like tea, it has a pleasing odor and is stimulating. It was used by the Indians and settlers as a tonic supposed to purify blood. It was also employed to treat wounds. *Ledum palustre* contains, among other things, tannin and valeric acid *(see both)*.

**LACTALBUMIN** • Albumin Milk. A componenet of skim milk protein. Exact function is not known, but may aid in stabilization of fat particles. Alpha-lactalbumin has been associated as of this writing with stress reduction; anticancer with human alpha-lactalbumin, immunomodulation and antimicrobial activity after protein breakdown. May cause an allergic reaction in those allergic to milk. ASP

**LACTALBUMIN PHOSPHATE** • A protein in milk that may cause allergy. *See* Lactalbumin. NIL

**LACTASE ENZYME PREPARATION FROM *ASPERGILLIUS NIGER*** • GRAS status pending.

**LACTASE ENZYME PREPARATION FROM *SACCHAROMYCES FRAGILIS* or *KLUVEROMYCES LACTIS*** • An enzyme that breaks down lactose *(see)*. There is no reported use of the chemical and there is no toxicology information available. GRAS. NUL

**LACTASE ENZYME PREPARATION FROM *KLYVEROMYCES LACTICS*** • Breaks down lactose. GRAS

**LACTASE PREPARATION FROM *CANDIDA PSEUDOTROPICALIS*** • Lactase enzyme preparation from *Candida pseudotropicalis,* a yeast for use in hydrolyzing lactose to glucose and galactose. EAF

**LACTIC ACID** • Butyl Lactate. Ethyl Lactate. Odorless, colorless, usually a syrupy product normally present in blood and muscle tissue as a product of the metabolism of glucose and glycogen. Present in sour milk, beer, sauerkraut, pickles, and other food products made by bacterial fermentation. It is produced commercially by fermentation of whey, cornstarch, potatoes, and molasses. Used as an acidulant in beverages, candy, olives, dried egg whites, cottage cheese, confections, bread, rolls, buns, cheese products, frozen desserts, sherbets, ices, fruit jelly, butter, preserves, jams (sufficient amounts may be added to compensate for the deficiency of fruit acidity), and in the brewing industry. Also used in infant-feeding formulas. Used in blackberry, butter, butterscotch, lime, chocolate, fruit, walnut, spice, and cheese flavorings for beverages, ice cream, ices, candy, baked goods, gelatins, puddings, chewing gum, toppings, pickles, and olives (24,000 ppm). Also used in skin fresheners. It is caustic in concentrated solutions when taken internally or applied to the skin. In cosmetic products, it may cause stinging in sensitive people, particularly in fair-skinned women. The final report to the FDA of the Select Committee on GRAS Substances stated in 1980 that it should continue its GRAS status with no limitations other than good manufacturing practices. ASP. E

**LACTIC YEASTS** • Obtained from milk. *See* Lactic Acid.

**LACTITOL** • A reduced-calorie sweetener derived from milk sugar. Internationally, it is approved for use in many countries, including the European Union (EU), Canada, Japan, Israel, and Switzerland. GRAS status has been applied for in the United States. E *See* lactose.

**LACTOFEN** • A pesticide used on soybeans. FDA tolerance is 0.05 ppm.

**LACTOFERRIN** • Bioactive milk protein that is said to play a role in the immune system response and helps protect the body against infections. Besides the stimulation of the immune system, scientific studies have revealed that lactoferrin also prevents the growth of pathogens, exerts antibacterial and antiviral properties, controls cell and tissue damage caused by oxidation, and facilitates iron transport. On August 22, 2003, the FDA announced that aLF Ventures, Salt Lake City, Utah, had consulted with the agency about aLF Ventures' plans to market lactoferrin as a component of an antimicrobial spray. This spray can be applied to uncooked beef carcasses to fight *E. coli* 0157:H7, an organism that can cause severe gastrointestinal disease in humans. The FDA informed aLF Ventures that it does not question their decision to market lactoferrin, an antimicrobial protein found in cow's milk and beef. Although aLF Ventures was not required to seek approval from the FDA before it marketed lactoferrin, aLF Ventures provided to the FDA scientific data supporting the firm's conclusion that lactoferrin is "generally recognized as safe" (GRAS) and safe for the general population as well as for individuals who are allergic to milk. "Innovative technology is a critical building block in preserving the strong foundation of the U.S. food supply," said Dr. Lester Crawford, Deputy Commissioner of the Food and Drug Administration. "We must continue to encourage scientific research and new technology to maintain this nation's safe food supply." In its notice submitted to the FDA, aLF Ventures noted that the amount of added lactoferrin that remains on the beef after spraying is comparable to the amount of lactoferrin that is naturally occurring in the beef. Data was also submitted to the U.S. Department of Agriculture (USDA) regarding the effectiveness of lactoferrin against *E. coli* 0157:H7. The USDA is the agency responsible for addressing labeling issues with lactoferrin-treated beef.

**LACTOFLAVIN** • *See* Riboflavin.

**LACTOSE** • Milk Sugar. Saccharum Lactin. D-Lactose. A slightly sweet-tasting, colorless sugar present in the milk of mammals (humans have 6.7 percent and cows 4.3 percent). Occurs as a white powder or crystalline mass as a by-product of the cheese industry. Produced from whey *(see)*. It is inexpensive and is widely used in the food industry as a culture medium, such as in souring milk, and as a humectant *(see)* and nutrient in infant or debilitated patient formula. Also used as a medical diuretic and laxative. Stable in air but readily absorbs odors. It is generally nontoxic. However, it was found to cause tumors when injected under the skin of mice in 50 milligram doses per kilogram of body weight. ASP

**LACTOSE HYDROLYZED** • A nutritive sweetener used in cheeses. *See* Lactose. NUL

**LACTYLIC ESTERS OF FATTY ACIDS** • Emulsifiers used in food products. *See* Esters and Fatty Acids. ASP

**LACTYLIC STEARATE** • Salt of stearic acid used as a dough conditioner to add volume and to keep baked products soft; it makes bread less sticky. *See* Stearic Acid for toxicity.

**LADY'S-MANTLE EXTRACT** • From the dried leaves and flowering shoots of *Alchemilla vulgaris*. A common European herb covered with spreading hairs, it has been used for centuries by herbalists to concoct love potions.

**LAKES, COLOR** • A lake is an organic pigment prepared by precipitating a soluble color with a form of aluminum, calcium, barium potassium, strontium, or zirconium, which then makes the colors insoluble. Not all colors are suitable for making lakes.

**LAMINARIA** • Seaweed from which algin is extracted. *See* Alginates. GRAS

**LAMINARIA JAPONICA BROTH and EXTRACT POWDER** • Used as a flavoring in meat products, poultry, fish, soups, gravies, and seasonings. GRAS

**LANALOOL** • Synthetic flavoring. GRAS

**LANOLIN** • Wool Fat. Wool Wax. A product of the oil glands of sheep. Used as a chewing-gum base component. Used in lipstick, liquid powder, mascara, nail polish remover, protective oil, rouge, eye shadow, foundation creams, foundation cake makeup, hair conditioners, eye creams, cold creams, brilliantine hairdressings, ointment bases, and emollients. A water-absorbing base material and a natural emulsifier, it absorbs and holds water to the skin. Chemically a wax instead of a fat. Contains about 25 to 30 percent water. Advertisers have found that the words "contains lanolin" help to sell a product and have promoted it as being able to "penetrate the skin better than other oils," although there is little scientific proof of this. Lanolin has been found to be a common skin sensitizer causing allergic contact skin rashes. It will not prevent or cure wrinkles and will not stop hair loss. It is not used in pure form today because of its allergy-causing potential. Products derived from it are less likely to cause allergic reactions. ASP

**LANTANA** • *See* Oregano.

**LARCH GUM** • Larch Turpentine. Venice Turpentine. Oleoresin *(see)* from *Larix decidua,* grown in middle and southern Europe. A yellow, sometimes greenish, tenacious, thick liquid with a pleasant aromatic odor, it has a hot, somewhat bitter taste. It becomes hard and brittle on prolonged exposure. It is used as a stabilizer, thickener, and texturizer.

**LARD and LARD OILS** • Pork Fat and Oils. It is the purified internal fat from the abdomen of the hog. It is a soft white unctuous mass, with a slight characteristic odor and a bland taste. It is used in packaging and in chewing-gum bases. Easily absorbed by the skin, it is used as a lubricant, emollient, and base in shaving creams, soaps, and various cosmetic creams. Insoluble in water. When lard was fed to laboratory animals in doses of from 2 to 25 percent of the diet, the male mice had a shortened life span and increased osteoarthritis. This was thought to be due to the large amounts of fat and not specifically to lard. The final report to the FDA of the Select Committee on GRAS Substances stated in 1980 that it should continue its GRAS status with no limitations other than good manufacturing practices. There is no reported use of the chemical and there is no toxicology information available. Lard is NUL and lard oil is NEW.

**LARD GLYCERIDE** • *See* Lard.

**LARIXINIC ACID** • *See* Maltol.

**LASALOCID** • An antibiotic used in beef, chicken, and lamb. Tolerance residue of 10.3 ppm in chicken skin, 0.7 ppm, in cattle liver, and 1.2 ppm in sheep muscle. Poison by ingestion and injection. An eye and skin irritant.

**LASOLOCID SODIUM** • An antibiotic feed additive. The tolerated residue in edible tissues of chicken is 0.05 ppm; 4.8 ppm in cattle liver.

**LASSO** • *See* Alachlor.

**LATEX** • Synthetic Rubber. Component of chewing-gum base. The milky, usually white juice or exudate of plants obtained by tapping. Used in beauty masks for its coating ability and in balloons, condoms, and gloves. Any of various gums, resins, fats, or waxes in an emulsion of water and synthetic rubber of plastic are now considered latex. Ingredients of latex compounds can be poisonous, depending upon which plant products are used. Can cause skin rash. In May 1991, the FDA cautioned doctors and manufacturers about potential allergic reactions to latex products. Allergic reactions caused the death of four patients undergoing medical procedures involving an inflatable latex cuff.

**LAUREL BERRIES** • *Laurus nobilis.* The fresh berries and leaf extract of the laurel tree. The berries are used as a flavoring for beverages and the leaf extract is a spice flavoring for vegetables. *See* Laurel Leaf Oil. GRAS. NIL

**LAUREL GALLATE** • An antioxidant, the laurel ester gallic acid. *See* Propyl Gallate.

**LAUREL LEAF OIL** • Derived from steam distillation of the leaves of *Laurus nobilis,* it is a yellow liquid with a spicy odor used as a flavoring additive. Moderately toxic by ingestion. A skin irritant. GRAS

**LAURIC ACID** • Dodecanoic Acid. A common constituent of vegetable fats, especially coconut oil and laurel oil. A white, glossy powder, insoluble in water, and used in the manufacture of miscellaneous flavors for beverages, ice cream, candy, baked goods, gelatins, and puddings. Its derivatives are widely used as a base in the manufacture of soaps, detergents, and lauryl alcohol (*see* Fatty Alcohols) because of their foaming properties. Has a slight odor of bay. A mild irritant but not a sensitizer. ASP

**LAURIC ALDEHYDE** • *See* Lauric Acid. ASP

**LAUROAMPHOACETATE** • A preservative. *See* Imidazole.

**LAUROAMPHODIACETATE** • A preservative. *See* Imidazole.

**LAUROAMPHODIPROPIONATE** • *See* Propionic Acid and Lauric Acid

**LAUROAMPHODIPROPIONIC ACID** • Preservative. *See* Lauric Acid and Propionic Acid.

**LAUROAMPHOHDROXYPROPYLSULFONATE** • *See* Imidazolin.

**LAUROAMPHOPROPINOATE** • *See* Lauric Acid and Propionic Acid.

**LAUROSTEARIC ACID** • *See* Lauric Acid.

**LAURYL ACETATE** • Dodecyl Acetate. Colorless liquid with fruity odor used in flavoring. ASP

**LAURYL ALCOHOL, SYNTHETIC** • *See* Fatty Alcohols.

*a*-**LAURYL-OMEGA-HYDROXYPOLY(OXYETHYLENE)** • Sanitation compound. May be used on beverage containers including milk containers and equipment.

**LAVANDIN ABSOLUTE AND CONCRETE** • *Lavandula officinalis. See* Lavandin Oil. EAF

**LAVANDIN OIL** • A flavoring from a hybrid related to the lavender plant, pale yellow liquid with a camphor-lavender smell. Used in berry and citrus flavorings for beverages, ice cream, ices, candy, baked goods, and chewing gum. A skin irritant. There is reported use of the chemical; it has not yet been assigned for toxicology literature. GRAS. EAF

**LAVENDER OIL** • *Lavandula officinalis.* The colorless liquid extracted from the fresh, flowery tops of the plant. Smells like lavender and is used in ginger ale flavoring for beverages. Lavender absolute is a fruit flavoring for beverages, ice cream, ices, candy, and baked goods. Lavender concrete is a fruit flavoring for beverages, ice cream, ices, candy, and baked goods. Lavender was once used to break up stomach gas. It can cause allergic reactions and has been found to cause adverse skin reactions when the skin is exposed to sunlight. GRAS. EAF

**LAVENDER, SPIKE** • *Lavandula latifolia.* The name lavender comes from the Latin *lavare,* to wash and refers to the Roman custom of scenting bath water with the leaves and flowers of this aromatic plant. Used in perfumes, soaps, and sachets. Antispasmodic, aromatic, carminative, cholagogue, diuretic, sedative, stimulant, stomachic, tonic, relaxant, antibacterial, antiseptic. Contains coumarin, triterpene, tannins, and flavonoid. One of the most popular medicinal herbs since ancient times; in Arab medicine, it is used as an expectorant and an antispasmodic. In European folk tradition it is used as a wound herb and a worm medicine for children. NUL

**LAVENDER OIL, SPIKE** • *Lavendula.* In aromatherapy, lavender oil is used to promote relaxation, relieve anxiety, and treat headaches. Traditional remedy for gassy stomach. EAF

**LEAD** • This metal can enter the body in two ways—by ingestion and inhalation. Lead can build up in the body even if you are exposed to small amounts for a long time. In general, the more lead in your body, the more likely harm will occur. It is one of the most hazardous of toxic metals because its poison is cumulative and its toxic effects are many and severe. Among these are leg cramps, muscle weakness, numbness, depression, brain damage, coma, and death. Obvious symptoms of lead toxicity may occur in some people with levels as low as 40 micrograms of lead per deciliter of blood. The good news is that the almost complete elimination of lead-soldered side seams in canned foods in a number of countries has contributed to a reduction in lead exposure. The FDA reports that the mean level in canned foods in the United States has decreased from 0.20 mg/kg in 1982–83 to 0.01 mg/kg since 1988–89. Most relevant to the concern about infant exposure to lead is that the concentration of lead in canned evaporated milk has decreased from 0.11 mg/kg in 1982–83 to undetectable levels (less than 0.01 mg/kg) since 1985–86. The lead content of drinking water may be greater than 100 micrograms per liter where lead pipes or lead solder are used in plumbing. The lead content of drinking water in Canada and the United States is generally below 5 micrograms per liter and averages 1 or 2 micrograms per liter. The World Health Organization recommends lead content of drinking water should not exceed 10 micrograms per liter. The FAO/WHO Expert Committee on Food Additives recommends PTWI *(see)* of 25 micrograms per kg of body weight for all age groups. The experts also said there is a need for continued epidemiological studies on the effects of lead on intellectual development in children. In particular, information is needed on whether a reduction in blood lead concentrations leads to reversal of lead-related intellectual deficits.

**LEAF ALCOHOL** • *See* 3-Hexen-1-ol.

**LEATHER MEAL, HYDROLYZED** • Used in feed. FDA tolerance, 1 percent by weight of feed.

**LEAVENING** • From the Latin *levare,* "to raise." It is a substance, such as yeast, acting to produce fermentation in dough or liquid. Leavening serves to lighten or enliven, such as baking soda when it produces a gas that lightens dough or batter.

**LECHEA CASPI or DE VACA** • A genus of herbs that have branched stems and have minute purplish flowers. ASP

**LECITHIN** • From the Greek, meaning "egg yolk." A natural antioxidant and emollient composed of units of choline, phosphoric acid, fatty acids, and glycerin *(see all).* Commercially isolated from eggs, soybeans, corn, and egg yolks and used as an antioxidant in prepared breakfast cereal, candy, sweet chocolate, bread, rolls, buns, and oleomargarine. Egg yolk is 8 to 9 percent lecithin. Hydroxylated lecithin is a defoaming component in yeast and beet sugar production. Lecithin with or without phosphatides (components of fat) is an emulsifier for sweet chocolate, milk chocolate, bakery products, frozen desserts, oleomargarine, rendered animal fat, or a combination of vegetable-animal fats. Also used in eye creams, lipsticks, liquid powders, hand creams and lotions, soaps, and many other cosmetics. Also a natural emulsifier and spreading additive. Nontoxic. The final report to the FDA of the Select Committee on GRAS Substances stated in 1980 that it should continue its GRAS status with no limitations other than good manufacturing practices. ASP. E

**LECITHIN, BENZOYL PEROXIDE MODIFIED** • Commercial lecithin is a naturally occurring mixture of the phosphatides of choline, ethanolamine, and inositol, with smaller amounts of other lipids. It is isolated as a gum following hydration of solvent-extracted soy, safflower, or corn oils. Lecithin is bleached, if desired, by hydrogen peroxide and benzoyl peroxide and dried by heating. ASP

**LECITHIN, ENZYME-MODIFIED** • EM Lecithin. In enzyme-modified lecithin, the middle-position fatty acid is removed with an enzyme. EM lecithin is used mainly for yeast-raised baked goods to extend shelf life, but it also improves volume with its ability to act as a dough-strengthening additive. EM lecithin can replace monoglycerides *(see)*. Its use in bread is becoming more popular with bakeries today. GRAS. EAF

**LECITHIN, HYDROGEN PEROXIDE MODIFIED** • *See* Lecithin, Benzyol Peroxide Modified. ASP

**LECITIHIN, HYDROXYLATED LECITHIN** • *See* Lecithin and Hydroxylated.

**LEEK OIL** • *Sempervivum tectorum.* Native to the mountains of Europe and to the Greek Islands, its longevity led to its being named *sempervivum,* which translated means "ever alive." It is used as flavoring. It has been used to treat shingles, gout, and to get rid of bugs. Its pulp was applied to the skin for rashes and inflammation, and to remove warts and calluses. The juice was used to reduce fever and to treat insect stings. The juice mixed with honey was prescribed for thrush, a fungal infection of the mouth, and an ointment made from the plant was used to treat ulcers, burns, scalds, and inflammation. There is reported use of the chemical; it has not yet been assigned for toxicology literature search. EAF

**LEGUMES** • Plants that include seeds in a pod, such as beans and peas. The Leguminosae family includes over eighteen thousand species and is one of the most economically important plant families in the world. They include the phytochemicals being studied as health factors. Phytochemicals from legumes are utilized as food additives, fungicides, and anticancer additives.

**LEMON** • Extract and Oil. The common fresh fruit. The lemon extract is used in flavorings for beverages, ice cream, ices, candy, baked goods, and icings. Lemon oil is a blueberry, loganberry, strawberry, butter, grapefruit, lemon, lime, orange, cola, coconut, honey, wine, rum, root beer, and ginger ale flavoring for beverages, ice cream, ices, candy, baked goods, gelatin desserts, chewing gum (1,900 ppm), condiments, meats, syrups, icings, and cereals. Lemon oil is suspected of being a cancer-causing additive. GRAS. ASP

**LEMON BALM** • Sweet Balm. Garden Balm. Used in perfumes and as a soothing facial treatment. An Old World mint cultivated for its lemon-flavored fragrant leaves. Often considered a weed, it has been used by herbalists as a medicine and to flavor foods and medicines. It reputedly imparts long life. Also used to treat earache and toothache.

**LEMON EXTRACT** • *See* Lemon Oil.

**LEMON JUICE** • *See* Lemon. EAF

**LEMON OIL** • Cedro Oil. Used in perfumes and food flavorings, it is the volatile oil expressed from the fresh peel. A pale yellow to deep yellow, it has a characteristic odor and taste of the outer part of fresh lemon peel. It can cause an allergic reaction and has been suspected of being a co-additive cause of cancer. Lemon oil is reportedly found in ninety-eight cosmetic formulations.

**LEMON OIL, TERPENELESS** • A lemon fruit, ginger, and ginger ale flavoring additive for beverages, ice cream, ices, candy, baked goods, gelatin desserts, chewing gum, and toppings. Terpene, which is removed to improve flavor, is a class of unsaturated hydrocarbons. *See* Lemon for toxicity. ASP

**LEMON PEEL** • From the outer rind, the extract is used as a flavor in medicines and in beverages, confectionery, and cooking. *See* Lemon for toxicity. ASP

**LEMON TERPENES** • Terpene *(see)* fraction obtained from cold-pressed lemon oil. Oily taste associated with lemons. NEW

**LEMON VERBENA EXTRACT** • Extract of *Lippia citriodora.* Flavoring in alcoholic beverages only. *See* Lemongrass Oil. ASP

**LEMONGRASS OIL** • Indian Oil of Verbena. Used in perfumes, especially those added to soap. It is the volatile oil distilled from the leaves of lemon grasses. A yellowish or reddish brown liquid, it has a strong odor of verbena. Also used in insect repellent. Used in lemon and fruit flavorings for beverages, ice cream, ices, candy, baked goods, gelatin desserts, and chewing gum. Death reported when taken internally; an autopsy showed lining of the intestines was severely damaged. ASP

**LEPIDINE** • Obtained by the distillation of cinchonine. *See* Quinoline. NIL

**LEUCINE** • L and DL forms. An essential amino acid *(see)* for human nutrition not manufactured in the body. It is isolated commercially from gluten, casein, and keratin *(see all).* The L form is a food additive that the FDA says can be 3.5 percent of table weight. Used in aspartame *(see)* tabs as a lubricant. It has a sweet taste. It has caused birth defects in experimental animals. ASP

**L-LEUCINE** • *See* Leucine. ASP

**LEVAMISOLE** • Ergamisol. A drug that appears to restore depressed immune function. Used as an animal drug and in animal feed to fight parasites. It is employed in treatment of beef, lamb, and pork. FDA limitations are 0.1 ppm in cattle, sheep, and swine. Poisonous by ingestion and other routes. Human systemic effects by ingestion include coma, skin rash and irritation, and fever. There was a great deal of controversy over the pricing of this drug in 1992, when it was revealed that while the veterinary drug cost $14, for a human cancer patient the cost was up to $1,500. The company that produces the drug explained that it backed fourteen hundred studies involving forty thousand patients, and that this was factored into the cost of the drug for humans.

**LEVULINIC ACID** • Crystals used as intermediate for plasticizers, solvents, resins, flavors, and pharmaceuticals. ASP

**LEVULOSE** • *See* Fructose. ASP

**L-GLUTAMIC ACID** • *See* Glutamic Acid.

**LICORICE** • Liquorice. Glycyrrhizin. Monoammonium Glycyrrhizinate. Ammoniated Glycyrrhizin. Extract, extract powder, and root. A black substance derived from a plant, *Glycyrrhiza glabra,* "sweet root," belonging to the Leguminosae and cultured from southern Europe to central Asia. It is used in fruit, licorice, anise, maple, and root beer flavorings for beverages, ice cream, ices, candy (29,000 ppm), baked goods, gelatin, chewing gum, and syrups. Licorice root is used in licorice and root beer flavorings for beverages, candy, baked goods, chewing gum (3,200 ppm), tobacco, and medicines. Some people known to have eaten licorice candy regularly and generously had raised blood pressure, headaches, and muscle weakness. It can cause asthma, intestinal upsets, and contact dermatitis. No known skin toxicity. Tentatively affirmed as GRAS in 1983. ASP

**LIGHT GREEN** • *See* FD and C Green No. 2.

**LIGNIN** • Sulfate. Ammonium. Calcium. Magnesium. Sodium and lignin from Abaca. Binding additive in animal feed from plant fibers. The FDA says it can be up to 4 percent of finished pellets in animal feed. It is also used on flakes and as a surfactant in molasses used in feeds. NUL

**LIGNIN SODIUM SULFONATE** • Lignosulfonates are noted for their versatility and applicability in a variety of uses. They're found in everything from concrete admixtures to animal feeds. They have nine specific regulatory approvals issued by the FDA and the U.S. Environmental Protection Agency (EPA). Can be a direct or indirect additive component of packaging in contact with food and also used as a defoaming ingredient. ASP

**LIGNOSULFONIC ACID** • *See* Lignin Sodium Sulfonate. ASP

**LIME ESSENCE** • *See* Lime Oil. ASP

**LIME JUICE** • Natural juice obtained from the whole fruit of *Citrus aurantifolia*. Known as Key lime, Mexican lime, or West Indian lime. ASP

**LIME OIL** • A natural flavoring extracted from the fruit of a tropical tree. Colorless to greenish. Used in grapefruit, lemon, lemon-lime, lime, orange, cola, fruit, rum, nut, and ginger flavorings for beverages, ice cream, ices, candy, baked goods, gelatin desserts, chewing gum (3,100 ppm), and condiments. Terpeneless (*see* Lemon Oil) lime oil is used in lemon, lime, lemon-lime, cola, pineapple, ginger, and ginger ale flavorings for beverages, ice cream, ices, candy, baked goods, gelatin desserts, chewing gum, and syrups. Also used in perfumery and as an antiseptic. A source of vitamin C. Can cause an adverse reaction when skin is exposed to sunlight. GRAS. There is reported use of the chemical, it has not yet been assigned for toxicology literature.

**LIME WATER** • Calcium hydroxide (*see*) solution. Clear, colorless, and odorless, it is strongly alkaline. Used to prepare many food additives such as emulsifiers and waterproofing compounds. *See* Calcium Stearate, for example.

**LIMESTONE, GROUND** • Flavoring additive. GRAS

**LIMINOIDS** • Found in citrus fruits, they seem to induce protective enzymes.

**LIMONENE** • D, L, and DL forms. A synthetic flavoring additive that occurs naturally in star anise, buchu leaves, caraway, celery, oranges, coriander, cumin, cardamom, sweet fennel, common fennel, mace, marigold, oil of lavandin, oil of lemon, oil of mandarin, peppermint, petitgrairn oil, pimento oil, orange leaf (absolute), orange peel (sweet oil), origanum oil, black pepper, peels of citrus, macrocarpa bunge, and hops oil. Used in lime, fruit, and spice flavorings for beverages, ice cream, ices, candy, baked goods, gelatin desserts, and chewing gum. A skin irritant and sensitizer. GRAS. It caused loss of weight and tumors in some experimental animals and therefore, the FAO/WHO *(see)* recommended its use be reduced and restricted to 75 nanograms per kilogram of body weight per day. For D and L limonene, the principal toxicological finding was that limonene worsens spontaneously occurring nerve damage in mature male rats with subsequent occurrence of kidney tumors. The committee concluded that "the postulated mechanism for *d*-limonene-induced neuropathy and renal tumors in the male rat was probably not relevant to humans." The ADI *(see)* was established based upon the significant decreases in the body weight gain associated with the administration of *d*-limonene to male and female rats and mice and female rabbits. It was based on the lowest NOEL *(see)* for this effect, which was 150 mg per kg of body weight per day administered by gavage in a two-year study of male rats. At its latest meeting, the committee concluded that the ADI should not be set on the basis of the highest dose level in the long-term rat study, where kidney damage in male rats precluded testing at higher doses. The committee noted that no toxicity, other than decreased weight gain, had been observed at nonfatal doses in female rats or in other species, and that current patterns of use indicate that most *d*-limonene consumption would be associated with natural sources. The committee therefore withdrew the previous ADI for *d*-limonene and allocated an "Acceptable Daily Intake not specified." D and L limonene are ASP while *d*-limonene is NUL.

**LINALOE WOOD OIL** • Bois de Rose Oil. A natural flavoring additive that is a colorless to yellow volatile essential oil distilled from a Mexican tree. It has a pleasant flowery scent and is soluble in most fixed oils. Used in berry, citrus, fruit, liquor, and ginger flavorings for beverages, ice cream, ices, candy, baked goods, and liquors. Also used in perfumes. May cause allergic reactions. EAF

**LINALOOL** • A synthetic flavoring that occurs naturally in basil, bois de rose oil, cassia, coriander, cocoa, grapefruit, grapefruit oil, oranges, peaches, tea, bay and bay leaf extract, ginger, lavender, laurel leaves, and other oils. Used in flavorings such as blueberry, chocolate, and lemon. It is a fragrant, colorless liquid. May cause allergic reactions and is mildly toxic by ingestion. ASP

**LINALOOL OXIDE** • Linalool oxide offers a floral woody earthy note with a camphoraceous undertone. It's a key component of lavender, lavandin, and geranium-type fragrances. ASP

**LINALYL ACETATE** • A colorless, fragrant liquid, slightly soluble in water, it is the most valuable constituent of bergamot and lavender oils, which are used in perfumery. It occurs naturally in basil, jasmine oil, lavandin oil, lavender oil, and lemon oil. It has a strong floral scent. Colorless, it is used in berry, citrus, peach, pear, and ginger flavorings for beverages, ice cream, ices, candy, baked goods, gelatin desserts, and chewing gum. GRAS. ASP

**LINALYL ANTHRANILATE** • A synthetic berry, citrus, fruit, and grape flavoring additive for beverages, ice cream, ices, candy, and baked goods. ASP

**LINALYL BENZOATE** • A synthetic flavoring, brownish yellow, with a roselike odor. Used in berry, citrus, fruit, and peach flavorings additive for beverages, ice cream, ices, candy, gelatin desserts, and baked goods. ASP

**LINALYL CINNAMATE** • A synthetic loganberry, floral, rose, fruit, grape, and honey flavoring additive for beverages, ice cream, ices, candy, and baked goods. ASP

**LINALYL FORMATE** • Formic Acid. A synthetic flavoring additive that occurs naturally in oil of lavandin. Used in berry, apple, apricot, peach, and pineapple flavorings for beverages, ice cream, ices, candy, and baked goods. *See* Formic Acid for toxicity. ASP

**LINALYL HEXANOATE** • Synthetic fruit flavoring additive for beverages, ice cream, ices, candy, and baked goods. ASP

**LINALYL ISOBUTYRATE** • Synthetic flavoring, colorless to slightly yellow, with a fruity odor. Used in berry, citrus, fruit, banana, black currant, cherry, pear, pineapple, plum, nut, and spice flavorings for beverages, ice cream, ices, candy, and baked goods. ASP

**LINALYL ISOVALERATE** • Synthetic flavoring, colorless to slightly yellow, with a fruity odor. Used in loganberry, apple, apricot, peach, pear, and plum flavorings for beverages, ice cream, ices, candy, gelatin desserts, and baked goods. ASP

**LINALYL OCTANOATE** • A synthetic citrus, rose, apple, pineapple, and honey flavoring additive for beverages, ice cream, ices, candy, gelatin desserts, and baked goods. ASP

**LINALYL PHENYLACETATE** • Artificial flavor. *See* Linalool. ASP

**LINALYL PROPIONATE** • Synthetic currant, orange, banana, pear, and pineapple flavoring additive for beverages, ice cream, ices, candy, and baked goods. ASP

**LINCOMYCIN** • Lincocin. An antibacterial introduced in 1965, it is used to treat respiratory tract, skin, soft tissue, gynecologic, and urinary tract infections; osteomyelitis, blood poisoning caused by streptococci, pneumococci, and staphylococci. FDA tolerance for residues are 0.1 ppm for edible tissues of chickens and swine, 0.1 ppm in milk. Potential adverse reactions may include blood problems, dizziness, headache, low blood pressure, sore tongue, ringing in the ears, nausea, vomiting, severe colitis, persistent diarrhea, abdominal cramps, itching around the anus, vaginitis, jaundice, rashes, hives, pain at injection site, and serious allergic reactions. Antidiarrheal medicines reduce oral absorption of lincomycin. Lincomycin may reduce the effectiveness of drugs to treat myasthenia gravis.

**LINDEN FLOWERS** • *Tilia glabra.* A natural flavoring extract from the flowers of the tree grown in Europe and the United States. Used in raspberry and vermouth flavorings for beverages (2,000 ppm). Also used in fragrances. Linden has been found to lower blood pressure and according to health practitioners, helps reduce mild anxiety. GRAS. EAF

**LINOLEAMIDE** • A releasing additive that prevents food from sticking to containers. *See* Linoleic Acid.

**LINOLEIC ACID** • An essential fatty acid *(see)* prepared from edible fats and oils. Component of vitamin F and a major constituent of many vegetable oils, for example, cottonseed and soybean. Used in emulsifiers and vitamins. Large doses can cause nausea and vomiting. When given in large doses to rats, weight loss and progressive secondary anemia developed. No known skin toxicity and, in fact, may have emollient properties. The final report to the FDA of the Select Committee on GRAS Substances stated in 1980 that it should continue its GRAS status with no limitations other than good manufacturing practices. GRAS. EAF

**LINOLENIC ACID** • Polyunsaturated acid produced in the body as a metabolite of linoleic acid. A nutrient used in the treatment of eczema. In the diet of Mediterranean people alpha-linolenic acid is believed to be important in the prevention of heart disease.

**LINSEED OIL** • Golden amber or brown oil with a peculiar odor and bland taste. Used in paints, varnishes, as a film, in printing inks, and for its protein. *See* flaxseed.

**LIPASE** • Any class of enzymes that break down fat to glycerol and fatty acids *(see both)*. It is used in the manufacture of cheeses. ASP

**LIPASE FROM ANIMAL TISSUE** • Most natural lipase products on the market today contain ground-up animal tissue. Lipases are enzymes that hydrolyze *(see* Hydrolysis) fats to glycerol and fatty acids. Lipase is abundant in the pancreas but also occurs in the intestines, fatty tissue, and milk. GRAS. NEW

**LIPASE FROM *ASPERGILLUS NIGER* or *ASPERGILLUS ORYZAE*** • Lipase, an enzyme, is derived from these fungi. It is used to hydrolyze *(see* Hydrolysis) fats to glycerol and fatty acids. GRAS. NEW

**LIPIDS** • Lipids are very diverse in both their respective structures and functions. These diverse compounds that make up the lipid family are so grouped because they are insoluble in water. They include fats, phospholipids, and steroids *(see all)*.

**LITHOLRUBINE BK** • Coloring. A synthetic azo dye, reddish in color, used solely for coloring the rind of hard cheeses. People who suffer from asthma, rhinitis, or the skin disease urticaria may have been reported to find their symptoms become worse following consumption of azo dyes. Hyperactivity, asthma, skin sensitivity, insomnia. Banned in Australia.

**LITSEA CUBEBA BERRY OIL** • An essential oil used for a lemon flavor, or a base note in citrus notes like orange. It can also be used to treat acne or put into face products for oily skin. It is used as an antiseptic, disinfectant, and insecticide as well as a sedative. EAF

**LIVER-STOMACH CONCENTRATE WITH INTRINSIC FACTOR COMPLEX** • A dietary supplement illegal in foods.

**LOAEL** • Lowest Observable Adverse Effect Level. Used to signify the lowest dose of a substance that causes an adverse effect in an experimental animal. *See also* NOEL.

**LOCUST BEAN GUM** • St. John's Bread. Carob Bean Gum. A thickener and stabilizer in cosmetics and foods. Also used in depilatories. A natural flavor extract from the seed of the carob tree cultivated in the Mediterranean area. The history of the carob tree dates back more than two thousand years when the ancient Egyptians used locust bean gum as an adhesive in mummy binding. It is alleged that the "locust" (through confusion of the locusts with carob) and wild honey, which sustained John the Baptist in the wilderness, was from this plant, thus the name St. John's Bread. The carob pods are used as feed for stock today because of their high protein content. Some health food enthusiasts also eat them for the same purpose. They are also used as a thickener and stabilizer. *See* Carob. Carob bean extract is used in raspberry, bitters, butter, butterscotch, caramel, chocolate, cherry, brandy, wine, maple, root beer, spice, vanilla, cream soda, and grape flavorings for beverages, ice cream, ices, candy, baked goods, gelatin desserts (600 ppm), icings, and toppings (1,000 ppm). The final report to the FDA of the Select Committee on GRAS Substances stated in 1980 that it should continue its GRAS status with limitations on amounts that can be added to food. ASP. E

**LOVAGE** • Smallage. *Levisticum officinale.* Flavoring obtained from the root of an aromatic herb native to southern Europe and grown in monastery gardens centuries ago for medicine and food flavoring. It has a hot, sharp, biting taste. The yellow-brown oil is extracted from the root or other parts of the herb. It has a reputation for improving health and inciting love; Czechoslovakian girls reportedly wear it in a bag around their necks when dating boys. Used in bitters, maple, and walnut flavorings for beverages, ice cream, ices, candy, baked goods, chewing gum, and table syrups. The extract is used in berry, butter, butterscotch, caramel, maple, meat, black walnut, and spice flavorings for the same foods as above, plus condiments and icings. The oil, yellow-brown and aromatic, is used in butter, butterscotch, caramel, coffee, fruit, licorice, liquor, maple, nut, walnut, and spice flavorings for the same food as is the extract. ASP

**LOW CALORIE** • Fewer than 40 calories per serving.

**LOW-CARB** • The newest craze, quickly taken up by food producers, is the low-carb diet. Books such as those by the late Robert Atkins, M.D., and the newer *The South Beach Diet* by Arthur Agatston, M.D., have promoted meat, eggs, and other fatty foods over carbohydrates *(see)*. While the phenomenon may not last too long, the shelves of the supermarkets are increasingly filled with products containing fewer carbohydrates. They achieve the "low-carbs" by doing such manipulations as replacing wheat flour with soy flour, adding extra fiber and high-fat ingredients, and replacing sugar with sugar alcohols *(see)*. The FDA as of this writing has not set standards for labeling products as "low-carb."

**LOW CHOLESTEROL** • 20 milligrams or less per serving.

**LOW CALORIE SWEETENERS** • *See* Intense Sweeteners.

**LOW FAT** • 3 grams or less per serving.

**LOW-FAT MILK** • *See* Milk.

**LOW SATURATED FAT** • 1 gram or less per serving.

**LOW SODIUM** • 140 milligrams or less per serving.

**LPE** • Lysophosphatidylethanolamine. A compound found in many plants and animal tissues, it is purified from egg yolks and soybeans. When applied before harvest, this compound accelerates the development of fruit flavor and color. It is also believed to make fruit last longer on grocers' shelves and in refrigerators. At this writing, it was being tested on cranberries, peaches, tomatoes, grapes, and cut flowers.

**LUNGMOSS** • Lungwort. *Sticta pulmonacea.* Any of several plants once thought helpful in pulmonary diseases. Used as a flavoring in foods. NIL

**LUPULIN EXTRACT** • Lupine. Hops. Extract of *Lupinus albus.* The seed has been used as a food since earliest times. A natural flavoring additive from a plant *(Humulus lupulus)* grown in Europe, Asia, and North America. Used in beer brewing. Formerly used as aromatic bitters and as a sedative. At one time veterinary usage was recommended for treatment of nymphomania. It contains lupulone, which is active against fungus and bacteria, and humulone, an antibiotic. It produces a light blue dye. GRAS. EAF

**LUTEIN** • Some uses may require a color listing. *See* Xanthophyll. GRAS. E

**LYCOPENE** • Red crystals, insoluble in water. The main pigment of tomato, paprika, grapefruit, and rose hips. Being studied as a compound to prevent heart disease and cancer. E

**LYSINE** • L form. An essential amino acid *(see)* isolated from casein, fibrin, or blood. It is used for food enrichment for wheat-based foods. Lysine improves their protein quality and results in improved growth and tissue synthesis. Employed in the fortification of specialty bread and cereal mixes up to 0.25 percent to 0.5 percent of the weight of flour. On the FDA list for further study since 1980. GRAS. ASP

**L-LYSINE** • *See* Lysine.

**LYSOPHOSPHOPHATIDYLETHANOLAMINE** • *See* LPE.

**LYSOZYME** • Found in animal tissue and used in cheese production to inhibit the growth of *Clostridium tyrobutyricum.* The use level is less than 40 mg of lysozyme per liter of cheese milk, resulting in a concentration of less than 400 mg of lysozyme per kg of cheese. In studies related to allergenic effects, the reactions produced by egg-white lysozyme in humans were less severe than those seen with other proteins such as albumin, which have a long history of use as food components. On the basis of available data, FAO/WHO *(see)* concluded that the low additional intake of lysozyme via cheese was not a hazard to consumer health, provided that the enzyme complied with the specifications.

# M

**MACE** • *Myristica fragrans.* Mace Oil and Oleoresin. Obtained by steam distillation from the ripe, dried seed of the nutmeg. Colorless to pale yellow, with the taste and odor of nutmeg. Used in bitters, meat, and spice flavorings for beverages, ice cream, ices, baked goods, condiments, and meats (2,000 ppm). The oil is used in chocolate, cocoa, coconut, cola, fruit, nut, spice, and ginger ale flavorings for beverages, ice cream, ices, candy, baked goods, chewing gum, condiments, and meats. The final report to the FDA of the Select Committee on GRAS Substances stated in 1980 that while no evidence in the available information on it demonstrates a hazard to the public at current use levels, uncertainties exist, requiring that additional studies be conducted. ASP

**MACE OIL** • *See* Mace. ASP

**MADURAMICIN AMMONIUM** • Cygro. An antiparasite medication used in chicken feed to prevent infection. FDA residue tolerances are: 0.24 ppm in muscle, 0.72 ppm in liver, and 0.48 ppm in fat. When used as a medication to treat infection, the residue tolerances are the same as in uncooked chicken, except for 0.48 ppm in uncooked chicken fat.

**MAGNESIA** • Slightly alkaline white powder taken from any one of several ores such as periclase. Named after Magnesia, an ancient city in Asia Minor. An antacid.

**MAGNESIUM** • Magnesium Acetate, Magnesium Phosphate, Magnesium Sulfate, Magnesium Oxide, Magnesium Silicate, Magnesium Chloride, Magnesium Carbonate, Magnesium Cyclaniate, Magnesium Stearate, and Magnesium Hydroxide. A silver white, light, malleable metal that occurs abundantly in nature and is widely used in combination with various chemicals as a powder. Magnesium acetate is used as a buffer and neutralizer in nonalcoholic beverages. GRAS. Magnesium phosphate, a white, odorless powder, and magnesium sulfate are used as mineral supplements for food, leavening additives, and pH control additives. Recommended daily allowances, according to the National Academy of Sciences, are 40 milligrams for infants, 100 to 300 milligrams for children, 350 milligrams for adult males and females. Magnesium sulfate is used also as a corrective in the brewing industry and for fertilizers. Magnesium silicate, a fine, white, odorless and tasteless powder, is used in table salt and vanilla powder as an anticaking additive; in table salt it is limited to 2 percent. Magnesium chloride is used for color retention and as a firming additive in canned peas. Magnesium carbonate is used as an alkali for sour cream, butter, ice cream, cacao products, and canned peas. It is also used as a drying additive and an anticaking additive. Magnesium carbonate is also used as a perfume carrier and coloring additive. It is a silver white, crystalline salt that occurs in nature as magnetite or dolomite. Can be prepared artificially and is also used in table salt, and as an antacid. Nontoxic to the intact skin but may cause irritation when applied to abraded skin. Magnesium chloride is used as a buffer and neutralizer in nonalcoholic beverages and is used for color retention and as a firming additive. GRAS. Magnesium citrate is a buffer and neutralizer in nonalcoholic beverages. Magnesium cyclamate was banned in 1969 as an artificial sweetener. Magnesium hydroxide is used as an alkali in dentifrices and skin creams, in canned peas, and as a drying additive and color retention additive for improved gelling in the manufacture of cheese. GRAS. Slightly alkaline, crystalline compound obtained by hydration of magnesia (see) or precipitation of seawater by lime. Toxic when inhaled. Harmless to skin and in fact soothes it. Magnesium oxide is used in canned peas, frozen desserts, and as a dietary supplement, and is considered GRAS. Magnesium phosphate is a nutrient supplement considered GRAS. Magnesium phosphide is a fungicide in animal feeds. Magnesium silicate is used in vanilla powder and is considered GRAS. Magnesium stearate, a soft, white powder, tasteless, odorless, and insoluble in water, is used as a dietary supplement, in food packaging, and as an emulsifying additive in cosmetics. Magnesium was reevaluated by the FDA in 1976 as not harmful in presently used current levels. However, the FAO/WHO (see) recommends further study of magnesium silicate because kidney damage in dogs has been reported upon ingestion. Magnesium carbonate, chloride, sulfate, stearate, phosphate, and silicate are all GRAS according to the final report to the FDA of the Select Committee on GRAS Substances and they should continue their GRAS status with no limitations other than good manufacturing practices.

**MAGNESIUM CAPRATE** • An anticaking agent and emulsifier. NUL
**MAGNESIUM CAPRYLATE** • An anticaking agent and emulsifier. NUL
**MAGNESIUM CARBONATE** • See Magnesium. GRAS. ASP. E
**MAGNESIUM CHLORIDE** • See Magnesium. GRAS. ASP
**MAGNESIUM CYCLAMATE** • Nonnutritive sweetener removed from the market September 1, 1969. Legal only in products complying with drug provision of the law. BANNED
**MAGNESIUM DIGLUTAMATE** • See Glutamic Acid. E
**MAGNESIUM FUMARATE** • Magnesium fumarate is a "nutrient dense" supplementary form of magnesium and an energy rich substrate-fumarate.

Magnesium as quantitative element is an essential part of animal nutrition, Fumarate is one of the key intermediates of the Krebs cycle, which contributes to efficient energy production in humans. Magnesium fumarate helps to increase body magnesium levels and thus enhance the benefits of magnesium to many areas that are concerned with energy and muscular performance. ATP is produced in the Krebs cycle of which fumarate is one of the key intermediates. Carbohydrates, lipids, and proteins cannot produce the sources of muscle contraction energy (ATP), without the presence of magnesium. NUL

**MAGNESIUM GLUCONATE** • A buffering additive in soda water. *See* Magnesium. ASP

**MAGNESIUM GLYCEROPHOSPHATE** • NUL

**MAGNESIUM HYDROXIDE** • Permitted as an optional ingredient in standardized food. *See* Magnesium. GRAS. ASP. E

**MAGNESIUM LACTATE** • Buffering and neutralizing additive in cacao products and in canned peas. *See* Magnesium.

**MAGNESIUM LAURATE** • An anticaking agent and emulsifier. NUL

**MAGNESIUM MYRISTATE** • An anticaking agent and emulsifier. NUL

**MAGNESIUM OLEATE** • An anticaking agent and emulsifier. NUL

**MAGNESIUM OXIDE** • Magnesia. White, odorless powder used as an alkali, anticaking additive, firming additive, free-flow additive, lubricant, neutralizing additive, nutrient, pH control additive, and releasing additive. It is used as a neutralizer in frozen dairy products, butter, cacao products, and canned peas. Inhalation can cause fever in humans. Also used as a dietary supplement. Has caused tumors in hamsters. *See* Magnesium. GRAS. ASP. E

**MAGNESIUM PHOSPHATE** • Di-, Tri-, Basic. A dietary supplement. GRAS. *See* Magnesium. Di- is ASP, Tri- is NUL. E

**MAGNESIUM PHOSPHIDE** • A fumigant used in animal feed and on processed foods. FDA residue tolerance is 0.01 ppm in processed foods and 0.1 ppm in animal feeds. A poison. Moderately toxic by inhalation. *See* Magnesium.

**MAGNESIUM SALTS OF FATTY ACIDS** • *See* Magnesium and Fatty Acids. ASP

**MAGNESIUM SILICATE** • An anticaking additive. *See* Magnesium. GRAS. ASP. E

**MAGNESIUM STEARATE** • Miscellaneous uses as a migratory substance from packaging materials, stabilizer, defoaming additive, anticaking additive. *See* Magnesium. GRAS. ASP

**MAGNESIUM SULFATE** • Nutrient supplement. *See* Magnesium. GRAS. ASP

**MAIDENHAIR FERN** • Venus Hair. Extract of the leaves of the fern *Adiantum capillus-veneris.* Used as a flavoring in alcoholic beverages only and to soothe irritated skin in herbal creams.

**MALATHION** • Derived from diethyl maleate and dimethyldithiophosphoric acid, it is an insecticide against such pests as aphids, the leaf-cutter bee, and the Mediterranean fruit fly. Toxic when absorbed through the skin and can damage transmission of nerve signals. In dehydrated citrus pulp for animal feed, the FDA allows a tolerance of 50 ppm; in nonmedicated cattle feed concentrate blocks from application of pesticide to paper used in packaging, the residue tolerance allowed in the blocks is 10 ppm.

**MALEIC ACID** • Made from benzene *(see)*, it is a strong irritant. Used in the manufacture of artificial resins and to retard rancidity of fats and oils which are said to keep three times longer than those without the acid.

**MALEIC HYDRAZIDE** • Regulates the growth of unwanted "suckers" on about 90 percent of the United States tobacco crop. It is also applied to 10 to 15 percent of domestic potatoes and onions to prevent sprouting after harvest. It is highly toxic to humans and has produced central nervous system disturbances and liver damage in experimental animals. It has led to liver and other tumors in some mice. However, other studies, including one done for the National Cancer Institute and published in 1969, report no carcinogenic effects. It has produced genetic damage in plant and animal systems, a fact that often signals a cancer-causing effect. The FDA residue tolerance for potato chips is 160 ppm from use as a preharvest pesticide.

**MALIC ACID** • A colorless, crystalline compound with a strong acid taste that occurs naturally in a wide variety of fruits, including apples and cherries. A flavoring additive and aid in aging wine. It has a strong acid taste. Used as an alkali in frozen dairy products, beverages, baked goods, confections, fruit, butter, and jelly and jam preserves "in an amount sufficient to compensate for the deficiency of fruit in artificially sweetened fruit." An alkali and antioxidant in cosmetics and ingredient of hair lacquer. Irritating to the skin and can cause allergic reaction when used in hair lacquers. The final report to the FDA of the Select Committee on GRAS Substances stated in 1980 that it should continue its GRAS status with no limitations other than good manufacturing practices. ASP. E

**MALLOW EXTRACT** • From the herb family. A moderate purplish red that is paler than magenta rose. Used in coloring and also as a source of pectin *(see)*.

**MALT EXTRACT** • Extracted from barley that has been allowed to germinate, then heated to destroy vitality, and dried. It contains sugars, proteins, and salts from barley. The extract is mixed with water and allowed to solidify. It is used as a nutrient and as a texturizer in cured meat and poultry. FDA limitations are 2.5 percent in cured meat. It is also widely used in the brewing industry. GRAS. NUL

**MALT SYRUP** • Component of caramel coloring. *See* Malt Extract. GRAS. ASP

**MALTITOL and MALTITOL SYRUP** • Obtained by the hydrogenate from maltose *(see)*. Used as a sugar substitute, it has 90 percent the sweetness of sugar and does contain calories. It is used in confections, baked goods, and candy coatings. In a cancer study in rats, changes were observed in the adrenal gland, which included increased incidence of both benign and malignant tumors of the adrenal glands in both sexes and a "slight increase" in breast cancer in female rats. FAO/WHO *(see)* did not consider these cancers to be related to treatment. The committee, however, recommended that the information database on adrenal overgrowth and tumors associated with polyols and other poorly absorbed carbohydrates *(see both)* be reviewed and that the mechanisms of appearance of these lesions and their toxicological significance be assessed at a future meeting. It also reportedly raises blood sugar and may have a laxative effect. E

**MALTODEXTRIN** • The sugar obtained by hydrolysis of starch. A combination of maltol *(see)* and dextrin *(see)* used as a texturizer and flavor enhancer in candies, particularly chocolate. Has less calories than *(see)* sucrose. The final report to the FDA of the Select Committee on GRAS Substances stated in 1980 that it should continue its GRAS status with no limitations other than good manufacturing practices. ASP

**MALTOL** • A white, crystalline powder with a butterscotch odor found in the bark of young larch trees, pine seeds, chicory, wood tars, and in roasted malt. It imparts a "freshly baked" odor and flavor to bread and cakes. Used as a synthetic chocolate, coffee, fruit, maple, nut, and vanilla flavoring additive for beverages, ice cream, ices, candy, baked goods, gelatin desserts, chewing gum, and jelly. ASP

**MALTOSE** • Malt Sugar. Colorless crystals derived from malt extract and used as a nutrient, sweetener, culture medium, and stabilizer. It is soluble in water and used as a supplement of sugar for diabetics. It is also used in brewing and as a stabilizer. It is nontoxic but it has been reported to cause tumors when injected under the skin of mice in doses of 500 milligrams per kilogram of body weight. NEW

**MALTYL ISOBUTYRATE** • Artificially synthesized flavor. *See* Maltol and Isobutyric Acid. ASP

**MANDARIN OIL** • Obtained by expression of the peel of a ripe mandarin orange, *Citrus reticulata.* Has a pleasant orangelike odor and is used in orange, tangerine, cherry, and grape flavoring for beverages, ice cream, ices, candy, baked goods, chewing gum, and gelatin desserts. GRAS. ASP

**MANEB** • A pesticide used on growing grapes. The residue tolerances are 28 ppm in raisins, 20 ppm in bran of barley, oats, rye, and wheat, and 1 ppm in flours of barley, oats, rye, and wheat. *See* Zinc.

**MANGANESE BACITRACIN** • An antibiotic in animal feed. *See* Bacitracin and Manganese Sources.

**MANGANESE CHLORIDE** • Dietary supplement. GRAS. *See* Manganese Sources. ASP

**MANGANESE CITRATE** • A light, pink-white, fine, granular solid. It is used as a nutrient. *See* Manganese Sources. GRAS. NUL

**MANGANESE GLUCONATE** • Dietary supplement. *See* Manganese Sources. GRAS. ASP

**MANGANESE GLYCEROPHOSPHATE** • Dietary supplement. *See* Manganese Sources. GRAS. NUL

**MANGANESE HYPOPHOSPHITE** • Dietary supplement. *See* Manganese Sources. GRAS. NUL

**MANGANESE SOURCES** • Manganese Acetate, Manganese Carbonate, Manganese Chloride, Manganese Citrate, Manganese Sulfate, Manganese Glycerophosphate, Manganese Hypophosphite, and Manganese Oxide. A mineral supplement first isolated in 1774, manganese occurs in minerals and in minute quantities in animals, plants, and in water. The chloride, citrate, gluconate, glycerate, hypophosphite, and sulfate are all used as dietary supplements and nutrients and are considered GRAS. Many forms are used in dyeing. Manganous salts are activators of enzymes and are necessary to the development of strong bones. They are used as nutrients and as dairy substitutes. Toxicity occurs by inhalation. Symptoms include languor, sleepiness, wakefulness, emotional disturbances, and Parkinson-like symptoms. Manganese chloride, citrate, glycerophosphate, and hypophosphite are all considered GRAS according to the final report of the Select Committee on GRAS Substances and should continue their GRAS status as nutrients with no limitations other than good manufacturing practices. However, manganese oxide, according to the committee, does not have enough known about it upon which to base an evaluation when it is used as a food ingredient.

**MANGANESE SULFATE** • Dietary Supplement. There is reported use of the chemical; it has not yet been assigned for toxicology literature. *See* Magnesia. GRAS. ASP

**MANGANOUS OXIDE** • A dietary supplement derived by reduction of the dioxide in hydrogen or by heating the carbonate without air. It is also used in ceramics, paints, bleaching tallow, animal feeds, and fertilizers. GRAS. NUL

**MANNITOL** • Widespread in plants but mostly prepared from seaweed. It is about 70 percent as sweet as sugar and it does contain calories. White, crystalline solid, odorless, and sweet tasting. Used as a texturizer in chewing gum, up to 31 percent, hard candy up to 5 percent, and pressed mints, 98 percent. It is also used in soft candy at 40 percent, frostings at 8 percent, jams and jellies at 15 percent. It has been used as a sweetener in "sugar-free" products but has calories and carbohydrates. The FDA says that "excess consumption may have a laxative effect: if ingested daily, it must carry that warning on the label." In 1982, the FDA reported that it does not cause cancer in rats. GRAS on an interim basis. ASP. E

**MANNOSE** • A carbohydrate occurring in some plants. It has a sweet taste.

**MAO INHIBITORS** • *See* Monoamine Oxidase Inhibitors.

**MAPLE, MOUNTAIN** • Flavoring.

**MARGARINE** • Oleomargarine. A butter substitute made from animal or vegetable fats or oils. If oils are used they are "hardened" into fats by the process of hydrogenation *(see)*. Skimmed milk, water, salt, coloring matter *(see* Carotene), artificial flavors, lecithin *(see),* and small amounts of vitamins are usually added. By federal regulations, margarine contains at least 80 percent fat.

**MARIGOLD, POT** • *Calendula officinalis*. A natural plant extract. The oil is used in various flavorings for beverages, ice cream, ices, candy, and baked goods. *See* Tagetes. GRAS. NIL

**MARJORAM, POT** • Sweet Marjoram. *Origanum marjorana* and *Origanum onites*. The natural extract of the flowers and leaves of two varieties of the fragrant marjoram plant. The oleoresin *(see)* is used in sausage and spice flavorings for condiments and meats. The seed is used in sausage and spice flavorings for meats (3,500 ppm) and condiments. Sweet marjoram is used in sausage and spice flavorings for beverages, baked goods (2,000 ppm), condiments, meats, and soups. The sweet oil is used in vermouth, wine, and spice flavorings for beverages, ice creams, ices, candy, baked goods, and condiments. Also used in hair preparations, perfumes, and soaps. Can irritate the skin. The redness, itching, and warmth experienced when applied to the skin are caused by local dilation of the blood vessels or by local reflex. May produce allergic reactions. Essential oils such as marjoram are believed to penetrate the skin easily and produce systemic effects. GRAS. EAF

**MARJORAM SEED** • *Majorana hortensis. Origanum marjorana*. Natural flavor isolated by physical methods This is a member of the mint family and is a cousin of oregano but with a milder, sweeter flavor. It gives Polish sausage its flavor. Sources are Egypt and the United States. NIL

**MARJORAM, SWEET** • *See* Marjoram, Pot. ASP

**MARSHMALLOW ROOT** • *See* Althea Root.

**MASSARANDUBA BALATA** • *Manilkara huberi*. Natural masticatory substances of vegetable origin from a tree. ASP

**MASSARANDUBA CHOCOLATE** • *Manilkara solimoesensis*. Used in chewing-gum base. ASP

**MASSOIA BARK OIL** • Flavoring harvested from trees in the wild. NUL

**MASTIC GUM** • A natural resin from a small tree, *Pistacia lentiscus,* found in Greece and other Mediterranean countries. It is used as a food ingredient in the Mediterranean region. Mastic gum has been used for centuries by traditional healers for stomach upsets and ulcers, and heartburn. In clinical trials, it has been found that even small doses (one pea-size dose of 1 mg per day) over a period of two weeks could have a positive impact on stomach and duodenal ulcers, also helping to relieve pain. NUL

**MATÉ EXTRACT** • Paraguay Tea Extract. St. Bartholomew's Tea. Jesuits' Tea. A natural flavoring extract from small gourds grown in South America where maté is a stimulant beverage. Among its constituents are caffeine, purines, and tannins. *See* Caffeine and Tannic Acid for toxicity. GRAS. ASP

**MATRICARIA EXTRACT** • Wild Chamomile Extract. Extract of the flower heads of *Matricaria chamomilla.* Used as a soothing tea and tonic internally, and externally as a soothing medication for contusions and other inflammation. *See* Tannic Acid. GRAS

**MATRICARIA OIL** • Chamomile Oil. Wild Chamomile Extract. The volatile oil distilled from the dried flower heads of *Matricaria chamomilla.* Used internally as a tonic and soothing tea and externally as a soothing medication for contusions and other inflammation. *See* Matricaria Extract.

**MATURING ADDITIVES** • *See* Bleaching Additives.

**MAYONNAISE** • The common salad dressing. Semisolid, made with eggs, vegetable oil, and vinegar or lemon juice.

**MCG** • Abbreviation for microgram, a metric measurement that is one millionth of a gram *(see).*

**MELAMINE** • Cyanuramide. Used in the manufacture of paper and paperboard for packaging materials. An experimental cancer-causing and tumor-causing additive. Moderately toxic by ingestion. An eye, skin, and mucous membrane irritant. Causes skin rash in humans.

**MELENGESTROL ACETATE** • A progesterone used to treat animals and to suppress ovulation when added to animal feed. Residue limitation is zero according to the FDA.

**MELISSA** • Essential oil. *See* Balm Oil. GRAS

**MELONAL** • *See* 2,6-Dimethyl-5-Heptenal.

**MENADIOL SODIUM DIPHOSPHATE** • *See* Vitamin K. NUL

**MENADIONE** • Vitamin $K_3$. A synthetic with properties of vitamin K. Dietary supplement. Extension of a petition has been filed to permit a limit of 1 mg per day. Its use was revoked March 22, 1963. No food additive regulation authorizing use of menadione in prenatal supplements or any other food products has been issued. However, menadione is permitted as a nutritional supplement in chicken and turkey feed for prevention of vitamin K deficiency and in swine feed. Used medically to prevent blood clotting and in food to prevent souring of milk products. Can be irritating to mucous membranes, respiratory passages, and the skin.

**MENHADEN OIL** • Hydrogenated and Partially Hydrogenated *(see).* Porgy Oil. Moss Bunker Oil. Obtained along the coast of Africa from the menhaden fish, which are a little larger than herrings. The fish glycerides of menhaden are reddish and have a strong fishy odor. Used as a nutrient. Also used in soaps and creams. GRAS. EAF

**MENTHA ARVENSIS OIL** • From *Mentha arvensis,* it is a colorless to yellow liquid with a minty odor used as a flavoring additive. GRAS. Has caused reproductive problems in experimental animals.

*p*-**MENTHA-1,8-DIEN-7-OL** • A synthetic citrus, fruit, mint, and vanilla flavoring additive for beverages, ice cream, ices, candy, and baked goods. It is found naturally in caraway. Can cause skin irritation. ASP

**MENTHADIENOL** • Although allowed as a food additive, there is no current reported use of the chemical, and therefore, although toxicology information may be available, it is not being updated, according to the FDA.

**CIS- AND TRANS-P-1(7),8-MENTHADIEN-2-YL** • Flavoring. NIL

**P-MENTHAN-2-ONE** • Flavoring. ASP

**P-MENTHA-8-THIOL-3-ONE** • Flavoring. ASP

**P-MENTH-1-ENE-9-AL** • Flavoring. NIL

**1-P-MENTHENE-8-THIOL** • Flavoring. EAF

**P-MENTH-1-EN-3-OL** • Flavoring. NIL

**P-MENTH-3-EN-1-OL** • Flavoring. NIL

**1-P-MENTHEN-9-YL ACETATE** • Flavoring. ASP

**MENTHOL** • A flavoring additive that can be obtained naturally from peppermint or other mint oils and can be made synthetically by hydrogenation *(see)* of thymol *(see)*. Used in butter, caramel, fruit, peppermint, and spearmint flavorings for beverages, ice cream, ices, candy, baked goods, chewing gum (1,100 ppm), and liquor. It is a local anesthetic. It is nontoxic in low doses, but in concentrations of 3 percent or more it exerts an irritant action that can, if continued too long, induce changes in all layers of the mucous membranes. It can also cause severe abdominal pain, nausea, vomiting, vertigo, and coma when ingested in its concentrated form. The lethal dose in rats is 2 grams per kilogram of body weight. GRAS. ASP

**1-MENTHOL-PROPYLENE** • Synthetic flavoring in baked foods, beverages, breakfast cereal, condiments, confectionery frostings, frozen dairy, fruit ices, gelatins, hard candy, imitation dairy, milk products, processed fruits, soft candy, soups, and snack foods. Declared GRAS by FEMA *(see)*.

**MENTHONE** • A synthetic flavoring additive that occurs naturally in raspberries and peppermint oil. Bitter, with a slight peppermint taste. Used in fruit and mint flavorings for beverages, ice cream, ices, candy, baked goods, and chewing gum. May cause gastric distress. There is reported use of the chemical; it has not yet been assigned for toxicology literature. ASP

**MENTHONE 1,2-GLYCEROL KETAL** • Flavoring. *See* Menthone. EAF

**L-MENTHONE 1,2-GLYCEROL KETAL** • Flavoring. *See* Menthone. EAF

**MENTHONE-8-THIOACETATE** • Flavoring. *See* Menthone. EAF

**3-L-MENTHOXYPROPANE-1,2-DIOL** • Flavoring. ASP

**MENTHYL ACETATE** • A natural flavoring additive that occurs naturally in peppermint oil. Colorless, with a mint odor. Used in fruit, mint, and spice flavorings for beverages, ice cream, ices, candy, baked goods, and chewing gum; also in perfumes and toilet waters. Mildly toxic by ingestion. A skin irritant. GRAS. ASP

**L-MENTHYL ETHYLENE GLYCOL CARBONATE D** • Flavoring. *See* Menthyl Acetate. EAF

**MENTHYL ISOVALERATE** • Flavoring. *See* Menthyl Acetate. ASP

**L-MENTHYL LACTATE** • Flavoring. See Menthyl Acetate. ASP

**1-MENTHYL METHYL ETHER** • A flavoring determined GRAS by FEMA. *See* Cyclohexane.

**L-MENTHYL 1,2-PROPYLENE GLYCOL CARBONATE** • Flavoring. *See* Menthyl Acetate. EAF

**MENTHYL PROPYLENE GLYCOL CARBONATE** • Flavoring. *See* Menthyl Acetate. EAF

**3-MERCAPTOHEXANOL** • Flavoring. *See* Hexanoic Acid. EAF

**3-MERCAPTOHEXYL ACETATE** • Flavoring. *See* Acetic Acid. EAF

**3-MERCAPTOHEXYL BUTYRATE** • Flavoring. *See* Butyric Acid. EAF

**3-MERCAPTOHEXYL HEXANOATE** • Flavoring. *See* Hexanoic Acid. EAF

**3-MERCAPTO-3-METHYL-1-BUTANOL** • Flavoring. EAF

**3-MERCAPTO-2-METHYL-1-BUTANOL** • Flavoring. EAF

**3-MERCAPTO-3-METHYLBUTYL FORMATE** • Flavoring. *See* Formic Acid. EAF

**3-MERCAPTO-2-METHYLPENTANAL** • Flavoring. Used in baked goods, breakfast cereals, fish products, gravies, nut products, processed vegetables, and soups. Declared GRAS by FEMA *(see)*. *See* 1-Pentanol. EAF

**2-MERCAPTO-2-METHYL-1-PENTANOL** • Flavoring. *See* 1-Pentanol. EAF

**3-MERCAPTO-2-METHYL-1-PENTANOL** • Flavoring. *See* 1-Pentanol. EAF

**4-MERCAPTO-4-METHYL-2-PENTANONE** • Flavoring. *See* 1-Pentanol. EAF

**2-MERCAPTOMETHYLPYRAZINE** • Flavoring. *See* Piperazine. ASP

**3-MERCAPTO-2-PENTANONE** • Flavoring. *See* 1-Pentanol. ASP

**1-MERCAPTO-2-PROPANONE** • Flavoring. *See* 1-Pentanol. EAF

**2-MERCAPTOPROPIONIC ACID 3-** • Antioxidants and reducing additives. Mercaptopropionic acid was found to be a potent inhibitor of respiration. ASP

**N-MERCAPTO METHYL PHTALIMIDE** • Phosphamidon. An organophosphate insecticide limited to 0.2 ppm tolerance by the FDA as a residue in meat by-products of cattle. *See* Organophosphates for toxicity.

**MESQUITE WOOD EXTRACT** • Prepared by stirring 1 pound of wood chips from mesquite (*Prosopis* spp.) in 400 gallons of 80 proof alcohol for two hours without heat. The final product is obtained by removing the chips with filtration. It is used primarily as an alternative to oak chips. Adults expected to consume alcoholic beverages containing mesquite wood extract have taste preferences for Southwestern cuisine. As is true with oak chip extract, the use of mesquite wood extract is self-limiting, with high concentrations resulting in an undesirable astringent taste. Based on the very low estimated human exposure to mesquite wood extract and the information regarding the similarity of mesquite wood extract to oak chip extract, as well as other information available to the FDA, the agency has no questions at this writing regarding the conclusion of the Givaudan Roure Flavors Corporation that mesquite wood extract is GRAS for use as a flavoring ingredient in alcoholic beverages. The agency has not, however, made its own determination regarding the GRAS status of the notified use of mesquite wood extract. As always, it is the continuing responsibility of Givaudan Roure Flavors Corporation to ensure that food ingredients that the firm markets are safe, and are otherwise in compliance with all applicable legal and regulatory requirements. EAF

**METALAXYL** • A fungicide used in animal feed, dried hops, potato chips, processed potatoes, soybean meal, sugar beet molasses, processed tomatoes, and wheat-milling fractions. The FDA limits residues to 7 ppm in citrus oil, 4 ppm in processed potatoes including potato chips, and 3 ppm in processed tomatoes.

**METALDEHYDE** • A polymer of acetaldehyde *(see)* used as a slug and snail poison on strawberries at the time of harvest. FDA residue tolerance is zero. Ingestion may cause severe abdominal pain, nausea, vomiting, diarrhea, fever, convulsions, and coma.

**METATARTARIC ACID** • Prevents the precipitation of tartaric acid crystals in wine. E

**METHACRYCLIC ACID-DIVINYL BENZENE COPOLYMER** • Used as a carrier for vitamin $B_{12}$ in nutritional supplements. ASP

**METHANEARSONIC ACID** • Used in or on cottonseed hulls used for animal feed. *See* Arsenic.

**METHANE DICHLORIDE** • Colorless, volatile liquid with the odor of chloroform used to dilute color and extract chemicals. It is used to decaffeinate coffee, fruits, hops, spices, and vegetables. The FDA permits residues of 30 ppm in spice oleoresins, 2.2 percent in hops extract, and 10 ppm in decaffeinated coffee. Moderately toxic by ingestion. An experimental cancer-causing and tumor-causing additive. Human systemic effects by ingestion and inhalation include numbness, altered sleep, convulsions, euphoria, and changes in cardiac rate. It causes birth defects in experimental animals and may be mutagenic in humans. It is an eye and severe skin irritant.

***p*-METHANE-3,8-DIOL** • A flavoring determined GRAS by FEMA *(see)*.

**METHANETHIOL** • Methyl Mercaptan. A pesticide and fungicide isolated from the roots of a plant. Occurs in the "sour" gas of West Texas, in coal tar, and in petroleum. Produced in the intestinal tract by action of bacteria.

Found in urine after ingestion of asparagus. Its odor may cause nausea and it may be narcotic in high concentrations.

**METHANOL** • Methyl Alcohol. Wood Alcohol. Wood Spirit. A solvent and denaturant obtained by the destructive distillation of wood. In the food industry, it is used to extract hops and spices. Flammable, poisonous liquid with a nauseating odor. Better solvent than ethyl alcohol. It is a softening additive for plastics. It is the raw material for making formaldehyde. It is on the Community-Right-To-Know List *(see)*. Methanol is highly toxic and readily absorbed from all routes of exposure. It possesses narcotic properties. Toxic effects are primarily on the nervous system. Symptoms include headache, dizziness, confusion, abdominal pain, lung problems, weakness, and coma. Ingestion can cause blindness and death. Lesser exposure causes blurring of vision, headache, and GI disturbances.

**METHDIATHION** • Insecticide. Residue tolerances are 0.03 ppm in milk, 0.05 ppm residue in fat, meat, and meat by-products of cattle, goats, hogs, poultry, and sheep.

**METHILANIN** • *See* Acimeton.

**METHIONINE** • D and DL Forms. An essential amino acid *(see)* that occurs in protein. Used as a dietary substance. It is attracted to fat and Rutgers University researchers patented a process to impregnate a carrier material with methionine for use in deep-frying cooking oil to impart a "fresh" potato or potato chip flavor to snack foods, soups, or salad dressings. Not to be used in baby foods. Used as a texturizer in cosmetic creams. Methionine is mildly toxic by injection and has caused birth defects in experimental animals. ASP

**METHIONINE HYDROXY ANALOG and ITS CALCIUM SALTS** • A nutrient for animal feeds. GRAS

**METHOPRENE** • A growth inhibitor that mimics juvenile hormone in insects. It is used in animal feed or mineral blocks for cattle. The FDA residue tolerances are: 22.7 to 45.4 mg per 100 pounds body weight; 0.05 ppm as residue in eggs and milk; 0.1 ppm as residue in meat and meat by-products of cattle, goats, hogs, and sheep; 0.3 ppm as residue in fat of cattle, goats, hogs, and sheep; 0.05 ppm as residue in fat and meat of poultry.

**2-METHOXY-3,6-DICHLOROBENZOIC ACID** • Banex. An herbicide used in animal feed and on sugarcane. The FDA residue tolerance is 2 ppm on sugarcane molasses and 2 ppm in sugarcane molasses when used for animal feed. In the EPA Genetic Toxicology Program *(see)*. Moderately toxic by ingestion.

**4-METHOXY-2-METHYL-2-BUTANETHIOL** • The FDA has not yet done a search of the toxicology literature concerning this additive.

***p*-METHOXY A-METHYLCINNAMALDEHYDE** • A flavoring. ASP

**2-METHOXY-4-METHYLPHENOL** • Creosol. A synthetic flavoring that occurs naturally in cassia and is used in fruit, rum, nut, and clove flavorings for beverages, ice cream, ices, candy, baked goods, and liqueurs. About the same toxicity as phenol, a highly caustic, poisonous compound derived from benzene.

**2-METHOXY-3 (S)-METHYLPYRAZINE** • A colorless liquid with the odor of roasted hazelnuts used as a flavoring additive in various foods. GRAS

**3-L-METHOXYPROPANE-1,2-DIOL** • A synthetic flavoring.

**1-METHOXY-4-PROPENYL BENZENE** • *See* Anethole.

**2-METHOXY-4-PROPENYL PHENOL** • *See* Isoeugenol.

**p-METHOXYACETOPHENONE** • Acetanisole. Crystalline solid with a pleasant odor. Soluble in alcohol and fixed oils and derived from the interaction of anisole and acetyl chloride with aluminum chloride and carbon disulfide. Used in perfumery as a synthetic floral odor and in flavoring.

**4-METHOXYACETOPHENONE** • Colorless to pale yellow solid with a hawthorn odor used as a flavoring additive in various foods. Moderately toxic by ingestion. Human systemic effect by inhalation was increased pulse rate. A skin irritant.

**0-METHOXYBENZALDEHYDE** • A synthetic flavoring additive that occurs naturally in cassia oil and used in spice and cinnamon flavorings for beverages, baked goods, and chewing gum. *See* Benzyl Acetate. ASP

**p-METHOXYBENZALDEHYDE** • Anisaldehyde. A synthetic flavoring additive that occurs naturally in hawthorn, fennel, oil of anise, star anise, and Tahiti vanilla beans. Used in raspberry, strawberry, butter, caramel, chocolate, apricot, cherry, peach, licorice, anise, nut, black walnut, walnut, spice, and vanilla flavorings for beverages, ice cream, ices, candy, baked goods, gelatin desserts, and chewing gum. *See* Benzyl Acetate. ASP

**METHOXYBENZENE** • *See* Anisole.

**p-METHOXY BENZYL ACETATE** • *See* Anisyl Acetate

**p-METHOXY BENZYL ALCOHOL** • *See* Anisyl Alcohol.

**p-METHOXYBENZYL FORMATE** • *See* Anisyl Formate.

**1-METHOXYCARBONYL-1-PROPEN-2-YL DIMETHYL PHOSPHATE** • Mevinphos. An organophosphate pesticide in dehydrated parsley as a result of application to the growing crop. FDA residue tolerance is 4 ppm. *See* Organophosphates for toxicity.

**p-METHOXYCINNAMALDEHYDE** • A flavoring. ASP

**METHOXYETHANOL** • *See* Ethanol.

**4 (p-METHOXYPHENYL)-2-BUTANONE** • A synthetic fruit, licorice, and anise flavoring additive for beverages, ice cream, ices, candy, baked goods, chewing gum, and gelatin desserts. A flavoring additive used in foods, it has a pale yellow color and a sweet floral odor. ASP

**1-(p-METHOXYPHENYL)-1-PENTEN-3-ONE** • A synthetic butter, cream, fruit, maple, nut, and vanilla flavoring additive for beverages, ice cream ices, candy, and baked goods. ASP

**1-(*p*-METHOXYPHENYL)-2-PROPANONE** • A synthetic flavoring additive that occurs naturally in star anise. Used in fruit and vanilla flavorings for beverages, ice cream, ices, candy, and baked goods. ASP

**2-METHOXYPYRAZINE** • A colorless to yellow liquid with a nutty, cocoalike odor used as a flavoring in a variety of foods. Skin and eye irritant. GRAS. ASP

***p*-METHOXYTOLUENE** • See Ylang-Ylang Oil.

**4-METHOXYTOLUENE-2,5-DIAMINE HCL** • A colorless liquid used in perfumery and flavorings. *See* Toluene.

**2-METHOXY-4-VINYLPHENOL** • Spicy, vanilla flavoring also used in fragrances to add spicy notes. ASP

**METHYL ABIETATE** • *See* Abietic Acid.

**METHYL ACETAMIDE** • *See* Methyl Acetate.

**METHYL ACETATE** • Acetic Acid. Colorless liquid that occurs naturally in coffee, with a pleasant apple odor. Used in perfume to emphasize floral odors, especially that of rose, and in toilet waters having a lavender odor. Also naturally occurs in peppermint oil. A flavoring used in fruit, rum, and nut flavorings for beverages, ice cream, ices, candy, baked goods, gelatin desserts, puddings, and liquor. Used as a solvent for many resins and oils. May be irritating to the respiratory tract and, in high concentrations, may be narcotic. Since it has an effective fat-solvent drying effect on skin, it may cause skin problems such as chafing and cracking. ASP

**4-METHYL ACETOPHENONE** • Colorless liquid with a fruit odor, it is used as a flavoring additive in various foods. Moderately toxic by ingestion. A human skin irritant. ASP

**METHYLACETOPYRONONE** • White crystalline powder used as a preservative in various foods. Poison by ingestion. Causes tumors in experimental animals. GRAS

**METHYL 5-ACETOXYHEXANOATE** • A flavoring in baked goods, beverages, chewing gum, condiments, frozen dairy, fruit ices, gelatins, hard candy, and other food products. Determined GRAS by FEMA *(see)*. *See* Hexanoic Acid.

**METHYL 1-ACETOXYCYCLOHEXYL KETONE** • A flavoring additive. The FAO/WHO *(see)* determined this substance needs further study. NIL

**METHYL ACRYLATE** • 2-Propanoic Acid, Methyl Ester. Derived from ethylene chlorohydrin, it is transparent and elastic. Used to coat paper and plastic film. Can be highly irritating to the eyes, skin, and mucous membranes. Convulsions occur if vapors are inhaled in high concentrations. GRAS for packaging. The final report to the FDA of the Select Committee on GRAS Substances stated in 1980 that there were insufficient relevant biological and other studies upon which to base an evaluation of it when used as a food ingredient. NUL

**METHYL ACRYLATE DIVINYLBENZENE, COMPLETELY HYDRO-LYZED, COPOLYMER** • Used in food processing. *See* Acrylamide. NUL

**METHYL ACRYLATE-DVB-(DEG-DIVINYLETHER), AMINOLYZED**

**METHYL ALCOHOL** • Solvent for spice oleoresins and in hops extract for beer. Clear, colorless liquid derived from carbon monoxide and hydrogen under pressure. Toxic by ingestion. Can cause blindness. Used in the manufacture of formaldehyde, acetic acid, and other compounds. Used to denature *(see)* alcohol. FDA tolerance for residues on spices is less than 50 ppm or less than 2.2 percent by weight. ASP

**METHYL AMYL KETONE** • *See* 2-Heptanone.

**METHYL ANISATE** • Anisic Acid. A synthetic fruit, melon, liquor, root beer, and spice flavoring additive for beverages, ice cream, ices, candy, and baked goods. ASP

**METHYL ANTHRANILATE** • Occurs naturally in neroli, ylang-ylang, bergamot, jasmine, and other essential oils. Colorless to pale yellow liquid with a bluish fluorescence and a grapelike odor. It is made synthetically from coal tar *(see)*. Used in loganberry, strawberry, orange, floral, rose, violet, cherry, grape, melon, liquor, wine, and honey flavorings for beverages, ice cream, ices, candy, baked goods, chewing gum (2,200 ppm), and liquors. Can irritate the skin. GRAS. ASP

**N-METHYL ANTHRANILIC ACID, METHYL ESTER** • *See* Methyl Anthranilate.

**A-METHYL BENZENE ACETATE** • A colorless liquid with a honey or jasmine odor, it is used as a flavoring additive in a variety of foods. Moderately toxic by ingestion and skin contact. ASP

**METHYL BENZOATE** • Essence of oil of Niobe. Made from methanol and benzoic acid *(see both)*. Colorless, transparent liquid with a pleasant fruity odor. Used in fruit rum, liquor, nut, spices, and vanilla flavorings for beverages, ice cream, ices, candy, and baked goods. Also used in perfumes. ASP

**METHYL BENZO CARBOXYLATE** • Colorless liquid with a fragrant odor used as a flavoring additive in various foods. Moderately toxic by ingestion. Mildly toxic by skin contact.

**METHYL-5-BENZOYL BENZIMIDAZOLE-2-CARBAMATE** • Vermirax. Telmin. Mebendazole. An antiworm medicine for animals. In the EPA Genetic Toxicology Program. Poison by ingestion. Causes mutations in animals.

**METHYL BROMIDE** • Prepared from the action of hydrobromic acid on methanol *(see)* it is used as a fumigant in warehouses and for extracting oils from nuts, seeds, and flours. Inhalation causes dizziness, headache, vomiting, abdominal pain, mental confusion, convulsions, pulmonary edema, coma, and death. Chronic exposure can cause central nervous system depression or kidney injury. FDA tolerance for various crops is from 5 to 200 ppm.

**METHYL-1-(BUTYL CARBAMOYL) 2-BENZIMIDAZOLYLCARBA-MATE** • BBC. Benylate. Benomyl. A fungicide used on apples, apricots, bananas, cherries, mangoes, nectarines, peaches, pears, pineapples, plums, raisins, and tomato products (concentrated). FDA residue tolerances are: 50 ppm in raisins and concentrated tomato products; 125 ppm in dried grape pomace and raisin waste; 70 ppm in dried apple pomace; 50 ppm in dried citrus pulp; 20 ppm in rice hulls. In EPA Genetic Toxicology Program *(see)*. Poison by ingestion. A human skin irritant. May cause birth defects.

**METHYL *p-tert*-BUTYLPHENYLACETATE** • A synthetic chocolate, fruit, and honey flavoring for beverages, ice cream, ices, candy, and baked goods. ASP

**METHYL BUTYRATE** • A synthetic flavoring additive that occurs naturally in apples. Colorless, used in fruit and rum flavorings for beverages, ice cream, candy, and baked goods. ASP

**METHYL CHLORIDE** • Chloromethane. Colorless gas or colorless liquid with a sweet taste, it is used as a spray pesticide in food storage and processing areas. It is not supposed to contact fatty foods. The FDA tolerance for modified hop extract for beer is up to 250 ppm. Poisonous, it can cause severe injury to liver and kidney.

**METHYL CINNAMATE** • White crystals, strawberrylike odor, and soluble in alcohol. Derived by heating methanol, cinnamic acid, and sulfuric acid. A synthetic strawberry, butter, cream, cherry, grape, peach, plum, and vanilla flavoring additive for beverages, ice cream, ices, candy, baked goods, chewing gum, and condiments See Cinnamic Acid. ASP

**METHYLCROTONIC ACID** • *See* Crotonic Acid. ASP

**2-METHYL-1,3-CYCLOHEXADIENE** • Synthetic flavoring. ASP

**1-METHYLCYCLOHEXADIONE** • Scent of the spruce beetle used as a flavoring and natural pesticide. ASP

**METHYL CYCLOHEXANECARBOXYLATE** • Flavor enhancer and flavoring. ASP

**2-METHYLCYCLOHEXANONE** • Flavoring. EAF

**3-METHYL-2-CYCLOHEXEN-1-ONE** • See 1-Methylcyclohexadione. EAF

**METHYL-2-DECENOATE** • Synthetic flavoring. *See* Decanoic Acid. NIL

**GAMMA-METHYLDECALACTON** • Flavoring. FAO/WHO says no average daily intake is known. EAF

**METHYL 2-DECENOATE** • Synthetic flavoring. *See* Decanoic Acid. NIL

**METHYL DISULFIDE** • A synthetic onion flavoring additive for baked goods, condiments, and pickle products. ASP

**2-METHYL-1,3-DITHIOLANE** • Flavoring liquid with a burned alliaceous odor. NIL

**METHYL ESTER OF FATTY ACIDS** • Produced from edible fats and oils. Used in dehydrating grapes to produce raisins. *See* Esters and Fatty Acids.

**METHYL ESTER OF HIGHER FATTY ACIDS** • Used in animal feed. *See* Fatty Acids.

**METHYL ESTER OF ROSIN PARTIALLY HYDROGENATED** • Used as a constituent of chewing-gum base. *See* Rosin and Hydrogenated.

**METHYL ESTERS OF FATTY ACIDS PRODUCED FROM EDIBLE FATS and OILS** • Used in dehydrating grapes to produce raisins. FDA tolerance is less than 3 percent of weight or less than 200 ppm in raisins.

**METHYL ESTERS OF HIGHER FATTY ACIDS** • Used in animal feed.

**METHYL ETHYL CELLULOSE** • A foaming, aerating, and emulsifying additive prepared from wood pulp or chemical cotton. Used in vegetable-fat whipped topping and as a emulsifying additive. Used as a bulk laxative but absorbed from the bowel. *See* Sodium Carboxymethyl Cellulose for toxicity.

**METHYL FORMATE** • Colorless liquid with a sweet odor used as a fumigant in raisins and dried currants. FDA residue tolerance of 250 ppm as formic acid *(see)* in raisins and dried currants.

**3-[(2-METHYL-3-FURYL)THIO]2-BUTANONE** • A flavoring determined GRAS by FEMA. *See* Butanone.

**METHYL GLUCOSIDE OF FATTY ACIDS OF EDIBLE COCONUT OIL** • Used in the manufacture of beet sugar and as an aid in crystallization of sucrose and dextrose. Used as a surfactant in molasses meant for animal feed. No known toxicity except that coconut is thought to contribute to cholesterol clogging of the arteries.

**METHYL HEPTANOATE** • A synthetic berry, grape, peach, and pineapple flavoring additive for beverages, ice cream, ices, candy, and baked goods.

**METHYL HEPTENONE** • *See* 6-Methyl-5-Hepten-2-One.

**6-METHYL-5-HEPTEN-2-ONE** • Methyl Heptenone. A synthetic flavoring additive that occurs naturally in oil of lavender and oil of lemon. Used in berry, citrus, banana, melon, pear, peach, and pineapple flavorings for beverages, ice cream, ices, candy, baked goods, and gelatin desserts. Moderately toxic by ingestion. A skin irritant.

**METHYL HEXENOATE** • A synthetic pineapple flavoring additive for beverages, ice cream, ices, candy, and baked goods.

**METHYL-*p*-HYDROXYBENZOATE** • Methylparaben. A preservative in beverages, baked goods, candy, and artificially sweetened jellies and preserves. Methylparaben may cause allergic skin reaction. On the FDA list of additives requiring further study. GRAS.E

**METHYL ISOBUTYL KETONE** • A synthetic fruit flavoring additive for beverages, ice cream, ices, candy, and baked goods. Used as solvent for cellulose and lacquer. Similar in toxicity to methyl ethyl ketone, which is irritating to the eyes and mucous membranes, but likely more toxic. Causes intestinal upsets and central nervous system depression.

**METHYL ISOBUTYRATE** • A synthetic fruit flavoring additive for beverages, ice cream, ices, candy, and baked goods.

**1-METHYL-4-ISOPROPYLCYCLOHEXADIENE-1,3** • A colorless liquid with a lemony odor, it is used as a flavoring additive in various foods. Moderately toxic by ingestion.

**METHYL LAURATE** • The ester of methyl alcohol and lauric acid. Derived from coconut oil. A synthetic flavoring additive for beverages, ice cream, ices, candy, and baked goods. It is also used in detergents, emulsifiers, wetting additives, stabilizers, resins, lubricants, and plasticizers.

**METHYL LINOLEATE** • The ester of methyl alcohol and linoleic acid, it is a colorless oil derived from safflower oil and used in detergents, emulsifiers, wetting additives, stabilizers, resins, lubricants, and plasticizers.

**METHYL MERCAPTAN** • A synthetic flavoring additive that occurs naturally in caseinate, cheese, skim milk, coffee, and cooked beef. Used in coffee flavorings for beverages, ice cream, ices, candy, and baked goods. *See* Methanethiol for toxicity.

**METHYL-2-METHYL BUTYRATE** • Colorless liquid with a sweet, apple-like odor used as a flavoring additive in various foods.

**METHYL MYRISTATE** • *See* Myristic Acid.

**METHYL b-NAPHTHYL KETONE** • Orange Crystals. 2′ Acetonaphthone. A synthetic flavoring additive used in berry, strawberry, citrus, fruit, grape, and vanilla flavorings for beverages, ice cream, ices, candy, baked goods, gelatin desserts, and chewing gum. *See* Methyl Isobutyl Ketone for toxicity.

**METHYL NICOTINATE** • *See* Niacin. EAF

**METHYL NONANOATE** • Synthetic flavoring that smells like coconut. ASP

**3-METHYL-2,4-NONANEDIONE** • A flavoring determined GRAS by the Expert Panel of the Flavor and Extract Manufacturers Association

**METHYL NONANOATE** • A synthetic berry, citrus, pineapple, honey, and cognac flavoring additive for beverages, ice cream, ices, candy, and baked goods.

**METHYL 2-NONENOATE** • A synthetic berry and melon flavoring additive for beverages, ice cream, ices, candy, and baked goods.

**METHYL 2-NONYNOATE** • A synthetic berry, floral, violet, fruit, and banana flavoring additive for beverages, ice cream, ices, candy, gelatin desserts, baked goods, and condiments.

**METHYL OCTANOATE** • A synthetic flavoring additive that occurs naturally in pineapple. Used in pineapple and berry flavorings for beverages, ice cream, ices, candy, and baked goods.

**METHYL 2-OCTYNOATE** • A synthetic flavoring additive used in berry, raspberry, strawberry, floral, violet, fruit, peach, liquor, and muscatel flavorings for beverages, ice cream, ices, candy, baked goods, gelatin desserts, chewing gum, and jellies.

**METHYL PELARGONATE** • Nonanoic Acid. Methyl Ester. The ester of ethyl alcohol and pelargonic acid used in perfume and flavorings.

**4-METHYL-2-PENTANONE** • A synthetic fruit flavoring for beverages, ice cream, ices, candy, and baked goods.

**2-METHYL-4-PHENYL-2-BUTYL ACETATE** • A synthetic fruit and tea flavoring additive for beverages, ice cream, ices, candy, and baked goods.

**a-METHYLBENZYL ALCOHOL** • A flavoring additive in foods and beverages derived from alcohol and benzoic acid *(see both)* and also appears naturally in a variety of foods. The FAO/WHO *(see)* found that in short-term toxicity studies, high rates of mortality were associated with dose levels of 1,000 mg and 2,000 mg per kg of body per day in mice and 2,000 mg per day in rats. It also adversely affected body weight, long-term survival rates, and caused birth defects. The committee said the intake of this compound from all sources is extremely low. On the basis of the evidence available, the committee concluded that the higher incidence of benign tumors in the kidneys of male rats was not relevant to humans. In view of the "limited database," the committee concluded that the available data could be used to set an ADI by application of a safety factor of 1,000 to the minimal-effect level of 93 mg per kg of body weight per day. Accordingly, an ADI of 0–0.1 mg per kg of body weight per day was allocated for this additive.

**1-(3-METHYL)BUTYL BENZOATE** • Amyl Benzoate. Isopentyl Benzoate. Used as a flavoring additive in various foods. Mildly toxic by ingestion. A skin irritant.

**METHYLCHLOROPINDOL** • Coccidiostat. An antibiotic drug for animals used on beef and in feed as well as cereal grains, chicken, fruits, goat, lamb, milk, pork, turkey, and vegetables. The FDA limits it to 0.2 ppm in cereal grains, vegetables, and fruits; 15 ppm in uncooked liver and kidney; 5 ppm in uncooked muscle of chickens and turkeys; and 3 ppm in uncooked kidney.

**3-METHYL-3-PHENYL GLYCIDIC ACID, ETHYL ESTER** • A synthetic strawberry flavoring. GRAS

**METHYL PHENYLACETATE** • Colorless liquid with a honeylike odor used in strawberry, chocolate, peach, and honey flavorings for beverages, ice cream, ices, baked goods, candy, gelatin desserts, chewing gum, and syrup. Also used in perfumery. Moderately toxic by ingestion and skin contact. *See* Phenyl Acetate.

**2-METHYL-4-PHENYLBUTYRALDEHYDE** • A synthetic nut flavoring additive for beverages, ice cream, ices, candy, and baked goods.

**3-METHYL-2-PHENYL BUTYRATE** • A synthetic fruit flavoring for beverages, ice cream, ices, and candy.

**METHYL 4-PHENYLBUTYRATE** • A synthetic strawberry, fruit, and honey flavoring additive for beverages, ice cream, ices, candy, and baked goods.

**METHYL PIPERAZINE** • Colorless liquid that absorbs water. Used as a surfactant *(see)*.

**METHYL PREDNISOLONE** • Medrol. Meprolone. A-MethaPred. Solu-Medrol. A hormone secreted by the adrenal gland that affects carbohydrate and protein metabolism. It was introduced as a medication in 1957 to treat severe inflammation or for immunosuppression or to decrease residual damage following spinal cord trauma. Used to treat cows. The FDA limits residue to 10 ppb in milk. Most adverse reactions are the result of dose- or length-of-time of administration. Potential adverse reactions include euphoria, insomnia, psychotic behavior, high blood pressure, swelling, cataracts, glaucoma, peptic ulcer, GI irritation, increased appetite, high blood sugar, growth suppression in children, delayed wound healing, acne, skin eruptions, muscle weakness, pancreatitis, hairiness, decreased immunity, and acute adrenal gland insufficiency. FDA tolerance in milk from treated cows is 10 ppb.

**METHYL SALICYLATE** • Salicylic Acid. Oil of Wintergreen. Found naturally in sweet birch, cassia, and wintergreen. Used in strawberry, grape, mint, walnut, root beer, sarsaparilla, spice, wintergreen, birch beer, and vanilla flavorings for beverages, ice cream, ices, candy, baked goods, chewing gum (8,400 ppm), and syrup. The volatile oil obtained by maceration. Toxic by ingestion. Use in foods restricted by the FDA.

**METHYL SILICONS** • Prepared by hydrolyzing *(see)* dimethyldichlorosilane or its esters, it is used to help compounds resist oxidation. *See* Silicones.

**METHYL SULFIDE** • A synthetic flavoring additive that occurs naturally in caseinate, cheese, coffee, coffee extract, and skim milk. Disagreeable odor. Used in chocolate, cocoa, fruit, and molasses flavorings for beverages, ice cream, ices, candy, baked goods, gelatin desserts, and syrups. Used also as a solvent for minerals.

**METHYL 9-UNDECENOATE** • A synthetic citrus and honey flavoring additive for beverages, ice cream, ices, candy, and baked goods.

**METHYL 2-UNDECYNOATE** • A synthetic floral and violet flavoring additive for beverages, ice cream, ices, candy, and baked goods.

**METHYL VALERATE** • A synthetic flavoring additive that occurs naturally in pineapple. Used in fruit flavorings for beverages, ice cream, ices, candy, and baked goods.

**2-METHYL VALERIC ACID** • A synthetic chocolate flavoring additive for candy.

**2-(5 — METHYL-5-VINYLTETRAHYDROFURAN-2-YL)PROPIONAL-DEHYDE** • Flavoring determined GRAS by FEMA *(see)*. See Furfural.

**METHYLACETALDEHYDE** • *See* Propionaldehyde.

**METHYLACETIC ACID** • *See* Propionic Acid.

**2-METHYLALLYL BUTYRATE** • A synthetic pineapple flavoring for beverages, ice cream, ices, candy, and baked goods.

***o*-METHYLANISOLE** • A synthetic fruit and nut flavoring for beverages, ice cream, ices, candy, and baked goods.

***p*-METHYLANISOLE** • A synthetic berry, maple, black walnut, walnut, and spice flavoring additive for beverages, ice cream, ices, candy, baked goods, gelatin desserts, puddings, condiments, and syrups.

**METHYLBENZYL ACETATE** • A synthetic flavoring additive, colorless, with a gardenia odor. Used in cherry and fruit flavorings for beverages, ice cream, ices, candy, baked goods, gelatin desserts, and chewing gum.

***a*-METHYLBENZYL ACETATE** • Acetic Acid. A synthetic berry and fruit flavoring additive for beverages, ice cream, ices, candy, baked goods, chewing gum, and toppings.

***a*-METHYLBENZYL BUTYRATE** • A synthetic berry and fruit flavoring additive for beverages, ice cream, ices, candy, and baked goods.

***a*-METHYLBENZYL ISOBUTYRATE** • A synthetic fruit flavoring additive for beverages, ice cream, ices, candy, and baked goods.

***a*-METHYLBENZYL FORMATE** • Formic Acid. A synthetic fruit and berry flavoring additive for beverages, ice cream, ices, candy, and baked goods. *See* Formic Acid for toxicity.

**2-METHYLBUTYRALDEHYDE** • A synthetic flavoring additive that occurs naturally in coffee and tea. Used in chocolate and fruit flavoring for beverages, ice cream, ices, candy, and baked goods.

**3-METHYLBUTYRALDEHYDE** • A synthetic flavoring additive that occurs naturally in coffee extract, oil of lavender, and peppermint oil. Used in butter, chocolate, cocoa, fruit, and nut flavorings for beverages, ice cream, ices, candy, baked goods, and gelatin desserts.

**2-METHYLBUTYRIC ACID** • A synthetic fruit flavoring additive for beverages, ice cream, ices, and candy.

**METHYLCELLULOSE** • Cellulose, Methyl Ether. A binder, thickener, dispersing, and emulsifying additive, it is prepared from wood pulp or chemical cotton by treatment with alcohol. Swells in water. Soluble in cold water and insoluble in hot. The commercial product has a methoxyl content of 29 percent. It is used as a bodying additive for beverages and canned fruits sweetened with artificial sweeteners; a thickener for kosher food products; a bulking additive for low-calorie crackers; a binder in nonwheat baked goods for nonallergic diets; a beer foam stabilizer; a condiment carrier; in food products for diabetics and low-calorie dietetic products; an edible film for food products; a leavening additive for prepared mixes; a clarifier for vinegar and beverages; and in imitation jellies and jams, processed cheese, confectionery, and toppings. It is a bulk laxative. Ingestion of large doses may cause flatulence, distension of the abdomen or intestinal obstruction, and may also affect the absorption of minerals or other drugs. A dose injected into the abdomen of rats causes cancer. Nontoxic on the skin. The final report to the FDA of the Select Committee on GRAS Substances stated in 1980 that there is no evidence in the available information that it is a hazard to the public when used as it is now and it should continue its GRAS status with limitations in the amounts that can be added to foods. *See* also Carboxymethyl Cellulose. GRAS.

**6-METHYLCOUMARIN** • White needlelike substance from benzene with a coconut odor. A synthetic flavoring additive used in butter, caramel, coconut, fruit, nut, root beer, and vanilla flavorings for beverages, ice cream, ices, candy, baked goods, gelatin desserts, puddings, and chewing gum. Unlike methylcoumarin, which is listed as GRAS by FEMA *(see)*, coumarin, once widely used in foods, is banned. Prolonged feeding of coumarin causes liver injury. Carcinogenic and allergenic. ASP

**METHYLCYCLOPENTENOLONE** • A synthetic flavoring additive used in berry, butter, butterscotch, caramel, maple, hazelnut, pecan, walnut, fruit, and vanilla flavorings for beverages, ice cream, ices, candy, baked goods, chewing gum, gelatin desserts, and syrups.

**METHYLENE CHLORIDE** • Dichloromethane. Methane Dichloride. Methylene Dichloride. Aerothene NM. Solaestine. Freon 30 Somethine. F-30. A colorless gas that compresses into colorless liquid of pleasant odor and sweet taste. A solvent in the microencapsulation of thiamin hydrochloride *(see)* intended for use in both dry beverages and dry gelatin mixes. One of the most commonly used solvents, it is used to remove caffeine from coffee and tea. The FDA estimates, based on coffee industry tests, that about 0.1 ppm remain in most brands decaffeinating this way. Once absorbed into the body, methylene chloride generates carbon monoxide. Because of public concern about methylene chloride, some brands are now using other methods of decaffeinating. Used as an anesthetic in medicine. High concentrations are narcotic. Damage to the liver, kidney, and central nervous system can occur, and persistent postrecovery symptoms after inhalation include headache, nervousness, insomnia, and tremor. Can be absorbed through the skin and is then converted to carbon monoxide which, in turn, can cause stress in the cardiovascular system. It is widely used as a degreaser; solvent for spices, waxes, oils, paint, and varnish thinner; as cleansers in many industries and work settings; in aerosols, including pesticides; in refrigeration and air-conditioning equipment. Methylene chloride enters your body when you breathe it in the air. Once it enters the body, methylene chloride generates carbon monoxide, which interferes with the blood's ability to pick up and deliver oxygen. The body responds to lack of oxygen by driving the heart to work harder. People with angina (chest pains) from coronary artery disease are extremely sensitive to carbon monoxide and may have increased chest pains from exposure to methylene chloride, even below the legal exposure limit (100 parts per million over an eight-hour workshift). It is also a skin irritant. Methylene chloride is considered to have "poor warning properties," since most people cannot smell it until it reaches a hazardous level (100–500 ppm). If you can smell it, you may be overexposed. Methylene chloride causes cancer in animals and is considered a potential cancer-causing additive in humans. The FAO/WHO said that epidemiological studies have not shown any carcinogenic effect of methylene chloride after occupational exposure. However, the committee noted that the power to detect excess risk in these studies was limited. On the basis of the available data, the committee concluded that the use of methylene chloride as an extraction solvent in food processing should be limited to use for spice oleoresins and the decaffeination of tea and coffee and for food additives that included residues of dichloromethane. FDA residue tolerances are: 30 ppm in spice oleoresins, less than 10 ppm in decaffeinated roasted coffee and decaffeinated instant coffee, and 2.2 percent as a residue in hops extract added before or during cooking of beer.

**5-METHYLFURFURAL** • A synthetic honey, maple, and meat flavoring for beverages, ice cream, ices, candy, and baked goods.

**2-METHYLOCTANAL** • A synthetic citrus flavoring additive for beverages, ice cream, ices, candy, and baked goods.

**METHYLPARABEN** • Methyl-*p*-Hydroxybenzoate. Preservative in jelly and preserves. Used in bubble baths, cold creams, eyeliners, and liquid makeup. It is an antimicrobial and preservative made of small, odorless, colorless crystals that have a burning taste. FDA residue tolerance in milk from cows treated with mastitis formulations is zero. Nontoxic in small amounts but can cause allergic skin reactions. See Methyl-*p*-Hydroxybenzoate. GRAS

**2-METHYLPENTANOIC ACID** • *See* 2-Methyl Valeric Acid.

***b*-METHYLPHENETHYL ALCOHOL** • A synthetic berry, rose, melon, and honey flavoring additive for beverages, ice cream, ices, candy, and baked goods.

**METHYLPROTOCATECHUIC ALDEHYDE** • *See* Vanillin.

**4-METHYLQUINOLINE** • A synthetic butter, honey, and nut flavoring additive for beverages, ice cream, ices, candy, and baked goods.

**2-METHYLRESORCINOL** • Orcin. An aromatic compound with white crystalline prisms derived from lichen; used in medicine and as a readditive for sugars and starches. *See* Resorcinol.

**METHYLTHEOBROMINE** • *See* Caffeine.

**2-METHYLUNDECANAL** • A synthetic flavoring additive, colorless, with a fatty odor. Used in a variety of foods.

**METOLACHLOR** • An odorless, preemergent herbicide. FDA residue tolerances are: 0.02 ppm in cattle, goats, sheep, hog fat, meat by-products, and in eggs; 0.05 ppm as residue in cattle, goat, hog, sheep liver; 0.1 ppm as residue in corn grain and cottonseed; 0.3 ppm as residue in sorghum grain; 0.2 ppm as residue in soybean; 2 ppm as residue in or on sorghum forage, fodder; and 8 ppm as residue in or on corn forage or fodder.

**METOSERPATE HYDROCHLORIDE** • An animal drug used in chicken. The FDA limits residue to 0.02 ppm in chicken. Crystals from benzene and cyclohexane. Used as a sedative. Poisonous by ingestion.

**METSULFURON METHYL** • A pre- and postemergent herbicide. FDA tolerances for residue in or on grain, green forage, hay, straw of barley and wheat, 0.05 to 20 ppm; 0.1 ppm as a residue in meat and meat by-products of cattle, hogs, and sheep; and 0.05 ppm as a residue in milk.

**MEXICAN SAGE** • *See* Oregano.

**MG** • Abbreviation for a milligram, a metric measurement that is one one-thousandth of a gram.

**MIBOLERONE** • Crystalline solid used as an animal feed drug. A male hormone, it used in dog food to increase growth. Caused adverse reproductive effects and birth defects in experimental animals.

***MICHELLA ALBA* EXTRACT** • Flavoring from an Asian tree related to the magnolia. EAF

**MICROCAPSULES** • Used for flavoring oils, these tiny vessels contain gelatin, arabinogalactan, silicon dioxide, glutaraldehyde, and octanal *(see all)*.

**MICROCRYSTALLINE CELLULOSE** • Used in frozen desserts. No longer listed as GRAS. Limited in standardized products. *See* Cellulose.

**MICROCRYSTALLINE WAX** • Obtained from crude oil, subsequent to the removal of paraffin. Its characteristics resemble those of the natural waxes closely, including its high melting point, high viscosity, flexibility at low temperatures, and high cohesion and adhesion. It is used as a substitute for other waxes in laminating paper and foils. E

**MICROPARTICULATED PROTEIN PRODUCT** • Thickener and texturizer in frozen dessert products. May not be used to replace milk fat in standardized frozen desserts. GRAS. NUL

**MIEHEI or *MUCOR PUSILLUS*** • Enzyme used to clot milk for making cheese.

**MILFOIL** • *See* Yarrow.

**MILK** • Milk may be a hidden ingredient in cream of rice, macaroni, filled candy bars, Ovaltine, junket, prepared flours, frankfurters, and other sausages. Some people are allergic to milk. *See also* Nonfat Dry Milk. The Food and Drug Administration ruled, starting January 1, 1998, lower-fat milk products must follow the same criteria as most other foods labeled "low fat." This means that such products as 2 percent milk, which contains about 5 grams of fat per serving, cannot be labeled "low fat" because the fat content is more than 3 grams per serving, which is the upper limit permitted in food products labeled "low fat." Actually, 2 percent milk has two-thirds the fat of whole milk. Milk with zero fat can be called "fat free" or "nonfat" instead of "skim" and 1 percent milk is "low fat." Whole milk normally contains 3.25 percent milkfat or 8 grams of fat per serving (a serving is defined as 1 cup).

**MILK-CLOTTING ENZYME FROM *ASPERGILLUS ORYZAE* RECOMBINANT** • Fungi additive used to tenderize meat and make cheese. Although it involves genetic alteration, the FDA has no safety concerns about it. EAF

**MILK-CLOTTING ENZYME FROM *BACILLUS CEREUS*** • Used to clot milk in cheese making. NUL

**MILK-CLOTTING ENZYME FROM *ENTOTHIA PARASITICA, MUCOR PUSILLUS*** • Used to clot milk for cheese making. ASP

**MILK-DERIVED LACTOFERRIN** • *See* Lactoferrin. GRAS

**MILK POWDER, WHOLE, ENZYME MODIFIED** • Enzyme-modified milk powder may be prepared with GRAS enzymes from reconstituted milk powder, whole milk, condensed or concentrated whole milk, evaporated milk, or milk powder. The lipolysis is maintained at a temperature that is optimal for the action of the enzyme until appropriate acid development is attained. The enzymes are then inactivated. The resulting product is concentrated or dried. ASP

**MILLET EXTRACT** • An extract of the seeds of *Panicum miliaceum.*

**MILLIGRAM (mg)** • A metric unit of weight equal to one-thousandth of a gram *(see).* Food labels list cholesterol and sodium in milligrams (mg) per serving.

**MILO STARCH** • See Modified Starch. The final report to the FDA of the Select Committee on GRAS Substances stated in 1980 that it should continue its GRAS status with no limitations other than good manufacturing practices.

**MIMOSA, ABSOLUTE** • *Acacia decurrens.* Black Wattle Flowers. Reddish yellow solid with a long-lasting, pleasant odor resembling ylang-ylang. Derived from trees, shrubs, and herbs native to tropical and warm regions. Mimosa droops and closes its leaves when touched. A natural flavoring additive used in raspberry and fruit flavorings for beverages, ice cream, ices, candy, and baked goods. May produce allergic skin reactions. EAF

**MINERAL OIL** • White Oil. A mixture of refined liquid hydrocarbons *(see)* derived from petroleum. Colorless, transparent, odorless, and tasteless. It is used as a defoaming component in the processing of beet sugar and yeast; as a coating for fresh fruits and vegetables; a lubricant and binder for capsules and tablets, supplying small amounts of flavor in spice condiments and vitamins. Also employed as a lubricant in food-processing equipment; a dough-divider oil; pan oil; and a lubricant in meat-packing plants. It is also used in confectionery as a sealant. When heated, it smells like petroleum. May inhibit absorption of digestive fats and it has a mild laxative effect. A human cancer-causing additive by inhalation. Causes birth defects if inhaled by humans and also causes testicular tumors in the fetus. An eye irritant. FDA tolerances include: 200 ppm in dried fruits and vegetables from use as a releasing additive in drying pans; less than 0.095 percent in meat from use as hot melt coating; less than 0.10 percent in egg white solids; and less than 0.06 percent as a releasing additive, binder, and/or lubricant in or on capsules or tablets containing concentrates of flavors, spices, condiments, and nutrients intended for addition to food. The FAO/WHO *(see)* requested in June 1998 that studies of the compositional factors in mineral oils that influence their absorption and toxicity be done in rats for at least one year. In addition, a one-year study of the potential effects on the immune system was requested. ASP

**MINTLACTONE** • Flavoring additive. See Pennyroyal Oil. EAF

**MISC** • FDA abbreviation for miscellaneous.

**MIXED CARBOHYDRASE and PROTEASE ENZYME PRODUCTS** • Enzymes. *See* Enzymes. GRAS

**MOCA** • Bis Amine. Curalin M. Packaging adhesive prohibited from indirect addition to human food from food contact surface. IARC, EPA Genetic Toxicology Program, and Community Right-To-Know List *(see all)* were concerned about this additive. Moderately toxic by ingestion. Caused cancer and tumors in experimental animals.

**MODIFIED CELLULOSE** • *See* Cellulose Gums.

**MODIFIED FIBERS** • Bran and cotyledon-source cereal fibers receive minimal processing compared with the concentrated, modified fibers. For the most part, the modified versions also come from cereal grains, but they are categorized separately because they are so different. Typically, these fibers are noncaloric, contain 90 percent or more total dietary fiber, are very bland, and have a very light color. Water-absorption properties are typically improved.

**MODIFIED SEA SALT** • Salts derived from seawater with a reduced sodium chloride content.

**MODIFIED STARCH** • Ordinary starch that has been altered chemically to modify such properties as thickening or jelling. Babies have difficulty in digesting starch in its original form. Modified starch is used in baby food on the theory that it is easier to digest. Questions about safety have arisen because babies do not have the resistance of adults to chemicals. Among chemicals used to modify starch are propylene oxide, succinic anhydride, 1-octenyl succinic anhydride, aluminum sulfate, and sodium hydroxide *(see all)*. On the FDA top priority list for reevaluation since 1980. Nothing new reported by the FDA since.

**MOENOMYCIN** • Bambermycin. Menomycin. An antibiotic produced by *Streptomyces roseoflavus* used as an animal feed drug for poultry, calves, and swine. An eye and skin irritant. Poison by ingestion. Moderately toxic by ingestion.

**MOLASSES EXTRACT** • *Saccharum officinarum.* Extract of sugarcane, a thick, brown, viscid syrup. Separated from raw sugar in the successive processes of sugar manufacture and graded according to its quality. It is a natural flavoring additive for candy, baked goods, ice cream, and medicines. GRAS. ASP

**MOLECULAR SIEVE RESINS** • Used in processing to trap small unwanted particles. NUL

**MOLYBDENUM** • A dietary supplement. The dark gray, powdered mineral is a trace element in animal and plant metabolism. Resembles chromium and tungsten in many of its properties. Low toxicity.

**MONOAMINE OXIDASE (MAO)** • An enzyme that acts in the nervous system to break down certain types of neurotransmitters (chemical messengers sent between nerve cells) such as dopamine, norepinephrine, and serotonin (see all).

**MONOAMINE OXIDASE INHIBITOR MEDICATIONS (MAOIs)** • A class of antidepressant medications usually prescribed for people who have certain forms of depression with symptoms including an increase in weight, appetite, or sleep. MAOIs may also be used for cases of mixed anxiety and depression, depression accompanied by pain, panic disorder, post-traumatic stress disorder, and bipolar depression. The drug works by raising the level of neurotransmitters by preventing their destruction by enzymes. People taking MAOIs must adhere to a special diet because of the interaction of the medications with certain foods. Foods that contain tyramine such as cheeses, yogurt, sour cream, beef or chicken livers, and red wines should be avoided. The combination of MAOIs and tyramine can shoot up blood pressure to dangerous levels. Symptoms include headache, increased or decreased heart rate, nausea and vomiting, sweating, fever or cold clammy skin, and chest pain.

**MONARDA SPECIES** • See Horsemint Leaves Extract.

**MONESIN** • Antibiotic isolated from Streptocyces cinnamonensis. Used in feed to combat parasites and fungus infections. It is also used to increase weight gain in cattle. FDA residue limits are: 0.05 ppm in edible tissues of cattle; 1.5 ppm in muscle tissue of chicken and turkey; 3 ppm as residue in skin with fat of chicken and turkey; and 4.5 ppm as residue in liver of chicken. Used as a medicated block for cattle; in liquid feed for cattle; in goat feed.

**4-MONOAMINOPHOSPHATIDE** • See Lecithin.

**MONOAMMONIUM GLUTAMATE** • Miscellaneous uses. See Glutamate and Ammonium. GRAS. ASP. E

**MONOAZO COLOR** • A dye made from diazonium and phenol, both coal-tar derivatives. See Coal Tar.

**MONOCALCIUM PHOSPHATE** • Calcium Phosphate, Monobasic. Buffer and neutralizing additive in self-rising cereal flours or meals. The FDA allows residues of up to 0.75 parts per 100 parts of flour; 4.5 parts including sodium bicarbonate per 100 parts of cereal product; 75 percent in phosphated flour, in self-rising cereal flours or meals; in fruit butters, jellies, and preserves; 0.1 percent in finished product of canned vegetables. *See* Calcium Phosphate. GRAS.

**MONOCHLORACETIC ACID** • A banned preservative. Any amount in beverages and other food will be considered adulterated by the FDA.

**MONO- and DIGLYCERIDES of FATS or OILS** • Mono- and diglycerides of edible fat-forming acids used as emulsifiers in oleomargarine. *See* Glycerides. GRAS. E

**MONOETHANOLAMINE** • Used in flume water for washing sugar beets prior to slicing. *See* Ethanolamine. ASP

**MONOGLYCERIDE CITRATE** • Aids the action of and helps dissolve antioxidant formulations that retard rancidity in oils and fats. *See* Citrate Salts for toxicity. ASP

**MONOGLYCERIDES DISTILLED** • Used to treat mastitis in dairy animals.

**MONOGLYCERIDES OF FATTY ACIDS** • Stabilizers in shortenings. *See* Fatty Acids.

**MONOGLYCEROL CITRATE** • A preservative. *See* Glycerols.

**MONOISOPROPYL CITRATE** • A sequestrant and plasticizer and antioxidant aid used in fats, lard, meat, oleomargarine, packaging materials, sausage, and shortening. *See* Isopropyl Citrate. GRAS. NUL

**MONOMER** • A molecule that by repetition in a long chain builds up a large structure or polymer *(see)*. Ethylene, the gas, for instance, is the monomer of polyethylene *(see)*.

**MONOPOTASSIUM GLUTAMATE** • Flavor enhancer and salt substitute used on meat. In EPA Genetic Toxicology Program *(see)*. Mildly toxic by ingestion. Human systemic effects by ingestion: headache. *See* Glutamate. GRAS. E

**MONOPOTASSIUM PHOSPHATE** • A derivative of edible fat. Used as an emulsifying additive in food products and as a buffer in prepared cereal. Cleared by the USDA's Meat Inspection Department to decrease the amounts of cooked-out juices in canned hams, pork shoulders, pork loins, chopped hams, and bacon. Monosodium phosphate is a urinary acidifier. The final report to the FDA of the Select Committee on GRAS Substances stated in 1980 that it should continue its GRAS status with no limitations other than good manufacturing practices.

**MONOSACCHARIDE LACTATE CONDENSATE** • The condensation product of sodium lactate and the sugars glucose, fructose, ribose, glucosamine, and deoxyribose.

**MONOSODIUM GLUTAMATE (MSG)** • Accent. Zest. The monosodium salt of glutamic acid *(see)*, one of the amino acids. Occurs naturally in seaweed, sea tangles, soybeans, and sugar beets. Used to intensify meat and spice flavorings in meats, condiments, pickles, soups, candy, and baked goods. Believed responsible for the so-called Chinese Restaurant Syndrome in which diners suffer from chest pain, headache, and numbness after eating a Chinese meal. Causes brain damage in young rodents and brain damage effects in rats, rabbits, chicks, and monkeys. Baby-food processors removed MSG from baby-food products. Depression, irritability, and other mood changes have been reported. On the FDA list of additives needing further study for mutagenic, teratogenic, subacute, and reproductive effects. Studies have shown that MSG administered to animals during the neonatal period resulted in reproductive dysfunction when both males and females became adults. Females treated with MSG had fewer pregnancies and smaller litters, while males showed reduced fertility. The final report to the FDA of the Select Committee on GRAS Substances stated in 1980 that while no evidence in the available information on it demonstrates a hazard to the public at current use levels, uncertainties exist requiring that additional studies be conducted. In 1995, a report from the Federation of American Societies for Experimental Biology (FASEB), an independent body of scientists that advises the FDA, identified two groups of people who may develop a condition, "MSG symptom complex." One group is those who may be intolerant to MSG when eaten in large quantities. The second is a group of people with severe, poorly controlled asthma. In addition to being prone to MSG symptoms these people may suffer temporary worsening of asthmatic symptoms after consuming MSG. The MSG dosage that produced reactions ranged from 0.5 grams to 2.5 grams. This report made the FDA propose that foods containing significant amounts of free glutamate (not bound in protein along with other amino acids) declare glutamate on the label. GRAS status has continued since 1980 while tests were being completed and evaluated.

**MONOSODIUM METHYLARSONATE** • Arsonate Liquid. Weed-E-Rad. An herbicide used on animal feed and cottonseed hulls. FDA residue limit is 0.9 ppm in cottonseed hulls when used for animal feed. Arsenic and its compounds are on the Community Right-To-Know List and in the EPA Genetic Toxicology Program *(see both)*. Moderately toxic by ingestion. A skin and eye irritant.

**MONOSODIUM PHOSPHATE** • Used as an emulsifier for cheeses, frozen eggs, and jellies. The FDA's tolerance is set at less than 5 percent. In medicine it is used as a laxative. GRAS

**MONOSODIUM PHOSPHATE DERIVATIVES OF DIGLYCERIDES** • Derived from edible fats or oils or edible fat-forming fatty acids and used as emulsifiers. GRAS

**MONOSTARCH PHOSPHATE** • A modified starch *(see)*. The final report to the FDA of the Select Committee on GRAS Substances stated in 1980 that there is no evidence in the available information that it is a hazard to the public when used as it is now and it should continue its GRAS status with limitations on amounts that can be added to food. E

**MONOTERPENES** • Found in parsley, carrots, broccoli, cabbage, cucumbers, squash, yams, tomatoes, eggplant, peppers, mint, basil, citrus fruits, they have some antioxidant properties. Have been found to inhibit cholesterol production and aid protective enzyme activity.

**MONOUNSAT FAT** • The listing on food labels for monounsaturated fat *(see)*.

**MONOUNSATURATED FATS** • The saturation of fat refers to the chemical structure of its fatty acids. Saturated fats, which are hard at room temperature—lard, suet, and butterfat are examples—consist primarily of fatty acids that contain a full load of hydrogen atoms. Monounsaturated fatty acids, however, can accept two additional hydrogen atoms. Fats that contain primarily monounsaturated fatty acids are liquid at room temperature but may become thickened when refrigerated. Polyunsaturated fats, which are liquid at room temperature, remain so even in the refrigerator and consist mainly of fatty acids that can hold four or more additional hydrogen atoms. Examples of polyunsaturated fats are safflower and corn oil. Examples of monounsaturated fats are olive oil, rapeseed oil, cashew oil, and avocado oil. Once thought to be neutral, monounsaturated fats may be beneficial for blood cholesterol levels. This concept evolved from epidemiological studies of populations who have a diet high in monounsaturated and a lower artery disease rate than populations eating a high saturated fat diet. Some even suggest that monounsaturated fats may be even better than polyunsaturates in preventing heart disease. Monounsaturated fats are manufactured normally by the body and are believed to be less likely to have some of the side effects thought to occur with polyunsaturates.

**MONTAN WAX FATTY ACIDS OXIDATIVELY REFINED, POLYHYDRIC ALCOHOL DIESTERS** • Permitted for coating on foods. *See* Fatty Acids. E

**MORANTEL** • Paratect. Suiminth. A worm medicine used to treat cattle that leaves residues in beef and milk. The FDA limits residues to 1.2 ppm to 4.8 ppm in cattle and to 0.4 ppm in milk.

**MORELLONE** • *See* 3-Benzyl-4-Heptanone.

**MORPHOLINE** • Salt Fatty Acid. Coating on fresh fruits and vegetables. Broad industrial uses. A cheap solvent for resins, waxes, and dyes. Also used as a corrosion inhibitor, antioxidant, plasticizer, viscosity improver, insecticide, fungicide, local anesthetic, and antiseptic. Irritating to the eyes, skin, and mucous membranes. It may cause kidney and liver injury and can produce sloughing of the skin. *See* Diethanolamine for potential cancer hazard. NIL

**MORPHOLINE STEARATE** • A coating and preservative. *See* Morpholine.

**MOSCHUS MOSCHIFERUS** • *See* Musk Tonquin.

**MOUNTAIN ASH EXTRACT** • The extract from the berries of a European tree or shrub, *Sorbus aucuparia,* used as an antioxidant. High in vitamin C, it has been used by herbalists to cure and prevent scurvy and to treat nausea.

**MOUNTAIN MAPLE EXTRACT** • Extract from a tall shrub or bushy tree found in the eastern United States. Used in chocolate, malt, and maple flavoring for beverages, ice cream, ices, candy, and baked goods. NUL

**MOUNTAIN MAPLE EXTRACT SOLID** • *Acer spicatum.* Flavoring that occurs in mountain maple tree sap; used in baked goods and candy. ASP

**MOXIDECTIN** • Cydectin. Antibacterial used for treatment and control of infections and infestations of certain internal and external parasites. The FDA allows a 0.5 percent solution as a pour-on for beef and nonlactating dairy cattle at 500 micrograms per kilogram of body weight. The ADI *(see)* is 4 mg/kg/day and residue tolerance in cattle is 50 ppb in muscle and 200 ppb in liver.

**MSG** • *See* Monosodium Glutamate.

**MUCILAGE** • A solution in water of the sticky principles of vegetable substances. Used as a soothing application to the mucous membranes.

**MUCOSA** • Mucous membrane lining the digestive tract.

**MUCOUS MEMBRANES** • The thin layers of tissues that line the respiratory and intestinal tracts and are kept moist by a sticky substance called mucous. These membranes line the nose and other parts of the respiratory tract, and are found in other parts of the body that have communication with air.

**MUGWORT** • The extract of the flowering herb, *Artemisia absinthium. See* Wormwood and Sesquiterpene Lactones.

**MUIRA PUAMA EXTRACT** • A wood extract used as an aromatic resin and fat.

**MULBERRY EXTRACT** • An extract of the dried leaves of various species of *Morus,* which produces a purplish black dye.

**MULLEIN FLOWERS** • The flowers from common mullein, *Verbascum thapsus.* Used as a flavoring in alcoholic beverages only. EAF

**MUSHROOM EXTRACT** • The extract of various species of mushrooms used as an oil and plasticizer.

**MUSK** • The dried secretion from preputial follicles of the northern Asian small hornless deer, which has musk in its glands. Musk is a brown, unctuous, smelly substance associated with attracting the opposite sex and is promoted by stores for such purposes. As musk ambrette it is used in fruit, cherry, maple, mint, nut, black walnut, pecan, spice, and vanilla flavorings for beverages, ice cream, ices, candy, baked goods, gelatin desserts, pudding, and chewing gum. Musk tonquin is used in fruit, maple, and molasses flavorings for beverages, ice cream, ices, candy, baked goods, and syrups. As musk ketone it is used in chewing gum and candy. At one time musk was a stimulant and nerve sedative in medicine. Can cause allergic reactions. GRAS

**MUSK AMBRETTE** • Found to have neurotoxic properties. This was first discovered in 1967 when mice were fed varying levels of musk ambrette. Since dietary consumption of musk ambrette is generally very low, the impact was discounted and no assessment was made of exposures from fragranced products. In 1985, after studies were published on the neurotoxic effect and it was determined that the musk ambrette was readily absorbed through the skin, the fragrance industry recommended that musk ambrette not be used in direct skin contact products. Musk ambrette had been used in fragranced products before the 1920s. It reportedly damages the myelin, the covering of nerve fibers. It can cause photosensitivity *(see)* and contact dermatitis. Musk ambrette is still used in food but not in cosmetics. ASP

**MUSK KETONE** • Among the nitro musks, musk ketone (MK) as a synthetic compound with a typical musk odor is widely used in cosmetics and is permitted as a food additive. Exposure to it, experiments in animals and with humam cells indicate, might increase the susceptibility to health hazards caused by carcinogens in humans. ASP

**MUSK TONQUIN** • *Moschus moshieferus.* Derived from Siberian deer musk. At the posterior part of its abdomen, there is a small sac situated immediately under the skin, which opens a little in front of the preputial orifice, and which is filled with a thick fluid, abounding particularly in the rutting season. This fluid, in the dried state, is musk. It is removed from the animal in its sac, and dried in this state for exportation. Synthetic musk tonquin is on the American market. GRAS. EAF

**MUSTARD** • Black, Brown, and Red. Pulverized dried, ripe seeds of the mustard plant *(Brassica nigra)* grown in Europe and Asia and naturalized in the United States. Used in mustard and spice flavorings for condiments (5,200 ppm) and meats (2,300 ppm). Used as an emetic. Has been used as a counterirritant on the skin. It has an intensely pungent odor that can be irritating. It is a strong skin blisterer and is used diluted as a counterirritant *(see)* and rubefacient *(see).* Can cause allergic reactions. May cause a sensitivity to light. On the FDA list of products to be studied for possible mutagenic, teratogenic, subacute, and reproductive effects. The final report to the FDA of the Select Committee on GRAS Substances stated in 1980 that it should continue its GRAS status with no limitations other than good manufacturing practices. ASP

**MUSTARD** • Yellow and White. The pulverized dried, ripe seeds of the mustard plant *(Brassica alba)* grown in Europe and Asia and naturalized in the United States. Used in sausage and spice flavoring for beverages, baked goods, condiments (8,200 ppm), meats, and pickles (3,800 ppm). Used as an emetic. The final report to the FDA of the Select Committee on GRAS Substances stated in 1980 that it should continue its GRAS status with no limitations other than good manufacturing practices. *See* Mustard, Black, for toxicity. ASP

**MUSTARD FLOUR** • Made from the preground seeds and is quite hot. It is used as a base in prepared mustards and many barbecue rubs. ASP

**MUSTARD OIL** • *See* Allyl Isothiocyanate. ASP

**MUSTARD, ORIENTAL** • As the name implies oriental mustard originated in China. This seed is golden yellow in color with seed diameter about 2 mm. Volatile oil is present at approximately 1 percent which gives oriental mustard a hot pungent taste with an inherent bitter note. Protein content is lower than in yellow mustard and there are no gums present in the bran. ASP

**MUTAGEN** • A substance that induces mutation *(see)*.

**MUTAGENIC** • Having the power to cause mutations. A mutation is a sudden change in the character of a gene that is perpetuated in subsequent divisions of the cells in which it occurs. It can be induced by the application of such stimuli as radiation, certain food chemicals, or pesticides. Certain food additives such as caffeine have been found to "break" chromosomes.

**MUTATION** • A change in the genetic material of the cell.

**MYCLOBUTANIL** • A systemic fungicide used on fruits. The FDA limits residue to 5 ppm in apple or grape pomace for feed; 10 ppm in grapes and raisins; 25 ppm in raisin waste; 0.05 ppm residue in meat, fat, and meat by-products of cattle, goats, hogs, poultry, and sheep; 0;3 ppm residue in liver of cattle, goats, hogs, poultry, and sheep; 0.02 ppm in eggs.

**MYCOBUTANOL** • A fungicide. The FDA allows 5 ppm residue in apples; 10 ppm residue in grapes; 10 ppm residue in raisins; 25 ppm in raisin waste; 0.05 ppm in meat, fat, and meat by-products of cattle, goats, hogs, poultry, and sheep; and 0.3 ppm residue in liver of cattle, goats, and hogs.

**MYCOPROTEIN** • A food made by continuous fermentation of the fungus *Fusarium gramineurum.* The fungus is grown in a large fermentation tower to which oxygen, nitrogen, glucose, minerals, and vitamins are continually added. After harvesting, the fungus is heat treated to reduce its RNA content to World Health Organization recommended levels before being filtered and drained. The resulting sheet of fungal mycelia is mixed with egg albumen which acts as a binder. Flavoring and coloring may also be added. The mycoprotein is then textured to resemble meat, before being sliced, diced, or shredded. A range of food products based on mycoprotein have been manufactured and sold in Europe. The line of mycoprotein products includes burgers, fillets, and nuggets; deli slices; and ready-to-eat meals in chilled and/or frozen formats. Mycoprotein is claimed to be a source of protein, fiber, biotin, iron, and zinc, and is low in saturated fat. GRAS

**MYRCENE** • A synthetic flavoring additive that occurs naturally in galbanum oil, pimenta oil, orange peel, palma rosa oil, and hop oil. Pleasant aroma. Used in fruit, root beer, and coriander flavorings for beverages, ice cream, ices, candy, and baked goods. A moderate skin and eye irritant. Found to cause birth defects in experimental animals. ASP

**MYRISTALDEHYDE** • A synthetic citrus and fruit flavoring additive for beverages, ice cream, ices, candy, baked goods, and gelatin desserts. ASP

**MYRISTIC ACID** • Used in shampoos, shaving soaps, and creams. A solid organic acid that occurs naturally in butter acids (such as nutmeg butter to the extent of 80 percent), oil of lovage, coconut oil, mace oil, cire d'abeille, in palm seed fats, and in most animal and vegetable fats. Used in butter, butterscotch, chocolate, cocoa, and fruit flavorings for beverages, ice cream, ices, candy, baked goods, and gelatin desserts. A human skin irritant. Causes mutations in laboratory animals. ASP

**MYRISTICA FRAGRANS** • *See* Mace and Nutmeg.

**MYRISTYL ALCOHOL** • *See* Fatty Alcohols. ASP

**MYROXYLON** • *See* Balsam Peru.

**MYRRH** • Extract, Gum, Oil. One of the gifts of the Magi, it is a yellowish to reddish brown, aromatic bitter gum resin that is obtained from various trees, especially from East Africa and Arabia. Used by the ancients as an ingredient of incense and perfumes and as a remedy for localized skin problems. The gum is used in fruit, liquor, tobacco, and smoke flavorings for beverages, baked goods, ice cream, ices, candy, chewing gum, and soups. The oil is used in honey and liquor flavorings for beverages, ice cream, ices, candy, and baked goods. The gum resin has been used to break up intestinal gas and as a topical stimulant. EAF

**MYRTLE LEAVES** • *Myrtus communis.* The extract of the leaves of *Myrtus communis,* a European shrub used in alcoholic beverages only. There is no reported use of the chemical and there is no toxicology information available. NUL

**MYRTLE OIL** • *Myrtus communis.* A native of the Mediterranean, the plant has been a symbol of innocence for many centuries. In fact, Aphrodite, the Greek goddess of beauty and love, apparently found refuge in a myrtle bush after she was created as a beautiful nude woman. The leaves and flowers were a major ingredient of "angel's water," a sixteenth-century skin-care lotion. Steam distillation is used on the leaves, twigs, and flowers. The most important constituents of myrtle oil (up to 0.8 percent in the leaves) are myrtenol, myrtenol acetate, limonene (23 percent), linalool (20 percent). It is used in folk medicine and reportedly relieves cramps. Used as a flavoring. Popular in aromatherapy and is said to be antibacterial. Myrtle should not be confused with wax myrtle *(Myrica cerifera)* or bog myrtle *(Myrica gale)* whose essential oils are toxic. EAF

**MYRTENOL** • Flavoring. A constituent of myrtle oil, it is the unsaturated primary alcohol. *See* Myrtle Oil. FAO/WHO *(see)* said it has no safety concern. ASP

**MYRTENYL ACETATE** • Flavoring. The FAO/WHO said it has no safety concern. NUL

**MYRTRIMONIUM BROMIDE** • *See* Quaternary Ammonium Compounds.

**NAPHTHA** • Obtained from the distillation of petroleum, coal tar, and shale oil. It is a common diluent *(see)* found in nail lacquer. Naphtha is an imprecise term because various fractions of petroleum may be called that. Among the common naphthas that are used as solvents are coal tar/naphtha and petroleum/naphtha. Naphthas are used as solvents for asphalts, road tars, pitches, paints, dry-cleaning fluids, in cleansing compounds, engraving and lithography, rubber cements, and naphtha soaps. Causes upper respiratory tract irritation. Although allowed as a food additive, there is no current reported use of the chemical, and, therefore, although toxicology information may be available, it is not being updated, according to the FDA. NUL

**NAPHTHALENE** • A coal-tar *(see)* derivative. Used to manufacture dyes, solvents, fungicides, smokeless powder, lubricants, as a moth repellent, and a topical and internal antiseptic. Naphthalene can enter your body through inhalation, skin absorption, ingestion, and eye and skin contact. It may produce damage to the eyes, liver, kidneys, skin, red blood cells, and the central nervous system. Has reportedly caused anemia in infants exposed to clothing and blankets stored in naphthalene mothballs. Can cause allergic contact dermatitis in adults and children.

**2-NAPHTHALENTHIOL** • Derived from naphthalene *(see)*, it has a disagreeable odor. It is used in the manufacture of food additives. ASP

**BETA-NAPHTHYL ANTHRANILATE** • A synthetic fruit and grape flavoring additive for beverages, ice cream, ices, baked goods, and candy. ASP

*b*-**NAPHTHYL ETHYL ETHER** • White crystals with an orange-blossom odor. Used in perfumes, soaps, and flavoring. ASP

**BETA-NAPHTHYL ISOBUTYL ETHER** • Fragarol. Flavoring. FAO/WHO says there is no safety concern but the EPA considers it a mutagen. *See a*-Pinene. ASP

*b*-**NAPHTHYL METHYL ETHER** • White crystals with a menthol odor. Used to perfume soaps. A synthetic berry, fruit, honey, and nut flavoring additive for beverages, ice cream, ices, chewing gum, candy, and baked goods.

**NARASIN** • An antibiotic in broiler chicken feed that is used to combat parasites and as a growth stimulant. It is derived from *Streptomyces aureofaciens. See* Antibiotics. ASP

**NARINGIN EXTRACT** • Naringin is in the flowers, fruit, and rind of the grapefruit tree. Most abundant in immature fruit. Extracted from grapefruit peel. Used in bitters, grapefruit, and pineapple flavorings for beverages, ice cream, ices, and liquors. GRAS. EAF

**NASTURTIUM EXTRACT** • The extract of the leaves and stems of *Tropaeolum majus*. A member of the mustard family, it has pungent, tasty leaves. It is very rich in vitamins A and C as well as containing vitamins B and $B_2$. It is soothing to the skin and supposedly has blood-thinning factors and increases the flow of urine.

**NAT** • FDA abbreviation for natural.

**NATAMYCIN** • *See* Pimaricin

**NATIONAL HEALTH and NUTRITION EXAMINATION SURVEY (NHANES)** • A series of surveys that include information from medical history, physical measurements, biochemical evaluation, physical examination, and dietary intake of population groups within the United States. The U.S. Department of Health and Human Services conducts the NHANES approximately every five years.

**NATIONAL TOXICOLOGY PROGRAM (NTP)** • Under the aegis of the National Institute of Environmental Health Sciences, the NTP tests chemicals for all federal agencies upon request. The program's staff also tests for cancer-causing additives.

**NATURAL** • The Federal Trade Commission requires that food advertised as "natural" may not contain synthetic or artificial ingredients and may not be more than minimally processed. For example, minimal processing includes such actions as washing or peeling fruits or vegetables; homogenizing milk; canning, bottling, and freezing food; baking bread; aging and roasting meats; and grinding nuts. It does not include processes that, in general, cannot be done in a home kitchen and involve certain types of chemicals or sophisticated technology; for example, chemically bleached foods will not qualify as minimally processed.

**NATURAL GAS** • A mixture of hydrocarbons obtained in petroleum-bearing areas. Its composition is 85 percent methane, 10 percent ethane, with the rest made up of propane, butane, and nitrogen. Used in making formaldehyde and other petrochemicals. NUL

**N-BUTANE** • *See* Butane.

**NDGA** • Illegal antioxidant. *See* Nordihydroguaiaretic Acid.

**NEO-DHC** • *See* Dihydrochalcones.

**NEOFOLINONE** • Occurs naturally in oil of lavender, orange leaf (absolute), palma rosa oil, rose, neroli, and oil of petitgrain. Used in citrus, honey, and neroli flavorings for beverages, ice cream, ices, candy, baked goods, chewing gum, gelatin desserts, and puddings.

**NEOHESPERIDINE DIHYDROCHALCONE** • Synthetic flavoring used in baked goods, beverages, breakfast cereals, cheese, chewing gum, condiments, egg products, fats/oils, fish products, frozen dairy, fruit ices, gelatins, gravies, hard candy, imitation dairy, instant coffee/tea, jams, meat products, milk products, nut products, grains, poultry, processed fruits, reconstituted vegetables, seasonings, snack foods, soft candy, soups, sugar substitutes, and sweet sauces. Declared GRAS by FEMA *(see)*. *See* Dihydrochalcones. EAF. E

**(d)-NEOMENTHOL** • A flavoring additive that occurs naturally in Japanese mint oil. Used in mint flavorings for beverages, ice cream, candy, and baked goods. *See* Menthol for toxicity. ASP

**NEOMYCIN SULFATE** • Biosol Veterinary. Otobiotic. Neomix Sulfate. Bactine First Aid Antibiotic. Campho-Phenique Triple Antibiotic Ointment. Mycitracin Plus Pain Reliever. Mycifradin. Myciguent. Neosporin Ointment. Neosulf. Introduced in 1951, it is one of the most widely used antibiotics for humans. The oral form is used to treat infectious diarrhea caused by *Escherichia coli (see)*. Among potential adverse reactions: headache, lethargy, ear problems, nausea, vomiting, kidney dysfunction, skin rashes, and hypersensitivity reactions. Interacts with Cephalothin, dimenhydrinate, oral anticoagulants (decreases vitamin K), IV loop diuretics, Cisplatin, methoxyflurane, and other aminoglycoside antibiotics. In animals it is used as a drug to treat cattle. FDA residue limitations are 0.25 ppm in calves and 0.15 ppm in milk.

**NEQUINATE** • An animal drug used to treat chickens. FDA residue limitation is 0.1 ppm in chickens. A coccidiostat *(see)* is added to chicken feed to inhibit or delay the onset of coccidiosis, a common and serious disease of many species that involves intestines and lungs. It has been reported in individuals with AIDS.

**NEOTAME** • On July 9, 2002, the U.S. Food and Drug Administration (FDA) announced its general use approval of neotame as a sweetener and flavor enhancer. Depending on its food application, neotame is approximately seven thousand to thirteen thousand times sweeter than sugar. It is a free-flowing, water soluble, white crystalline powder that is heat stable and can be used as a tabletop sweetener as well as in cooking applications. Used in foods and beverages, including but not limited to, chewing gum, carbonated soft drinks, refrigerated and nonrefrigerated ready-to-drink beverages, tabletop sweeteners, frozen desserts and novelties, puddings and fillings, yogurt-type products, baked goods and candies. It can also be used in both cooking and baking applications. In determining the safety of neotame, the FDA reviewed data from more than 113 animal and human studies. The safety studies were designed to identify possible toxic effects, such as cancer-causing, reproductive, and neurological effects. From its evaluation of the neotame database, the FDA was able to conclude that neotame is safe for human consumption. Some eminent scientists are wary about this sweetener as they were about another produced by the same company, aspartame *(see)*, labeling it, as they did aspartame, as toxic and carcinogenic. Neotame, like aspartame, contains aspartic acid, phenylalanine, and a methyl ester. Neuroscientists have found, in animal studies, that aspartic acid and glutamic acid load on the same receptors in the brain, cause identical brain lesions and neuroendocrine disorders, and act in an addictive fashion. People who are sensitive to processed free glutamic acid (MSG) experience similar reactions to aspartame, and people who are sensitive to aspartame experience similar reactions to MSG, providing that they ingest amounts of the substances that exceed their tolerances for MSG/aspartame. People who currently react to MSG and/or aspartame should expect to react similarly to neotame. Neotame is chemically similar to aspartame, but is broken down differently in the human digestive system. Foods containing neotame do not need to include a warning for people with phenylketonuria or PKU, as is required for foods containing aspartame. Both neotame and aspartame are made by the NutraSweet Company in Illinois. EAF

**NEROL** • A primary alcohol used in perfumes, especially in rose and orange blossom scents. Occurs naturally in oil of lavender, orange leaf, palma rosa oil, rose, neroli, and oil of petitgrain. It is colorless, with the odor of rose. Used in citrus, neroli, and honey flavorings for beverages, ice cream, ices, candy, baked goods, gelatin desserts, puddings, and chewing gum. Similar to turpentine in toxicity. ASP

**NEROLI BIGARADE OIL** • Used chiefly in cologne and in perfumes. Named for the putative discoverer, Anna Maria de La Trémoille, princess of Nerole (1670). A fragrant, pale yellow essential oil obtained from the flowers of the sour orange tree, *Citrus aurantium.* Used in berry, orange, cola, cherry, spice, and ginger ale flavorings for beverages, ice cream, ices, candy, baked goods, and chewing gum. GRAS. EAF

**NEROLIDOL** • A sesquiterpene alcohol. A straw-colored liquid with an odor similar to rose and apple. Occurs naturally in balsam Peru and oils of orange flower, neroli, sweet orange, and ylang-ylang. Also made synthetically. Used in flavoring. *See* Nerol. ASP

**NEROSOL** • *See* Nerol.

**NERYL ACETATE** • A synthetic citrus, fruit, and neroli flavoring for beverages, ice cream, ices, candy, and baked goods. ASP

**NERYL BUTYRATE** • A synthetic berry, chocolate, cocoa, citrus, and fruit flavoring additive for beverages, ice cream, ices, candy, and baked goods. ASP

**NERYL FORMATE** • Formic Acid. A synthetic berry, citrus, apple, peach, and pineapple flavoring additive for beverages, ice cream, ices, candy, and baked goods. *See* Formic Acid for toxicity. ASP

**NERYL ISOBUTYRATE** • A synthetic citrus and fruit flavoring additive for beverages, ice cream, ices, candy, and baked goods.

**NERYL ISOVALERATE** • A synthetic berry, rose, and nut flavoring additive for beverages, ice cream, ices, candy, and baked goods. ASP

**NERYL PROPIONATE** • A synthetic berry and fruit flavoring additive for beverages, ice cream, ices, candy, and baked goods. ASP

**NETSON** • *See* Acimeton.

**NETTLES** • A troublesome weed, with stingers, it has a long history and was used in folk medicine. Its flesh is rich in minerals and plant hormones. Used to make tomatoes resistant to spoilage, to encourage the growth of strawberries, and to stimulate the fermentation of humus. Hemp belongs to the nettle family.

**NEURAL TUBE DEFECT** • In simple terms, a neural tube defect (NTD) is a malformation of the brain or spinal cord (neurological system) during embryonic development. Infants born with spina bifida, where the spinal cord is exposed, can grow to adulthood but usually suffer from paralysis or other disabilities. Babies born with anencephaly, where most or all of the brain is missing, usually die shortly after birth. These NTDs make up about 5 percent of all U.S. birth defects each year. If all women of childbearing age consumed sufficient folic acid (either through diet or supplements), 50 percent to 70 percent of birth defects of the brain and spinal cord could be prevented, according to the U.S. Centers for Disease Control and Prevention. A leading CDC authority refers to folic acid as "the sleeping giant of preventive medicine" for its potential to eliminate much of the risk of NTDs—if only it were consumed in the right quantities by the right people at the right time.

**NEURON** • The basic nerve cell of the central nervous system containing a nucleus within the cell body, an axon (a trunklike projection containing neurotransmitters), and dendrites (spiderlike projections that send and receive messages).

**NEUROTENSIN** • A peptide of thirteen amino acid derivatives that helps to regulate blood sugar by its effects on a number of hormones, including insulin and glucagon. It is also thought to play a part in pain suppression.

**NEUROTRANSMITTERS** • Molecules that carry chemical messages between nerve cells. Neurotransmitters are released from a nerve cell, diffuse across the minute distance between two nerve cells (synaptic cleft) and bind to a receptor at another nerve site.

**NEUTRALIZING ADDITIVE** • A substance, such as ammonium bicarbonate or tartaric acid *(see both),* used to adjust the acidity or alkalinity of certain foods. *See* pH.

**NEW** • The U.S. Food and Drug Administration's designation that there is reported use of the substance, and an initial toxicology literature search is in progress.

**NHANES** • Abbreviation for National Health and Nutrition Examination Survey *(see).*

**NIACIN** • Nutrient. Nicotinic Acid. Nicotinamide. White or yellow crystalline powder, it is an essential nutrient that participates in many energy-yielding reactions and aids in the maintenance of a normal nervous system. It is a component of the vitamin B complex. Added to prepared breakfast cereals, peanut butter, baby cereals, enriched flours, macaroni, noodles, breads, rolls, cornmeal, corn grits, and farina. Niacin is distributed in significant amounts in liver, yeast, meat, legumes, and whole cereals. Recommended daily intake is 18 to 19 milligrams for men and 13 to 15 milligrams for women. Nicotinic acid is a component of the vitamin B complex. The final report to the FDA of the Select Committee on GRAS Substances stated in 1980 that it should continue its GRAS status with no limitations other than good manufacturing practices. ASP

**NIACINAMIDE** • Nicotinamide. Vitamin $B_3$. A dietary supplement. Also used as a skin stimulant. A white or yellow crystalline, odorless powder used to treat pellagra, a vitamin-deficiency disease, and in the assay of enzymes for substrates. No known skin toxicity. The final report to the FDA of the Select Committee on GRAS Substances stated in 1980 that it should continue its GRAS status with no limitations other than good manufacturing practices. ASP

**NIACINAMIDE ASCORBATE** • A complex of ascorbic acid *(see)* and niacinamide *(see)*. Used as a dietary supplement. *See* Niacin.

**NICARBAZIN** • Nicoxin. Nicrazin. An animal drug used in chicken feed to inhibit or delay coccidiosis *(see)*. FDA residue limitations are 4 ppm in uncooked muscle, liver, skin, and neck of chickens.

**NICKEL** • Metal that occurs in the earth. Lustrous, white, hard metal that is used as a catalyst for the hydrogenation *(see)* of fat. Nickel may cause dermatitis in sensitive individuals and ingestion of large amounts of the soluble salts may cause nausea, vomiting, and diarrhea. Food is the major source of nickel exposure, with an average intake for adults estimated to be approximately 100 to 300 micrograms per day. The final report to the FDA of the Select Committee on GRAS Substances stated in 1980 that it should continue its GRAS status with no limitations other than good manufacturing practices. A number of nickel compounds cause cancer including nickel acetate, nickel chloride, nickel hydroxide, and nickel carbonate. *See* Nickel Sulfate. ASP

**NICKEL SULFATE** • Occurs in the earth's crust as a salt of nickel. It has a sweet, astringent taste. Used as a mineral supplement. It acts as an irritant and causes vomiting when swallowed in larger doses. Its systemic effects include blood vessel, brain, and kidney damage, and nervous depression. Also listed as a cancer-causing agent by inhalation. The lethal dose varies widely. The dose in guinea pigs is 62 milligrams per kilogram.

**NICOTINAMIDE** • *See* Niacin.

**NICOTINAMIDE-ASCORBIC ACID COMPLEX** • A dietary supplement in multivitamin preparations. NIL

**NICOTINIC ACID** • *See* Niacin.

**NIGER GUTTA** • *Ficus platyphylla.* The coagulated latex from a tree that is mixed with chicle *(see)* to make chewing gum. ASP

**NIL** • The U.S. Food and Drug Administration's designation that although listed as added to food, there is no current reported use of the substance, and therefore, although toxicology information may be available in PAFA *(see)*, it is not being updated.

**NIOSH** • Abbreviation for National Institute of Occupational Safety and Health. Congress set up this institute in 1970 to play a key role in helping protect workers and their health on the job. The agency was to conduct occupational-health research; to inspect manufacturers' plants at employers' and workers' requests, and for its own studies; and to recommend standards for safe exposure to hazardous substances. NIOSH is supposed to work closely with OSHA, the organization responsible for setting the legally permitted exposures to hazards in the workplace. NIOSH, through its investigations into plant conditions and studies of already available data, provides OSHA with the scientific background needed to determine these rules. When a workplace crisis arises, the two agencies often work in tandem to find out how the workers were harmed and to help the industry correct the problem. Under the law, NIOSH documents summarizing its findings about a hazard should be used by OSHA to help in setting health and safety regulations for the industry.

**NISIN PREPARATION** • Crystals from *Streptococcus lactis* used as a preservative and antimicrobial additive in cheese spreads, semolina, clotted cream, and tapioca puddings and similar products. Also used in surface treatment of hard, semihard, and semisoft cheese, and dried and cured sausages. The FDA limits residue to 250 ppm in the finished product. It is also used in canned vegetables and fruit. GRAS. ASP. E. The European Parliament said in 2003 that nisin should not be used because it could cause resistance to antibiotics in humans. This review should be undertaken now, and as long as the safety of these additives cannot be scientifically guaranteed, they should be banned.

**NISPERO** • Sapodilla. An evergreen tree that often reaches a height of sixty feet or more. In southern Mexico, this species is tapped for its ingredient for chewing gum. EAF

**NITAPYRIN** • An insecticide. The FDA limits residues in cottonseed to 1.0 ppm; in the fat, meat, and meat by-products of cattle, goats, hogs, poultry, and sheep to 0.05 ppm.

**NITARSONE** • A feed additive.

**NITER** • *See* Nitrate.

**NITRATE** • Potassium and Sodium. Potassium nitrate, also known as saltpeter and niter, is used as a color fixative in cured meats. Sodium nitrate, also called Chile saltpeter, is used as a color fixative in cured meats. Both nitrates are used in matches and to improve the burning properties of tobacco. They combine with natural stomach saliva and food substances (secondary amines) to create nitrosamines, powerful cancer-causing additives. Nitrosamines have also been found in fish treated with nitrates. Researchers at the Michael Reese Medical Center's Department of

Pathology in Chicago induced cancer in mice by giving single doses of one three-thousandth (0.3 microgram) of a gram of nitrosamine for each gram of the animal's weight. This is in contrast to the way other researchers have induced cancer in laboratory animals with nitrosamines by using repeated small doses or single large doses. The tumors that developed were analogous to human liver tumors. Nitrosamines caused pancreatic cancer in hamsters, similar to human pancreatic cancers. Nitrates have caused deaths from methemoglobinemia (it cuts off oxygen to the brain). Because nitrates are difficult to control in processing, they are being used less often. However, they are still employed in long curing processes, such as for country hams, as well as dried, cured, and fermented sausages. In the early 1970s, baby-food manufacturers voluntarily removed nitrates from their products. The U.S. Department of Agriculture, which has jurisdiction over meats, and the FDA, which has jurisdiction over processed poultry, has asked manufacturers to show that the use of nitrates is safe. Efforts to ban nitrates have failed because manufacturers claim there is no good substitute for them. Nitrates change into nitrites on exposure to air. Our major intake of nitrates in foodstuffs comes primarily from vegetables or water supplies that are high in nitrate content, or from nitrates used as additives in meat curing. Nitrates are natural constituents of plants. They occur in very small amounts in fruits but are high in certain vegetables—spinach, beets, radishes, eggplant, celery, lettuce, collards, and turnip greens—as high as more than 3,000 ppm. The two most important factors responsible for large accumulations of nitrates in vegetables are the high levels of fertilization with nitrate fertilizers and the tendency of the species to accumulate nitrate. Nitrites and/or nitrates are food additives when combined in curing premixes with spices and/or other flavoring or seasoning ingredients that contain or constitute a source of secondary or tertiary amines, including but not limited to essential oils, disodium inosinate, disodium guanylate, hydrolysates of animal or plant origin (such as hydrolyzed vegetable protein), oleoresins of spices, soy products, and spice extractives. Such food additives may be used only after the establishment of an authorizing food additive regulation. A food additive petition supported by data demonstrating that nitrosamines are not formed in curing premixes containing such food additives is required to establish safety. ASP

**NITRITE** • Potassium and Sodium. Potassium nitrite is used as a color fixative in the more than $125 billion a year cured-meat business. Sodium nitrite has the peculiar ability to react chemically with the myoglobin molecule and impart red-bloodedness to processed meats, to convey tanginess to the palate, and to resist the growth of *Clostridium botulinum* spores. It is used as a color fixative in cured meats, bacon, bologna, frankfurters, deviled ham, meat spread, potted meats, spiced ham, Vienna sausages, smoke-cured tuna fish products, and in smoke-cured shad and salmon. Nitrite combines with natural stomach and food chemicals (secondary amines) to create nitrosamines, powerful cancer-causing additives. The U.S. Department of Agriculture, which has jurisdiction over processed meats, and the FDA, which has jurisdiction over processed poultry, asked manufacturers to show that the use of nitrites was safe and that nitrosamines were not formed in the products as preliminary tests showed in bacon. Processors claimed there was no alternate chemical substitute for nitrite. They said alternate processing methods could be used, but the products would not look or taste the same. Baby-food manufacturers voluntarily removed nitrites from baby foods in the early 1970s. The FDA found that adding vitamin C to processed meats prevents or at least retards the formation of nitrosamines. In May 1978, the USDA announced plans to require bacon manufacturers to reduce their use of nitrite from 150 to 120 ppm and to use preservatives that retard nitrosamine formation. Processors would have been required to keep nitrosamine levels to 10 ppm under the interim plan. But in August 1978 a new concern about nitrite was raised. The USDA and the FDA issued a joint announcement that the substance had been directly linked to cancer by a Massachusetts Institute of Technology study. That work was later disputed. In 1982, amyl and butyl nitrites used by homosexual men were linked to Kaposi's sarcoma and other abnormalities of the immune system. Researchers at the Michael Reese Medical Center linked infinitesimal amounts of nitrite to cancer in young laboratory mice, especially in the liver and lungs. Dr. Koshlya Rijhsinghani and her colleagues gave single doses of one three-thousandth (0.3 microgram) of a gram of nitrosamine for each gram of the animal's weight. This method differs from the way other researchers have induced cancer in mice with nitrosamines by repeated small doses of single large doses. Nitrosamines also produce cancer in hamsters similar to pancreatic cancers in humans. In 1980, the FDA revoked its proposed phase-out because manufacturers said there was no adequate substitute for nitrites. In 1977 Germany banned nitrites and nitrates except in certain species of fish. However, a Committee on Nitrite and Alternative Curing Additives in Food, formed by the National Research Council in the United States, concluded that there was no single additive or process that could replace nitrite completely: "Several chemical and physical treatments appear to be comparable in inhibiting outgrowth of *Clostridium botulinum* spores in types of meat products but none confers the color and flavor that consumers have come to expect in nitrite-cured meats." Until the all-purpose additive comes along or until consumer preference changes, the best compromise probably will be continued use of nitrite in conventional amounts with vitamins C and E added to block formation of nitrosamines, or the use of smaller amounts of nitrite in combination with biological acidification, irradiation, or the chemicals potassium sorbate, sodium hypophosphite, or fumarate esters, the committee said. To reduce nitrosamines in bacon, the U.S. Department of Agriculture requires meat packers to add sodium ascorbate or sodium erythorbate (vitamin C) to the curing brine. This offers only a partial barrier because ascorbate is soluble in water and its activity in fat is limited. Vitamin E, however, inhibits nitrosation in fatty tissues. The committee suggested that both C and E be added to provide more complete protection. If you must eat nitrite-laced meats, include a food or drink high in vitamin C at the same time—for example, orange juice, grapefruit juice, cranberry juice, or lettuce. In 2003, the FDA put in abeyance *(see)* a request by the U.S. Department of Commerce to permit sodium nitrite in white fish. ASP

**NITRO-** • A prefix denoting one atom of nitrogen and two of oxygen. Nitro also denotes a class of dyes derived from coal tars. Nitro dyes can be absorbed through the skin. When absorbed or ingested they can cause a lack of oxygen in the blood. Chronic exposure may cause liver damage. *See* FD and C Colors.

**NITROCELLULOSE** • Any of several esters *(see)* obtained as white fibrous flammable solids by adding nitrate to cellulose, the cell walls of plants. Used in food processing and in skin protective creams, nail enamels, and lacquers.

**NITROFURANS** • Nitrofuran antibiotics have been banned in Europe but are administered to poultry in New Zealand. Some shrimp and prawns from Southeast Asia, and freshwater catfish from Canada have been found to have nitrofuran residues. Nitrofurans are a group of chemicals which are banned for use in Europe, the United States, and Canada in food-producing animals. Consumption of foods contaminated with nitrofurans may pose a human health risk related to the inherent toxicity of the drug and the potential to cause allergies and cancer. However, a number of flavorings are derived from furans *(see)*.

**NITROFURAZONE** • Aldomycin. Furacillin. Coxistat. Nitrofurazone. A once widely used antibiotic in animal feed for pigs and poultry. The FDA withdrew permission for its use in 1991. A human sensitizer. IARC review and EPA Genetic Toxicology Program *(see both)*. Potential adverse reactions include kidney toxicity, redness, itching, burning, water retention, severe blistering, and allergic skin rash. It is also listed as a cancer-causing agent.

**3-([5-NITROFURFURYLIDENE] AMINO)2-OXAZOLIDONE** • Bifuron. Corizium. Diafuron. Enterotoxon. Furazone. Furazolidone. Furoxone. A widely used antiprotozoal *(see)* drug in animals, particularly for pigs. It is also a human medication for diarrhea and enteritis caused by *Giardia lamblia* and *Vibrio cholerae*. Taken by mouth, it works inside the intestines to counteract cholera, colitis, and/or diarrhea caused by the bacteria. Potential adverse reactions include joint pain, fever, itching, skin rash or redness, nausea, vomiting, diarrhea, stomach pain, headache, and sore throat. Severe high blood pressure and other side effects may occur if combined with MAO inhibitors *(see)*, ephedrine, and tricyclic antidepressants with this drug. Severe high blood pressure and other undesirable side effects may occur if the following are eaten or drunk while taking this drug: aged cheese, caviar, yeast or protein extracts, fava or broad beans; smoked or pickled meat, poultry, or fish; fermented sausages (bologna, pepperoni, salami, summer sausage) or other fermented meat; or any overripe fruit. You should not drink dark beer, red wine, sherry, or liqueurs. If the human medication is taken, the above foods and drinks are to be avoided for at least two weeks after stopping furazolidone. The FDA says that residues must be zero in meat sent to market, but who can do adequate testing for its presence all the time?

**NITROGEN** • A gas that is 78 percent by volume of the atmosphere and essential to all living things. Odorless. Used as a preservative for cosmetics, in which it is nontoxic. In high concentrations, it can asphyxiate. Toxic concentration in humans is 90 ppm; in mice, 250 ppm. GRAS. ASP. E

**NITROGEN OXIDES** • Nitrous Oxide *(see)*, Nitric Oxide, Nitrogen Dioxide, Nitrogen Trioxide, Nitrogen Pentoxide. Bleaching additive for cereal flour, nitrogen dioxide is a deadly poison gas. Short exposure may cause little pain or discomfort but several days later, fluid retention and inflammation of the lungs can cause death. About 200 ppm can be fatal. There is no reported use of the chemical and there is no toxicology information available, according to the FDA. NUL

**3-NITRO-4-HYDROXYPHENYLARSONIC ACID** • Roxarsone. Tufts of pale yellow needles used to control intestinal infections and to improve growth and feed efficiency. FDA limits are 0.5 ppm as arsenic in muscle meat and eggs of chickens as residue; 2 ppm as arsenic in edible by-products, turkey, and swine; 0.5 ppm as arsenic in muscle tissue and by-products other than liver and kidney. *See* Arsenic.

**NITROMIDE with SULFANITRAN** • A feed additive used in chicken feed. Both ingredients are antibacterials. FDA tolerance is zero residue for nitromide in uncooked edible chicken.

**4-NITROPHENYLARSONIC ACID** • Nitarsone. An animal feed drug used to combat intestinal parasites chiefly affecting turkeys, chickens, and other birds. The FDA says the feed additive is not to be used at a level in excess of the amount reasonably required to accomplish the intended effect. An arsenic compound, it is on the Community Right-To-Know List *(see)*. Poison by ingestion.

**NITROSYL CHLORIDE** • Nonexplosive, very corrosive, reddish yellow gas, intensely irritating to the eyes, skin, and mucosa. Used as a bleaching additive for cereal flour. Inhalation may cause pulmonary edema and hemorrhage. NIL

**NITROUS OXIDE** • Laughing Gas. A whipping additive for whipped cosmetic creams and a propellant in pressurized cosmetic containers. Slightly sweetish odor and taste. Colorless. Used in rocket fuel. Less irritating than other nitrogen oxides but narcotic in high concentrations and it can asphyxiate. GRAS. ASP. E

**NNS** • FDA abbreviation for nonnutritive sweetener.

**NOAEL** • No Observed Adverse Effect Level. *See* NOEL.

**NOBELITIN** • A substance found in citrus fruit that has been found to have anticancer properties in laboratory studies.

**NOEL** • Test results that show a given dose of a substance has a No Observed Effect Level or sometimes called a No Observed Adverse Effect Level. The safety factor usually has a value of one hundred in the case of a NOEL derived from long-term animal study, on the assumption that humans are ten times as sensitive as the test animal used and that there is a tenfold range of sensitivity within the human population.

**NONADIENAL** • Cucumber Aldehyde or Alcohol. A flavoring additive used in various foods. A moderate skin irritant. ASP

*g*-**NONALACTONE** • Aldehyde C-18. Prunolide. Coconut Aldehyde. A synthetic berry, coconut, fruit, and nut flavoring additive for beverages, ice cream, ices, candy, baked goods, gelatin desserts, chewing gum, and icings. ASP

**NONALOL** • *See* Nonyl Alcohol.

**NONANAL** • Pelargonic Aldehyde. Colorless liquid with an orange-rose odor. A synthetic flavoring that occurs naturally in lemon oil, rose, sweet orange oil, mandarin, lime, orris, and ginger. Used in lemon and fruit flavorings for beverages, ice cream, ices, candy, baked goods, chewing gum, and gelatin desserts. A severe skin irritant. *See* Aldehyde. ASP

**1,3-NONANEDIOL ACETATE** • Colorless to slightly yellow mixture of isomers used in synthetic berry and fruit flavorings for beverages, ice cream, ices, candy, and baked goods. *See* Nonanoic Acid and Acetic Acid. ASP

**1,4-NONANEDIOL DIACETATE** • Synthetic flavoring with a fresh, green cucumber odor. NIL

**NONANNOYL 4-HYDROXY-3-METHOXY BENZYLAMIDE** • Perlargonyl Vanillylamide. A synthetic spice flavoring additive for candy, baked goods, and condiments.

**NONANOIC ACID** • Pelargonic Acid. Nonoic acid. Nonglic Acid. Occurs in the oil of pelargonium plants such as the geranium. Used in berry, fruit, nut, and spice flavorings for beverages, ice cream, ices, candy, baked goods, and shortenings. Can be very irritating to the skin. ASP

**2-NONANOL** • *See* Nonyl Alcohol. ASP

**3-NONANON-1-YL-ACETATE** • A synthetic berry, rose, fruit, and cheese flavoring additive for beverages, ice cream, ices, candy, and baked goods. NIL

**2-NONENAL** • *See* Isoamyl Nonanoate. ASP

**CIS-2-NONEN-1-OL** • Synthetic flavoring with a melonlike odor. ASP

**NONFAT DRY MILK** • The solid residue produced by removing the water from defatted cow's milk. Comparisons between whole and dry milk: 100 grams fluid whole milk contains 68 calories; 87 grams of water; 3.5 grams of protein; 3.9 grams of fat; 0.7 gram of ash; 4.9 grams of carbohydrates; 118 milligrams of calcium; 93 milligrams of phosphorus; 0.1 milligram of iron; 50 milligrams of sodium; 140 milligrams of potassium; 160 international units of vitamin A; 0.04 milligram of vitamin $B_1$; 0.17 milligram of $B_2$; 0.1 milligram of nicotinic acid; and 1 milligram of vitamin C. Total calories for one cup of milk is 166. Nonfat dry milk has 362 calories per 100 grams; 3.5 grams of water; 35.6 grams of protein; 1 gram of fat; 7.9 grams of ash; 52 grams of total carbohydrates; 1,300 milligrams of calcium; 1,030 milligrams of phosphorus; 0.6 milligrams of iron; 77 milligrams of sodium; 1,130 milligrams of potassium; 40 international units of vitamin A; 0.35 milligrams of vitamin $B_1$; 196 milligrams of vitamin $B_2$; 1.1 milligrams of nicotinic acid; and 7 milligrams of vitamin C. The total calories for a tablespoon of dry nonfat milk is 28. *See* Milk.

**NONNUTRITIVE SWEETENERS** • Sugar substitutes that contain no calories. Saccharin and cyclamates *(see both)* are examples.

**NONYL ACETATE** • An ester produced by the reaction of nonyl alcohol and acetic acid *(see)*. Pungent odor suggestive of mushrooms but when diluted it resembles the odor of gardenias. Used for beverages, ice cream, ices, candy, and baked goods. ASP

**NONYL ALCOHOL** • Nonalol. A synthetic flavoring, colorless to yellow with a citronella oil odor. Occurs in oil of orange. Used in butter, citrus, peach, and pineapple flavorings for beverages, ice cream, ices, candy, and chewing gum. Also used in the manufacture of artificial lemon oil. In experimental animals it has caused central nervous system and liver damage. ASP

**NONYL CARBINOL** • *See* 1-Decanol.

**NONYL ISOVALERATE** • A synthetic fruit and hazelnut flavoring additive for beverages, ice cream, ices, candy, and baked goods. ASP

**γ-NONYL LACTONE** • Yellowish to almost colorless liquid with a coconutlike odor. Used in flavors. *See* Nonyl Alcohol.

**NONYL NONANOATE** • Nonyl Pelargonate. Liquid with a floral odor used in flavors, perfumes, and organic synthesis. *See* Nonyl Alcohol.

**NONYL OCTANOATE** • Synthetic flavoring. An oily liquid with a sweet, rose, mushroom odor. NIL

**NOOTKATONE** • From a cypress tree grown in northwest Washington State and British Columbia. It is named after the Nootka people who populated the area. It smells like cedar. It is used in flavorings. ASP

**NOPINENE** • *See* b-Pinene.

**NORBIXIN** • From the seeds of *Bixa orellana* used in a suspension of vegetable oil for coloring in food. *See* Annatto. E

**NORDIHYDROGUAIARETIC ACID (NDCA)** • An antioxidant used in brilliantines and other fat-based cosmetics. Occurs in resinous exudates of many plants. White or grayish white crystals. Lard containing 0.01 percent NGDA stored at room temperature for nineteen months in diffuse daylight showed no appreciable rancidity or color change. It was used as an antioxidant in prepared pie-crust mix, candy, lard, butter, ice cream, and pressure-dispensed whipped cream. Canada banned the additive in food in 1967 after it was shown to cause cysts and kidney damage in a large percentage of rats tested. The FDA removed it from the GRAS list in 1968 and prohibited its use in products over which it has control. The U.S. Department of Agriculture, which controls antioxidants in lard and animal shortenings, banned it in 1971. BANNED

**NOREPINEPHRINE** • Noradrenaline. A hormone released by the adrenal gland, it possesses the ability to stimulate epinephrine but has minimal inhibitory effects. It has little effect on the lungs' smooth muscles and metabolic processes and differs from epinephrine in its effect on the heart and blood vessels.

**NORFLURAZON** • An herbicide used in feed and hops used for animal feed. FDA tolerance limits are 1 ppm in dried citrus molasses, 3 ppm in citrus pulp, and 0.1 ppm in milk, fat, meat, and meat by-products of cattle, goats, hogs, poultry, and sheep.

**NORVALINE** • A protein amino acid *(see)* soluble in hot water and insoluble in alcohol. *See* Valeric Acid.

**NOTE** • A distinct odor or flavor. Top note is the first note normally perceived when a flavor is smelled or tasted; usually volatile and gives "identity." Middle or main note is the substance of the flavor, the main characteristic. Bottom note is what is left when top and middle notes disappear. It is the residue when the aroma or flavoring evaporates.

**NOVATONE** • *See* Acetanisole.

**NOVOBIOCIN** • Albamycin. An antibiotic from *Streptomyces niveus,* it is used in animal feed for beef, chicken, duck, and turkey. FDA residue limitations are 0.1 in milk, 1 ppm in cattle, chickens, turkeys, and ducks. Moderately toxic by ingestion.

**NUL** • The U.S. Food and Drug Administration's designation that there is no reported use of the substance and there is no toxicology information available in PAFA *(see)*.

**NTP** • Abbreviation for National Toxicology Program *(see)*.

**NUCLEIC ACIDS** • Originally isolated from the cell nuclei, they are carriers and mediators of genetic information. There are two types, DNA (deoxyribonucleic acid) and RNA (ribonucleic acid). DNA has one less oxygen molecule in its component sugar ribose and is double-stranded. The messages carried by DNA are carried out by RNA. The two types are components of all cells so that any food in which cells are concentrated are rich sources of nucleic acids. Organ meats, poultry, and fish are examples. Butter, fat, fruits, milk, nuts, vegetables, and carbohydrates are low in nucleic acids. *See* Purines, Disodium Guanylate, and Disodium Inosinate.

**NUTMEG** • Nutmeg is not a nut, but the kernel of an apricotlike fruit. A natural flavoring extracted from the dried ripe seed of *Myristica fragrans.* Used in cola, vermouth, sausage, eggnog, and nutmeg flavorings for beverages, ice cream, ices, baked goods (2,000 ppm), condiments, meats, and pickles. The oil is used in loganberry, chocolate, lemon, cola, apple, grape, muscatel, rum, sausage, eggnog, pistachio, root beer, cinnamon, dill, ginger, mace, nutmeg, and vanilla flavorings for beverages, ice cream, ices, candy, baked goods, chewing gum, condiments, meats, syrups, and icings. In common household use since the Middle Ages, nutmeg is still a potentially toxic substance. Ingestion of as little as three whole seeds or 5 to 15 grams of grated spice can cause flushing of the skin, irregular heart rhythm, absence of salivation, and central nervous system excitation, including euphoria and hallucinations. GRAS. ASP

**NUTMEG OLEORESIN** • Nutmeg is the dried, ripe seed, and mace is the dried aril which envelops the shell containing the seed of trees of *Myristica* species, principally *Myristica fragrans.* The ground seed is the spice nutmeg; the ground arillus is the spice mace. Oil of nutmeg and oil of mace are the essential oils obtained by steam distillation of nutmeg and mace, respectively. Nutmeg and mace owe their characteristic aroma to these essential oils. Mace oleoresin is a butterlike product obtained by pressing. A similar product, nutmeg butter, can be pressed from nutmeg *(see).* ASP

**NUTR** • FDA abbreviation for nutrient.

**NUTRACEUTICALS** • One term used to describe substances in or parts of a food that may be considered to provide medical or health benefits.

**NUTRASWEET** • *See* Aspartame.

**NUTRS** • FDA abbreviation for nutritive sweetener.

**NUTRIENT CONTENT CLAIM** • Descriptor. A claim on a food product that directly or by implication characterizes the level of a nutrient in the food such as "low fat" or "high in oat bran." Nutrient content claims are also known as descriptors.

**NYSTATIN** • Mycostatin. Nadostine. Nilstat. Nystex. O-V Statin. Yellow to light tan powder with a cereallike odor, it is used in animal feed for poultry and pigs. The FDA requires zero residue in eggs, swine, and poultry. Antifungal medication introduced in 1954. It is used in human medicine to treat oral, vaginal, and intestinal infections caused by *Candida albicans* (Moniliales) and other *Candida* species. In cream or ointment it is used to treat infant eczema, itching around the anus or vagina, and localized forms of candidiasis. Potential adverse reactions include nausea, vomiting, and diarrhea. Skin applications may cause occasional contact dermatitis from preservatives in some formulations. Nystatin is in the EPA Genetic

Toxicology Program. Moderately toxic by ingestion. Causes birth defects in experimental animals.

# O

**OAK BARK EXTRACT** • *Quercus alba.* Oak Chip Extract. The extract from the white oak used in bitters and whiskey flavorings for beverages, ice cream, ices, candy, whiskey (1,000 ppm), and baked goods. Contains tannic acid *(see)* and is exceedingly astringent. The Indians used it in a wash for sore eyes and as a tonic. ASP

**OAKMOSS, ABSOLUTE** • Any one of several lichens, *Evernia* spp., that grow on oak trees and yield a resin for use as a fixative *(see)* in perfumery. Stable green liquid with a long-lasting characteristic odor. Soluble in alcohol. Used in fruit, honey, and spice flavorings for beverages, ice cream, ices, candy, baked goods, gelatin desserts, condiments, and soups. A common allergen in aftershave lotions. ASP

**OAKMOSS, CONCRETE** • *Evernia prunasti.* Oakmoss concrete is prepared by hydrocarbon solvent extraction of the lichen *Evernia prunasti* collected mainly from oak trees in Yugoslavia, France, Italy, Corsica, Morocco, Hungary, and various central European countries. The lichen is often soaked in lukewarm water twenty-four hours prior to extraction. Oakmoss concrete is a solid, waxy, dark green mass with a phenolic woody, slightly tarlike but delicate and pleasant odor, reminiscent of seashore, forest, bark, wood, green foliage, and tannery. Strong sensitizing potential. *See* Oakmoss, Absolute. EAF

**OAK WHITE, CHIPS EXTRACT** • *See* Oak Bark Extract. ASP

**OAK WOOD, ENGLISH** • *Quercus robur.* Used as a coloring in alcoholic beverages only. ASP

**OATS** • Whole grain oats contain more soluble fiber than other whole grains such as wheat, corn, or rye. They contain more protein and lipids than other grains. Oats contain naturally occurring phytochemicals that have been associated with protection from a variety of chronic diseases. Whole grains contain naturally occurring phytoestrogens, which have been linked to decreased risk of hormone-related diseases such as breast cancer. Oats were discovered to lower cholesterol in 1963. They are also a good source of selenium, iron, calcium, manganese, magnesium, zinc, and copper.

**OAT BRAN** • The broken coat of oats, *Avena sativa. See* Oats and Oat Flour.

**OAT EXTRACT** • The extract of the seeds of oats, *Avena sativa. See* Oat Flour.

**OAT FLOUR** • Flour from the cereal grain that is an important crop grown in the temperate regions. Light yellowish or brown to weak greenish or yellow powder. Slight odor; starchy taste. Makes a bland ointment for cosmetic treatments, including soothing baths.

**OAT GUM** • A plant extract used as a thickener and stabilizer in foods and cosmetics. Also an antioxidant in butter, creams, and candy up to 1.5 percent. It is used as a thickener and stabilizer in pasteurized cheese spread and cream cheese. In foods, it can cause an allergic reaction including diarrhea and intestinal gas. NUL

**OATMEAL** • Meal obtained by grinding of oats from which the husks have been removed.

**OBESITY or OVERWEIGHT** • Although precise definitions vary among experts, overweight has been traditionally defined as 10 to 20 percent above an optimal weight for height, derived from statistics. Some scientists argue that the amount and distribution of an individual's body fat is a significant indicator of health risk and therefore should be considered in defining overweight. Abdominal fat has been linked to more adverse health consequences than fat in the hips or thighs. Thus, calculations of waist-to-hip ratio are preferred by some health experts to help determine if an individual is overweight.

**OCIMENE** • A terpene obtained from sweet basil oil. Used in flavors and perfumes. ASP

**OCIMUM BASILICUM** • *See* Basil Extract.

**OCOTEA CYMBA RUM OIL** • An oil obtained by steam distillation from the wood of a Brazilian tree. Used chiefly as a source of safrole *(see),* a natural oil, and as a substitute for sassafras *(see).*

**OCTADECANOIC ACID** • Abracol S.L.G. Dermagine. Distearin. Orbon. Stearic Acid, Monoester with Glycerol. Pure white or cream-colored, waxlike solid used as a coating additive, emulsifier, lubricant, solvent, and texturizer in baked goods, shortening, fruits, ice cream, nuts, peanut butter, puddings, and whipped toppings. *See* Stearic Acid. ASP

**9-OCTADECENOIC ACID** • *See* Oleic Acid.

**1-OCTADECANOL** • *See* Stearic Acid.

**9-OCTADECENAL** • A flavoring determined GRAS by the Expert Panel of the Flavor and Extract Manufacturers Association.

**OCTAFLUOROCYCLOBUTANE** • A nonflammable gas. A refrigerant, propellant, and aerating additive in foamed or sprayed food products. Used alone or in combination with carbon dioxide or nitrous oxide *(see both).* Nontoxic when used alone. NIL

**OCTAHYDROCOUMARIN** • One of the newer flavoring additives. See Coumarin. ASP

**OCTALACTONE** • D and G. *See* Lactic Acid. ASP

**OCTANAL** • Octanaldehyde. Found in many essential oils *(see)* including a number of citrus oils, it is a colorless to light yellow liquid with an orange odor. It is used as a flavoring additive in many foods. Mildly toxic by ingestion. ASP

**2,3-OCTANEDIONE** • A flavoring determined GRAS by FEMA *(see)*.

**OCTANOIC ACID** • Colorless, oily liquid with a bad odor derived from coconut, it is used as an antimicrobial additive in other food additives and as a defoaming additive, flavoring additive, and lubricant. It is used in baked goods, soft candies, cheese, fats, frozen dairy desserts, gelatins, meat products, oils, packaging materials, puddings, and snack foods. Mildly toxic by ingestion and a skin irritant, it has caused mutations in experimental animals. FDA residue limits are 0.0013 percent in baked goods; 0.04 percent in frozen dairy desserts; 0.005 percent in meat products; 0.005 percent in soft candies; 0.016 percent in snack foods; and 0.001 percent in other food categories when used in accordance with good manufacturing practices. GRAS as an indirect additive. ASP

**N-OCTANOIC (CAPRYLIC) ACID** • Preservative and other miscellaneous uses. Can be up to 0.013 percent in baked products; 0.04 percent in cheeses; 0.005 percent in fats and oils; 0.016 percent in snack foods; 0.001 percent in all other food categories. Used in a lye peeling solution for fruits and vegetables and is a component of sanitizing solution. GRAS in cheese wraps. *See* Caprylic Acid.

**1-OCTANOL** • Caprylic Alcohol. Used in the manufacture of flavorings. Occurs naturally in oil of lavender, oil of lemon, oil of lime, oil of lovage, orange peel, and coconut oil and has a penetrating, aromatic scent. May cause skin rash. ASP

**3-OCTANOL** • Colorless liquid with a strong nutty odor; used as a flavoring additive in various foods. It is a moderate skin and eye irritant. ASP

**2-OCTANONE** • A synthetic fruit and cheese flavoring additive for beverages, ice cream, ices, candy, and baked goods.

**3-OCTANONE** • A synthetic flavoring that occurs naturally in oil of lavender. Used in citrus, coffee, peach, cheese, and spice flavorings for beverages, ice cream, ices, candy, and baked goods. ASP

**1-OCTEN-3-OL** • A synthetic fruit and spice flavoring additive for beverages, ice cream, ices, candy, baked goods, condiments, and soups. ASP

**1-OCTENYL SUCCINIC ANHYDRIDE** • A starch modifier incorporating up to 3 percent of the weight of the product. Limited to 2 percent in combination with aluminum sulfate *(see)*.

**OCTODECANOIC ACID** • *See* Stearic Acid.

**OCTOXYNOL** • Waxlike emulsifiers, dispersing additives, and detergents derived from phenol *(see)* and used as a surfactant. The numbers from -1 to -70 after the additive signify the viscosity.

**OCTYL ACETATE** • Acetic Acid. Octyl Ester. A colorless liquid with an orange-jasmine scent, it is used as a flavoring additive in various foods. Moderately toxic by ingestion. ASP

**OCTYL ALCOHOL, SYNTHETIC** • Caprylic Alcohol. Colorless, viscous liquid soluble in water and insoluble in oil. Used as a solvent in the manufacture of food additives. Occurs naturally in the oils of lavender, lemon, lime, lovage, orange peel, and coconut. It has a penetrating aromatic scent. Moderately toxic by ingestion. A skin irritant. Has caused mutations in experimental animals. NUL

***n*-OCTYL BICYCLOHEPTENE DI CARBOXIMIDE** • Dimethyl Carbate. Pyrodone. Octacide 264. A widely used insecticide in various foods. FDA residue tolerance is 10 ppm. Moderately toxic by ingestion and skin contact. Has caused adverse reproductive effects in experimental animals. Large doses can cause central nervous system stimulation followed by depression.

**OCTYL BUTYRATE** • Butyric Acid. A synthetic strawberry, butter, citrus, fruit, cherry, melon, peach, pineapple, pumpkin, and liquor flavoring additive for beverages, ice cream, ices, candy, and baked goods. ASP

**OCTYL FORMATE** • Formic Acid. A synthetic flavoring, colorless with a fruity odor. Used in citrus and fruit flavorings for beverages, ice cream, ices, candy, and baked goods. *See* Formic Acid for toxicity. ASP

**OCTYL GALLATE** • A salt of gallic acid made from the tannins of nutgalls or from *Penicilliun glaucum* or *Aspergillus niger,* it is used as an antioxidant in margarine with a limit of 0.02 percent set by the FDA. Mildly toxic by ingestion. When heated to decomposition emits acrid smoke and irritating fumes. *See* Gallates. ASP. E

**OCTYL HEPTANOATE** • A synthetic citrus, coconut, and fruit flavoring for beverages, ice cream, ices, candy, and baked goods. ASP

**OCTYL ISOBUTYRATE** • Isobutyric Acid. A synthetic citrus, fruit, melon, peach, liquor, and wine flavoring additive for beverages, ice cream, ices, candy, and baked goods. ASP

**OCTYL ISOVALERATE** • Isovaleric Acid. A synthetic berry, butter, citrus, apple, cherry, grape, honey, and nut flavoring additive for beverages, ice cream, ices, candy, and baked goods. NIL

**OCTYL OCTANOATE** • Octanoic Acid. A synthetic citrus, grape, and pineapple flavoring additive for beverages, ice cream, ices, candy, and baked goods. NIL

**OCTYL PHENYLACETATE** • Phenylacetic Acid. A synthetic berry, apple, banana, grape, peach, pear, and honey flavoring additive for beverages, ice cream, ices, candy, and baked goods. NIL

**OCTYL PROPIONATE** • Propionic Acid. A synthetic berry, citrus, and melon flavoring additive for beverages, ice cream, ices, candy, and baked goods. ASP

**ODORLESS LIGHT PETROLEUM HYDROCARBONS** • Liquids with a faint odor used as coating additives, defoamers, and in insecticide formulations for beet sugar, eggs, fruits, pickles, vegetables, vinegar, and wine. *See* Petroleum.

**OIL OF NIOBE** • *See* Methyl Benzoate.

**OIL OF SASSAFRAS, SAFROLE FREE** • This flavoring without the saf-role is permitted in foods. Oil of Sassafras that is used to correct disagreeable odors in cosmetics is 80 percent safrole. May produce allergic reactions in sensitive persons. Banned in foods.

**OITICICA OIL** • Rosewood Oil. The tree grows wild and only in Brazil. The oil is extracted from oiticica nuts. Its use is limited and is employed as a substitute for tung oil or linseed oil when the price of either of these products prohibit their use. NUL

**OLEAMIDE** • An additive that prevents sticking to pans. *See* Oleic Acid.

**OLEANDOMYCIN HYDROCHLORIDE** • An antibiotic produced by *Streptomyces antibioticus* used in animal feed for chickens, swine, and turkeys. Moderately toxic by ingestion. The FDA requires zero residue in chickens, turkeys, and swine for market.

**OLEIC ACID** • Obtained from various animal and vegetable fats and oils. Colorless. On exposure to air, it turns a yellow to brown color and develops a rancid odor. Used as a defoaming additive; as a synthetic butter, cheese, and spice flavoring additive for beverages, ice cream, ices, candy, baked goods, and condiments; as a lubricant and binder in various foods; and as a component in the manufacture of food additives. It caused tumors when injected under the skin of rabbits in 3,120-milligram doses per kilogram of body weight and when painted on the skin of mice in 62-milligram doses per kilogram of body weight. The final report to the FDA of the Select Committee on GRAS Substances stated in 1980 that it should continue its GRAS status with no limitations other than good manufacturing practices. ASP

**OLEIC ACID DERIVED FROM TALL OIL FATTY ACIDS** • Used as a component in the manufacture of food-grade additives on fresh citrus fruit and in processing beet sugar and yeast. *See* Oleic Acid and Tall Oil. ASP

**OLEINIC ACID** • *See* Oleic Acid.

**OLEORESIN** • A natural plant product consisting of essential oil and resin extracted from a substance, such as ginger, by means of alcohol, ether, or acetone. The solvent alcohol, for example, is percolated through the ginger. Although the oleoresin is very similar to the spice from which it is derived, it is not identical because not all the substances in the spice are extracted. Oleoresins are usually more uniform and more potent than the original product. The normal use range of an oleoresin is from one-fifth to one-twentieth the corresponding amount for the crude spice. Certain spices are extracted as oleoresins for color rather than for flavor. Examples of color-intensifying oleoresins are those from paprika and turmeric.

**OLESTRA** • Sucrose Polyester. Olean. A fat substitute developed by Procter and Gamble that cannot be digested. It has no calories. It is aimed at replacing conventional fats in french fries and baked desserts. It is a mixture of esters *(see)* of sucrose *(see)* prepared by the reaction of sucrose with edible fatty acids *(see)*. It occurs as a solid, soft gel, or liquid at room temperature depending on the fatty acids used. It looks, cooks, and tastes like ordinary fat, but adds no fat or calories to foods with which it is cooked. Potato chips made with Olean, for example, contain no fat and only 75 calories versus 10 grams of fat and 150 calories in regular chips. Use of olestra in foods requires addition of specific amounts of vitamins A, D, E, and K to these foods. Olestra may cause abdominal cramping and loose stools in some individuals and the FDA requires this observation to be on the labels of all foods made with olestra. Henry Blackburn, M.D., of the University of Minnesota, writing an editorial in the April 11, 1996, issue of the *New England Journal of Medicine* wrote he was concerned that olestra would be used for a long time by millions of people without good direct evidence that its use "would benefit them, reduce weight among the obese, prevent weight gain among those at risk for conditions associated with obesity, or reduce caloric intake substantially in representative population—all purported reasons for adding Olestra to the food supply." He said there is no regulatory requirement as there is for drugs that the petitioner demonstrate a benefit. He said members of the committee that approved olestra expressed the view that the gastrointestinal symptoms associated with it were at most an "annoyance," not a serious health problem, and required only a warning label on the product. He wrote that this shifts the responsibility to the public when experts knowingly approved a "gastrointestinal hazard." The American Medical Association, on the other hand, noted that approximately 150 studies, including 43 clinical trials, had been conducted with olestra in advance of FDA approval, making it "one of the most thoroughly tested foodstuffs to come to market in America." The FDA is amending the food additive regulations to remove the requirement for the label statement prescribed specifically for savory snack products that contain olestra. This action is in response to a petition filed by the Procter and Gamble Co., the developer of olestra. The regulation became effective August 5, 2003. The change meant that manufacturers no longer need to display the 1996 label statement on products containing olestra informing consumers that olestra may cause abdominal cramping and loose stools in some individuals, that it inhibits the body's absorption of vitamins A, D, E, and K and other nutrients, and that these vitamins have been added to compensate for olestra's effects on these nutrients. Consumers will now see an asterisk after each of these added fat-soluble vitamins listed in the ingredient statement of products containing olestra. The asterisk will reference the statement, "Dietarily insignificant." The FDA approved olestra in 1996 for use in savory snacks like potato chips, cheese puffs, and crackers. As part of that approval, the FDA required manufacturers to add vitamins A, D, E, and K to olestra-containing foods to compensate for olestra's effects on these fat-soluble vitamins. The FDA still requires manufacturers to continue adding vitamins A, D, E, and K to such products. EAF

**OLIBANUM EXTRACT** • Frankincense Extract. The extract of *Boswellia carteri* of various species. The volatile, distilled oil from the gum resin of a plant found in Ethiopia, Egypt, and Arabia. It was one of the gifts of the Magi. It is used in cola, fruit, and spice flavorings for beverages, ice cream, ices, candy, and baked goods. EAF

**OLIBANUM, GUM** • The dried, gummy exudation obtained from various species of Burseraceae trees. The main species are *Boswellia carteri, Boswellia frererana, Boswellia papyrifera,* and many others. Main producing countries are Somalia, Ethiopia, southeast Arabia, and India. It is used as a thickener and stabilizer in beverages, candies, chewing gums, confectioneries, dairy products, gelatins, nut products, puddings and canned vegetables. Recent studies have found positive influence of olibanum on rheumatism. In classical Indian medicine, gum olibanum is used as an anti-inflammatory remedy. EAF

**OLIBANUM OIL** • Processed olibanum gum *(see)*. EAF

**OLIBANUM, RESINOID** • Processed olibanum gum *(see)*. *See also* Frankincense. EAF

**OLIVE OIL** • A monounsaturated fat *(see)*. Superior to mineral oils in penetrating power. It is a pale yellow or greenish fixed oil obtained from ripe olives grown around the Mediterranean Sea. May cause allergic reactions. Has been reported to be beneficial to blood cholesterol.

**OMEGA-3 FATTY ACIDS** • Found in fish oils, reported to lower fats in the blood and thus reduce the risk of coronary artery disease. The FDA had denied a claim for omega-3 fatty acids in reducing the risk of coronary heart disease because studies relating fish intake and risk of coronary heart disease were "conflicting and inconsistent." The FDA said the most compelling evidence was a well-controlled study that showed fish consumption may reduce the chance of death from a second heart attack. However, these studies did not establish that the effects were due specifically to omega-3 fatty acids. Data revealed that omega-3 may raise blood LDL (the bad kind of cholesterol) of people with high blood fats and may interfere with blood glucose control in diabetics. *See* Fish Oil.

**ONION EXTRACT** • Extract of the bulbs of onion, *Allium cepa,* discovered in Asia. Used in meat, onion, and spice flavorings for beverages, ice cream, ices, baked goods, condiments, meats, and pickles. Skin irritant. When heated to decomposition it emits acrid smoke and irritating fumes. GRAS

**ONION OIL** • A volatile oil with a strong and permanent odor. ASP

**OPOPANAX GUM** • Bisabol. An odorous, myrrh-type gum resin from southern European or African herbs. Once used in medicine. Now used as a flavoring. EAF

**OPONANAX OIL** • An odorous gum resin formerly used in medicine and believed to be obtained from Hercules Allheal. A fragrance ingredient. EAF

**ORANGE B** • Dull orange crystals derived from coal tar. Coloring for casing of frankfurters and sausages. The color additive was limited to not more than 150 ppm by weight of finished food. In 1978, the FDA said use could result in exposure of consumers to beta-naphthylamine, a known cancer-causing additive. Although it was permanently listed by the FDA, the only manufacturer of it stopped making it. See FD and C Colors. ASP

**ORANGE BITTER, FLOWERS and PEEL** • Essential oil is used as a flavoring. GRAS. ASP

**ORANGE BLOSSOMS** • Orange blossoms, absolute, is a natural flavoring derived from the fruit of the bitter plant species. Used in citrus and fruit flavorings for beverages, ice cream, ices, candy, baked goods, and chewing gum. The flowers provide a natural flavoring extract for citrus and cola flavorings for beverages (2,000 ppm). The orange leaf extract is used as a natural fruit flavoring for beverages, ice cream, ices, and baked goods. Orange peel bitter oil is expressed from the fresh fruit and is used in orange and fruit flavorings for beverages, ice cream, ices, candy, gelatin desserts, chewing gum, and liquors. GRAS. ASP

**ORANGE CRYSTALS** • *See* Methyl *b*-Naphthyl Ketone.

**ORANGE FLOWER, BITTER OIL** • *See* Nerol. ASP

**ORANGE LEAF** • *See* Orange Blossoms. ASP

**ORANGE OIL** • Sweet Orange Oil. Yellow to deep orange, highly volatile, unstable liquid with a characteristic orange taste and odor expressed from the fresh peel of the ripe fruit of the sweet orange plant species. Used in orange and fruit flavorings for beverages, ice cream, ices, candy, baked goods, gelatin desserts, and chewing gum. Inhalation or frequent contact with oil of orange may cause severe symptoms such as headache, dizziness, and shortness of breath. May cause allergic reaction in the hypersensitive. Omitted from hypoallergenic cosmetics. ASP

**ORANGE PEEL, BITTER OIL** • *See* Orange Blossoms. ASP

**ORANGE PEEL, SWEET EXTRACT** • From the fresh rind of the fruit. Sweetish, fragrant odor; slightly bitter taste. Used in orange and ginger ale flavorings for beverages, ice cream, ices, candy, and baked goods. GRAS. ASP

**ORANGE PEEL, SWEET OIL (TERPENELESS)** • From the fresh rind of the fruit. Sweetish, fragrant odor; slightly bitter taste. Used in orange and fruit flavoring for beverages, ice cream, ices, candy, baked goods, gelatin desserts, and puddings. ASP

**ORANGE, SWEET and LEAF, FLOWER, PEEL** • Used as a flavoring. *See* Orange Blossoms and Orange Oil. ASP

**OREGANO** • Mexican Oregano. Mexican Sage. Origanum. The wild marjoram *(see)* plant, but spicier, ordinarily found in Eurasia. Used in loganberry, cherry, sausage, root beer, and spice flavorings for beverages, baked goods, condiments (2,800 ppm), and meats. *See* Origanum Oil for toxicity. GRAS. ASP

**ORGANIC** • The term usually means produce grown without pesticides, herbicides, or synthetic fertilizers on land that has been free of such chemicals for one to seven years. It also means animals supposedly not subjected to antibiotics, hormones, or other additives.

**ORGANOPHOSPHATES** • Compounds containing phosphorus that belong to several groups including:

- Phospholipids or phosphatides, which are widely distributed in plants and animals. Lecithin is an example.
- Esters of phosphinic and phosphonic acids, which are used as plasticizers, insecticides, resin modifiers, and flame retardants.
- Pyrophosphates, which are the basis for many insecticides that inhibit cholinesterase, an enzyme necessary for nerve transmission. Tetraethyl pyrophosphate (TEPP), which is highly toxic, was developed during World War II.
- The phosphoric esters of glycerol, glycol, and other fatty alcohols that are used in fertilizers.

Organophosphates, pesticides, and insecticides can be extremely toxic. They can kill quickly or slowly depending on the amount of exposure. Most are easily absorbed through the skin, eyes, stomach, and lungs. Among the organophosphate pesticides in use are azinphosmethyl, carbophenothion, demeton, diazinon, dichlorvos, dicrotophos, dimethoate, endothion, EPN, fensulfothion, fenthion, Hinosan, methyl demeton, methyl parathion, mevinphos, mipafox, monocrotophos, naled, parathion, phorate, phosphamidon, Phostex, tetraethyl pyrophosphate (TEPP), thiometon, and trichlorfon. Organophosphorous compounds are now being studied for delayed neurotoxicity. It can occur in factory workers exposed during the production of organophosphorous chemicals, which are used as plasticizers, lubricants, fire retardants, and pesticides.

**ORIGAN** • *See* Oregano.

**ORIGANOL** • *See* 4-Carvomenthenol.

**ORIGANUM OIL** • The volatile oil is obtained by steam distillation from a flowering herb. Yellowish red to dark brown, with a pungent odor. Used in vermouth, sausage, root beer, and spice flavorings for beverages, ice cream, ices, candy, baked goods, condiments, and meats. A teaspoonful can cause illness and less than an ounce has killed adults. GRAS. ASP

**ORIZANOL** • The ester of ferulic acid and terpene alcohol widely found in plants used in flavorings. *See* Cinnamate.

**ORMETOPRIM** • A feed additive. The FDA tolerance for residue in edible tissues of chickens, ducks, turkeys, salmoids, and catfish is 0.1 ppm.

**ORRIS** • Orris Root Oil. White Flag. Love Root. Made from the roots of the plant. Yellowish, semisolid, and fragrant oil. Distilled for use in raspberry, blackberry, strawberry, violet, cherry, nut, and spice flavorings for beverages, ice cream, ices, candy, baked goods, gelatin desserts, chewing gum, and icings. *See* Orris Root Extract. EAF

**ORRIS ROOT EXTRACT** • Obtained from dried orris root. Has an intense odor and is used in perfumery. Used in chocolate, fruit, nut, vanilla, and cream soda flavorings for beverages, ice cream, ices, candy, baked goods, gelatin desserts, and chewing gum. Causes frequent allergic reactions. EAF

**ORTHOPHENYL PHENOL** • Preservative. *See* Phenol. E

**ORYZALIN** • Surflan. Dirimal. An herbicide used in peppermint and spearmint. The FDA limits it to 0.1 ppm in peppermint and spearmint oil.

**OSHA** • Occupational Safety and Health Administration, U.S. Department of Labor. An agency that establishes workplace safety and health regulations.

**OSMANTHUS, ABSOLUTE** • A widely distributed genus of evergreen shrubs or trees, family Oleaceae, with inconspicuous bisexual flowers, and sometimes foliage resembling holly. Used in flavoring and perfumery. EAF

**OSTEOPOROSIS** • A skeletal disease, in which the bones lose mass and density, the pores in bones enlarge, and the bones generally become fragile. Osteoporosis often is not diagnosed until a fracture occurs, most commonly in the spine, hip, or wrist. The National Osteoporosis Foundation says about 1.5 million such fractures occur each year in the United States.

**OTHER CARB** • The listing for other carbohydrates on food labels. *See* Carbohydrates.

**OURICURY WAX** • The wax exuded from the leaves of a Brazilian palm tree. The hard brown wax has the same properties and uses as carnauba wax (*see*).

**OXALIC ACID** • Occurs naturally in many plants and vegetables, particularly in the Oxalis family; also in many molds. Some plants such as rhubarb, spinach, and amaranthus are high in it. Oxalic acid has the ability to bind some metals such as calcium and magnesium and has therefore been suspected of interfering with the metabolism of these minerals.

**OXAMYL** • A pesticide. The FDA residue tolerance in pineapple bran is 6 ppm.

**OXAZOLINE** • A series of synthetic waxes that are versatile and miscible with most natural waxes and can be applied to the same uses.

**OX BILE** • Oxgall. Emulsifier from the fresh bile of male castrated bovines. Brownish green or dark green; viscous. Characteristic odor. Bitter, disagreeable taste. Used in dried egg whites up to 0.1 percent. The final report to the FDA of the Select Committee on GRAS Substances stated in 1980 that it should continue its GRAS status with no limitations other than good manufacturing practices. ASP

**OXFENDAZOL** • Crystals from chloroform and methanol, it is used in a suspension to kill worms in cattle. FDA tolerance is 0.8 ppm in cattle liver.

**OXIDIZED POLYETHYLENE** • The resin produced by exposing polyethylene *(see)* to air. It is used as a protective coating or component of protective coatings for fresh avocados, bananas, beets, coconuts, eggplant, garlic, grapefruit, lemons, limes, mangoes, muskmelons, onions, oranges, papaya, peas (in pods), pineapple, plantain, pumpkin, rutabaga, squash (acorn), sweet potatoes, tangerines, turnips, watermelon, Brazil nuts, chestnuts, filberts, hazelnuts, pecans, and walnuts (all nuts in shells). E

**OXIDIZED TALLOW** • A defoaming component used in yeast and beet sugar production in reasonable amounts required to inhibit foaming. *See* Tallow Flakes.

**OXIDIZER** • A substance that causes oxygen to combine with another substance. Oxygen and hydrogen peroxide are examples of oxidizers.

**OXIDES OF NITROGEN** • Used as a bleaching additive in flour. *See* Nitrogen.

**OXIRANE (CHLOROMETHYL)-, POLYMER WITH AMMONIA, REACTION PRODUCT** • Food processing additive to make a product more alkaline. NUL

**3-OXOBUTANAL, DIMETHYL ACETAL** • Artificial flavoring. NIL

**3-OXODECANOIC ACID GLYCERIDE** • Artificial flavoring. NUL

**3-OXODODECANOIC ACID GLYCERIDE** • Artificial flavoring. NUL

**3-OXOHEXADECANOIC ACID GLYCERIDE** • Artificial flavoring. NUL

**3-OXOHEXANOIC ACID DIGLYCERIDE** • Artificial flavoring. NUL

**3-OXOOCTANOIC ACID GLYCERIDE** • Artificial flavoring. NUL

**2-OXOPENTANEDIOIC ACID** • Synthetic flavoring. FAO/WHO *(see)* says there is no safety concern. EAF

**2-OXO-3-PHENYLPROPIONIC ACID** • Synthetic flavoring. EAF

**3-OXOTETRADECANOIC ACID GLYCERIDE** • Synthetic flavoring. NUL

**OXIDIZED STARCH** • *See* Modified Starch. E

**OXYFLUORFEN** • Orange solid used as an herbicide in cottonseed oil, mint oil, and soybean oil. Limitation of 0.25 ppm in the oils.

**OXYGEN** • Non-metallic gas used in the manufacture of food additives. E

**OXYSTEARIN** • A mixture of the glycerides *(see)* of partially oxidized stearic acids *(see)* and other fatty acids *(see)*. Occurs in animal fat and used chiefly in manufacture of soaps, candles, cosmetics, suppositories, pill coatings. Tan, waxy. Used as a crystallization inhibitor in cottonseed and soybean cooking. In salad oils up to 0.125 percent. Also used as a defoamer in the production of beet sugar and yeast. The Select Committee of the Federation of American Societies for Experimental Biology advising on food additives recommended further study of this additive. The final report to the FDA of the Select Committee on GRAS Substances stated in 1980 that while no evidence in the available information on it demonstrates a hazard to the public at current use levels, uncertainties exist, requiring that additional studies be conducted. GRAS status has continued since 1980 while tests were being completed and evaluated. ASP

**OXYTETRACYCLINE** • An antibiotic substance used in feed to increase growth and found in edible tissue of chickens and turkeys. The FDA permits a residue in the birds of up to 3 ppm in liver and 1 ppm in uncooked muscle, fat, and skin of chickens and turkeys. It is used in combination with carbomycin *(see)* in the drinking water of chickens. It is used in tablet form for cattle. Because it is an antimicrobial, it may cause sensitivity to light, nausea, inflammation of the mucous membranes of the mouth, and diarrhea. *See* Antibiotics.

**OZOKERITE** • Ceresin. A naturally occurring waxlike mineral; a mixture of hydrocarbons. Colorless or white when pure; horrid odor. Upon refining, it yields a hard, white, microcrystalline wax known as ceresin *(see)*. An emulsifier and thickening additive used in lipstick and cream rouge.

**OZONE** • A colorless gas or dark blue liquid used as an antimicrobial additive in bottled water. Under the EPA Genetic Toxicology Program *(see)*. Toxic effects are from inhalation. GRAS. EAF

# P

**P-4000** • 5-Nitro-2-propoxyaniline. Substance that is four thousand times sweeter than sugar without an aftertaste. Used in some European countries but banned in the United States because of potential toxic effects. BANNED

**PABA** • *See* para-Aminobenzoic Acid.

**PAFA** • Stands for the U.S. Food and Drug Administration's Priority-based Assessment of Food Additives.

**PALATONE** • *See* Maltol.

**PALE CATECHU** • *See* Catechu Extract.

**PALM KERNEL OIL** • The oil from the fruit of the oil palm *Elaeis guineensis.* A fatty solid with a sweet, nutty flavor. Used as a coating additive, emulsifying additive, and texturizer in confectionery products and margarine. GRAS

**PALM OIL** • Palm Butter. Palm Tallow. Yellow-brown, buttery, edible solid at room temperature. Oil palms are native to central Africa and Malaysia. A fatty mass with a faint violet odor. Used as a shortening, as a substitute for tallow, and in making soaps and ointment.

**PALM OIL GLYCERIDE** • *See* Palm Oil.

**PALMA ROSA OIL** • Geranium Oil. The volatile oil obtained by steam distillation from a variety of partially dried grass grown in East India and Java. Used in rose, fruit, and spice flavorings for ice cream, ices, candy, and baked goods. Believed as toxic as other essential oils, causing illness after ingestion of a teaspoonful and death after ingestion of an ounce. A skin irritant. GRAS

**PALMAMIDE MEA** • A mixture of ethanolamides of the fatty acids derived from palm oil *(see)*.

**PALMITAMIDE** • A substance that keeps food from sticking to a container. Used in packaging material. *See* Palmitic Acid.

**PALMITATE** • Salt of palmitic acid *(see)* occurs in palm oil, butter fat, and most other fatty oils and fats.

**PALMITIC ACID** • A mixture of solid organic acids obtained from fats consisting chiefly of palmitic acid with varying amounts of stearic acid *(see)*. It is white or faintly yellow and has a fatty odor and taste. Palmitic acid occurs naturally in allspice, anise, calamus oil, cascarilla bark, celery seed, butter acids, coffee, tea, and many animal fats and plant oils. It forms about 21 percent of cow's milk. Obtained from palm oil, Japan wax, or Chinese vegetable tallow. Used in butter and cheese flavorings for seasoning preparations. ASP

**PALMITOYL HYDROLYZED ANIMAL PROTEIN** • *See* Hydrolyzed Protein.

**PALMITOYL HYDROLYZED MILK PROTEIN** • The condensation product of palmitic acid chloride and hydrolyzed milk protein. *See* Hydrolyzed and Milk.

**PANCREATIC EXTRACT** • *See* Pancreatin.

**PANCREATIN** • Hi-Vegi-Lip. Pancreatin Enseals. A preparation of pancreatic hormones used to aid digestion of starches, fats, and proteins. Potential adverse reactions include nausea and diarrhea. Antacids may negate pancreatin's beneficial effects. Should be used cautiously in people who are allergic to pork. GRAS. NUL

**PANSY EXTRACT** • The extract obtained from *Viola tricolor*. Flavoring in alcoholic beverages only. Also used as a coloring in cosmetics. NUL

**PANTHENOL** • Dexpanthenol. Vitamin B Complex Factor. A viscous, slightly bitter liquid used as a medicinal supplement in foods to aid digestion and in liquid vitamins. It is good for human tissues.

*d*-**PANTOTHENAMIDE** • Vitamin B Complex. Vitamin $B_5$. Made synthetically from the jelly of the queen bee, yeast, and molasses. Cleared as a source of pantothenic acid in foods for special dietary use. Pantothenic acid (common sources are liver, rice bran, and molasses) is essential for metabolism of carbohydrates, fats, and other important substances. Nerve damage has been observed in patients with low pantothenic acid. It helps release energy from carbohydrates in the breakdown of fats. Children and adults need from 5 to 10 milligrams per day. *See* Calcium Pantothenate. NIL

**PANTOTHENIC ACID** • Vitamin $B_5$. A necessity in human diets. It helps metabolize fats and proteins. Nontoxic.

*d*-**PANTOTHENYL ALCOHOL** • The final report to the FDA of the Select Committee on GRAS Substances stated in 1980 that it should continue its GRAS status with no limitations other than good manufacturing practices. *See* Calcium Pantothenate. NUL

**PANTOTHENYL ETHYL ETHER** • The ethyl ether of the B vitamin panthenol *(see).*

**PANTOTHENYL ETHYL ETHER ACETATE** • The ester of acetic acid and the ethyl ether of the B vitamin panthenol *(see).*

**PAPAIN** • A proteinase enzyme for meat tenderizing. Prepared from papaya, a fruit, and *Carica papaya,* grown in tropical countries. Used for clearing beverages. Added to enriched farina to reduce cooking time. Used medically to prevent adhesions. It is deactivated by cooking, but because of its protein digesting ability it can dissolve necrotic material with disastrous results. The usual grade used in food digests about thirty-five times its weight of lean meat. It may cause allergic reactions. Has caused birth defects in experimental animals. The final report to the FDA of the Select Committee on GRAS Substances stated in 1980 that it should continue its GRAS status with no limitations other than good manufacturing practices.

**PAPAYA** • A fruit grown in tropical countries. It contains an enzyme, papain, used as a meat tenderizer and medicinally to prevent adhesions. It is deactivated by cooking. Because of its protein-digesting ability, it can dissolve necrotic (dead) material. It may cause allergic reactions. *See* Papain. ASP

**PAPRIKA** • The finely ground pods of dried, ripe, sweet pepper, *Capsicum annuum.* The strong, reddish orange powder is used in sausage and spice flavorings for baked goods (1,900 ppm), condiments, meats (7,400 ppm), and soups (7,500 ppm). The oleoresin *(see)* is used in fruit, meat, and spice flavorings for beverages, ice cream, ices, candy, baked goods, condiments, and meats. Both paprika and paprika oleoresins are used as red coloring. Permanently listed since 1966 for use in foods consistent with good manufacturing practices. They do not require certification. GRAS. ASP. E

**PAPRIKA OLEORESIN** • Used as a color additive. *See* Paprika. GRAS. ASP

**PARA-AMINOBENZOIC ACID** • The colorless or yellowish acid found in vitamin B complex. It is used medicinally to treat arthritis. However, it can cause allergic eczema *(see)* and sensitivity to light in susceptible people, whose skin may react to sunlight by erupting with a rash, sloughing, and/or swelling.

**PARABENS** • Butylparaben. Heptylparaben. Methylparaben. Propylparaben. Parahydroxybenzoate. The parabens are the most commonly used preservatives in the United States as a preservative in surface treatment of dried meat products, cereal- or potato-based snacks and coated nuts, etc. The parabens have a broad spectrum of antimicrobial activity—relatively nonirritating, nonsensitizing, and nonpoisonous—are stable over the pH *(see)* range in cosmetics, and are sufficiently soluble in water to be effective in liquids. The typical paraben preservative system contains 0.2 percent methyl- and 0.1 percent propylparaben. Methyl- and propylparaben are esters of parahydroxybenzoic acid. Neither occurs in nature. In foods, parabens function as preservatives that prevent the growth of molds and yeasts. They are used in baked goods, sugar substitutes, artificially sweetened jams, mincemeats, milk preparations, soft drinks, packaged fish, meat, poultry, jellies, fats, oils, and frozen dairy desserts. Methyl- and propylparabens are used at 1,000 ppm in tomato pulp, puree, ketchup, pickles, and relishes. It had been reported that methylparaben caused birth defects in offspring of mice and rats fed 550 milligrams per kilogram of body weight daily during pregnancy, and in hamsters fed 300 milligrams under the same conditions. The European Parliament said in 2003 that parabens should be reevaluated because they have been found to cause cell proliferation in the forestomach and developmental toxicity. In April 2003, the Scientific Committee on Food notes that in the event that the parabens are still used in food, the Committee cited its statement of October 2000, that the temporary acceptable daily intake (ADI) should be withdrawn if no further data are submitted. As these data have not been submitted in the last thirty months, the conditional authorization for parabens should be withdrawn. Then in 2004, a study published in the Journal of Applied Toxicology (2004, 25:5) reported parabens are a cause for concern. British researchers found traces of it in twenty women who had breast tumors. It is believed parabens act like the female hormone estrogen. In high levels, estrogen can cause some women to develop breast cancers. There were also reports that parabens may contribute to the notable drop in sperm count in European men. There is pressure by some members of the EU and scientists in other countries to ban the use of parabens in underarm deodorants, in particular, and in foods, if possible. *See* Methylparaben, Butylparaben, and propyl-p-hydroxyrenzoate.

**PARAFFIN AND SUCCINIC DERIVATIVES SYNTHETIC** • Coating on fresh citrus, muskmelons, and sweet potatoes. *See* Paraffin Wax and Succinic Acid. ASP

**PARAFFIN WAX** • A colorless, somewhat translucent, odorless mass with a greasy feel. Used as a defoaming component in yeast and sugar beet production. Not digested or absorbed in the intestines. Used to cover food products. A component of chewing-gum base. Obtained from the distillate of wood, coal, petroleum, or shale oil. Easily melts over boiling water. Pure paraffin is harmless to the skin, but the presence of impurities may give rise to irritations and eczema. *See also* Wax. ASP

**PARAFORMALDEHYDE** • Preservative used to control fungus in maple-tree tap holes (residue limit of 2 ppm of formaldehyde in maple syrup).

**PARALDEHYDE** • Made from acetaldehyde *(see)*. Used in processing food additives. It is a sedative and hypnotic that can be habit forming. Used in baked goods, beverages, breakfast cereal, chewing gum, confectionery frostings, egg products, fats and oils, fruit ices, hard candy, instant coffee, milk products, seasonings, and soft candy. Declared GRAS by FEMA *(see)*. EAF

**PARAMIPHOS-METHYL** • A pesticide. The FDA allows a residue of 60 ppm in or on rice hulls and 50 ppm in or on rice milling fractions and in or on wheat milling fractions.

**PARAQUAT** • Defoliant and herbicide used in animal feed for goats, cattle, swine, and lambs. The FDA limits residue to up to 0.2 ppm in dried hops, 3 in mint hay, 6 in sunflower seed hulls. Paraquat is in the EPA Genetic Toxicology Program *(see)*. Poison by ingestion and skin contact. Causes ulceration of the digestive tract, diarrhea, vomiting, renal damage, jaundice, edema, hemorrhage, lung damage, and death from suffocation. When heated to decomposition, emits toxic fumes.

**PARATHION** • A deep brown to yellow liquid, it is an organophosphate *(see)* insecticide and acaricide. Highly toxic by skin contact, inhalation, or ingestion. It interferes with the transmission of nerve signals. Repeated exposure may, without warning, be increasingly hazardous. *See* Organophosphates.

**PARMESAN CHEESE, REGGIANO CHEESE** • A hard, dry cheese with a sharp flavor that is cured for several years. It is used as a flavoring.

**PARSLEY, LEAVES, OIL, and OLEORESIN** • The aromatic leaves of the annual herb *Petroselinum* ssp., cultivated everywhere, are used in spice flavorings for beverages, meats, soups, baked goods, and condiments. Parsley oil is obtained by steam distillation of the ripe seeds of the herb. The oleoresin *(see)* is used in spice flavorings for condiments. Parsley may cause the skin to break out with a rash, redden, and swell when exposed to light. It may also cause an allergic reaction in the sensitive. GRAS. ASP

**PARSLEY SEED OIL** • See Parsley, Leaves, Oil, and Oleoresin.

**PARTIALLY DELACTOSED WHEY (PDW)** • Used increasingly as a substitute for nonfat dry milk, which is more expensive. PDW is used in processed cheese foods and spreads. It is the result of the partial removal of lactose *(see)* from the milk ingredient whey *(see)*.

**PARTIALLY DEMINERALIZED and DELACTOSED WHEY** • Removal of some minerals as well as lactose from whey. *See* Partially Delactosed Whey.

**PARTIALLY HYDROGENATED VEGETABLE OIL** • Used in margarine, crackers, fried foods, and baked goods. *See* Hydrogenation and Trans Fatty Acids.

**PARVE** • *See* Kosher.

**PASSIONFLOWER** • Extract of the various species of *Passiflora incarnata*. Indians used passionflower for swellings, relieving sore eyes, and to induce vomiting. It is used as a flavoring. It has been shown that an extract of the plant depresses the motor nerves of the spinal cord. NUL

**PATCHOULY OIL** • Patchouli Oil. Essential oil obtained from the leaves of an East Indian shrubby mint, *Pogostemon* spp. Yellowish to greenish brown liquid, with the pleasant fragrance of summer flowers. Used in cola, fruit, nut, and spice flavorings for beverages, ice cream, ices, candy, baked goods, and chewing gum. May produce allergic reactions. EAF

**PATENT BLUE V** • Color. Information on the metabolism of the color is lacking, according to FAO/WHO. Long-term and reproduction studies in the rat did not reveal any significant toxicological effects. A long-term study in a second species is required as well as a short-term study in a non-rodent species. These have not been supplied.

**PCBs** • *See* Polychlorinated Biphenyls.

**PD** • Substance for which a petitition has been filed but denied because of lack of proof of safety. Substances in this category are illegal and may not be used in foods.

**PEACH ALDEHYDE** • *See* Undecalactone.

**PEACH EXTRACT** • *See* Peach Juice Extract.

**PEACH JUICE EXTRACT** • The liquid obtained from the pulp of the peach *Prunus persica.* It is used as a natural flavoring. Nontoxic.

**PEACH KERNEL OIL** • Persic Oil. A light yellow liquid expressed from the seed. Smells like almonds. Used as a natural flavoring in conjunction with other natural flavorings. GRAS

**PEACH LEAVES** • Flavoring for alcoholic beverages only. *See* Peach Juice Extract. NUL

**PEANUT OIL** • Arachis Oil. Greenish yellow, with a pleasant odor. Prepared by pressing shelled and skinned seeds of the peanut. A solvent in salad oil, shortening, mayonnaise, and confections. Also used in conjunction with natural flavorings. Peanut butter is about 50 percent peanut oil suspended in peanut fibers. It may migrate from cotton in dried food packaging. Used in the manufacture of soaps, baby preparations, hair-grooming aids, nail driers, shampoos, and as a solvent for ointments and liniments; also in night creams and emollients. It is used as a substitute for almond and olive oils in cosmetic creams, brilliantines, antiwrinkle oils, and sunburn preparations. The oil acts as a mild cathartic and as a protective for the gastrointestinal tract when corrosive poisons have been swallowed. The final report to the FDA of the Select Committee on GRAS Substances stated in 1980 that it should continue its GRAS status with no limitations other than good manufacturing practices. A study done by the Department of Nutrition, University of California, Davis, found in 1997 that crude peanut oil caused allergic reactions in 10 percent of allergic subjects studied and should be avoided. Refined peanut oil did not pose a risk to the subjects. Check with your physician before trying if you are allergic to peanut oil. ASP

**PEANUT STEARINE** • Natural flavoring. *See* Peanut Oil. GRAS. ASP

**PEANUTAMIDEMEA** • Loramine Wax. *See* Peanut Oil.

**PEANUTAMIDEMIPA** • A mixture of isopropanolamides of the fatty acids derived from peanut oil *(see).*

**PECAN SHELL POWDER** • A coloring additive used in cosmetics. Employed medicinally by the American Indians. It is the nut from a hickory of the southern central United States with rough bark and hard but brittle wood. Edible.

**PECTINS** • Pectin is found in roots, stems, and fruits of plants and forms an integral part of such structures. It is a coarse or fine powder, practically odorless, with a gluey taste. Richest source of pectin is lemon or orange rind, which contains about 30 percent of this polysaccharide. Used as a stabilizer, thickener, and bodying additive for artificially sweetened beverages, syrups for frozen products, ice cream, ice milk, confections, fruit sherbets, water ices, French dressing, fruit jelly, preserves, and jams to compensate for a deficiency in natural pectin. Used in foods as a "cementing additive." Also used as an antidiarrheal medicine. The final report to the FDA of the Select Committee on GRAS Substances stated in 1980 that it should continue its GRAS status with no limitations other than good manufacturing practices. ASP. E

**PECTINASE** • Enzyme used as a clarifying additive *(see)* in wine and juice from *Aspergillus niger* or *Bacillus subtilis.*

**PEGU CATECHU EXTRACT** • *See* Catechu Extract.

**PELARGONALDEHYDE** • *See* Nonanal.

**PELARGONIC ACID** • Nonanoic Acid. A synthetic flavoring additive that occurs naturally in cocoa and oil of lavender. Used in berry, fruit, nut, and spice flavorings. Used in peeling solution for fruits and vegetables. A strong irritant.

**PELARGONIC ALDEHYDE** • *See* Pelargonic Acid.

**PELARGONYL VANILLYLAMIDE** • *See* Pelargonic Acid.

**PENDARE** • *Couma macrocarpa. Couma utilis.* A flavoring from tropical South American trees. *See* Coumarin. ASP

**PENDIMETHALIN** • Prowl. Stomp. An herbicide. FDA tolerance is 0.1 ppm as a residue in or on corn fodder or forage, grain, potatoes, sorghum, soybeans, or sunflower seeds.

**PENICILLINASE FROM *BACILLUS SUBTILIS*** • An enzyme from a mold used in processing. NUL

**PENICILLINS** • Amoxicillin. Ampicillin. Azlocillin. Bacampicillin. Carbenicillin. Cloxacillin. Dicloxacillin. Methicillin. Mezlocillin. Nafcillin. Oxacillin. Penicillin G, V. Piperacillin. Ticarcillin. A group of beta-lactam antibiotics produced by several species of mold and/or semisynthetically. There are many kinds and they offer a broad clinical spectrum of activity. They act by inhibiting bacterial enzymes involved in making cell walls. Used to treat animal infections and in animal feed to prevent infections and to encourage growth, particularly in chickens, lamb, swine, turkey, pheasants, and quail. The FDA limits residues to 0.05 ppm in cattle. Limitation of zero in chickens, pheasant, quail, swine, sheep, eggs, milk, and foods in which milk has been used. Limitation of 0.01 ppm in turkeys. In EPA

Genetic Toxicology Program *(see)*. Human reproductive effects by ingestion: abortion. Human systemic effects by intramuscular route: skin rash. Has been implicated in aplastic anemia.

**PENICILLIUM ROQUEFORTII** • Mold used to make cheeses. NUL

**PENNYROYAL OIL, AMERICAN** • Squaw Mint. *Hedeoma pulegiodes.* An extract of the flowering herb *Mentha pulegium.* Used since ancient days as a medicine, scent, flavoring, and food. Obtained from the dried flower tops and leaves, it contains tannin, which is soothing to the skin. Used in mint flavorings for beverages, ice cream, ices, candy, and baked goods. Formerly used as an aromatic perspirant, to stimulate menstrual flow, for flatulence, as an abortion inducer, and as a counteractant for painful menstruation. Brain damage has been reported following doses of less than one teaspoon. Nausea, vomiting, bleeding, circulatory collapse, confusion, restlessness, and delirium have been reported. EAF

**PENNYROYAL OIL, EUROPEAN** • *Mentha pulegium.* EAF

**PENTACHLOROPHENOL** • Chloropben. Santophen. Dark-colored flakes with a characteristic odor used as a preservative in packaging materials. FDA limit of 50 ppm in treated wood. International Agency for Research on Cancer (IARC) *(see)* review and on EPA Extremely Hazardous List, Community Right-To-Know List and EPA Genetic Toxicology Program *(see all)*. Human poison by ingestion. A suspected human cancer-causing additive. Causes birth defects in experimental animals. Skin irritant. Acute poisoning causes weakness with difficult breathing and changes in blood pressure and urinary output. Can cause death.

**PENTADECALACTONE** • Angelica Lactone. Exaltolide. It is obtained from the fruit and root of a plant grown in Europe and Asia. A synthetic berry, fruit, liquor, wine, nut, and vanilla flavoring additive for beverages, ice cream, ices, candy, baked goods, gelatin desserts, and alcoholic beverages. ASP

**PENTADECANOLIDE** • *See* Pentadecalactone.

**2-PENTADECANONE** • An essential oil found in wild tomatoes and in pheromones of fruit flies and other insects that attract mates. EAF

**PENTADESMA BUTTER** • Kanya Butter. The vegetable fat extracted from the nut of *Pentadesma butyracea. See* Shea Butter.

**PENTADIENAL** • Synthetic flavoring. FAO/WHO *(see)* says there is no safety concern. ASP

**PENTAERYTHRITOL ESTER OF MALEIC ANHYDRIDE MODIFIED WOOD ROSIN** • Coating on citrus fruit. Pentaerythritol is a resin made by treating acetaldehyde *(see)* with formaldehyde *(see)* in a solution of calcium hydroxide.

**PENTAERYTHRITOL ESTER OF PARTIALLY HYDROGENATED WOOD ROSIN** • Hard, amber-colored solid used as a coating for citrus fruits and in chewing-gum bases. *See* Rosin.

**PENTANAL** • *See* Valeraldehyde.

**PENTANE** • The aliphatic hydrocarbon derived from petroleum. Used as a solvent. Narcotic in high doses.

**2,3-PENTANEDIONE** • A synthetic flavoring additive that occurs naturally in coffee. Used in strawberry, chocolate, butterscotch, butter, caramel, fruit, rum, and cheese flavorings for beverages, ice cream, ices, candy, baked goods, gelatin desserts, and puddings.

**2-PENTANETHIOL** • *n*-Amyl Mercaptan. A liquid with a strong, unpleasant odor used in the manufacture of food additives. Mild irritant to skin and mucous membranes. EAF

**PENTANOIC ACID** • *See* Valeric Acid.

**1-PENTANOL** • Pentyl Alcohol. *n*-Amyl Alcohol. Liquid with a mild, pleasant odor, slightly soluble in water. Used as a solvent. Irritating to the eyes and respiratory passages, and absorption may cause a lack of oxygen in the blood. ASP

**2-PENTANONE** • A synthetic flavoring that occurs naturally in apples. Used in fruit flavorings for beverages, ice cream, ices, candy, and baked goods. Moderately toxic by ingestion. Mildly toxic by skin contact and inhalation. In humans, inhalation may cause headache, nausea, and irritation of the respiratory passages, eyes, and skin. ASP

**4-PENTENOIC ACID 9** • A synthetic butter and fruit flavoring additive for beverages, ice cream, ices, candy, baked goods, and margarine. ASP

**1-PENTEN-3-ONE** • Synthetic flavoring with a powerful, penetrating odor. ASP

**2-PENTENYL ACETATE** • Synthetic flavoring. A clear colorless to slightly yellow liquid with a herbaceous odor. Used in baked goods, beverages, breakfast cereals, chewing gum, frozen dairy desserts, hard candy. Declared GRAS by FEMA *(see)*. *See* Acetic Acid. EAF

**PENTYL ALCOHOL** • *See* Amyl Alcohol.

**2-PENTYL-1-BUTEN-3-ONE** • Synthetic flavoring. Pale yellow liquid; musty, mushroom odor. *See* Octanoic Acid. NIL

**PENTYL BUTYRATE** • *See* Amyl Butyrate. EAF

**2-TERT-PENTYLCYCLOHEXYL ACETATE** • An alcohol used in the manufacture of fragrances and flavorings. NUL

**2-PENTYLFURAN** • Flavoring from soybeans. ASP

**PENTYL 2-FURYL KETONE** • Artificial flavoring. *See* Furfural. ASP

**2-PENTYL-3-METHYL-2-CYCLOPENTEN-1-ONE** • Dihydrojasmone. Synthetic flavoring used in bergamot, citrus, fern, fougere, floral, green natural, green, and herbal scents and flavorings. NUL

**2-PENTYLPYRIDINE** • Synthetic flavoring on the FAO/WHO *(see)* list to be evaluated.

**PEPPER, BLACK** • A pungent product obtained from the dried, unripe berries of the East Indian pepper plant, *Piper nigrum*. Used in sausage and spice flavorings for beverages, baked goods, condiments, meats, soups, and pickles. Black pepper oil is used in meat and spice flavorings for beverages, ice cream, ices, candy, baked goods, condiments, and meats. Black pepper oleoresin *(see)* is used in sausage and pepper flavorings for beverages, ice cream, ices, candy, baked goods, condiments, and meats. Pepper was formerly used as a carminative to break up intestinal gas, to cause sweating, and as a gastric additive to promote gastric secretion. Has insecticidal properties. GRAS. ASP

**PEPPER BLACK, OIL** • *Piper nigrum.* The oil is extracted by steam from dried unripe berries Usually comes from India. The pepper plant is a perennial vine with dark green leaves, creeping up to 6 meters (20 feet), but commercially is limited to 3–4 meters (10–12 feet). It produces three kinds of oil (pepper black, pepper white, and pepper green) taken from the peppercorns that sprout after the small white flowers. The pepper black oil is a green-yellow color and distilled from the dried immature peppercorns and has a hot and spicy scent. ASP

**PEPPER, BLACK OLEORESIN** • *Piper nigrum.* Yellow semisolid liquid. Biting, pungent flavor. *See* Pepper Black, Oil

**PEPPER, CAYENNE** • *See* Cayenne Pepper. EAF

**PEPPER, RED** • *See* Cayenne Pepper. GRAS. EAF

**PEPPER TREE OIL** • *See* Schinus Molle Oil.

**PEPPER, WHITE** • The pungent product obtained from the undecorticated (with the outer covering intact) ripe berries of the pepper plant. Used in sausage and spice flavorings for beverages, baked goods, condiments, meats, and soups. White pepper oil is used in spice flavorings for baked goods. White pepper oleoresin *(see)* is used in spice flavorings for meats. *See* Pepper, Black. GRAS

**PEPPER, WHITE OIL** • *Piper nigrum.* ASP

**PEPPERMINT EXTRACT** • *See* Peppermint Oil.

**PEPPERMINT LEAVES** • *See* Peppermint Oil. EAF

**PEPPERMINT OIL** • *Mentha × piperita.* The oil made from the dried leaves and tops of a plant common to Asian, European, and American gardens, *Mentha × piperita.* Used in chocolate, fruit, cordial, crème de menthe, peppermint, nut, and spice flavorings for beverages, ice cream, ices, candy (1,200 ppm), baked goods, gelatin desserts, chewing gum (8,300 ppm), meats, liquors, icings, and toppings. Peppermint has been used as a carminative to break up intestinal gas and as an antiseptic. It can cause allergic reactions such as hay fever and skin rash. Two patients who consumed large quantities of peppermint candy over a long period developed irregular heart rhythms. GRAS. ASP

**PEPPERMINT PLANT** • A hardy perennial, which can grow two to three feet tall, including the flowering spikes. It grows pale lilac flowers in the summer around late July if not clipped down. This mint plant has a strong aroma of peppermint. Mint is also used for medicinal use and flavoring purposes. This plant will spread underground by growing root shoots in early spring and the plants can become prolific. The fresh mint leaves are used as a flavoring in beverages and the dry leaves in hot teas. NUL

**PEPSIN** • A digestive enzyme found in gastric juice that helps break down protein. Allowed up to 0.1 percent by weight in enriched farina. The product, also used to aid digestion, is obtained from the glandular layer of the fresh stomach of a hog. Slightly acid taste and a mild odor. GRAS. ASP

**PEPTIDE** • Two or more amino acids chained together in head-to-tail links. Generally larger than simple amino acids or the monoamines, the largest peptides discovered thus far have forty-four amino acids. Neuropeptides signal the body's endocrine glands to balance salt and water. Opiate peptides can help control pain and anxiety. The peptides work with amino acids.

**PEPTONES** • Secondary protein derivatives formed during digestion—the result of gastric and pancreatic juices acting upon protein. Peptones are used as a foam stabilizer for beer and as a processing aid in baked goods, confections, and frostings. Determined to be GRAS in 1982. EAF

**PERACETIC ACID** • Peroxyacetic Acid. A starch modifier prepared from acetaldehyde (see). It is 40 percent acetic acid and highly corrosive. Acrid odor; explodes violently on heating to 110 degrees. NUL

**PERFLUOROHEXANE** • Used to cool or freeze chickens.

**PERILLALDEHYDE** • Isolated from Perilla arguta, it is used as a sweet flavoring additive. ASP

**PERILLA OIL** • Light yellow oil derived from the seeds of Perilla ocimoides, grown in Japan and Korea. It is used as a substitute for linseed oil and as an edible oil in Asia. It is also used in the manufacture of varnishes. There is reported use of the chemical, it has not yet been assigned for toxicology literature. EAF

**PERILLA LEAF OIL** • Used as a flavoring in baked goods, beverages, chewing gum, confectionery frostings, fish products, frozen dairy, gelatins, and imitation dairy. Declared GRAS by FEMA (see).

**PERILLYL ACETATE** • Synthetic flavoring derived from tangerine rind. It is an almost colorless or pale yellowish oily liquid with a warm herbaceous spicy odor. ASP

**PERIODIC ACID** • Derived from iodine (see) and is used as an oxidizer in processing of food additives. EAF

**PERLITE** • A filtering aid. The final report to the FDA of the Select Committee on GRAS Substances stated in 1980 it should continue its GRAS status with no limitations other than good manufacturing practices.

**PEROXIDE** • Benzoyl, Calcium, and Hydrogen. Benzoyl peroxide is used as a bleaching additive for flours, oils, and cheese. Calcium peroxide or dioxide is odorless, almost tasteless. Used as a dough conditioner and oxidizing additive for bread, rolls, and buns. Formerly used as an antiseptic. Hydrogen peroxide *(see)* or dioxide is used as a bleaching and oxidizing additive, a modifier for food starch, and a preservative and bactericide for milk and cheese. Bitter taste. May decompose violently if traces of impurities are present. A strong oxidant that can injure skin and eyes. On the FDA list of additives to be studied for mutagenic, teratogenic, subacute, and reproductive effects.

**PERSIC OIL** • *See* Apricot and Peach Kernel Oil.

**PERUVIAN BALSAM** • *See* Balsam Peru. GRAS

**PEST** • FDA abbreviation for pesticide other than a fumigant.

**PESTICIDE** • A broad class of crop protection chemicals including four major types: insecticides used to control insects; herbicides used to control weeds; rodenticides used to control rodents; and fungicides used to control mold, mildew, and fungi. In addition consumers use pesticides in the home or yard to control termites and roaches, clean mold from shower curtains, stave off crabgrass on the lawn, kill fleas and ticks on pets, and disinfect swimming pools, to name just a few "specialty" pesticide uses. Some pesticides are immediately toxic to humans. Others take a long time to produce cancer and other illnesses.

**PETITGRAIN OIL** • The volatile oil obtained from the leaves and twigs and unripe fruit of the bitter orange tree. Brownish to yellow with a bittersweet odor. Used in loganberry, violet, apple, banana, berry, grape, peach, pear, honey, muscatel, nut, ginger, and ginger ale flavorings for beverages, ice cream, ices, candy, baked goods, gelatin desserts, chewing gum, and condiments. GRAS. EAF

**PETITGRAIN OIL (LEMON, MANDARIN, TANGERINE)** • Fragrant essential oils from a variety of citrus trees. Used in citrus and fruit flavorings for beverages, ice cream, ices, candy, and baked goods. GRAS. ASP

**PETROLATUM** • Crude or Mineral Oil. Vaseline. Petroleum Jelly. Paraffin Jelly. A purified mixture of semisolid hydrocarbons from petroleum. Yellowish to light amber or white, unctuous mass, practically odorless and tasteless, almost insoluble in water. A releasing additive and sealant for confections. A coating for fruits, vegetables, and cheese. A defoaming additive in yeast and beet sugar production. Used in baking products, as a lubricant in meatpacking plants, and used in dried egg albumin. Defoaming additive, lubricant, polishing additive, protective coating, release (nonstick) additive, and sealing additive in bakery products, beet sugar, confectionery, egg white solids, dehydrated fruits, and dehydrated vegetables. The FDA limits petrolatum to 0.15 percent in bakery products, 0.2 percent in confectionery, 0.02 percent in dehydrated fruits and vegetables, 0.1 percent in egg white. May contain FDA-approved antioxidants. When ingested, it produces a mild laxative effect. Not absorbed but may inhibit digestion. It is generally nontoxic. ASP

**PETROLEUM** • Hydrocarbons, Naphtha, Waxes. A highly complex mixture of paraffinic, naphthalenic, and aromatic hydrocarbons containing some sulfur and trace amounts of nitrogen and oxygen compounds. Believed to have originated from both plant and animal sources millions of years ago. By cracking petroleum into fractions, the gases butane, ethane, and propane are obtained, as well as naphtha, gasoline, kerosene, fuel oils, gas oil, lubricating oils, paraffin wax, and asphalt. A defoaming additive in processing beet sugar and yeast and a coating on cheese and raw fruits and vegetables. Used as a coating on eggshells; in froth-flotation cleaning of vegetables; as a float on fermentation fluids as in the manufacture of vinegar, wine, and pickle brine; as a component of pesticide formulations; in modified hops extract of beer; and in many other formulations. Formerly used for bronchitis, tapeworms, and externally for arthritis and skin problems. Many petroleum products are reported to be cancer-causing additives. ASP

**PETROLEUM NAPHTHA** • Solvent used as coating on fresh citrus. *See* Petroleum. NIL

**PETROLEUM WAX** • Antifoaming additive used in beet sugar and yeast. Used in chewing-gum base and other foods, as a coating on cheese, fruits, and vegetables, and as a component of microcapsules for spice flavor for frozen pizza. *See* Petroleum. ASP

**PETROLEUM WAX, SYNTHETIC** • Coating on cheese and raw fruits and vegetables. Also used as an antifoaming additive in beet sugar and yeast.

**pH** • The scale used to measure acidity and alkalinity. pH is the hydrogen (H) ion concentration of a solution; *P* stands for the power of the hydrogen ion. The pH of a solution is measured on a scale of 14. A truly neutral solution, neither acidic nor alkaline, such as water, is 7. Acid is less than 7. Alkaline is more than 7. The pH of blood is 7.3; vinegar is 2.3.; lemon juice is 2.2; and lye is 13. Skin and hair are naturally acidic. Soap and detergents are alkaline. ASP

**PHAFFIA** • The Food and Drug Administration (FDA) amended its color additive regulations in 2000 to provide for the use of phaffia yeast as a color additive in the feed of salmonid fish to enhance the color of their flesh. In 2003, the United Kingdom register of Organic Food Standards board meeting said it could not endorse the use of phaffia yeast without further evidence of its health benefits and, ideally, a common view from the industry. EAF

***a*-PHELLANDRENE** • A synthetic flavoring additive that occurs naturally in allspice, star anise, angelica root, bay, dill, sweet fennel, black pepper, peppermint oil, and pimenta. Isolated from the essential oils of the eucalyptus plant. Used in citrus and spice flavorings for beverages, ice cream, ices, candy, and baked goods. Can be irritating to, and is absorbed through, the skin. Ingestion can cause vomiting and diarrhea. ASP

**PHENETHYL ACETATE** • A fragrance and flavoring ingredient. *See* Acetic Acid. ASP

**PHENETHYL ALCOHOL** • 2-Phenethyanol. It occurs naturally in oranges, raspberries, and tea. A synthetic fruit flavoring additive that is used in strawberry, butter, caramel, floral, fruit, and honey flavorings for beverages, ice cream, ices, candy, baked goods, chewing gum, and gelatin desserts. It is a sensitizer. It is a strong local anesthetic and has caused central nervous system injury in mice. ASP

**PHENETHYLAMINE** • Stimulant in chocolate. ASP

**PHENETHYL ANTHRANILATES** • A synthetic butter, caramel, fruit, honey, and grape flavoring additive for beverages, ice cream, ices, candy, and baked goods. *See* Coal Tar. ASP

**PHENETHYL BENZOATE** • A synthetic fruit and honey flavoring additive for beverages, ice cream, ices, candy, chewing gum, and baked goods. *See* Coal Tar. ASP

**PHENETHYL BUTYRATE** • A synthetic butter, strawberry, caramel, floral, apple, peach, pineapple, and honey flavoring additive for beverages, ice cream, ices, candy, and baked goods. See Coal Tar. ASP

**PHENETHYL CINNAMATE** • A synthetic fruit flavoring additive for beverages, ice cream, ices, candy, puddings, and baked goods. *See* Coal Tar. ASP

**PHENETHYL FORMATE** • Formic Acid. A synthetic berry, apple, apricot, banana, cherry, peach, pear, plum, and honey flavoring additive for beverages, ice cream, ices, candy, and baked goods. *See* Coal Tar. ASP

**PHENETHYL 2-FUROATE** • Synthetic flavoring. NIL

**PHENETHYL HEXANOATE** • Synthetic flavoring. *See* Hexanoic Acid. ASP

**PHENETHYL ISOBUTYRATE** • A synthetic flavoring additive, slightly yellow, with a rose odor. Used in strawberry, floral, rose, apple, peach, pineapple, honey, and cheese flavorings for beverages, ice cream, ices, candy, and baked goods. Mildly toxic by ingestion. *See* Coal Tar. ASP

**PHENETHYL ISOTHIOCYANATE PEITC** • A naturally occurring compound found in some cruciferous vegetables. It is being studied as an agent to prevent cancer. It is added as a nutrient to some health foods. It is also widely used in baked goods, beverages, breakfast cereal, chewing gum, confectionery frostings, egg products, fats and oils, fish products, frozen dairy, gelatins, gravies, hard candy, imitation dairy, processed vegetables, seasonings, snack food, soft candy, and soups. Decalred GRAS by FEMA. EAF

**PHENETHYL ISOVALERATE** • A synthetic apple, apricot, peach, pear, and pineapple flavoring additive for beverages, ice cream, ices, candy, baked goods, and chewing gum. Mildly toxic by ingestion. *See* Coal Tar.

**PHENETHYL MERCAPTAN** • Synthetic flavoring. EAF

**1-PHENYLETHYLMERCAPTAN** • A flavoring determined GRAS by FEMA *(see)*. *See* Benzene.

**2-PHENETHYL 2-METHYL BUTYRATE** • Colorless liquid with a floral-fruity odor used as a flavoring additive in various foods. ASP

**PHENETHYL OCTANOATE** • Synthetic flavoring. Colorless oily liquid; mild fruity winelike odor. ASP

**PHENETHYL PHENYLACETATE** • A synthetic fruit and honey flavoring additive for beverages, ice cream, ices, candy, maraschino cherries, and baked goods. *See* Coal Tar. ASP

**PHENETHYL PROPIONATE** • A synthetic fruit and honey flavoring additive for beverages, ice cream, ices, candy, and baked goods. *See* Coal Tar. ASP

**PHENETHYL SALICYLATE** • A synthetic apricot and peach flavoring additive for beverages, ice cream, ices, candy, and baked goods. *See* Coal Tar. ASP

**PHENETHYL SENECIOATE** • A synthetic liquor and wine flavoring additive for beverages, ice cream, ices, candy, and alcoholic beverages. *See* Coal Tar. ASP

**PHENETHYL TIGLATE** • A synthetic fruit and nut flavoring additive for beverages, ice cream, ices, candy, and baked goods. *See* Coal Tar. ASP

**PHENOL** • Obtained from coal tar *(see)*, it is used in the manufacture of many food additives and processing aids. Ingestion of even small amounts of phenol may cause nausea, vomiting, circulatory collapse, paralysis, convulsions, coma, respiratory failure, and cardiac arrest. It is an antiseptic and general disinfectant. ASP

**PHENOL-FORMALDEHYDE** • Used in treatment of food or potable water. *See* Formaldehyde and Phenol. NUL

**PHENOXYACETIC ACID** • A synthetic fruit and honey flavoring additive for beverages, ice cream, ices, candy, and baked goods. Used to soften calluses and corns. A mild irritant. ASP

**2-PHENOXYETHYL ISOBUTYRATE** • A synthetic fruit flavoring, colorless, with a roselike odor. Used in beverages, ice cream, ices, candy, and baked goods.

**PHENYL ACETATE** • A synthetic flavoring additive prepared from phenol and acetic chloride. Used in berry, butter, caramel, floral, rose, fruit, hony, and vanilla flavorings for beverages, ice cream, ices, candy, and baked goods. Phenol is highly toxic. Death from 1.5 grams has been reported. EAF

**PHENYLALANINE** • L form. An essential amino acid *(see)* considered essential for growth in normal human beings and not synthesized by the body. It is associated with phenylketonuria (PKU), an affliction that, if not detected soon after birth, leads to mental deterioration in children. Restricting phenylalanine in diets results in improvement. Whole egg contains 5.4 percent and skim milk 5.1 percent. The FDA asked for further study of this amino acid as a food additive in 1980.

**DL-PHENYLALANINE** • The D form occurs naturally in microbial products. The DL form occurs in water or alcohol and has a sweetish taste. *See* Phenylalanine. ASP

**L-PHENYLALANINE** • *See* Phenylalanine. ASP

**4-PHENYL-2-BUTANOL** • A synthetic fruit flavoring for beverages, ice cream, ices, candy, and baked goods. ASP

**2-PHENYL-2-BUTENAL** • Synthetic flavoring. *See* 4-Phenyl-2-Butanol. ASP

**4-PHENYL-3-BUTEN-2-OL** • A synthetic fruit flavoring for beverages, ice cream, ices, candy, and baked goods. ASP

**4-PHENYL-3-BUTEN-2-ONE** • A synthetic chocolate, cocoa, fruit, cherry, nut, and vanilla flavoring additive for beverages, ice cream, ices, candy, baked goods, gelatin desserts, and shortenings. ASP

**4-PHENYL-2-BUTYL ACETATE** • A synthetic fruit and peach flavoring additive for beverages, ice cream, ices, candy, and baked goods. *See* Acetic Acid for toxicity. ASP

**PHENYL CARBOXYL ISOBUTYRATE** • See *a-a*-Dimethylbenzyl Isobutyrate. ASP

**PHENYL DISULFIDE** • Synthetic flavoring, clear and colorless. ASP

**2-PHENYL-3(2-FURYL)-PROP-2-ENAL** • Synthetic flavoring. ASP

**PHENYL 2-FUROATE** • A synthetic chocolate and mushroom flavoring additive for beverages, candy, and gelatin desserts.

**I-PHENYL-3-METHYL-3-PENTANOL** • A synthetic fruit flavoring additive for beverages, candy, and gelatin desserts. ASP

**PHENYL PELARGONATE** • Liquid, insoluble in water. Used in flavors, perfumes, bactericides, and fungicides.

**2-PHENYL-4-PENTENAL** • Synthetic flavoring. ASP

**3-PHENYL-4-PENTENAL** • Synthetic flavoring. ASP

**1-PHENYL-1,2-PROPANEDIONE** • Synthetic flavoring with a strong plastic odor. ASP

**I-PHENYL-1-PROPANOL** • A synthetic fruit and honey flavoring additive for beverages, ice cream, ices, candy, and baked goods. ASP

**3-PHENYL-1-PROPANOL** • A synthetic flavoring that occurs naturally in tea. Used in strawberry, apricot, peach, plum, hazelnut, pistachio, cinnamon, and walnut flavorings for beverages, ice cream, ices, candy, baked goods, liqueurs, and chewing gum.

**PHENYLACETALDEHYDE** • An oily, colorless liquid with a harsh odor. Upon dilution, emits the fragrance of lilacs and hyacinths. Derived from phenethyl alcohol *(see)*. A synthetic raspberry, strawberry, apricot, cherry, peach, honey, and spice flavoring for beverages, ice cream, ices, candy, baked goods, and chewing gum. Used also in perfumes. Less irritating than formaldehyde *(see),* but a stronger central nervous system depressant. In addition, it sometimes produces fluid in the lungs upon ingestion. ASP

**PHENYLACETALDEHYDE 2,3-BUTYLENE CLYCOL ACETAL** • A synthetic floral and fruit flavoring additive for candy *See* Phenylacetaldehyde for toxicity.

**PHENYLACETALDEHYDE DIMETHYL ACETAL** • A colorless liquid with a strong odor used as a synthetic fruit, apricot, cherry, honey, and spice flavoring additive for beverages, ice cream, ices, candy, baked goods, and chewing gum. Moderately toxic by ingestion.

**PHENYLACETALDEHYDE GLYCERYL ACETAL** • Synthetic floral and fruit flavoring additive for beverages, candy, ice cream, and ices. *See* Phenylacetaldehyde and Acetic Acid for toxicity.

**PHENYLACETIC ACID** • Synthetic flavoring additive that occurs naturally in Japanese mint, oil of neroli, and black pepper. Used in butter, chocolate, rose, honey, and vanilla flavorings for beverages, ice cream, ices, candy, baked goods, gelatin desserts, chewing gum, liquors, and syrups. Also used in the manufacture of penicillin. Moderately toxic by ingestion. Causes birth defects in experimental animals. ASP

**p-PHENYLENEDIAMINE** • Most permanent home and beauty parlor dyes contain this chemical or a related one such as 4-nitro-o-phenylenediamine. Also called oxidation dyes, amino dyes, para dyes, or peroxide dyes. PPD was first introduced in 1890 for dyeing furs and feathers. It comes in about thirty shades and is used as an intermediate in coal-tar dyes. May produce eczema, bronchial asthma, gastritis, skin rash, and death. Can cross-react with many other chemicals, including azo dyes used for temporary hair colorings. Can also produce photosensitization. It has reportedly caused cancer in some animal experiments and not in others.

**2-PHENYLETHYL ISOVALERATE** • *See* Phenethyl Isovalerate.

**2-PHENYLPROPIONALDEHYDE** • A synthetic berry, rose, apricot, cherry, peach, plum, and almond flavoring additive for beverages, ice cream, ices, candy, and baked goods.

**3-PHENYLPROPIONALDEHYDE** • A synthetic flavoring additive, slightly yellow, with a strong floral odor. Used in berry, rose, apricot, cherry, peach, plum, and almond flavorings for beverages, ice cream, ices, candy, and baked goods.

**2-PHENYLPROPIONALDEHYDE DIMETHYL ACETAL** • A synthetic berry, floral, rose, fruit, honey, mushroom, nut, and spice flavoring additive for beverages, ice cream, ices, candy, baked goods, chewing gum, and condiments. *See* Acetic Acid for toxicity.

**3-PHENYLPROPYL ACETATE** • A synthetic flavoring, colorless, with a spicy floral odor. Used in berry, fruit, and spice flavorings for beverages, ice cream, ices, candy, baked goods, chewing gum, and condiments. Propyl acetate may be irritating to skin and mucous membranes and narcotic in high concentrations

**2-PHENYLPROPYL BUTYRATE** • A synthetic flavoring used in beverages, ice cream, ices, candy, and baked goods. No specific flavorings listed.

**3-PHENYLPROPYL CINNAMATE** • Synthetic butter, caramel, chocolate, cocoa, coconut, grape, and spice flavoring additive for beverages, ice cream, ices, candy, and baked goods.

**3-PHENYLPROPYL FORMATE** • Formic Acid. A synthetic currant, raspberry, butter, caramel, apricot, peach, and honey flavoring additive for beverages, ice cream, ices, candy, and baked goods. *See* Formic Acid for toxicity.

**3-PHENYLPROPYL HEXANOATE** • A synthetic fruit flavoring for beverages, ice cream, ices, candy, and baked goods.

**2-PHENYLPROPYL ISOBUTYRATE** • A synthetic fruit flavoring for beverages, ice cream, ices, and candy.

**3-PHENYLPROPYL ISOBUTYRATE** • A synthetic apple, apricot, peach, pear, pineapple, and plum flavoring additive for beverages, ice cream, ices, candy, and baked goods.

**3-PHENYLPROPYL ISOVALERATE** • A synthetic butter, caramel, apple, pear, and nut flavoring additive for beverages, ice cream, ices, candy, and baked goods.

**3-PHENYLPROPYL PROPIONATE** • A synthetic apricot flavoring for beverages, ice cream, ices, candy, and baked goods.

**2-3(3-PHENYLPROPYL) TETRAHYDROFURAN** • A synthetic fruit, honey, and maple flavoring additive for beverages, ice cream, ices, candy, gelatin, puddings, and chewing gum.

**PHORATE** • Thimet. Vegfru. An insecticide used in animal feed. On EPA Extremely Hazardous Substances List and EPA Genetic Toxicology Program *(see both)*. Poison by ingestion. Causes mutations in experimental animals and interferes with nerve signals.

**PHOSALONE** • An insecticide used to kill insects and mites. FDA residue tolerance resulting from application on dried apple pomace is 85 ppm; on dried prunes, 40 ppm; on raisins, 20 ppm; on dried citrus pulp, 12 ppm; on dried grape pomace, 45 ppm; and on tea, 8 ppm. *See* Organophosphates.

**PHOSPHATE** • Salt of ester of phosphoric acid *(see)*. Used as an emulsifier and texturizer and sequestering additive *(see)* in foods. Sodium phosphate is used in evaporated milk up to 0.1 percent of weight. Carbonated beverages contain phosphoric acid. Without sufficient phosphate there is abnormal parathyroid (gland) function, bone metabolism, intestinal absorption, malnutrition, and kidney malfunction. Chemicals that interfere with phosphate action include detergents, mannitol *(see)*, vitamin D, and aluminum hydroxide *(see)*, a leavening additive. Ingestion of large amounts of phosphates can cause kidney damage and may adversely affect the absorption of other minerals.

**PHOSPHATE, AMMONIUM** • Dibasic and Monobasic. *See* Ammonium Phosphate.

**PHOSPHATE, CALCIUM HEXAMETA-** • *See* Calcium Hexametaphosphate.

**PHOSPHATE, CALCIUM, MONOBASIC and TRIBASIC** • *See* Calcium Phosphate.

**PHOSPHATE, POTASSIUM** • Monobasic and Dibasic. *See* Potassium Phosphate.

**PHOSPHATED DISTARCH PHOSPHATE** • The final report to the FDA of the Select Committee on GRAS Substances stated in 1980 that there is no available evidence that it is a hazard to the public when used as it is now and it should continue its GRAS status with limitations on amounts that can be added to food. *See* Modified Starches. E

**PHOSPHATIDYLSERINE** • PS. A naturally occurring phospholipid nutrient, it is essential to the functioning of all the cells of the body, but is most concentrated in the brain. Low levels of phosphatidylserine in the brain are associated with impaired mental function and depression. PS was only available from animal sources (brain), and occurred in commercial lecithins only in trace amounts; however, a plant source for PS has been developed. The FDA has allowed the claim in 2003 for this dietary supplement that "consumption of phosphatidylserine may reduce the risk of dementia (cognitive dysfunction) in the elderly" with the added "FDA concludes that there is little scientific evidence supporting this claim."

**PHOSPHOLIPIDS** • Phosphatides. Complex fat substances found in all living cells. While fats are typically composed of three fatty acids, phospholipids have two fatty acids. Phospholipids are a major component of cell membranes. Lecithin is an example.

***n*-(PHOSPHONOMETHYL)GLYCINE** • An herbicide used in animal feed, imported olives, palm oil, soybean oil, dried tea, and instant tea. The FDA's residue allowances: 30 ppm in molasses, sugarcane; 0.1 ppm in palm oil; 0.1 ppm in olives; 1 ppm in dried tea; 4 ppm in instant tea. Moderately toxic by ingestion.

**PHOSPHORIC ACID** • A colorless, odorless solution made from phosphate rock. Mixes with water and alcohol. A sequestering additive *(see)* for rendered animal fat or a combination of such fat with vegetable fat. Also used as an acidulant and flavoring in soft drinks, jellies, frozen dairy products, bakery products, candy, cheese products, and in the brewing industry. Concentrated solutions are irritating to the skin and mucous membranes. The final report to the FDA of the Select Committee on GRAS Substances stated in 1980 that it should continue its GRAS status with no limitations other than good manufacturing practices. ASP. E

**PHOSPHOROUS CHLORIDE** • Phosphate derivative used as a starch modifier and a chlorinating additive. Intensely irritating to the skin, eyes, and mucous membranes. Inhalation may cause fluid in the lungs.

**PHOSPHOROUS OXYCHLORIDE** • Phosphoryl Chloride. Colorless, clear, strongly fuming vapors, used as a starch modifier and as a solvent and chlorinating additive. Inhalation may cause pulmonary edema. NUL

**PHOSPHOROUS SOURCES** • Calcium Phosphate, Magnesium Phosphate, Potassium Glycerophosphate, and Sodium Phosphate. Mineral supplements for cereal products, particularly breakfast foods such as farina. Phosphorus was formerly used to treat rickets and degenerative disorders. *See* Phosphate.

**PHOTOSENSITIVITY** • A condition in which the application or ingestion of certain chemicals, such as propylparaben *(see),* causes skin problems—including rash, hyperpigmentation, and swelling—when the skin is exposed to sunlight.

**PHTHALATES** • Salts of phthalic acid *(see)* used to make food packaging. Their use has increased steadily since the 1950s. By the mid-1980s, worldwide production was estimated at 2.7 million tons per year. In recent years phthalate esters emissions have become a major environmental and health concern. Many European countries—including Austria, Belgium, Denmark, England, Germany, the Netherlands, and Spain—have recommended a ban on PVC toys that contain phthalate esters. At issue are health concerns about phthalates. Phthalates also are used extensively in medical and food packaging products. Phthalate esters vary in their toxicity, but the most widely used phthalate, DEHP [di(-ethylhexyl)phthalate] has been linked in animal studies to damage to kidneys and liver and has been labeled as a probable human carcinogen. It can be passed through skin and mouth or by inhalation. Children are at particular risk since many toys (such as chewable items) are made from PVC. Millions of pounds of DEHP have been released into land and water in the United States. Phthalate esters are now widespread environmental pollutants and concern about their use has been mounting because some of the phthalates have been shown to damage the testes and decrease sperm production. Butyl benzyl phthalate (BBP) and di-n-butyl phthalate (DBP) also act like estrogens. Phthalates in the environment are regarded as endocrine disrupters, although the Phthalate Esters Panels of the Chemical Manufacturers Association denies this. The British Ministry of Agriculture, Fisheries, and Food found that there were phthalates in infant formulas but below tolerable daily intakes (TDI) but that as "a matter of prudence phthalate levels should be reduced in infant formulae." May be cancer-causing. In 1998, a panel including a former surgeon general was formed to study the safety of phthalates. Food packaging concerns have been focused on the use of phthalate plasticizers in many inks, coatings, and packaging films. These plasticizers are used to add flexibility to resins, such as nitrocellulose. Phthalates can migrate into food from plastics, inks, or coatings. Levels greater than a few parts per million of phthalates can be transferred. While manufacturers assure us that the leaching of phthalates into our foods is minuscule and harmless and scientists continue to puzzle over phthalates, it is wise not to use flexible wrap containing phthalates to cover dishes to be heated in the microwave. Wax paper in the meantime may be a better choice.

**PHTHALIC ACID** • Obtained by oxidation of various benzene derivatives, it can be isolated from the fungus *Gibberella fujikuroi*. It is used in the manufacture of plastics and dyes. Moderately irritating to the skin and mucous membranes. *See* Phthalates.

**PHTHALIC ANHYDRIDE** • White crystalline needles derived from naphthalene *(see)*. Used as a hardener for resins and a plasticizer. Also used in many dyes, chlorinated products, insecticides, and polyesters. A skin irritant. *See* Phthalates.

**PHTHALIMIDOMETHYL-O,O-DIMETHYL  PHOSPHORODITHI-OATE** • APPA. Kemolate. Prolate. Smidan. A widely used insecticide in cottonseed oil. FDA residue tolerance is 0.2 ppm in cottonseed. EPA Extremely Hazardous Substance List *(see)*. A human poison by ingestion. *See* Phthalates.

**PHYTIC ACID** • Occurs in nature in the seeds of cereal grains and is derived commercially from corn. It is used to chelate heavy metals, as a rust inhibitor, in metal cleaning, and in the treatment of hard water. Nontoxic, although those allergic to corn may have a reaction.

**PHYTOCHEMICAL** • Phytochemicals are substances found in edible fruits and vegetables that may be ingested by humans daily in gram quantities and that exhibit a potential for modulating the human metabolism in a manner favorable for reducing risk of cancer.

**PICHIA PASTORIS YEAST** • *See* Yeast.

**PICLORAM** • Crystalline solid made from picolinic acid, it is used as an herbicide and defoliant. It is toxic by ingestion and inhalation. Its use has been restricted in the United States. The FDA permits tolerances of 3 ppm in milled fractions (except flour) of barley, oats, and wheat resulting from application to the growing crop; 1 ppm in flour of barley and wheat; 0.2 ppm as residue in fat, meat by-products, and meat of cattle, goats, hogs, and sheep; 0.05 ppm as residue in milk and eggs; and 0.5 as residue in oat, barley, and wheat grains.

**PICRAMIC ACID** • 4,6-Dinitro-2-Aminophenol. A red crystalline acid obtained from phenol *(see)* and used chiefly in making azo dyes *(see)*. Highly toxic material. Readily absorbed through intact skin. Vapors absorbed through respiratory tract. Produces marked increase in metabolism and temperature, profuse sweating, collapse, and death. May cause skin rash, cataracts, and weight loss.

**PILEWORT EXTRACT** • An extract of *Ranunculus ficaria*, the coarse, hairy, perennial figwort of the eastern and central United States. It was once used to treat tuberculosis.

**PIMARICIN** • Natamycin. Natacyn. Myprozine. A fungicide produced from *Streptomyces natalensis* from soil near Pietermaritzburg, South Africa. It is applied to surface cuts and slices of cheese where standards permit to inhibit mold. FDA residue tolerance is 200 to 300 ppm. A drug used to treat fungal infections of the eye or eyelid in humans. Potential adverse reactions include swelling around the eyes and "black eyes" from blood gathering there. *See* Antibiotics. Moderately toxic by ingestion. Natamycin is used in human medicine and resistance is absolutely to be avoided. The European Parliament's Committee on Food said that it will review the safety and need for the use of these substances. ASP. E

**PIMENTA LEAF OIL** • Jamaica Pepper. Allspice. Derived from the dried ripe fruit of an evergreen shrub grown in the West Indies and Central and South America. Used in raspberry, fruit, nut, and spice flavorings for beverages, ice cream, ices, candy, baked goods, gelatin desserts, chewing gum, condiments, and meat products. Moderately toxic by ingestion. A severe skin irritant. GRAS. ASP

**PINE BARK, WHITE, SOLID EXTRACT** • Extract from *Pinus strobus*, used as a flavoring. EAF

**PINE CONE EXTRACT** • Extract from the cones of *Pinus sylvestris*. *See* Pine Needle Oil.

**PINE MOUNTAIN OIL** • *See* Pine Needle Oil and Pine Needle Dwarf Oil. EAF

**PINE NEEDLE DWARF OIL** • *Pinus mugo*. Pine Mountain Oil. The volatile oil obtained by steam distillation from a variety of pine trees, *Pinus mugo*. Colorless with a pleasant pine smell. Used in citrus, pineapple, and liquor flavorings for beverages, ice cream, ices, candy, and baked goods. There is reported use of the chemical; it has not yet been assigned for toxicology literature. EAF

**PINE NEEDLE OIL** • Pine Mountain Oil. An extract of various species of *Pinus* used as a natural flavoring in pineapple, citrus, and spice flavorings. Ingestion of large amounts can cause intestinal hemorrhages. EAF

**PINE SCOTCH OIL** • Volatile oil obtained by steam distillation from the needles of a pine tree. Colorless or yellowish, with an odor of turpentine. Used in various flavorings for beverages, candy, and baked goods. *See* Turpentine for toxicity. EAF

**PINE TAR** • A product obtained by distillation of pinewood. A blackish brown, viscous liquid, slightly soluble in water. Used as an antiseptic in skin diseases. May be irritating to the skin. *See* Pine Tar Oil.

**PINE TAR OIL** • The extract from a variety of pine trees. A synthetic flavoring obtained from a species of pinewood. Used in licorice flavorings for ice cream, ices, and candy. Also used as a solvent, disinfectant, and deodorant. As an oil from twigs and needles. Irritating to the skin and mucous membranes. Bomyl acetate, a substance obtained from various pine needles, has a strong pine odor. It can cause nausea, vomiting, convulsions, and dizziness if ingested. In general, pine oil in concentrated form is an irritant to human skin and may cause allergic reactions. In small amounts it is nontoxic. ASP

**PINEAPPLE EXTRACT** • *See* Pineapple Juice.

**PINEAPPLE JUICE** • The common juice from the tropical plant. Contains a protein-digesting and milk-clotting enzyme, bromelin *(see)*. An anti-inflammatory enzyme, it is used in cosmetic treatment creams. It is also used as a texturizer.

*a*-**PINENE** • A synthetic pine oil flavoring additive that occurs naturally in angelica root oil, anise, star anise, asafoetida oil, coriander, cumin, fennel, grapefruit, juniper berries, oils of lavender and lime, mandarin orange leaf, black pepper, peppermint, pimenta, and yarrow. It is the principal ingredient of turpentine *(see)*. Used chiefly in the manufacture of camphor. Used in lemon and nutmeg flavorings for beverages, ice cream, ices, candy, baked goods, and condiments. Also used as a chewing-gum base. Readily absorbed from the gastrointestinal tract, the skin, and the respiratory tract. It is a local irritant, central nervous system depressant, and an irritant to the bladder and kidney. Has caused benign skin tumors from chronic contact. ASP

**2-PINENE** • See *a*-Pinene.

*b*-**PINENE** • A synthetic flavoring that occurs naturally in black currant buds, coriander, cumin, black pepper, and yarrow. Used in citrus flavorings for beverages, ice cream, ices, candy (600 ppm), and baked goods (600 ppm). Also cleared for use in chewing-gum base. *See a*-Pinene for toxicity. ASP

**PINUS PUMILO OIL** • *See* Pine Needle Dwarf Oil.

**PINOCARVEOL** • Synthetic flavoring from pine. NIL

**PIPERAZINE** • Adipate and Citrate. Entacyl. Antepar. Bryrel. Pin-Tega Tabs. Pipril. Ta-Verm. Vermirex. Vermizine. An anthelmintic ingredient that paralyzes worms, causing their expulsion by normal movement of the human intestines. Adverse reactions include uncoordination, numbness, seizures, memory problems, headache, dizziness, eye problems, nausea, vomiting, diarrhea, abdominal cramps, hives, skin rashes, joint pain, fever, bronchospasm, and anemia. NUL

**PIPERIDINE** • A synthetic flavoring that occurs naturally in black pepper. Used in beverages, candy, baked goods, meats, soups, and condiments. Soapy texture. Has been proposed for use as a tranquilizer and muscle relaxant. ASP

**PIPERINE** • Celery Soda. A synthetic flavoring additive that occurs naturally in black pepper, it is used as a pungent brandy flavoring. It is also used as a nontoxic insecticide. Believed to be more toxic than the commercial pyrethrins. ASP

**PIPERITENONE** • A synthetic flavoring additive that occurs naturally in Japanese mint. Used in beverages, ice cream, ices, candy, and baked goods. Used to give dentifrices a minty flavor and to give perfumes their peppermint scent. NIL

**PIPERONAL** • Heliotropin. A synthetic flavoring and perfume additive that occurs naturally in vanilla and black pepper. White crystalline powder with a sweet floral odor. Used in strawberry, cola, cherry, rum, maple, nut, and vanilla flavorings in beverages, ice cream, ices, baked goods, gelatin puddings, and chewing gum. Ingestion of large amounts may cause central nervous system depression. Has been reported to cause skin rash. ASP

**PIPERONYL ACETATE** • A synthetic fruit flavoring additive for beverages, ice cream, ices, candy, and baked goods. *See* Piperonal for toxicity. ASP

**PIPERONYL ALDEHYDE** • *See* Piperonal.

**PIPERONYL BUTOXIDE** • Butoxide. Pyburthrin. Butocide. A light brown liquid, a widely used insecticide in animal feed, dried foods, milled fractions derived from cereal grains, and packaging materials. It is used in combination with pyrethrins *(see)* in oil solutions, emulsions, powders, or aerosols. The FDA permits residues of up to 10 ppm in milled fractions derived from cereal grains, in dried foods, and in animal feed. International Agency for Research on Cancer (IARC) review and on the Community Right-To-Know List. No evidence, as yet, that it is a cancer-causing additive, but it is poisonous by skin contact. Moderately toxic by ingestion. Large doses have caused vomiting and diarrhea in humans. Has shown adverse reproductive effects in experimental animals.

**PIPERONYL ISOBUTYRATE** • A synthetic fruit and cheese flavoring for beverages, ice cream, ices, candy, and baked goods. *See* Piperonal for toxicity. ASP

**PIPERONYL PIPERIDINE** • *See* Piperine.

**PIPSISSEWA LEAVES EXTRACT** • *Chimaphila unbellata.* Love-in-Winter. Prince's Pine. Extracted from the leaves of an evergreen shrub. Used in root beer, sarsaparilla, wintergreen, and birch beer flavorings for beverages and candy. Its leaves have been used as an astringent, diuretic, and tonic. The Cree name means "to break up"—bladder stones, that is. There is reported use of the chemical, it has not yet been assigned for toxicology literature. GRAS. EAF

**PLANT ESTROGENS** • A host of estrogens have been identified in plants. Although they are considerably less active than those in animals, chronic exposure may lead to the accumulation of levels that are active in humans.

**PLANT STEROLS** • Vitamin D precursors found in broccoli, cabbage, cucumbers, squash, yams, tomatoes, eggplant, peppers, soy products, and whole grains. They cause cells to differentiate. GRAS

**PLANTAIN EXTRACT** • The extract of various species of plantain. The starchy fruit is a staple throughout the tropics and is used for bladder infections by herbalists. It is a natural astringent and antiseptic with soothing and cooling effects on blemishes and burns.

**PLANTAROME** • *See* Yucca Extract.

**PLASTICIZERS** • Substances when migrating from food packaging material include acetyl tributyl citrate, butyl stearate, and epoxidized soybean oil.

**PLUM EXTRACT** • The extract of the fruit of the plum tree *Prunus* × *domestica*. The Indians boiled the wild plum and gargled with it to cure mouth sores.

**POLOXAMER 331** • A thick liquid used as a dough conditioner, foam control additive, solubilizing additive in flavor concentrates, as a detergent, and in a wash for poultry. The FDA limits it to equal weight in flavor concentrations and to 0.5 percent in poultry baths; 5 grams per hog in debarring machines; and 0.5 percent by weight of flour

**POLY-** • A prefix meaning "many."

**POLYACRYLAMIDE** • The polymer of acrylamide monomers, it is a white solid, water soluble, that is used as a thickening additive, suspending additive, and as an additive to adhesives. In modified form it is used to clarify (*see* Clarifying Additive) cane sugar. Used as a film former in the imprinting of soft-shell gelatin capsules. Used in washing fruits and vegetables. Highly toxic and irritating to the skin. Causes central nervous system paralysis. Can be absorbed through unbroken skin. *See* acrylamides. ASP

**POLYACRYLIC ACID** • *See* Acrylic Resins. ASP

**POLYALKYL ACRYLATE** • Used in the production of petroleum wax. *See* Petroleum. EAF

**POLYAMINE-EPICHLORHYDRIN RESIN** • A petition was filed to use this as a fixing additive in an enzyme derived from the bacillus *Steptomyces olivaceus*. The FDA put the petition in abeyance *(see)* in 2003.

**POLYAMINO SUGAR CONDENSATE** • The condensation product of the sugars fructose, galactose, glucose, lactose, maltose, mannose, rhamnose, ribose, or xylose, with a minute amount of amino acids such as alanine, arginine, aspartic acid, glutamic acid, glycine, histidine, hydroxyproline, isoleucine, leucine, lysine, methionine, phenylalanine, proline, pyroglutamic acid, serine, threonine, tyrosine, or valine. *See* Amino Acids.

**POLYBUTENE** • Indopol. Polybutylene. A plasticizer. A polymer *(see)* of one or more butylenes obtained from petroleum oils. Used in lubricating oil, adhesives, sealing tape, cable insulation, films, and coatings. May asphyxiate.

**POLYCHLORINATED BIPHENYLS (PCB)** • Clear, amber-colored, or dark oily liquids. They may have a faint smell like motor oil, and some contain chlorobenzenes, which make them smell like mothballs. Widely used since the 1930s because of their excellent electrical and insulating abilities, PCBs were banned in 1978 by the Environmental Protection Agency. The toxic effects were first noted when more than twelve hundred people in Japan were poisoned by eating food cooked in oil heavily contaminated with PCBs. Soon afterward, studies showed that PCBs caused cancer in test animals. PCBs, unfortunately, remain in the environment for a long time because they do not break down. Research at the University of Maryland reported in 1998 said children exposed to dioxins *(see)* and PCBs prenatally or during infancy can suffer behavioral, memory, and learning problems. The Maryland investigators suggest that the underlying mechanism may be thyroid hormone disruption. Even moderate impairment of thyroid hormone function has been associated with various problems in behavior and intellectual development, and certain thyroid diseases are associated with attention deficit hyperactivity disorder and language disorders. Studies of adults exposed to dioxin and PCBs show no marked neurological effects. The Maryland research was funded by the university and by the American Thyroid Association.

**POLYDEXTROSE** • A reduced-calorie bulking additive developed by Pfizer, Inc., and approved for use in foods by the FDA in June 1981. It includes glucose, citric acid, and sorbitol. The FDA says it is not a substitute for saccharin *(see)* or a general sweetener but that it can replace sucrose *(see)* as a bulking additive in frozen desserts, cakes, and candies and reduce calories in some products as much as 50 percent. According to Pfizer, it is a one-calorie-per-gram bulking additive capable of replacing higher calorie—4 to 9 calories per gram—ingredients such as sucrose, carbohydrates, and fats in many food products. ASP. E

**POLY(DIVINYLBENZENE-COETHYLSTYRENE** • Packaging. *See* Styrene and Benzene. EAF

**POLY(DIVINYLBENZENE-COTRIMETHYL(VINYLBENZYL)AM-MONIUM CHLORIDE)** • Packaging. *See* Benzene and Ammonium Chloride. EAF

**POLYESTER-POLYURETHANE RESIN-ACID DIANHYDRIDE ADHE-SIVE** • A petition for its use in pouches containing fatty foods was put in abeyance *(see)* by the FDA in 2003.

**POLYETHOXYLATED ALKYLPHENOL** • Dodecyl, Nonyl, and Octyl. Components of a commercial detergent for raw foods, followed by water rinsing. The only symptoms shown in animals poisoned with this substance is gastrointestinal irritation.

**POLYETHYLENE** • A polymer *(see)* of ethylene; a product of petroleum gas or dehydration of alcohol. One of a group of lightweight thermoplastics that have a good resistance to chemicals, low moisture absorption, and good insulating properties. Used as a chewing-gum base ingredient and as a film former and sheets for packaging. Also used as roughage replacement in feedlot rations for cattle. No known skin toxicity, but implants of large amounts in rats caused cancer. Ingestion of large oral doses has produced kidney and liver damage.

**POLYETHYLENE GLYCOL** • 400–2,000 molecular weight. PEG. Defoaming additive in processed beet sugar and yeast. Improves resistance to moisture and oxidation. ASP

**POLYETHYLENE GLYCOL (600) DIOLEATE** • Polyethylene glycol esters of mixed fatty acids from tall oil; polyethylene glycol (400 through 6,000). An additive in nonnutritive artificial sweeteners; a component of coatings and binders in tablet food; improves resistance to oxidation and moisture. *See* Polyols. ASP

**POLYGLYCERATE 60** • *See* Glycerides.

**POLYGLYCEROL** • Prepared from edible fats, oils, and esters of fatty acids. Derived from corn, cottonseed, palm, peanut, safflower, sesame, and soybean oils, lard, and tallow.

**POLYGLYCEROL ESTER OF FATTY ACIDS** • Several partial or complete esters of saturated and unsaturated fatty acids with a variety of derivatives of polyglycerols. E

**POLYGLYCERYL-4 COCOATE** • *See* Coconut Oil and Polyglycerol.

**POLYGLYCEROL POLYRICINOLEATE** • *See* Riconoleate. E

**POLYGLYCERYL-10 DECALINOLEATE** • *See* Polyglycerol and Linoleic Acid.

**POLYGLYCERYL-10 DECAOLEATE** • *See* Oleic Acid and Polyglycerol.

**POLYGLYCERYL-2 DIISOSTEATE** • *See* Isostearic Acid and Polyglycerol.

**POLYGLYCERYL-6 DIOLEATE** • *See* Oleic Acid and Glycerin.

**POLYGLYCERYL-6 DISTEARATE** • *See* Stearic Acid and Glycerin.

**POLYGLYCERYL-3 HYDROXYLAURYL ETHER** • *See* Fatty Alcohols and Glycerin.

**POLYGLYCERYL-4 ISOSTEARATE** • *See* Isostearic Acid and Glycerin.

**POLYGLYCERYL-2 LANOLIN ALCOHOL ETHER** • *See* Lanolin and Glycerin.

**POLYGLYCERYL-LAURYL ETHER** • *See* Fatty Alcohols and Glycerin.

**POLYGLYCERYL-3, -4 OLEATE** • Oily liquid prepared by adding alcohol to coconut oil or other triglycerides with a polyglyceryl. Used in foods, drugs, and cosmetics as fat emulsifiers. In addition, they may also be used as lubricants, plasticizers, gelling additives, and dispersants.

**POLYGLYCERYL-3, -4, or -8 OLEATE** • Ester of oleic acid and glycerin (*see both*).

**POLYGLYCERYL-2 or -4 OLEYL ETHER** • Ether of oleyl alcohol and glycerin (*see both*).

**POLYGLYCERYL-3-PEG-2 COCOAMIDE** • *See* Coconut Oil and Glycerin.

**POLYGLYCERYL-2-PEG-4 STEARATE** • An ether of peg-4 stearate and glycerin. *See* Stearic Acid and Glycerin.

**POLYGLYCERYL PHTHALATE ESTERS OF COCONUT OIL FATTY ACIDS** • *See* Coconut Oil and Fatty Acids. EAF

**POLYGLYCERYL-2-SESQUIISOSTEARATE** • A mixture of esters of isostearic acid and glycerin *(see both)*.

**POLYGLYCERYL-2-SESQUIOLEATE** • A mixture of ester of oleic acid and glycerin *(see both)*.

**POLYGLYCERYL SORBITOL** • A condensation product of glycerin and sorbitol *(see both)*.

**POLYGLYCERYL-3, -4, or -8 STEARATE** • An ester of stearic acid and glycerin *(see both)*.

**POLYGLYCERYL-10 TETRAOLEATE** • An ester of oleic acid and glycerin *(see both)*.

**POLYGLYCERYL-2 TETRASTEARATE** • *See* Stearic Acid and Glycerin.

**POLYISOBUTENE** • *See* Polybutene.

**POLYISOBUTYLENE** • Soft to hard, elastic, light, white solid, odorless and tasteless. Used as a chewing substance in gum. *See* Resin, Isobutylene. ASP

**POLYISOBUTYLENE 317** • Ranging from diglycerol to triacontaglycerol. Prepared from edible fats, oils, and fatty acids, hydrogenated or nonhydrogenated *(see* Hydrogenation). Derived from corn, cottonseed, palm, peanut, safflower, sesame, and soybean oils, lard, and tallow. Used as lubricants, plasticizers, gelling additives, humectants, surfactants, dispersants, and emulsifiers in foods.

**POLYLIMONENE** • A general fixative derived from citrus oils. It is used in candy (4,500 ppm), chewing gum, and baked goods (1,000 ppm). It can be a skin irritant and sensitizer. *See* Limonene. ASP

**POLYMALEIC ACID** • Used in the processing of sugar. *See* Maleic Acid. ASP

**POLYMALEIC ANHYDRIDE, SODIUM SALT** • Used in the processing of sugar. *See* Maleic Acid. EAF

**POLYMER** • A substance or product formed by combining many small molecules (monomers). The result is essentially recurring long-chain structural units that have tensile strength, elasticity, and hardness. Examples of polymers (literally, "having many parts") are plastics, fibers, rubber, and human tissue.

**POLYMIXIN B** • A generic term for antibiotics obtained from fermentation of various media by strains of *Bacillus polymyxa*. Used as a bactericide in yeast culture for beer. May cause renal irritation and damage.

**POLYOLS** • Alcohol compounds that absorb moisture. They have a low molecular weight: polyols with a weight above 1,000 are solids and less toxic than those with weight 600 or below. The latter are liquid, and although higher in toxicity, large doses are required to kill animals. Such deaths in animals have been found to be due to kidney damage. *See* Propylene Glycol and Polyethylene Glycol as examples.

**POLYOXYALKALENE GLYCOL** • Defoaming additive in beet sugar production.

**POLYOXYETHYLENE COMPOUNDS** • Nonionic emulsifiers used in hand creams and lotions. Usually oily or waxy liquids.

**POLYOXYETHYLENE (600) DIOLEATE** • A defoamer. NEW

**POLYOXYETHYLENE GLYCOL** • Ester of edible cottonseed oil and fatty acids. Solubilizing additive in pickles.

**POLYOXYETHYLENE GLYCOL (600) MONORICINOLEATE** • De-foaming component used in processing beet sugar and yeast.

**POLYOXYETHYLENE (600)MONORICINOLEATE** • Plasticizer. *See* Polyoxyethylene and Ricinoleic Acid. ASP. E

**POLYOXYETHYLENE (40) MONOSTEARATE** • Defoaming additive in processed foods; emulsifier for frozen desserts. Application to the skin of mice has been shown to cause skin tumors. The compound has been fed to animals and does not appear to produce tumors on its own, but there is a suggestion that it allows cancer-causing additives to penetrate more quickly. On the FDA list for further study for long- and short-term effects since 1980.

**POLYOXYETHYLENE (20) SORBITAN MONOOLEATE** • Emulsifier and defoamer in the production of beet sugar; a dietary vitamin and mineral supplement. Used in dill oil in spiced green beans, icing, frozen custard, iced milk, fruit, and sherbet. The FDA asked for short-term, mutagenic, teratogenic, subacute, and reproductive effects in 1980 and has not reported any findings since. E

**POLYOXYETHYLENE (20) SORBITAN MONOPALMITATE** • An emulsifier, flavor-dispersing additive, and defoaming additive. Used in whipped cream, beverages, confectionery, and soup. The FDA asked for further study of the safety of this additive in 1980 and has reported nothing about it since. E

**POLYOXYETHYLENE (20) SORBITAN MONOSTEARATE** • Polysorbate 60. An emulsifier and flavor-dispersing additive in shortening and edible oils. Used in whipped vegetable-oil topping, cake, and cake mixes; cake icing or filling; sugar-type confection coatings; coconut spread; beverage mixes; confectionery; chicken bases; gelatin desserts; dressings made without egg yolks; solid-state, edible vegetable fat-water emulsions used in substitutes for milk or cream; dietary vitamin supplements; foaming additives in nonalcoholic beverage mixes to be added to alcoholic beverages; and a wetting and dispersing additive for powdered processed foods. The FDA asked for further study of this additive in 1980.

**POLYOXYETHYLENE (20) SORBITAN TRISTEARATE** • Emulsifier, defoaming additive, and flavor-dispersing additive. Used in cakes and cake mixes, including doughnuts, whipped mixes, and vegetable oil toppings; cake icings and fillings; ice cream; frozen custard, ice milk, fruit sherbet, and nonstandardized frozen desserts; solid-state, edible vegetable fat-water emulsions used as milk and cream substitutes in coffee; and wetting and dispersing additives in processed powdered food. E

**POLYOXYETHYLENE STEARATE** • A mixture of stearate (*see* Stearic Acid) and ethylene oxide, it is a waxy solid once added to bread to make it "feel fresh." It was fed to rats as one-fourth of their diets and resulted in the formation of bladder stones, and subsequently a number of tumors. Banned in 1952. The European Parliament said in 2003 that this synthetic stabilizing agent can contain harmful by-products (ethylene oxide, mono- and diethyleneglycols). Its use should therefore be banned. E

**POLYPHOSPHATES** • Polyphosphates are legally permitted additives that are widely used to aid processing or to improve eating quality of many foods, particularly meat and fish products. Phosphates are also used in making baking powder and cola drinks, and great quantities are used in fertilizers and detergents. Phosphates are present normally in all living things and are an essential component of our diet. A phosphate is a salt of phosphoric acid; when a number of simple phosphate units are linked to form a more complex structure, this is known as a polyphosphate. The phosphates used in foods may be simple phosphates, pyrophosphates containing two phosphate units, tripolyphosphates containing three units, or polyphosphates containing more than three phosphate units. The main value of polyphosphates lies in improving the retention of water by the protein in fish. The manner in which they do this is not clearly understood, but their effect is mainly on the surface of the fish. Other substances such as common salt give similar results but with undesirable flavor effects. E

**POLYPROPYLENE GLYCOL** • Defoaming additive for yeast and beet sugar. ASP

**POLYSACCHARIDES** • Carbohydrates that are organic compounds consisting of carbon, hydrogen, and oxygen. The polysaccharides include starch, dextrin, glycogen, and cellulose.

**POLYSORBATE 60 and POLYSORBATE 80** • Both are emulsifiers that have been associated with the contaminant 1,4 dioxane, known to cause cancer in animals. The 60 is a condensate of sorbitol with stearic acid, and the 80 is a condensate of sorbitol and oleic acid (*see all*). The 60 is waxy, soluble in solvents, and is used as an emulsifier, stabilizer, wetting, and dispersing additive for powdered processed foods, and a foaming additive for beverage mixes. It is added to chocolate coatings to prevent cocoa-butter substitutes from tasting greasy. It is found in frozen and gelatin desserts, cakes, cake mixes, doughnuts, and artificial chocolate coatings, nondairy whipped cream and creamers, powdered convenience foods, salad dressings made without egg yolks, and vitamin supplements. The 80 is a viscous liquid with a faint caramel odor and is used as an emulsifier, stabilizer, and humectant. It prevents oil from separating from nondairy whipped cream and helps nondairy coffee whiteners to dissolve. It is also found in baked goods, ice cream, frozen custard, shortenings, and vitamin and mineral supplements. FDA residue tolerances in various products are from less than 0.1 percent to 4.5 percent. Polysorbate 40 is also widely used as an emulsifier of essential oils in water. ASP

**POLYSORBATE 80 WITH CARRAGEENAN** • *See* Polysorbates and Carrageenan.

**POLYSORBATES** • 1 through 85. These are widely used emulsifiers and stabilizers. For example, polysorbate 20 is a viscous, oily liquid derived from lauric acid. Used in vitamins, pickle products, mineral preparations, in special diet foods, alone or in combination with sorbitan. They are also used as dispersing additives in gelatin desserts and mixes; and up to 10 ppm in finished table salt. They are used in creaming mixtures for cottage cheese and low-fat cottage cheese and as a surfactant and wetting additive for natural and artificially colored barbecue sauces. It is a stabilizer of essential oils in water. It is used as a nonionic surfactant *(see)*. ASP. The European Parliament said in 2003 that polysorbates are used as preservatives in cakes, cheeses, and wines, for example. Extended use may be assumed to cause damage to health; it is therefore important that their use be subject to review. Polysorbates contain harmful residues (ethylene oxide, ethylene glycols), can increase the absorption of fat-dissolving substances, and modify the digestion of various substances.

**POLYSTYRENE** • Used in the manufacture of resins. Reported to be an unintentional additive when tea and coffee are drunk from polystyrene cups. Colorless to yellowish, oily liquid with a penetrating odor. Obtained from ethylbenzene by removing the hydrogen or by chlorination. Sparingly soluble in water; soluble in alcohol. May be irritating to the eyes and mucous membranes and, in high concentrations, may be narcotic.

**POLYSTYRENE CROSS-LINKED CHLOROMETHYLATED, THEN LAMINATED** • Packaging. *See* Polystyrene. ASP

**POLYUNSAT FAT** • Listing on food labels for polyunsaturated fats *(see)*.

**POLYUNSATURATED FATS** • The saturation of fat refers to the chemical structure of its constituent fatty acids. Polyunsaturates are liquid at room temperature and consist mainly of fatty acids that can hold four or more additional hydrogen atoms. *See* Monounsaturated Fats.

**POLYVINYL ACETATE** • Used in chewing-gum base. ASP

**POLYVINYL ALCOHOL 9** • Synthetic resins used to dilute the color of eggshells and used in lipstick, setting lotions, and various creams. A polymer is prepared from polyvinyl acetates by replacement of the acetate groups with the hydroxyl groups. Dry, unplasticized polyvinyl alcohol powders are white to cream-colored and have different viscosities. Solvent in hot and cold water but certain ones require alcohol-water mixtures. The FDA requires no penetration of polyvinyl alcohol through eggshell. An experimental cancer-causing and tumor-inducing additive. International Agency for Research on Cancer (IARC) *(see)* review. NIL

**POLYVINYL BUTYRAL** • Condensation of polyvinyl alcohol and butyraldehyde *(see both)*. It is a synthetic flavoring found in coffee and strawberry. May be an irritant and narcotic.

**POLYVINYL CHLORIDE (PVC)** • Chloroethylene Polymer. Derived from vinyl chloride *(see)*, it consists of a white powder or colorless granules that are resistant to weather, moisture, acids, fats, petroleum products, and fungus. It is widely used for everything from plumbing to raincoats. The use of PVC as a plastic wrap for food, including meats, and for human blood, has alarmed some scientists. Human and animal blood can extract potentially harmful chemicals from the plastic. The chemicals are added to polyvinyl chloride to make it flexible, and they migrate from the plastic into the blood and into the meats in amounts directly proportional to the length of time of storage. The result can be contamination of the blood, causing lung shock, a condition in which the patient's blood circulation to the lungs is impeded. PVC is also used in cosmetics and toiletries in containers, nail enamels, and creams. PVC has caused tumors when injected under the skin of rats in doses of 100 milligrams per kilogram of body weight.

**POLYVINYL ETHYL ETHER** • *See* Polyvinyl Alcohol 9.

**POLYVINYL IMIDAZOLINIUM ACETATE** • The polymer of vinyl imidazolinium acetate. *See* Polyvinylpyrrolidone

**POLYVINYL METHYL ETHER** • *See* Polyvinyl Alcohol.

**POLY(2-VINYLPYRIDICINE-CO-STYRENE)** • A coating for nutrients for cattle. *See* Polyvinylpyrrolidone and Styrene.

**POLYVINYL POLYPYRROLIDONE** • Purified vinylpyrrolidone. Used in clarifying sparkling wine. *See* Polyvinylpyrrolidone. ASP E

**POLYVINYLPYRROLIDONE (PVP)** • A faintly yellow, solid plastic resin resembling albumin. Used in dietary products. Also a clarifying additive in vinegar, beer, and wine. Limitation of 6 pounds per 1,000 gallons in wine. FDA requires that it be removed by filtration. The FDA residue tolerance is less than 10 ppm in beer, less than 40 ppm in vinegar and 60 ppm in wine from use as a clarifying additive; and less than 60 ppm as a tableting adjuvant in nonnutritive sweeteners and in flavor, vitamin, and mineral concentrates in tablet form. Ingestion may produce gas and fecal impaction or damage to lungs and kidneys. It may last in the system several months to a year. Strong circumstantial evidence indicates thesaurosis—foreign bodies in the lungs—may be produced in susceptible individuals from concentrated exposure to PVP in hairsprays. Modest intravenous doses in rats caused them to develop tumors. The European Parliament said in 2003 that these substances can contain residues of vinylpyrrolidone, a substance which is considered cancerogenous in animals. E1201 has been assessed as not classifiable by WHO's International Agency for Research on Cancer (IARC). ASP. E

**POMEGRANATE BARK EXTRACT** • A flavoring from the dried bark, stem, or root of the tree *Punica granatum,* grown in the Mediterranean region and elsewhere. Contains about 20 percent tannic acid *(see)*; rind of fruit contains 30 percent. Formerly used to expel tapeworms. Overdose can cause nausea, vomiting, and diarrhea. GRAS. EAF

**PONCEAU 4R** • Coloring. *See* Cochineal. E

**POPLAR EXTRACT** • Balm of Gilead. Extract of the leaves and twigs of *Populus nigra.* In ancient times, the buds were mashed to make a soothing salve that was spread on sunburned skin, scalds, scratches, inflamed skin, and wounds. They were also simmered in lard for use as an ointment and for antiseptic purposes. The leaves and bark were steeped by American colonists to make a soothing tea. It supposedly helped allergies and soothed reddened eyes. Used as a flavoring in alcoholic beverages only. NUL

**POPPY SEED** • The seed of the poppy *Papaver somniferum.* Used as a natural spice for flavoring for baked goods (8,600 ppm). GRAS. ASP

**POT MARIGOLD** • *See* Marigold, Pot. GRAS

**POT MARJORAM** • *See* Marjoram, Pot. GRAS

**POTASSIUM** • The healthy human body contains about nine grams of potassium. Most of it is found inside body cells. Potassium plays an important role in maintaining water balance and acid-base balance. It participates in the transmission of nerve impulses and in the transfer of messages from nerves to muscles. It also acts as a catalyst in carbohydrate and protein metabolism. Potassium is important for the maintenance of normal kidney function. It has a major effect on the heart and all the muscles of the body.

**POTASSIUM ACETATE** • Colorless, water-absorbing crystals or powder, odorless or with a faint acetic aroma and a salty taste. Used as a buffer and antimicrobial preservative. Very soluble in water. Also used medicinally to treat irregular heartbeat and as a diuretic. The GRAS designation was removed by the FDA in the 1990s. NIL. E

**POTASSIUM ACID PYROPHOSPHATE** • *See* Sodium Acid Pyrophosphate. NUL

**POTASSIUM ACID TARTRATE** • Salt of tartaric acid. Colorless with a pleasant odor. An acid and buffer, it is the acid constituent of some baking powders. Used in effervescent beverages. It is also used in some confectionery products. Formerly a cathartic. GRAS. ASP

**POTASSIUM ADIPATE** • Antioxidant primarily used in low salt foods. No adverse effects reported. *See* Adipic Acid. E

**POTASSIUM ALGINATE** • A stabilizer *(see)*. *See* Alginates. GRAS. E

**POTASSIUM ALUM** • *See* Alum.

**POTASSIUM ALUMINUM SILICATE** • *See* Aluminum and Silicate. E
**POTASSIUM ASPARTAME** • *See* Aspartame.
**POTASSIUM ASPARTATE** • The potassium salt of aspartic acid *(see)*.
**POTASSIUM BENZOATE** • A preservative used in margarine and wine.
The FDA limits the amount to 0.1 percent or if used in combination with
sorbic acid *(see)* to 0.2 percent in margarine and 0.1 percent in wine. *See*
Benzoic Acid. ASP E
**POTASSIUM BICARBONATE** • Carbonic Acid, Monopotassium Salt.
Colorless, odorless, transparent crystals or powder, slightly alkaline, salty
taste. Considered a miscellaneous and/or general-purpose food additive, it
is present in fluids and tissues of the body as a product of normal metabolic
processes. Soluble in water. It is used in baking, soft drinks, and in low-pH
liquid detergents. The final report to the FDA of the Select Committee on
GRAS Substances stated in 1980 that it should continue its GRAS status
with no limitations other than good manufacturing practices. ASP
**POTASSIUM BISULFATE** • Derived by heating potassium sulfiate with
sulfuric acid. Used in wine processing and to make potassium bitartrate.
GRAS
**POTASSIUM BISULFITE** • Same uses as for sodium sulfite *(see)* in ale,
beer, and fruit-pie mix. Not to be used in foods containing vitamin $B_1$, raw
fruit and vegetables, including fresh potatoes (not frozen, canned, or dehydrated). The final report to the FDA of the Select Committee on GRAS
Substances stated in 1980 that there is no evidence in the available information that it is a hazard to the public when used as it is now and it should
continue its GRAS status with limitations on the amounts that can be added
to food. *See* Sulfites. ASP
**POSTASSIUM BORATE** • Boric Acid, Potassium Salt. A crystalline salt
used as an oxidizing ingredient and as a preservative in flour. *See* Borates
for toxicity. NUL
**POTASSIUM BROMATE** • The compound is added as an improving additive in bread. The expected result is to obtain a fine spongelike quality with
the action of oxygen. This method is used in Great Britain, the United
States, and Japan. Legal allowance of potassium bromate is below 50 ppm
in white flour and 75 ppm in whole wheat flour. Very toxic when taken
internally. Burns and skin irritation have been reported from its industrial
uses. In toothpaste it has been reported to have caused inflammation and
bleeding of gums. In 1980, the Ames Test *(see)* found it to be a mutagen.
The FAO/WHO *(see)* said in 1993 that new data about potassium bromate
showed long-term toxicity and carcinogenicity including kidney tumors,
tumors of the lining of the stomach, and thyroid tumors in rats and slightly
increased kidney tumors in hamsters. On the basis of the new safety data
and the new data on residual bromate in bread, the committee concluded the

use of potassium bromate as a flour treatment additive was not appropriate. The previous acceptable level of treatment of flours for bread-making was therefore withdrawn. The FDA has taken no action at this writing to restrict the use of this additive. ASP

**POTASSIUM BROMIDE** • A preservative used in washing fruits and vegetables. Used medicinally as a sedative and antiepileptic. In large doses it can cause central nervous system depression. Prolonged intake may cause bromism. Bromism's main symptoms are headache, mental inertia, slow heartbeat, gastric distress, skin rash, acne, muscular weakness, and occasionally violent delirium. Bromides can cross the placental barrier and have caused skin rashes in the fetus. ASP

**POTASSIUM CAPRATE** • A cleansing ingredient. *See* Capric Acid. NUL

**POTASSIUM CAPRYLATE** • Source of potassium added to food. NUL

**POTASSIUM CARBONATE** • Salt of Tartar. Pearl Ash. Inorganic salt of potassium. Odorless, white powder soluble in water but practically insoluble in alcohol. Used as an alkali in combination with potassium hydroxide *(see)* for extracting color from annatto *(see)* seed. Also used in confections and cocoa products. Formerly employed as a diuretic to reduce body water and as an alkalizer. Irritating and caustic to human skin and may cause dermatitis of the scalp, forehead, and hands. The final report to the FDA of the Select Committee on GRAS Substances stated in 1980 that it should continue its GRAS status with no limitations other than good manufacturing practices. ASP. E

**POTASSIUM CASEINATE** • The potassium salt of milk proteins used in ice cream, frozen custard, ice milk, and fruit sherbets. *See* Casein. ASP

**POTASSIUM CHLORIDE** • A colorless, crystalline, odorless powder with a salty taste. A yeast food used in the brewing industry to improve brewing and fermentation and in the jelling industry. Small intestinal ulcers may occur with oral administration. Large doses ingested can cause gastrointestinal irritation, purging, weakness, and circulatory collapse. Used as a substitute for sodium chloride *(see)* in low-sodium dietary foods. The final report to the FDA of the Select Committee on GRAS Substances stated in 1980 that it should continue its GRAS status with no limitations other than good manufacturing practices. ASP. E

**POTASSIUM CITRATE** • A transparent or white powder, odorless, with a cool, salty taste. Used as a buffer in confections and in artificially sweetened jellies and preserves. It is a urinary alkalizer and gastric antacid. The final report to the FDA of the Select Committee on GRAS Substances stated in 1980 that it should continue its GRAS status with no limitations other than good manufacturing practices. E

**POTASSIUM COCOATE** • *See* Coconut Oil. ASP

**POTASSIUM COCO-HYDROLYZED PROTEIN** • *See* Proteins.

**POTASSIUM CORNATE** • The potassium salt of fatty acids derived from corn oil. *See* Corn Oil.

**POTASSIUM CYCLAMATE** • Nonnutritive sweetener removed from the GRAS list in 1969 and is now illegal in foods. BANNED

**POTASSIUM 2-(1-ETHOXY)ETHOXYPROPANOATE** • Synthetic flavoring. NIL

**POTASSIUM FERROCYANIDE** • Coloring. Human studies, according to FAO/WHO have demonstrated that high levels were toxic to the kidney in the single short-term study available but no kidney function tests were performed. May be harmful by inhalation/ingestion/skin absorption. May cause irritation. E

**POTASSIUM FUMARATE** • Acidifier. *See* Fumaric Acid. NUL

**POTASSIUM GIBBERELLATE** • The salt of gibberellic acid, a plant growth-promoting hormone. White crystalline powder that absorbs water. Used as an enzyme activator in fermented malt beverages. The FDA limits it to 2 ppm in treated barley malt and 0.5 ppm in the finished beverage. EAF

**POTASSIUM GLUCONATE** • The potassium salt of gluconic acid *(see)* used as a buffering additive that helps keep soda water bubbling. Mildly toxic by ingestion. The final report to the FDA of the Select Committee on GRAS Substances stated in 1980 that it should continue its GRAS status with no limitations other than good manufacturing practices. NUL. E

**POTASSIUM GLYCEROPHOSPHATE** • Nutrient additive. *See* Glycerides. GRAS. EAF

**POTASSIUM HYDROGEN SULFITE** • *See* Sulfites. E

**POTASSIUM HYDROXIDE** • Caustic Potash. An alkali used to extract color from annatto seed, a peeling additive for tubers and fruits, also in cacao products. Occasionally used to prevent the growth of horns in calves. Prepared industrially by electrolysis of potassium chloride *(see)*. Extremely corrosive, and ingestion may cause violent pain, bleeding, collapse, and death. When applied to the skin of mice, moderate dosages cause tumors. May cause skin rash and burning. The FDA banned household products containing more than 10 percent potassium hydroxide. GRAS. ASP. E

**POTASSIUM HYPOPHOSPHATE** • The final report to the FDA of the Select Committee on GRAS Substances stated in 1980 that it should continue its GRAS status with no limitations other than good manufacturing practices. *See* Phosphate. NUL

**POTASSIUM HYPOPHOSPHITE** • Used in processing additives. Can be explosive. *See* Phosphorous. EAF

**POTASSIUM IODATE** • Oxidizer. Dough Conditioner. *See* Potassium Iodide and Iodine Sources. ASP

**POTASSIUM IODIDE** • Potassium Salt. A dye remover and an antiseptic. Used in table salt as a source of dietary iodine. It is also in some drinking water. May cause allergic reactions. GRAS. ASP

**POTASSIUM LACTATE** • Flavoring. *See* Lactic Acid. GRAS. ASP. E

**POTASSIUM LAURATE** • The potassium salt of lauric acid *(see)*. NUL

**POTASSIUM LAURYL SULFATE** • A water softener. *See* Sodium Lauryl Sulfate.

**POTASSIUM MALATE** • *See* Malic Acid. E.

**POTASSIUM METABISULFITE** • Potassium Pyrosulfite. White or colorless, with an odor of sulfur dioxide *(see)*, it is an antioxidant, preservative, and antifermentative in breweries and wineries. Should not be used in meats or foods recognized as sources of vitamin $B_1$. Also used for bleaching straw and as an antiseptic, preservative, antioxidant, and a developing additive in dyes. Low toxicity. The final report to the FDA of the Select Committee on GRAS Substances stated in 1980 that there is no available evidence that it is a hazard to the public when used as it is now and it should continue its GRAS status with limitations on the amounts that can be added to foods. *See* Sulfites. ASP. E

**POTASSIUM-*n*-METHYLDITHIO-CARBAMATE** • A bacteria-killing component in controlling microorganisms in sugarcane mills. Carbamates are used to prevent sprouting in potatoes and other products by stopping cell division, something we call mutations. Carbamate mutations may lead to birth defects and to cancer. The final report to the FDA of the Select Committee on GRAS Substances stated in 1980 that there is no available evidence that it is a hazard to the public when used as it is now and it should continue its GRAS status with limitations on the amounts that can be added to food. FDA residue tolerances are less than 3.5 ppm in sugarcane being processed, less than 4.1 ppm. in terms of weight of raw cane or beets, and less than 200 ppm in cured cod roe. ASP

**POTASSIUM MYRISTATE** • The potassium salt of myristic acid *(see)*. EAF

**POTASSIUM NITRATE** • *See* Nitrate. ASP. E

**POTASSIUM NITRITE** • *See* Nitrite. NUL. E

**POTASSIUM OCTOXYNOL-12 PHOSPHATE** • The potassium salt of a mixture of esters of phosphoric acid and octoxynol *(see both)*.

**POTASSIUM OLEATE** • Miscellaneous additive. *See* Potassium and Oleic Acid. NUL

**POTASSIUM PALMITATE** • The potassium salt of palmitic acid *(see)*. NUL

**POTASSIUM PECTINATE** • *See* Pectin and Potassium. EAF

**POTASSIUM PERMANGANATE** • Dark purple or bronzelike, odorless crystals with a sweet, antiseptic taste, used as a starch modifier. Dilute solutions are mildly irritating; highly concentrated solutions are caustic. EAF

**POTASSIUM PERSULFATE** • White crystals, soluble in water or alcohol. Derived from potassium sulfate. Used as a flour-maturing additive, for modification of starch, and as an antiseptic. Sprayed on fresh citrus as a coating. Strong irritant. NIL

**POTASSIUM PHOSPHATE** • Monobasic, Dibasic, and Tribasic. Used as a yeast food in the brewing industry and in the production of champagne and other sparkling wines. Used in frozen eggs as a color preservative. Has been used medicinally as a urinary acidifier. The final report to the FDA of the Select Committee on GRAS Substances stated in 1980 that it should continue its GRAS status with no limitations other than good manufacturing practices. ASP. E

**POTASSIUM POLYMETAPHOSPHATE** • The final report to the FDA of the Select Committee on GRAS Substances stated in 1980 that it should continue its GRAS status with no limitations other than good manufacturing practices. *See* Potassium Phosphate for uses. NUL

**POTASSIUM PROPIONATE** • Preservative, antimold and antirope agent. Propionates occur naturally in some foods, notably cheese, and are naturally present in the body. Propionate is formed every day in our intestines when dietary fiber is fermented. It is subsequently absorbed into the bloodstream. It has been estimated that 5 to 10 percent of the population may have various food sensitivities or intolerance. Of this group, 30 to 40 percent may be affected by propionate, but not in isolation. Sensitivity to propionate always occurs in conjunction with sensitivity to other chemicals, either naturally occurring or added to food. E

**POTASSIUM PYROPHOSPHATE** • Colorless, deliquescent crystals or granules, used as a sequestering, peptizing, and dispersing additive and in soaps and detergents. Low toxicity. The final report to the FDA of the Select Committee on GRAS Substances stated in 1980 that it should continue its GRAS status with no limitations other than good manufacturing practices. ASP

**POTASSIUM SALTS OF FATTY ACIDS** • In foods as binders, emulsifiers, and anticaking additives. *See* Fatty Acids. NEW

**POTASSIUM SILICATE** • Soluble Potash Glass. Colorless or yellowish, translucent to transparent, glasslike particles. It is used for inorganic protective coatings, in detergents, as a catalyst, and in adhesives. The final report to the FDA of the Select Committee on GRAS Substances stated in 1980 that it should continue its GRAS status with no limitations other than good manufacturing practices.

**POTASSIUM SORBATE** • Sorbic Acid Potassium Salt. White crystalline powder used as a preservative; a mold and yeast inhibitor; and a fungistat in beverages, baked goods, chocolate, and soda fountain syrups, fresh fruit cocktail, tangerine puree (sherbet base), salads (potato, macaroni, coleslaw, gelatin), cheesecake, pie fillings, cake, cheeses in consumer-size packages, and artificially sweetened jellies and preserves. Low oral toxicity but may cause irritation of the skin. GRAS. ASP. E

**POTASSIUM STEARATE** • Stearic Acid Potassium Salt. White powder with a fatty odor. Used as a chewing-gum base. Strongly alkaline. A defoaming additive in brewing. ASP

**POTASSIUM SULFATE** • Does not occur free in nature but is combined with sodium sulfate. Colorless or white crystalline powder, with a bitter taste. Used as a flavoring in foods. A water corrective used in the brewing industry. Used as a salt substitute; also used as a fertilizer and a cathartic. Large doses can cause severe gastrointestinal bleeding. to the skin. GRAS. ASP. E

**POTASSIUM SULFITE** • *See* Sulfites. EAF

**POTASSIUM TARTRATES** • Acidifier. No adverse reaction reported. E

**POTASSIUM TRICHLOROISOCYANURATE** • A sanitizer. *See* Arsenic.

**POTASSIUM TRIPOLYPHOSPHATE** • A white crystalline solid that is used in water-treating compounds, cleaners, and fertilizers; widely used as a sequestering additive *(see)* in processed foods. The final report to the FDA of the Select Committee on GRAS Substances stated in 1980 that it should continue its GRAS status with no limitations other than good manufacturing practices. ASP

**POTATO PROTEIN** • Potato protein is a coproduct from the potato starch industry. The product has a high protein content (85 percent) and a balanced amino acid level. GRAS

**POTATO STARCH** • A flour prepared from potatoes ground to a pulp and washed of fibers. Swells in hot water to form a gel on cooling. May cause allergic skin reactions and stuffy nose in the hypersensitive. The final report to the FDA of the Select Committee on GRAS Substances stated in 1980 that it should continue its GRAS status with no limitations other than good manufacturing practices. ASP

**POTENTIATOR** • A flavor ingredient with little flavor of its own that augments or alters the flavor response, such as sodium glutamate and sodium inosinate.

**PPB** • Abbreviation for parts per billion.

**PPG** • Abbreviation for propylene glycol *(see)*.

**PPG BUTETH-260 THROUGH 5100** • Emulsifiers. *See* Butyl Alcohol.

**PPG BUTETH ETHER-200** • Emulsifier. Polymer *(see)* prepared from butyl alcohol with propylene glycol *(see both)*

**PPG-4-CETETH-1, -5, or -10** • *See* Cetyl Alcohol.

**PPG-8-CETETH-5, -10, or -20** • *See* Cetyl Alcohol.

**PPG-10-CETYL ETHER** • *See* Cetyl Alcohol.

**PPG-30-CETYL ETHER** • A liquid nonionic surfactant *(see)*. *See* Cetyl Alcohol.

**PPG-20-DECYLTETRADECETH-10** • *See* Decanoic Acid.

**PPG-24 or -66 GLYCERETH-24 or -12** • *See* Glycerin.

**PPG-27 and -55 GLYCERYLETHER** • *See* Glycerin and Propylene Glycol.

**PPG-ISOCETYL ETHER** • *See* Cetyl Alcohol.

**PPG-3-ISOSTEARETH-9** • *See* Stearyl Alcohol and Propylene Glycol.

**PPG-2, -5, -10, -20, or -30 LANOLIN ALCOHOL ETHERS** • *See* Lanolin Alcohol.

**PPG-30 LANOLIN ETHER** • Derived from lanolin alcohols *(see)*.

**PPG-9 LAURATE** • *See* Lauric Acid.

**PPG-20-METHYL GLUCOSE ETHER** • *See* Propylene Glycol and Glucose.

**PPG-3-MYRETH-11** • *See* Polyethylene Glycol and Myristic Acid.

**PPG-4 MYRISTYL ETHER** • *See* Fatty Alcohols.

**PPG-30 or -50 OLEYL ETHER** • *See* Oleic Acid.

**PPG-6-C12-18 PARETH** • A mixture of synthetic alcohols. *See* Fatty Alcohols.

**PPG-9-STEARETH-3** • *See* Stearyl Alcohol.

**PPG-11 or -15 STEARYL ETHER** • *See* Propylene Glycol and Stearyl Alcohol.

**PPM** • Abbreviation for parts per million.

**PRECIPITATE** • To separate out from solution or suspension. A deposit of a solid separated out from a solution or suspension as a result of a chemical or physical change.

**PRECURSOR** • A biologic process in which a substance turns into another active or more mature substance. Beta-carotene is a precursor of vitamin A, because the body can use it to make vitamin A.

**PREDNISOLONE** • Metacortandrolone. Cortalone. Delta-Cortef. Introduced in 1955, prednisolone is related chemically to cortisol. It is used to treat inflammation in cattle. FDA residue tolerance for milk is zero. It is used to treat severe inflammation, as an immunosuppressant, in the treatment of ulcerative colitis, and in proctitis in humans. Most adverse reactions are the result of dose or length of time of administration. Potential adverse reactions include euphoria, insomnia, psychotic behavior, high blood pressure, swelling, cataracts, glaucoma, peptic ulcer, GI irritation, increased appetite, high blood sugar, growth suppression in children, delayed wound healing, acne, skin eruptions, muscle weakness, pancreatitis, hairiness, decreased immunity, and acute adrenal gland insufficiency. When withdrawn, there may be rebound inflammation, fatigue, weakness, joint pain, fever, dizziness, lethargy, depression, fainting, a drop in blood pressure upon arising from a seated or prone position, shortness of breath, loss of appetite, and high blood sugar.

**PREDNISONE** • Deltacortisone. Introduced in 1955 and related chemically to cortisone, a hormone secreted by the adrenal gland, prednisone is widely used to treat severe inflammation, as an immunosuppressant, and to treat acute attacks of multiple sclerosis, arthritis, and irritable-bowel syndrome in humans. It is used to treat cattle and horses for inflammation. The FDA has a zero tolerance in milk. Under International Agency for Research on Cancer (IARC) *(see)* review. Most adverse reactions are the result of dose or length of time of administration. In humans, potential adverse reactions from medication include euphoria, insomnia, psychotic behavior, high blood pressure, swelling, cataracts, glaucoma, peptic ulcer, GI irritation, increased appetite, high blood sugar, growth suppression in children, delayed wound healing, acne, skin eruptions, muscle weakness, pancreatitis, hairiness, decreased immunity, irregular menstruation, male infertility, and acute adrenal gland insufficiency. When withdrawn, there may be rebound inflammation, fatigue, weakness, joint pain, fever, dizziness, lethargy, depression, fainting, a drop in blood pressure upon arising from a seated or prone position, shortness of breath, loss of appetite, and high blood sugar. Sudden withdrawal may be fatal. Contraindicated in systemic fungal infections. Prednisone has been implicated in aplastic anemia and is an experimental tumor inducer.

**PREDONIN** • *See* Prednisone.

**PREEMPT** • *See* CF-3.

**PREGELATINIZED STARCH** • When starch and water are heated, the starch molecules burst and form a gelatin. The final report to the FDA of the Select Committee on GRAS Substances stated in 1980 that it should continue its GRAS status with no limitations other than good manufacturing practices.

**PRENYL THIOACETATE** • Synthetic pine flavoring. EAF

**PRES** • FDA abbreviation for preservative.

**PRESERVATIVES** • About one hundred "antispoilants," which retard or prevent food from going "bad," are in common use. Preservatives for fatty products are called antioxidants. Preservatives used in bread are labeled mold or rope inhibitors. They include sodium propionate and calcium propionate *(see both)*. Preservatives to prevent mold and fungus growth on citrus fruits are called fungicides. Among the most commonly used preservatives are sodium benzoate *(see)* to prevent the growth of microbes on cheese and syrups, sulfur dioxide *(see)* to inhibit discoloration in fruit juice concentrates, and nitrates and nitrites that are used to "cure" processed meats. In many instances a product might show no visible evidence of microbial contamination and yet contain actively growing, potentially harmful germs.

**PRICKLY ASH BARK** • A natural cola, maple, and root beer flavor extract from a prickly aromatic shrub or small tree, *Zanthoxylum* spp., bearing yellow flowers. Used in beverages, candy, and baked goods. GRAS. NIL

**PRIMATOL** • Prometon. Aatrex. Zeazine. Weedex A. Widely used herbicide on cropland. Moderately toxic by ingestion. Induces tumors and causes adverse reproductive effects in experimental animals. A skin and severe eye irritant.

**PRIMULA EXTRACT** • The extract of various species of *Primula* taken from the rhizome and roots of the primrose or cowslip. It has been used as an expectorant, diuretic, and worm medicine. In some sensitive persons, it may cause a rash.

**PROCAINE PENICILLIN** • An antibiotic used as an injection in animals. FDA tolerance in uncooked edible tissue of cattle is 0.05 ppm, and in uncooked edible tissue of turkey, 0.01 ppm. Zero tolerance in milk and uncooked edible tissue of chicken, pheasants, quail, swine, sheep, and eggs.

**PROFENOFOS** • A pesticide used in feed. FDA tolerances are 6 ppm in or on cottonseed hulls; 15 ppm in soap stocks. As a residue in meat by-products of goats, cattle, hogs, poultry, and sheep, the FDA allows a residue of 0.05 ppm.

**PROFLURALIN** • Yellow-orange crystals used as an herbicide. FDA residue tolerances are 0.3 as a residue in or on soybean hay; 0.1 ppm in or on cottonseed, pod vegetables, and sunflower seeds; and 0.02 ppm as residue in or on eggs or milk, meat, fat, and meat by-products of cattle, hogs, goats, poultry, and sheep.

**PROGESTERONE** • Corlutin. Cyclogest. Luteal Hormone. Synovex. Gesterol 50. Progestaject. A progestin drug that suppresses ovulation, possibly by inhibiting pituitary gonadotropin secretion. It forms a thick cervical mucus. Used to treat absent menstruation or abnormal uterine bleeding in humans. Used in cattle and sheep to regulate reproductive cycles. Not allowed in veal calves. Potential adverse reactions in humans include nausea, vomiting, depression, high blood pressure, dizziness, migraine, lethargy, blood clots, swelling, bloating, and abdominal cramps. May cause breakthrough bleeding, altered menstrual flow, painful or absent menstruation, enlargement of benign tumors of the uterus, cervical erosion, abnormal secretions, and vaginal candidiasis. There may be jaundice; high blood sugar; dark spots appearing on the skin; breast tenderness, enlargement, or secretion; and decreased libido. Contraindicated in persons with blood-clot disorders, cancer of the breast, undiagnosed abnormal vaginal bleeding, and in pregnancy. The FDA limits residues from progesterone treatment in animals to 3 ppb in muscle, 12 ppb in fat, 9 ppb in kidney, and 6 ppb in liver of steers and calves and 3 ppb in muscle, and 15 ppb for fat, kidney, and liver of lambs. International Agency for Research on Cancer (IARC) *(see)* review. A cancer and tumor inducer in experimental animals. May cause birth defects.

**PROLINA** • A soy protein that can be made into fat-free whipped cream. *See* Soybean.

**PROLINE** • L Form. An amino acid *(see)* used as a food supplement but classified as nonessential. Usually isolated from wheat or gelatin. L-proline is the naturally occurring form and DL-proline is the synthetic. GRAS. ASP

**PROMOTION** • An intermediate stage of cancer development during which initiated *(see)* cells, in the presence of promoters, move further along the pathway to cancer. The promotion stage may take several decades in humans.

**PROPANE** • A gas heavier than air; odorless when pure. It is used as a fuel and refrigerant. Cleared for use in combination with octafluorocyclobutane in a spray propellant and as an aerating additive for foamed and sprayed foods. Cleared for use in a spray propellant and as an aerating additive for cosmetics in aerosols. May be narcotic in high concentrations. The final report to the FDA of the Select Committee on GRAS Substances stated in 1980 that it should continue its GRAS status with no limitations other than good manufacturing practices. NUL

**1,2-PROPANEDITHIOL** • *See* Propylene Glycol. NIL

**2-PROPANETHIOL** • Gas that smells like a skunk. EAF

**PROPAN-1.2-DIOL ESTERS OF FATTY ACIDS** • *See* Esters of Fatty Acids and Propylene Glycol. E

**PROPANE-1.2-DIOL ALGINATE** • *See* Alginates.

**4-PROPENYL-2,6-DIMETHOXYPHENOL** • Synthetic flavoring.

**PROPENYLGUAETHOL** • Synthetic flavoring. ASP

**PROPENYL PROPYL DISULFIDE** • Onion oil *(see)*. NIL

**PROPIANALDEHYDE** • A colorless liquid aldehyde. Used in the manufacture of plastics and as a disinfectant and preservative. In animals causes liver damage and high blood pressure. ASP

**PROPANOIC ACID** • *See* Propionic Acid. ASP

**PROPARQUITE** • A pesticide applied to growing crops to kill mites. FDA residue tolerance is 80 ppm in dried apple pomace and 40 ppm in dried citrus pulp and dried grape pulp. Less than 100 ppm can kill fish if it gets in water.

**PROPAZINE** • Propasin. Prozinex. An herbicide used on animal feed to control weeds. Moderately toxic by ingestion. Caused tumors in experimental animals.

**PROPELLANT** • A compressed gas used to expel the contents of containers in the form of aerosols. Chlorofluorocarbons were widely used because of their nonflammability. The strong possibility that they contribute to depletion of the ozone layer of the upper atmosphere has resulted in prohibition of their use for this purpose. Other propellants used are hydrocarbon gases, such as butane and propane, carbon dioxide, and nitrous oxide. The materials dispersed include shaving cream, whipping cream, and cosmetic preparations.

**(Z)-4-PROPENYLPHENOL** • A flavoring determined GRAS by the Expert Panel of the Flavor and Extract Manufacturers Association. *See* Phenol.

**PROPETAMPHOS** • A pesticide used as a spot, crack, and crevice treatment to kill parasites.

**PROPIOMAZINE** • Propionylpromethazine. A sedative and hypnotic used in human medicine. A tranquilizer used to treat stress in pigs.

**PROPIONALDEHYDE** • Propanal. A synthetic flavoring additive that occurs naturally in apples and onions. Used in fruit flavorings for beverages, ice cream, ices, candy, and baked goods. Suffocating odor. May cause respiratory irritation. Moderately toxic by ingestion. ASP

**PROPIONATE** • Propionate is formed every day in our intestines when dietary fiber is fermented. It is subsequently absorbed into the bloodstream. It has been estimated that 5 to 10 percent of the population may have various food sensitivities or intolerance. Of this group, 30 to 40 percent may be affected by propionate, but not in isolation. Sensitivity to propionate always occurs in conjunction with sensitivity to other chemicals, either naturally occurring or added to food. Foods permitted to contain propionates include bread, biscuits, cakes, pastries, and other flour products. Calcium propionate is an approved preservative in bread and helps to keep the bread fresh. Potassium propionate and sodium propionate are also approved preservatives. By inhibiting the growth of mold and other microorganisms, propionates allow consumers the convenience of keeping soft, fresh bread in the home without having to purchase it every day. Although both calcium propionate and sodium propionate are equally effective antimicrobial agents, calcium propionate is the form commonly used throughout the world as a preservative in bread production. In finished bread products, it can act as a calcium enricher, contributing to total calcium in the diet, and its use in bread in preference to sodium propionate will result in slightly lower sodium levels in the bread. In contrast, sodium propionate is favored over calcium propionate in cake production since added calcium can interfere with the leavening, or rising action, of the cake.

**PROPIONIC ACID** • Propanoic Acid. Occurs naturally in apples, strawberries, tea, and violet leaves. An oily liquid with a slightly pungent, rancid odor. Can be obtained from wood pulp, waste liquor, and by fermentation. Used in butter and fruit flavorings for beverages, ice cream, ices, candy, baked goods; and cheese flavorings for beverages, ice cream, ices, candy, baked goods, and cheese (600 ppm). Also used as an inhibitor and preservative to prevent mold in baked goods and processed cheeses. Its salts have been used as antifungal additives to treat skin mold. May cause migraine in those susceptible to migraines, and contact with the chemical may cause skin irritations in bakery workers. Large oral dose in rats is lethal. GRAS. ASP. E

**2-PROPIONYLPYRROLINE** • A flavoring in baked goods, beverages, breakfast cereal, imitation dairy, grains, soft candy, and many other food products. Determined GRAS by the Expert Panel of the Flavor and Extract Manufacturers Association. *See* Pyrrole. NIL

**2-PROPIONYL-2-THIAZOLINE** • A flavoring determined GRAS by the

Expert Panel of the Flavor and Extract Manufacturers Association. *See* Propionic Acid. ASP

**PROPIOPHENONE** • Fixative in perfumes and used in additive processing. ASP

**PROPYL ACETATE** • Colorless liquid, soluble in water, derived from propane and acetate *(see both)*. It has the odor of pears. A synthetic currant, raspberry, strawberry, apple, cherry, peach, pineapple, and rum flavoring additive for beverages, ice cream, ices, candy, and baked goods. Also used as a solvent for resins. It may be irritating to the skin and mucous membranes and narcotic in high doses. ASP

**PROPYL ALCOHOL** • Obtained from natural gas and fusel oil. Alcoholic and slightly overpowering odor. Occurs naturally in cognac green oil, cognac white oil, and onion oil. A synthetic fruit flavoring for beverages, ice cream, ices, candy, and baked goods. Used instead of ethyl alcohol as a solvent for shellac, gums, resins, and oils; as a denaturant *(see)* for alcohol in perfumery. Not a primary irritant, but because it dissolves fat, it has a drying effect on the skin and may lead to cracking, fissuring, and infections. No adverse effects have been reported from local application as a lotion, liniment, mouthwash, gargle, or sponge bath. Mildly irritating to the eyes and mucous membranes. Ingestion may cause symptoms similar to that of ethyl alcohol *(see)*. ASP

*p*-**PROPYL ANISOLE** • A synthetic flavoring additive, colorless to pale yellow, with an anise odor. Used in licorice, root beer, spice, vanilla, wintergreen, and birch beer flavorings for beverages, ice cream, candy, and baked goods. Moderately toxic by ingestion. Caused mutations in experimental animals. ASP

**PROPYL BENZOATE** • A synthetic fruit flavoring additive for beverages, ice cream, ices, candy, and baked goods. NIL

**PROPYL BUTYRATE** • Contains propyl alcohol and butyric acid. A synthetic strawberry, banana, pineapple, plum, tutti-frutti, liquor, and rum flavoring additive for beverages, ice cream, ices, candy, and baked goods. *See* Propyl Alcohol and Butyric Acid for toxicity. ASP

**PROPYL CINNAMATE** • Cinnamic Acid. A synthetic berry, floral, rose, apple, grape, and honey flavoring additive for beverages, ice cream, ices, candy, baked goods, and gelatins. ASP

**PROPYL 2,4-DECADIENOATE** • Synthetic flavoring. NIL

**4-PROPYL-2,6-DIMETHOXYPHENOL** • Synthetic flavoring. *See* Onion Oil. NIL. ASP

**PROPYLENE CHLOROHYDRIN** • Colorless liquid used in manufacture of propylene oxide. Toxic by ingestion and skin absorption. NUL

**PROPYL FORMATE** • Formic Acid. A synthetic berry, apple, and rum flavoring additive for beverages, ice cream, ices, candy, and baked goods. *See* Formic Acid for toxicity.

**PROPYL 2-FURANACRYLATE** • A synthetic coffee and honey flavoring additive for beverages and candy.

**PROPYL 2-FUROATE** • A synthetic chocolate and mushroom flavoring additive for candy, baked goods, and condiments. ASP

**PROPYL GALLATE** • A fine, white, odorless powder with a bitter taste used as an antioxidant for foods, fats, and oils and for potato flakes, mashed potatoes, and mayonnaise. Also used in lemon, lime, fruit, and spice flavorings for beverages, ice cream, ices, candy, baked goods, and gelatin desserts. Used in pressure-sensitive adhesives as the food contact surface of labels and or tapes applied to food. Can cause stomach or skin irritation especially in people who suffer from asthma or are sensitive to aspirin. Reaffirmed as GRAS in the FDA's reevaluation in the following amounts: 0.02 percent maximum in fat or oil content of food; maximum of 0.015 percent in food prepared by the manufacturer. ASP. E

**PROPYL HEPTANOATE** • A synthetic berry, coffee, fruit, cognac, and rum flavoring additive for beverages, ice cream, ices, candy, liqueurs, and baked goods. ASP

**PROPYL HEXANOATE** • A synthetic pineapple flavoring additive for beverages, ice cream, ices, and candy. ASP

**PROPYL-*p*-HYDROXYRENZOATE** • Propylparaben. A preservative used in beverages, candy, baked goods, and artificially sweetened jellies and preserves. Also used in fruit flavorings for beverages, ice cream, ices, candy, and baked goods. Less toxic than benzoic acid *(see)* or salicylic acid *(see)*. Experimental animals showed no kidney or liver damage. On the FDA list for further study for short-term mutagenic, subacute, teratogenic, and reproductive effects. GRAS. ASP. E

**PROPYL ISOVALERATE** • A synthetic strawberry, apple, banana, and peach flavoring additive for beverages, ice cream, ices, candy, and baked goods. ASP

**PROPYL MERCAPTAN** • A synthetic berry and onion flavoring additive for baked goods and pickles. ASP

**PROPYL METHOXYBENZENE** • *See p*-Propyl Anisole.

**PROPYL PHENYLACETATE** • A synthetic butter, caramel, rose, fruit, and honey flavoring additive for beverages, ice cream, ices, candy, and baked goods. ASP

**PROPYL PROPIONATE** • Propyl alcohol and propionic acid. A synthetic banana, cherry, melon, peach, prune, apple, plum, and rum flavoring additive for beverages, ice cream, ices, candy, and baked goods. Colorless, thick liquid prepared from glycerol *(see* Glycerin) and used as an anticaking additive, antioxidant, dough conditioner, humectant, solvent, stabilizer, detergent, texturizer, thickener, and wetting additive. Used in alcoholic beverages, confections, flavorings, frostings, frozen dairy products, pork, nut products, poultry, seasonings, and wine. The FDA limits it to 5 percent in alcoholic beverages; 24 percent in confections and frostings; 2.5 percent in frozen dairy products; 97 percent in seasonings and flavorings; 5 percent in nuts and nut products; and 2 percent in all other foods when used in accordance with good manufacturing practices. Limitation of 40 ppm in wine. EPA Genetic Toxicology Program. Caused birth defects in experimental animals. ASP

**PROPYLENE GLYCOL** • 1,2-Propanediol. A clear, colorless, viscous liquid, slightly bitter tasting. In food, it is used in confectionery, chocolate products, ice cream emulsifiers, shredded coconut, beverages, baked goods, toppings, icings, and meat products to prevent discoloration during storage. Defoaming additive in processed beet sugar and yeast. Used in antifreeze in breweries and dairy establishments. It is the most common moisture-carrying vehicle other than water itself in cosmetics. Its use is being reduced and replaced by safer glycols such as butylene and polyethylene glycol. Large oral doses in animals have been reported to cause central nervous system depression and slight kidney changes. The final report to the FDA of the Select Committee on GRAS Substances stated in 1980 that it should continue its GRAS status with no limitations other than good manufacturing practices. ASP

**PROPYLENE GLYCOL ALGINATE** • Kelcloid. The propylene glycol ester of alginic acid *(see),* derived from seaweed. Used as a stabilizer, filler, and defoaming additive in food. Cleared for use in French dressing and salad dressing under food standard regulations. Used as a stabilizer in ice cream, frozen custard, ice milk, fruit sherbet, and water ices, it is permitted up to 0.5 percent of the weight of the finished product. Can cause allergic reactions. The final report to the FDA of the Select Committee on GRAS Substances stated in 1980 that there is no available evidence that it is a hazard to the public when used as it is now and it should continue its GRAS status with limitations on amounts that can be added to food. ASP

**PROPYLENE GLYCOL DIBENZOATE** • Preservative. *See* Benzoic Acid. ASP

**PROPYLENE GLYCOL MONO- and DIESTERS OF FATS and FATTY ACIDS** • Emulsifiers. ASP

**PROPYLENE GLYCOL MONOSTEARATE** • Cream-colored wax that disperses in water and is soluble in hot alcohol. It is used as a lubricating additive and emulsifier; also a dough conditioner in baked goods. Employed as a stabilizer of essential oils. Slightly more toxic than propylene glycol *(see)* in animals and in large doses produces central nervous system depression and kidney injury. The final report to the FDA of the Select Committee on GRAS Substances stated in 1980 that it should continue its GRAS status with no limitations other than good manufacturing practices.

**PROPYLENE GLYCOL STEARATE** • Cream-colored wax. Disperses in water, soluble in hot alcohol. Widely used lubricating ingredient and emulsifier and stabilizer of essential oils. ASP

**PROPYLENE OXIDE** • Propene Oxide. Colorless, liquid starch modifier. FDA tolerance residues are less than 25 percent for treatment of starch; 700 ppm as propylene glycol in dried prunes and glacéed fruit; and 300 ppm in cocoa gums and processed nut meats (except peanuts). NIL

**3-PROPYLIDENEPHTHALIDE** • Synthetic fruit and spice flavoring additive for beverages, ice cream, ices, candy, and baked goods.

**PROPYLPARABEN** • Propyl-*p*-Hydroxybenzoate. Developed in Europe, the esters of *p*-hydroxybenzoic acid are widely used in the cosmetics industry as preservatives and bacteria and fungus killers. They are active against a variety of organisms, are neutral, low in toxicity, slightly soluble, and active in all solutions, alkaline, neutral, or acid. Used medicinally to treat fungus infections. Can cause contact dermatitis. Less toxic than benzoic or salicylic acid *(see both)*. GRAS

**PROPYLPARASEPT** • *See* Propylhydroxybenzoate.

*a*-**PROPYLPHENETHYL ALCOHOL** • A synthetic fruit flavoring additive for beverages, ice cream, ices, candy, and puddings. Toxicity similar to ethanol *(see)*.

**PROPYLPYRIDINE** • A flavoring determined GRAS by the Expert Panel of the Flavor and Extract Manufacturers Association.

**2-PROPYLPYRAZINE** • Synthetic nutty flavoring. EAF

**PROSTAGLANDINS** • PGA, PGB, PGC, PGD. Taglandin F2-a. Lutalyse. A group of extremely potent hormonelike substances present in many tissues. Prostaglandins are a group of about twenty lipids that are modified fatty acids. There are more than sixteen known with effects such as dilating or constricting blood vessels, stimulation of intestinal or bronchial smooth muscle, uterine stimulation, and antagonism to hormones and influencing fat metabolism. Various prostaglandins in the body can cause fever, inflammation, and headaches. Prostaglandins or drugs that affect prostaglandins are used medically in humans to induce labor, prevent and treat peptic ulcers, control high blood pressure, in the treatment of bronchial asthma, and to induce delayed menstruation. They are used in animals to induce labor and to induce abortion attached to a five-membered ring. Aspirin inhibits prostaglandin synthesis, leading to reduced inflammation.

**PROTEASES** • Enzymes from *Aspergillus flavus* or *Aspergillus niger; Aspergillus oryzae* or *Bacillus amyloliquefacients* or *Bacillus licheniformis* or *Bacillus subtilis.* Used as meat tenderizers and in sausage curing, dough conditioning, and beer-haze removal. All EAF.

**PROTECTIVE COATINGS** • Antioxidants and preservatives that are used in goat cheeses and fresh fruits and vegetables to retard spoilage. The coatings may expose consumers to hidden antibiotics or coal-tar products. Among the coating additives used are anoxomer, calcium disodium and disodium EDTA, coumarone-indene resin, ethoxyquin, morpholine, natamycin, petroleum naphtha, polyacrylamide, synthetic paraffin and succinic derivatives, and terpene resin *(see all)*. Citrus fruits, squash, grapes, sweet potatoes, asparagus, melons, papaya, plantain, turnips, watermelons, and nuts are commonly coated.

**PROTEIN** • Chemically, a protein is a complex nitrogenous compound made up of amino acids in peptide linkages. Dietary proteins are involved in the synthesis of tissue protein and other special metabolic functions. In anabolic processes they furnish the amino acids required to build and maintain body tissues. As an energy source, proteins are equivalent to carbohydrates in providing 4 calories per gram. Proteins perform a major structural role in all body tissues and in the formation of enzymes, hormones, and various body fluids and secretions. Proteins participate in the transport of some lipids, vitamins, and minerals and help maintain the body's homeostasis.

**PROTEIN ANIMAL HYDROLYZED** • *See* Hydrolyzed Animal Protein. ASP

**PROTEIN CONCENTRATE, WHOLE FISH** • Dietary supplement.

**PROTEIN FATTY ACID CONDENSATES** • *See* Amides.

**PROTEIN HYDROLYSATES** • Used as flavor enhancers,

**PROTEIN HYDROLYZED UNSPECIFIED** • *See* Hydrolyzed Protein. ASP

**PROTEIN, MILK HYDROLYZED** • *See* Hydrolyzed Whey Protein. NUL

**PROTEIN, VEGETABLE, HYDROLYZED** • *See* Hydrolyzed Vegetable Proteins.

**PROVITAMIN A** • *See* Carotene.

**PRUSSIATE OF SODA, YELLOW** • Salt of hydrocyanic acid derived from ammonia. Anticaking additive in salt. Hydrocyanic acid is toxic by ingestion, inhalation, and skin absorption.

**PRUSSIC ACID** • Hydrocyanic Acid. Occurs in some plants but is usually derived by reacting ammonia and air with methane or natural gas or from coal and ammonia. It is used in the manufacture of cyanide, acrylates, and pesticides. Toxic by ingestion. *See* Cyanide.

**PS** • Substance for which prior sanction has been granted by FDA for specific uses.

**PSEUDOPINENE** • A synthetic flavoring additive used in various foods. Mildly toxic by ingestion. See *a*-Pinene.

**PSYLLIUM** • *Plantago psyllium* is a cultivated weed and has been used as a laxative since the early 1930s. It absorbs water and expands to increase bulk and moisture content of the stool to encourage bowel movement. Psyllium contains a soluble fiber that studies have shown can lower cholesterol levels. General Mills introduced the first psyllium cereal, Benefit, in April 1989. Heartwise was introduced in August of that year. Procter and Gamble, which makes the psyllium laxative Metamucil, had asked the FDA to prohibit General Mills from making claims that its cereal could reduce cholesterol. Procter and Gamble contended psyllium was a drug, not a food, and thus the cereal could only be marketed after extensive tests to prove to regulators that it is safe and effective in performing as claimed. Procter and Gamble is barred from making claims about Metamucil's ability to reduce cholesterol.

General Mills withdrew Benefit from the market in December 1989 citing poor sales. Heartwise is the only major brand of cereal containing a significant amount of psyllium, 3 grams in a one-ounce serving. Bran Buds is made by Kellogg but has less psyllium. Allergic reactions occurred in some people who ate the cereal Heartless, made by the Kellogg company; reactions ranged from itchy eyes and runny noses to severe difficulty in breathing. In September 1989 the FDA sent a letter to Kellogg raising new questions about its use of psyllium which has been used for decades in bulk laxatives like Metamucil and Fiberall. On October 30, 1990, the FDA published proposed regulations in the Federal Register that would require a warning label on over-the-counter drugs containing water-soluble fibers, including psyllium, which is not absorbed systemically. The FDA ruled in February 1998 that labels on food containing soluble fiber from psyllium seed, including some breakfast cereals, may claim that these products may reduce the risk of coronary artery disease when eaten as part of a diet low in saturated fat and cholesterol. As psyllium can be hard to swallow, the new labels are also required to recommend that people eating these types of foods drink plenty of liquid.

**PSYLLIUM SEED HUSK** • A stabilizer from the seed of the fleaseed plant used in frozen desserts up to 0.5 percent of the weight of the finished product. *See* Psyllium. NUL

**PTEROYLGLUTAMIC ACID** • Dietary supplement. Isolated from yeast.

**PTWI** • Provisional Tolerable Weekly Intake.

**PULEGONE** • Found in oils of plants, principally pennyroyal. Pleasant odor, midway between camphor and peppermint. Used in peppermint flavorings for beverages, ice cream, ices, candy, and baked goods. *See* Pennyroyal Oil for toxicity. ASP

**PULLULAN** • Pullulan is an extracellular bacterial polysaccharide produced from starch by aureobasidium. A slowly digested carbohydrate in humans. GRAS

**PULPS** • From wood, straw, bagasse, or other natural sources. A source of cellulose in food. The wood is treated with a mixture containing mainly sodium hydroxide *(see)*. Treatment removes the fibrous lignin—the resinous substance that binds the fiber that lines the cells of wood. An indirect human food additive from packaging. The FDA's reevaluation in 1976 labeled pulps GRAS. NUL

**PURINES** • Components of nucleic acid, they are widely distributed in nature. Important purines are uric acid, adenine, guanine, and xanthine. Uric acid is the form of purines excreted in human urine. Caffeine is a stimulant purine. Some of the richest food sources of purines are anchovies, asparagus, organ meats, mushrooms, and sardines. Foods with low purines include bread, cereals, fats, cheese, eggs, fruits, milk, and nuts.

**PYCNOGENOL** • An extract of the French maritime pine tree, it is a rich source of antioxidant flavonoids *(see)*. It reportedly reduces free radicals *(see)* in the body.

**PYRANTEL TARTRATE** • An antiworm medicine used in feed and as a veterinary medicine. The FDA's residue tolerance is 10 ppm in swine liver and kidney and 1 ppm in swine muscle.

**PYRAZINES** • Synthetic flavorings. During peanut roasting, pyrazine compounds correlate highly with roasted flavor and aroma. Also have the aroma of roasted coffee. *See* Piperazine. EAF

**PYRAZINE ETHANETHIOL** • Synthetic flavoring. ASP

**PYRAZINE METHYL SULFIDE** • Synthetic flavoring. ASP

**PYRETHRINS** • Thick liquids from the pyrethrum flowers. Used in household insecticidal sprays and powders and deodorant sprays. Also used in paper bags for shipping cereals. Residues from packaging materials and equipment and storage areas may be only 1 ppm on dried foods, cereal grains, and dried prunes. Insecticides labeled nontoxic to human beings and pets usually contain pyrethrins.

**PYRIDINE** • Occurs naturally in coffee and coal tar. Disagreeable odor; sharp taste. Used in chocolate flavorings for beverages, ice cream, ices, candy, and baked goods. Also used as a solvent for organic liquids and compounds. Once used to treat asthma, but may cause central nervous system depression and irritation of the skin and respiratory tract. After prolonged administration, kidney and liver damage may result. Pyridine is absorbed from the respiratory and gastrointestinal tract. Small oral doses in humans have produced loss of appetite, nausea, fatigue, and mental depression. ASP

**2-PYRIDINEMETHANETHIOL** • Synthetic meat flavoring. Tastes like lamb. ASP

**PYRIDOXINE** • *See* Pyridoxine Hydrochloride. NIL

**PYRIDOXINE DIOCTENCIATE** • Vitamin $B_6$ Hydrochloride. Texturizer. A colorless or white crystalline powder present in many foodstuffs. A coenzyme that helps in the metabolism of amino acids *(see)* and fats. Also soothing to the skin. Nontoxic.

**PYRIDOXINE HYDROCHLORIDE** • Vitamin $B_6$. A colorless or white crystalline powder added to evaporated milk base in infant foods. Present in many foodstuffs. Especially good sources are yeast, liver, and cereals. A coenzyme that helps in the metabolism of ammo acids *(see)* and fat. Permits normal red blood cell formation. The final report to the FDA of the Select

Committee on GRAS Substances stated in 1980 that it should continue its GRAS status with no limitations other than good manufacturing practices. The FDA is doing a toxicology search on this additive. ASP

**PYRIDOXINE TRIPALMITATE** • Vitamin B$_6$ Tripalmitate. *See* Pyridoxine Hydrochloride.

**PYRIDOXOL HYDROCHLORIDE** • Vitamin B$_6$. Dietary supplement and nutrient used in baked goods, beverages and beverage bases, cereals, dairy products, meat products, plant-protein products, and snack foods.

**PYROLIGNEOUS ACID and EXTRACT** • A yellow acid. Consists of 6 percent acetic acid *(see)* and small concentrations of creosote, methyl alcohol, and acetone *(see)*. It is obtained by the destructive distillation of wood. Used as a synthetic flavoring in butter, butterscotch, caramel, rum, tobacco, smoke, and vanilla flavorings for beverages, ice cream, ices, candy, baked goods, puddings, and meats (300 ppm). The extract is used largely for smoking meats (300 ppm) and in smoke flavorings for baked goods (200 ppm) and alcoholic beverages. It is corrosive and may cause epigastric pain, vomiting, circulatory collapse, and death. ASP

**PYROMUCIC ALDEHYDE** • *See* Furfural.

**PYROPHOSPHATE** • Salt of pyrophosphoric acid. It increases the effectiveness of antioxidants in creams and ointments. In concentrated solutions it can be irritating to the skin and mucous membranes.

**PYROPHYLLITE** • Aluminum Silicate Monohydrate. Obtained naturally from clay or synthesized, it is used as an anticaking and coloring additive in powders. Used as a carrier or pelleting aid in animal feed. Nontoxic.

**PYRORACEMIC ACID** • *See* Pyruvic Acid.

**PYRROLE** • Colorless liquid with a mild, nutty odor used as a flavoring additive in various foods. GRAS when used at a level not in excess of the amount reasonably required to accomplish the intended effect. ASP

**PYRROLIDINE** • Colorless to pale yellow liquid used as an intermediate in insecticides and fungicides. Used to inhibit citrus decay. Also used as a curing agent for epoxy resins. Toxic by ingestion and inhalation. ASP

**1-PYRROLINE** • *See* Pyrrole. EAF

**PYRUVALDEHYDE** • A synthetic flavoring, yellowish, with a pungent odor. Formed as an intermediate in the metabolism or fermentation of carbohydrates and lactic acid *(see)*. Used in coffee, honey, and maple flavorings for beverages, ice cream, ices, candy, and baked goods. ASP

**PYRUVIC ACID** • An important intermediate in fermentation and metabolism, it occurs naturally in coffee and when sugar is metabolized in muscle. It is reduced to lactic acid *(see)* during exertion. Pyruvic acid is isolated from cane sugar. It is a synthetic flavoring used in coffee and rum flavorings for beverages, ice cream, ices, candy, chewing gum, and baked goods. Has been used as a paste in the treatment of deep burns. ASP

# Q

**QUACK GRASS** • A couch grass, a pernicious weed in cultivated fields. *See* Dog Grass Extract.

**QUASSIA EXTRACT** • Bitter Ash. Bitterwood. Yellowish white to bright yellow chips. Bitter alkaloid obtained from the wood of *Quassia amara,* a tree bearing bright scarlet flowers grown in Jamaica, the Caribbean Islands, and South America. Named for a black slave who discovered its medicinal value in the mid-eighteenth century. Slight odor, bitter taste. Used in bitters, citrus, cherry, grape, liquor, root beer, sarsaparilla, and vanilla flavorings for beverages, baked goods, and liquors. Used to poison flies, to imitate hops, and as a bitter tonic and remedy for roundworms in children. EAF

**QUATERNARY AMMONIUM CHLORIDE COMBINATION** • The additive contains the following compounds: *n*-dodecyl dimethyl benzyl ammonium chloride; *n*-dodecyl dimethyl ethylbenzyl ammonium chloride; *n*-hexadecyl dimethyl benzyl ammonium chloride; *n*-octadecyl dimethyl benzyl ammonium chloride; *n*-tetradecyl dimethyl benzyl ammonium chloride; *n*-tetradecyl dimethyl ethylbenzyl ammonium chloride. The additive is used as an antimicrobial agent in raw sugar cane juice. NUL

**QUATERNARY AMMONIUM COMPOUNDS** • A wide variety of preservatives, surfactants, germicides, sanitizers, antiseptics, and deodorants. They are used in processing sugarcane and in beet sugar mills. Benzalkonium chloride *(see)* is one of the most popular. Quaternary ammonium compounds are synthetic derivatives of ammonia, a natural product that occurs in animal metabolism.

**QUEBRACHO BARK EXTRACT** • Extract of a native Argentine tree, used in fruit, rum, and vanilla flavorings for beverages, ice cream, candy, ices, and baked goods. Closely related to the tranquilizer reserpine. Once promoted as an aphrodisiac, it can cause low blood pressure, nausea, abdominal distress, weakness, and fatigue. ASP

**QUERCETIN** • Widely distributed in the plant kingdom especially in rinds and barks and in clover blossoms and ragweed pollen. Used therapeutically to protect blood vessels. Used in food additives to form epoxy resins.

**QUERCITRON** • Inner bark of a species of oak tree common in North America. Its active ingredient, isoquercitrin, is used in forming resins. Allergic reactions have been reported. *See* Rutin.

**QUERCUS ALBA** • *See* Oak Bark Extract.

**QUICK GRASS** • Triticum. *See* Dog Grass Extract.

**QUILLAIA** • China Bark Extract. Soapbark. *See* Quillaja Extract.

**QUILLAJA EXTRACT** • Soapbark. Quillay Bark. Panama Bark. China Bark. The extract of the inner dried bark of a tree grown in South America, *Quillaja saponaria.* Used in fruit, root beer, and spice flavorings for beverages, ice cream, and candy. Formerly used to treat bronchitis and externally as a detergent. ASP. E

**QUINCE SEED** • The seed of a plant, *Cydonia* spp., grown in southern Asia and Europe for its fatty oil. Thick jelly produced by soaking seeds in water. Used in fruit flavorings for beverages, ice cream, ices, and baked goods. Used medicinally as a demulcent. Has been largely replaced by cheaper substitutes. It may cause allergic reactions. GRAS. NIL

**QUININE BISULFATE** • Most important alkaloid of cinchona extract *(see)* from trees that grow wild in South America and are cultivated in Java. Very bitter. Used in bitters flavoring for beverages and not to exceed 83 ppm in soda. Used to treat fever and as a local anesthetic and analgesic. *See* Quinine Extract. NIL

**QUININE EXTRACT** • An extract of cinchona bark *(see* Cinchona Extract), which grows wild in South America. White crystalline powder, almost insoluble in water. It is used as a local anesthetic in hair tonics and sunscreen preparations. Used in bitters in limited amounts as flavoring for beverages. When taken internally, it reduces fever. It is also used as a flavoring additive in numerous over-the-counter cold and headache remedies as well as "bitter lemon" and tonic water, which may contain as much as 5 milligrams per 100 milliliters. Cinchonism, which may consist of nausea, vomiting, disturbances of vision, ringing in ears, and nerve deafness, may occur from an overdose of quinine. If there is a sensitivity to quinine, such symptoms can result from drinking tonic water. Quinine more commonly causes a rash. The FAO/WHO said the amount of quinine in drinks was not of concern to most, but that some consumers show a hyperreactivity to quinine, and therefore, its presence in foods and beverages should be noted.

**QUININE HYDROCHLORIDE** • A synthetic flavoring additive derived from cinchona bark *(see)* and used in bitters, citrus, and fruit flavorings for beverages. Same medical use as quinine sulfate *(see)*. *See* Quinine Extract for toxicity. ASP

**QUININE SULFATE** • A synthetic flavoring additive derived from cinchona bark *(see)* and used in bitters flavoring for beverages. Also used medicinally to treat malaria, as an analgesic, and as a local anesthetic. ASP

**QUINOLINE** • A coal-tar derivative used in the manufacture of dyes. Also a solvent for resins. Made either by the distillation of coal tar, bones, and alkaloids or by the interaction of aniline *(see)* with acetaldehyde and formaldehyde *(see both)*. Absorbs water. Also used as a preservative for anatomical specimens. *See* Coal Tar for toxicity. *See also* FD and C Colors. NIL

**QUINOLINE YELLOW** • *See* Quinoline. E

**QUIZALOFOPETHYL** • White crystals used as an herbicide in animal feed. FDA residue tolerances are: 0.2 ppm in soybean hulls; 0.5 ppm in soybean meal; 1.0 ppm in soybean soap stock; 0.5 on soybeans; 0.2 ppm in eggs; 0.1 in eggs; 0.05 ppm in milk fat; 0.05 in fat of cattle, goats, hogs, and sheep; 0.02 ppm in meat of cattle, goats, hogs, and sheep; 0.05 ppm; 0.05 ppm as residues in fat, meat, and meat by-products of cattle, goats, hogs, and sheep; and 1.0 as residues on cottonseed.

# R

**RACEMIC ACID** • *See* Tartaric Acid.

**RADIATION OF FOOD** • *See* Irradiation of Food.

**RADISH EXTRACT** • Extract of *Raphanus sativus*. The small seeds of the radish remain viable for years. Has been used as a food since ancient times.

**RAISIN-SEED OIL** • Dried grapes or berries used in lubricating creams. *See* Grape-Seed Oil.

**RALGRO** • Zeranol. Used to increase growth in cattle and sheep. The FDA limits residue to zero in cattle and sheep. Has adverse reproductive effects in experimental animals.

**RAPESEED OIL, HYDROGENATED** • Brownish yellow oil from a turnip-like annual herb of European origin. Widely grown as a forage crop for sheep in the United States. Canada sought clearance to sell rapeseed in the U.S. market, but it was barred because it contains erucic acid, which was cited in the early 1970s as a possible source of heart problems based on the results of tests on rats. New varieties of the seeds, canola, have been developed that have low erucic acid levels. Now rapeseed oil is used in American salad oils, peanut butter, and some cake mixes. A distinctly unpleasant odor. Can cause acnelike skin eruptions. When rats were fed a diet high in rapeseed oil over a lifetime, they showed significantly greater degenerative changes in the liver and a higher incidence of kidney damage than animals fed other vegetable oils. *See* Erucic Acid. GRAS. ASP

**RAPESEED OIL, FULLY HYDROGENATED** • A stabilizer used in peanut butter. GRAS. ASP

**RAPESEED OIL, FULLY HYDROGENATED, SUPERGLYCERINATED** • An emulsifier used in shortenings for cake mixes. *See* Rapeseed Oil, Hydrogenation, and Glycerin. GRAS. NEW

**RAPESEED OIL, LOW ERUCIC ACID** • Miscellaneous additive that may be used in many products except in infant formula. May be declared on the label as canola oil. *See* Erucic Oil. NUL

**RAPESEED OIL, UNSAPONIFIABLES** • Fraction of rapeseed oil *(see)* that is not changed into a fatty alcohol when it is saponified (heated with an alkali and acid). GRAS except in infant formula.

**RASPBERRY EXTRACT** • *See* Raspberry Juice.

**RASPBERRY JUICE** • Juice from the fresh ripe fruit grown in Europe, Asia, the United States, and Canada. Used as a flavoring for lipsticks, food, and medicines. It has astringent properties.

**rBST** • Abbreviation for recombinant bovine somatotropin. *See* Bovine Somatotropin and IGF-I.

**RDA** • Recommended Dietary Allowances of the Food and Nutrition Board, National Academy of Sciences, National Research Council. The Recommended Daily Dietary Allowance was started in the 1940s to safeguard the public's health. The RDAs were estimates of the nutritional needs of adults and children developed by the FDA to be used as the legal standards for labeling foods in regard to nutritional content.

**READDITIVE** • A chemical that reacts or participates in a reaction; a substance that is used for the detection or determination of another substance by chemical or microscopical means. The various categories of readditives are colorimetric—to produce color-soluble compounds; fluxes—to lower melting point; oxidizers—used in oxidation; precipitants—to produce insoluble compounds; reducers—used in reduction (*see*); solvents—used to dissolve water-insoluble compounds.

**RECOMBINANT DNA** • The DNA formed by combining segments of DNA from different types of organisms. Recombinant DNA technology is one technique of genetic engineering.

**RECOMBINANT DNA TECHNOLOGY** • A broad range of techniques involving the manipulation of genetic material of organisms, including technologies by which scientists isolate genes from one organism and insert them into another. The term is often used synonymously with genetic engineering and to describe DNA sequences isolated from and transferred between organisms by genetic engineering techniques.

**RECOMMENDED DIETARY ALLOWANCES (RDA)** • The former listing of amounts of certain of nutrients needed to maintain health. These have been replaced by Daily Values (see pages 15–16 in introduction) on labels. *See* RDA.

**RED** • See FD and C Red (Nos. 3, 4, 40, and Citrus Red).

**RED ALGAE** • Seaweed. GRAS

**RED PEPPER** • Cayenne Pepper. A condiment made from the pungent fruit of the plant. Used in sausage and pepper flavorings. May be an irritant and also cause allergic reactions. Used medically as a topical pain killer.

**RED RASPBERRY LEAF EXTRACT** • An extract of the leaves of the red raspberry. Used as a flavoring.

**RED 2G** • Color used in Europe. E

**RED SAUNDERS** • Red Sandalwood. Flavoring in alcoholic beverages only.

**REDUCED** • Product has been nutritionally altered and contains at least 25 percent less of a nutrient such as fat or salt or 25 percent fewer calories than the regular product.

**REDUCED-LACTOSE WHEY** • *See* Whey and Reducing Additive. GRAS

**REDUCED-MINERALS WHEY** • Obtained by removing a portion of the minerals from whey. Used as a texturizer, nutritional extender, nutritive sweetener, formulation, and processing aid. *See* Whey and Reducing Additive. GRAS

**REDUCING ADDITIVE** • A substance that decreases, deoxidizes, or concentrates the volume of another substance. For instance, a reducing additive is used to convert a metal oxide to the metal itself. It also means a substance that adds hydrogen additives to another; for example, when acetaldehyde is converted to alcohol in the final step of alcoholic fermentation. It is used in foods to keep metals from oxidizing and affecting the taste or color of fats, oils, salad dressings, and other foods containing minerals.

**REDUCTION** • The process of reducing by chemical or electrochemical means. The gain of one or more electrons by an ion or compound. It is the reverse of oxidation.

**REG** • Food additive for which a petition has been filed and regulation issued.

**REGENERATED CELLULOSE** • Miscellaneous use with resins. *See* Cellulose.

**RELEASE AGENTS** • Substances migrating from food-packaging include linoleamide, oleamide, and palmitamide.

**RELEASING ADDITIVE** • A compound such as butter or an oil that prevents a product from sticking to the sides of a container. Also refers to a chemical that permits easy removal of the meat of a clam or other crustacean.

**RENNET** • Rennin (animal derived) and chymosin preparation (fermentation derived). Enzyme from the lining membranes of the stomach of suckling calves. Used for curdling milk in cheese making and in junket. Sometimes as a digestant. Reaffirmed GRAS in 1982. ASP

**RESIN, ACRYLAMIDE — ACRYLIC ACID** • A clarifying additive in beet sugar and sugarcane juice. The acid is used in the synthesis of this acrylic resin.

**RESIN, COUMARONE — INDENE** • A chewing-gum base and protective coating for citrus fruit. Coumarone is derived from coal tar and is used with a mixture of indene chiefly in the synthesis of coumarone resins.

**RESIN FROM FORMALDEHYDE, ACETONE and TETRAETHYLENE-PENTAMINE** • Used to coat film in touch with food. NUL

**RESIN, ISOBUTYLENE** • Polyisobutylene. A chewing-gum base made from the chemical used chiefly in manufacturing synthetic rubber.

**RESIN, METHACRYLIC and DIVINYL BENZENE** • A compound of fine particle size, weakly acidic. Used as an absorbent for Vitamin $B_{12}$ in nutritional supplement products.

**RESIN, PETROLEUM HYDROCARBON** • A chewing-gum base synthesized from fuel oil.

**RESINS** • The brittle substance, usually translucent or transparent, formed from the hardened secretions of plants. Among the natural resins are damar, elemi, and sandarac *(see all)*. Synthetic resins include polyvinyl acetate, various polyester resins, and sulfonamide resins *(see all)*. Toxicity depends upon ingredients used. *See* Gums.

**RESIN, TERPENE** • Alpha and Beta Pinene. A chewing-gum base and coating for fresh fruits and vegetables. Pinene *(see)* has the same toxicity as turpentine.

**RESORCINOL** • A preservative, antiseptic, and antifungal additive. Obtained from various resins. A sweetish taste. Irritating to the skin and mucous membranes. May cause allergic reactions, particularly of the skin. The FDA issued a notice in 1992 that resorcinol has not been shown to be safe and effective for stated claims in over-the-counter products. ASP

**RETINOIDS** • Derived from retinoic acid, vitamin A, it is used to treat acne and other skin disorders. *See* Vitamin A.

**RETINOL** • Vitamin A *(see)*.

**RETINYL PALMITATE** • The ester of vitamin A and palmitic acid sometimes mixed with vitamin D *(see all)*.

**RHAMNOSE, L** • Occurs in poison sumac, *Rhus toxicodendron*. Combined with sugar in many other plants. It is used in the manufacture of food additives. ASP

**RHATANY ROOT** • A flavoring. The dried root of *Krameria triandra* from Peru and Brazil. A flavoring additive. Used as a cosmetic astringent. *See* Krameria Extract. EAF

**RHIZOPUS ORYZAE** • An enzyme used in production of dextrose (sugar) from starch.

**RHODENAL** • *See* Citronellal.

**RHODINOL** • A synthetic flavoring additive isolated from geranium rose oil *(see)*. It has the strong odor of rose and consists essentially of geraniol and citronellol *(see both)*. Used in strawberry, chocolate, rose, grape, honey, spice, and ginger ale flavorings for beverages, ice cream, ices, candy, baked goods, gelatin desserts, chewing gum, and jelly. ASP

**RHODINYL ACETATE** • Acetic Acid. An acidulant and synthetic flavoring, colorless to slightly yellow, with a light, fresh, roselike odor. Used in berry, coconut, apricot, floral, rose, and honey flavorings for beverages, ice cream, ices, candy, and baked goods. A skin irritant. ASP

**RHODINYL BUTYRATE** • Butyric Acid. A synthetic raspberry, strawberry, and fruit flavoring additive for beverages, ice cream, ices, candy, baked goods, and chewing gum. ASP

**RHODINYL FORMATE** • Formic Acid. Synthetic flavoring with a roselike odor. Used in raspberry, rose, apple, cherry, plum, pear, and pineapple flavorings for beverages, ice cream, ices, candy, baked goods, and gelatin desserts. *See* Formic Acid for toxicity. ASP

**RHODINYL ISOBUTRYATE** • Isobutyric Acid. A synthetic raspberry, floral, rose, apple, pear, pineapple, and honey flavoring additive for beverages, ice cream, ices, candy, baked goods, and gelatin desserts. ASP

**RHODINYL ISOVALERATE** • Isovaleric Acid. A synthetic berry, floral, rose, and fruit flavoring additive for beverages, ice cream, ices, candy, and baked goods. ASP

**RHODINYL PHENYLACETATE** • Phenylacetic Acid. A synthetic flavoring used in beverages, ice cream, ices, candy, and baked goods. ASP

**RHODINYL PROPIONATE** • Propionic Acid. A synthetic berry, rose, plum, and honey flavoring additive for beverages, ice cream, ices, candy, and baked goods. ASP

**RHODYMENIA PALMATA** • *See* Dulse.

**RHUBARB** • The root of *Rheum rhaponticum* used as a flavoring in alcoholic beverages only. Has been used as a laxative. ASP

**RHYNCHOSIA PYRAMIDALIS** • A large, tropical twining plant with yellow flowers. Used as a flavoring.

**RIBOFLAVIN** • Vitamin $B_2$. Lactoflavin. Formerly called vitamin G. Riboflavin is a factor in the vitamin B complex and is used in emollients. Every plant and animal cell contains a minute amount. Good sources are milk, eggs, and organ meats. It is necessary for healthy skin and respiration, protects the eyes from sensitivity to light, and is used for building and maintaining human body tissues. A deficiency leads to lesions at the corner of the mouth and to changes in the cornea. Recommended Daily Requirements for infants is 4,000 micrograms per day and for adults 1,300 micrograms. Its yellow to orange-yellow color is used to dye eggshells. It is permanently listed as a food color. It does not require certification. Riboflavin and its more soluble form, riboflavin-5-phosphate, are added as enrichment to dry baby cereals, poultry stuffing, peanut butter, prepared breakfast cereals, enriched flour, enriched cornmeal, enriched corn grits, enriched macaroni, and enriched breads and rolls. GRAS. ASP. E

**RIBOFLAVIN-5-PHOSPHATE** • A more soluble form of riboflavin *(see)*. The final report to the FDA of the Select Committee on GRAS Substances stated in 1980 that it should continue its GRAS status with no limitations other than good manufacturing practices. EAF

**RIBONUCLEIC ACID (RNA)** • Found in both the nucleus and cytoplasm of the cell, it is the material that contains directions for the genetic code of the cell, DNA.

**D-RIBOSE** • *See* Ribose, D-.

**RIBOSE, D-** • Ribose occurs naturally in all living cells. It is a simple sugar that begins the metabolic process for ATP production *(see)*. Prepared by hydrolysis of yeast *(see)*. ASP

**RIBOTIDE** • A flavor enhancer developed by the Japanese.

**RICE BRAN OIL** • Oil expressed from the broken coat of rice grain. Used as a coating for candy. Nontoxic.

**RICE BRAN WAX** • The wax obtained from the broken coat of rice grain.

Used as a coating additive, as a chewing-gum base, and a releasing additive *(see)*. NIL

**RICE, MILLED** • Rice with the bran removed. ASP

**RICE STARCH** • The finely pulverized grains of the rice plant used as an anticaking additive, thickener, and gelling additive. May cause an allergic reaction. The final report to the FDA of the Select Committee on GRAS Substances stated in 1980 that it should continue GRAS status with no limitations other than good manufacturing practices. ASP

**RICINOLEIC ACID** • A mixture of fatty oils found in the seeds of castor beans. Castor oil contains 80 to 85 percent ricinoleic acid. The oily liquid is used in soaps, flavorings, antifungal additives, and in contraceptive jellies. It is believed to be the active laxative in castor oil.

**RICINOLEATE** • Salt of ricinoleic acid found in castor oil.

**RIGHT-TO-KNOW** • *See* Community Right-To-Know List established by the Environmental Protection Agency and other government and civic organizations.

**RNA** • Ribonucleic Acid. A nucleic acid that is found in the cytoplasm and also in the nucleus of some cells. One function of RNA is to direct the manufacture of proteins.

**RNI** • Canadian Recommended Nutrient Intake.

**ROBENIDINE** • Crystals from ethanol *(see)*. Used to treat parasites in chickens. The FDA limits 0.2 ppm in skin and fat of chickens and 0.1 ppm in other chicken tissues. Moderately toxic by ingestion.

**ROCHELLE SALT** • Potassium Sodium Tartrate. Translucent crystals or white crystalline powder with cooling saline taste. Used in the manufacture of baking powder and in the silvering of mirrors.

**RONNEL** • Used in cattle feed. A systemic pesticide. *See* Organophosphates.

**ROSA ALBA** • *See* Rose, Absolute.

**ROSA CANINA** • *See* Rose Hips Extract.

**ROSA CEMTIFOLIA** • *See* Rose, Absolute.

**ROSE, ABSOLUTE** • Same origin as for rose Bulgarian *(see)*. Used as a berry, rose, fruit, and nut flavoring additive for beverages, ice cream, ices, candy, and baked goods. except for allergic reactions. GRAS. EAF

**ROSE BENGAL** • A bluish red, fragrant liquid taken from the rose of the Bengal region of the Asian subcontinent. Nontoxic.

**ROSE BUDS, FLOWERS** • Flavoring. *See* Rose Extract. GRAS. NUL

**ROSE BULGARIAN** • True Otto Oil. Attar of Roses. Rose Otto Bulgaria. One of the most widely used perfume ingredients, it is the essential oil, steam-distilled from the flowers of *Rosa × damascena*. The rose flowers are picked early in the morning when they contain the maximum amount of perfume and are distilled quickly after harvesting. Bulgaria is the main source of supply, but Russia, Turkey, Syria, and Indochina also grow them.

The liquid is pale yellow and has warm, deep floral, slightly spicy, and extremely fragrant red-rose smell. Used as a flavoring additive in loganberry, raspberry, strawberry, orange, rose, violet, cherry, grape, peach, honey, muscatel, maple, almond, pecan, and ginger ale flavorings for beverages, ice cream, ices, candy, baked goods, gelatin desserts, chewing gum, and jellies. Also used in coloring matter, and as a flavoring in pills. May cause allergic reactions. GRAS

**ROSE EXTRACT** • An extract of the various species of rose, it is used in raspberry and cola beverages and in fragrances, except for allergic reactions. GRAS

**ROSE FLOWERS** • *See* Rose Extract. NUL

**ROSE GERANIUM** • Distilled from any of several South African herbs grown for their fragrant leaves. May cause allergic reactions. GRAS

**ROSE HIPS EXTRACT** • Hip berries. Extract of the fruit of various species of wild roses, it is rich in vitamin C and is used as a natural flavoring. Widely used by organic food enthusiasts. GRAS. EAF

**ROSE LEAVES EXTRACT** • Derived from the leaves of the genus *Rosa*. Used in raspberry and cola beverages. NUL

**ROSE OIL** • Attar of Roses. The fragrant, volatile, essential oil distilled from fresh flowers. Colorless or yellow with a strong fragrant odor and taste of roses. Nontoxic but may cause allergic reactions. *See* Rose Bulgarian. EAF

**ROSE OTTO BULGARIA** • *See* Rose Bulgarian.

**ROSE WATER, STRONGER** • *Rosa × centifolia*. The watery solution of the odoriferous constituents of roses, made by distilling the fresh flowers with water or steam. Nontoxic but may cause allergic reactions. NIL

**ROSELLE** • *Hibiscus sabdariffa*. An herb cultivated in the East Indies, it is used for making tarts and jellies, and gives a tart taste to acid drinks. It is also used as a natural red food coloring for soft drinks, tea-type products, punches, apple jelly, and pectin jelly, but it is not stable in carbonated beverages. GRAS. EAF

**ROSEMARY EXTRACT** • Garden Rosemary. A flavoring and perfume from the fresh aromatic flowering tops of the evergreen shrub, *Rosemarinus officinalis* grown in the Mediterranean region. Light blue flowers and gray-green leaves. Used for beverages, condiments, and meat. It is also used in citrus, peach, and ginger flavorings for beverages, ice cream, ices, candy, baked goods, condiments, and meats. Also being studied as a natural antioxidant. A teaspoonful of the oil may cause illness in an adult, and an ounce may cause death. GRAS. EAF

**ROSEMARY OIL** • The oil obtained from the flowering tops of *Rosemarinus officinalis*. *See* Rosemary Extract. ASP

**ROSEMARY OLEORESIN** • Dark brownish yellow semisolid with the fresh leaf fragrance of rosemary used as a scent of new-mown hay. ASP

**ROSIDINHA** • Sideroxylon. A large green genus of tropical trees, family Sapotaceae having hard wood and somewhat bell-shaped flowers with a few seeded berries. Used as a flavoring. ASP

**ROSIN AND ROSIN DERIVATIVES** • Colophony. Softener for chewing gum from *Pinus* spp. Also used as a coating for citrus fruit. It is a pale yellow residue left after distilling off the volatile oil from the oleoresin obtained from various species of pine trees chiefly produced in the United States. Also used in the manufacture of varnishes and fireworks. It can cause contact dermatitis. NUL

**ROSIN, GUM, GLYCEROL ESTER** • A softener for chewing gum. *See* Rosin and Glycerol. ASP

**ROSIN, LIMED** • Made by heat fusing of rosin and calcium hydroxide *(see)* with good oil and solvent solubility, and mainly used for manufacturing. Used as a coating in contact with food. NIL

**ROSIN, METHYL ESTER, PARTIALLY HYDROGENATED** • Used in the manufacture of food additives and as a softener for chewing gum. ASP

**ROSIN, PARTIALLY DIMERIZED, CALCIUM SALT, or PARTIALLY (CATALYTICALLY) HYDROGENATED** • A coating for fresh citrus fruit. *See* Rosin and Hydrogenated. ASP

**ROSIN, POLYMERIZED GLYCEROL ESTER, PARTIALLY HYDROGENATED GLYCEROL ESTER, or PARTIALLY DIMERIZED GLYCEROL ESTER** • A softener for chewing gum. *See* Rosin and Glycerol. ASP

**ROSIN, TALL OIL, GLYCEROL ESTER** • The natural product rosin is a complex mixture of mutually soluble organic compounds. There are three general methods of producing rosins commercially, these methods (and their products) being: solvent extraction of pure stump wood (wood rosin); tapping of gum from the living tree (gum rosin); separation from tall oil (tall oil rosin). The three rosins, freed of extraneous impurities and refined, differ somewhat quantitatively and in color but all three may be glycinerated to produce the glycerol ester. See Tall Oil and Glycerol. ASP

**ROSIN, WOOD, GUM or WOOD PARTIALLY HYDROGENATED, PENTAERYTHRITOL** • A coating for fresh citrus fruit. *See* Rosin and Maleic Acid. ASP

**ROSMARINUS OFFICINALIS** • *See* Rosemary Extract.

**ROXARSONE** • An antibacterial for control of enteric infections and to improve growth and feed efficiency. Used in chicken and swine feeds, in drinking water of chickens, turkey, and swine.

**RUBBER, NATURAL, SMOKED SHEET, and LATEX SOLIDS** • *Hevea brasiliensis.* Rubber as well as rubber-based adhesives are common causes of contact dermatitis. The natural gum obtained from the rubber tree is not allergenic; the offenders are the chemicals added to natural rubber gum to make it a useful product. Such chemicals are accelerators, antioxidants, stabilizers, and vulcanizers, many of which can cause allergies. A petition to employ single-use rubber threads in processing and packaging of foods, including meat and poultry, was put in abeyance *(see)* by the FDA in 2003. ASP

**RUBBER, BUTADIENE STYRENE** • Latex. A chewing-gum base.

**RUBBER, SMOKED SHEET** • A chewing-gum base. *See* Rubber, Natural.

**RUE OIL** • A spice additive obtained from the fresh aromatic blossoming plants grown in southern Europe and Asia, *Ruta graveolens.* The oil has a fatty odor and is used in baked goods. It is obtained by steam distillation and is used in fragrances and in blueberry, raspberry, coconut, grape, peach, rum, cheese, and spice flavorings for beverages, ice cream, ices, candy, baked goods, and condiments. Formerly used in medicine to treat disorders and hysteria. It may cause photosensitivity. In 1976 the FDA confirmed rue as GRAS in all categories of food at a maximum use level of 2 ppm. The final report to the FDA of the Select Committee on GRAS Substances stated in 1980 that there is no evidence in the available information that it is a hazard to the public when used as it is now and it should continue its GRAS status with limitations on amounts that can be added to food.

**RUM** • An alcoholic beverage from fermented molasses. Flavoring for candied fruits. EAF

**RUM ETHER** • A synthetic flavoring, consisting of water, ethanol, ethyl acetate, methanol, ethyl formate, acetone, acetaldehyde, and formaldehyde *(see all)*. Used in butter, liquor, and rum flavorings for beverages, ice cream, ices, candy, baked goods, gelatin, chewing gum, and alcoholic beverages (1,600 ppm). ASP

**RUTIN** • Pale yellow crystals found in many plants, particularly buckwheat. Used as a dietary supplement for blood or lymph vessel fragility. There is reported use of the chemical; it was not assigned for toxicology literature in 1999 and is still EAF.

**RYE FLOUR** • Used in powders. Flour made from hardy annual cereal grass. Seeds are used for feed and in the manufacture of whiskey and bread. May cause allergic reactions.

# S

**SACCHARIDE HYDROLYSATE** • A mixture of sugars derived from using an alkali and water on a mixture of glucose and lactose *(see)*.

**SACCHARIDE ISOMERATE** • *See* Saccharide Hydrolysate.

**SACCHARIN** • An artificial sweetener in use since 1879. It is three hundred times as sweet as natural sugar. Used as a sweetener. Odorless or with a faint aromatic odor. It was used with cyclamates in the experiments that led to the ban on cyclamates. The FDA proposed restricting saccharin to 15 milligrams per day for each kilogram of body weight or one gram a day for a 150-pound person. Then, on March 9, 1977, the FDA announced the use of saccharin in foods and beverages would be banned because the artificial sweetener had been found to cause malignant bladder tumors in laboratory animals. The ban was based on the findings of a study sponsored by the Canadian government that found that seven out of thirty-eight animals developed tumors, three of them malignant. In addition, one hundred offspring were fed saccharin, and fourteen of them developed bladder tumors. In contrast, one hundred control rats were not fed saccharin and only two developed tumors. At the time of the FDA's announcement, 5 million pounds of saccharin were being consumed per year, 74 percent of it in diet soda, 14 percent in dietetic food, and 12 percent as a tabletop replacement for sugar. There was an immediate outcry, led vociferously by the Calorie Control Council, an organization made up of commercial producers and users of saccharin. The FDA, urged by Congress, then delayed the ban. The moratorium on prohibiting the use of saccharin has been extended indefinitely. Since 1977, however, saccharin containers carry labels warning that saccharin may be hazardous to your health. Saccharin has exhibited mutagenic activity (genetic changes) in the early-warning Ames Test *(see)* for carcinogens. When administered orally to mice, mutagenic activity was demonstrated in the urine of these animals as well as in tissue tests. Highly purified saccharin was not mutagenic in tissue tests, but the urine of mice fed saccharin was. Congress's Office of Technology Assessment, in view of the evidence to date, strongly endorsed the scientific basis of the FDA's proposed ban. "This review of animal studies leads to the conclusion that saccharin is a carcinogen for animals," the FDA panel said. Clouding the degree of risk, however, is that up to 20 ppm of unknown chemical impurities contaminated those doses fed the rats in the Canadian study that led to the FDA's original move. The impurities themselves proved mutagenic in the Ames Test. On November 6, 1978, the Committee of the Institute of Medicine and National Research Council concluded that saccharin is a potential carcinogen in humans. The extremely low potency of saccharin as a carcinogen was emphasized by the committee. However, they expressed special concern that children under ten years of age were consuming diet sodas and other saccharin-containing products in increasing amounts. Exposure in children, the committee noted, may have special significance because of the long time required for some cancers to develop. There were some "worrisome data" regarding consumption by women of childbearing age, children, and teenagers. The concern about fetal exposure grew out of earlier findings of increased bladder cancers in male rats fed high-saccharin diets or born to mothers that were on high-saccharin diets during pregnancy. The committee concluded that it is most likely that saccharin itself is the carcinogenic additive, rather than any impurities that may be associated with its manufacture. The fight to keep saccharin on the market spotlighted the Delaney Amendment, which prohibits known carcinogens from being added to food, and a move to weaken that amendment persists. In 1969, Britain banned saccharin except as an artificial sweetener. In 1950, France banned it except as a nonprescription drug. Germany restricts its use to certain foods and beverages, which must state on the label that it is in the product. In 1997, the Caloric Control Council, a trade group, successfully requested the National Toxicology Program to review new data to lead to a delisting of saccharin as a carcinogen. In 2003, the FDA continued its approval of saccharin use. NUL. E

**SACCHARIN, SODIUM SALT** • *See* Saccharin. ASP. E

**SAFFLOWER GLYCERIDE** • *See* Safflower Oil.

**SAFFLOWER OIL** • The edible oil expressed from the seed of an Old World herb that resembles a thistle, with large, bright red or orange flowers. Widely cultivated for its oil, which thickens and becomes rancid on exposure to air. It is used in salad oils and shortenings, and as a vehicle for medicines. As a dietary supplement it is alleged to be a preventative in the development of atherosclerosis—fat-clogged arteries. A drug consisting of the dried flowers of safflower is used in medicine in place of saffron *(see)*. American safflower (American saffron) is no longer authorized for use.

**SAFFRON** • Crocus. Vegetable Gold. Spanish or French Saffron. The dried stigma of the crocus, *Crocus sativus,* cultivated in Spain, Greece, France, and Iran. Orange-brown; strong, peculiar aromatic odor; bitterish, aromatic taste. Almost entirely employed for coloring and flavoring. It has been permanently listed for use in foods since 1966. It does not require certification. Used in bitters, liquors, and spice flavorings for beverages, baked goods, meats, and liquors. Cleared by the USDA Meat Inspection Department for coloring sausage casing, oleomargarine, shortening, and for marking ink. The extract is used in honey and rum flavorings for beverages, ice cream, ices, candy, baked goods, and condiments, and it goes into yellow coloring. Formerly used to treat skin diseases. GRAS. ASP

**SAFROLE and ANY OIL CONTAINING SAFROLE** • Illegal. Found in certain natural oils such as star anise, nutmeg, and ylang-ylang, it is a stable, colorless to brown liquid with an odor of sassafras and root beer. Used in the manufacture of heliotropin *(see)* and in expensive soaps and perfumes. Used as a beverage flavoring until it was banned in 1960. The toxicity of this fragrance ingredient is being questioned by the FDA. It is an animal liver carcinogen. BANNED

**SAFROLE-FREE EXTRACT OF SASSAFRAS** • A flavoring in food. *See* Sassafras Extract. ASP

**SAGE** • Spanish. Greek. The flowering tops and leaves of the shrubby mints. Spices include Greek sage and Spanish sage. The genus is *Salvia,* so named for the plant's supposed healing powers. Greek sage is used in fruit and spice flavorings for beverages, baked goods, and meats (1,500 ppm). Greek sage oil, obtained by steam distillation, is used in berry, grape, liquor, meat, crème de menthe, nutmeg, and sage flavorings for beverages, ice cream, ices, candy, baked goods, chewing gum, condiments, meats, and pickles. Greek sage oleoresin *(see)* is used in sausage and spice flavorings for condiments and meats. Spanish sage oil is used in fruit and spice flavorings for beverages, ice cream, ices, candy, baked goods, condiments, and meats. It is also used as a meat preservative. Greek sage is used in medicine. Used by herbalists to treat sore gums, mouth ulcers, and to remove warts. Arabs believed it prevents dying. GRAS. ASP

**SAIGON CINNAMON** • *See* Cinnamon.

**SAIGON CINNAMON LEAF OIL** • *See* Cinnamon.

**SAINT JOHN'S BREAD** • *See* Locust Bean Gum. GRAS

**SAINT JOHN'S WORT FLOWERS, LEAVES, and CAULIS** • *Hypericum perforatum.* Amber. Blessed. Devil's Scourge. God's Wonder Herb. Grace of God. Goatweed. Hypericum. Klamath Weed. A perennial native to Britain, Europe, and Asia, it is now found throughout North America. The plant contains volatile oil, tannin, resin, pectin and glycosides *(see all)*. It was believed to have infinite healing powers derived from the saint, the red juice representing his blood. It was used as an antivenereal. It is used to treat pains and diseases of the nervous system, arthritic pains, and injuries. An infusion made from its leaves is used for stomach disorders, diarrhea, depression, and bladder problems, and to remove threadworms in children. It is now being studied by researchers from the National Cancer Institute and various universities as a potential treatment for cancer and AIDS. The FDA listed Saint John's wort as an "unsafe herb" in 1977. The FDA issued a notice in 1992 that Saint John's wort has not been shown to be safe and effective as claimed in OTC digestive-aid products. That does not mean, however, that it cannot be used for other purposes. NIL

**SALAD OIL** • Any edible vegetable oil. Dermatologists advise rubbing salad oils or fats on the skin, particularly on babies and older persons.

**SALATRIM** • Short and Long Chain Acid Triglyceride Molecules. This is a family of reduced-calorie fats that are only partially absorbed in the body. It contains 5 calories per gram. It is used in such products as Hershey's reduced-fat, semisweet chocolate-flavor baking chips. GRAS

**SALICARIA EXTRACT** • Spiked Loosestrife. Extract of the flowering herb *Lythrum salicaria,* which has purple or pink flowers. Used since ancient Greek times as an herb that calms nerves and soothes skin.

**SALICIN** • A chemical derived from the bark of several species of willows and poplar trees. Aspirin and other salicylates are derived from salicin or made synthetically.

**SALICYLALDEHYDE** • Salicylic Aldehyde. A synthetic flavoring made by heating phenol (very toxic) and chloroform. Occurs naturally in cassia bark. Clear, bitter, almondlike odor, burning taste. White to slightly pink, crystalline, bitter powder. Gives a sensation of warmth on the tongue. Soluble in hot water. Used in butter flavorings for beverages, ice cream, ices, candy, baked goods, chewing gum, condiments, and liqueurs. Used chiefly in perfumery. Used as an analgesic, fungicide, and antiinflammatory to soothe the skin. Lethal dose in rats is 1 gram per kilogram of body weight. ASP

**SALICYLATES** • Amyl. Phenyl. Benzyl. Menthyl. Glyceryl. Dipropylene Glycol Esters. Salts of Salicylic Acid. Those who are sensitive to aspirin may also be hypersensitive to FD and C Yellow No. 5, a salicylate, and to a number of foods that naturally contain salicylate, such as almonds, apples, apple cider, apricots, blackberries, boysenberries, cherries, cloves, cucumbers, currants, gooseberries, grapes, nectarines, oil of wintergreen, oranges, peaches, pickles, plums, prunes, raisins, raspberries, strawberries, and tomatoes. Foods with added salicylates for flavoring may be ice cream, bakery goods (except bread), candy, chewing gum, soft drinks, Jell-O, jams, cake mixes, and wintergreen flavors.

**SALICYLIC ACID** • Occurs naturally in wintergreen leaves, sweet birch, and other plants and has a sweetish taste. Synthetically prepared by heating phenol with carbon dioxide, it is used as a preservative in food products. It is also used as a fungicide in the treatment of animals. Residues are prohibited in milk. EPA Genetic Toxicology Program (see). It is used in making aspirin. It can be absorbed through the skin. Absorption of large amounts may cause vomiting, abdominal pain, increased respiration, acidosis, mental disturbances, and skin rashes in sensitive individuals. It is poisonous by ingestion. Causes birth defects in experimental animals. ASP

**SALICYLIC ETHER** • See Ethyl Salicylate.

**SALICYLIDES** • Any of several crystalline derivatives of salicylic acid (see) from which the water has been removed.

**SALINOMYCIN** • Coxistac. An antiparasite drug used in chicken feed.

**SALMONELLA** • Named for the American veterinarian Dr. D. E. Salmon, it is a bacteria that occurs in the intestinal tract and tissues of infected humans and animals. Many of the more than twelve hundred different types can cause food poisoning, entering the food supply through meats or animal products from infected animals or from contamination by an infected animal or person. One of the most common food-borne illnesses in the United States, the symptoms are diarrhea, abdominal cramps, fever, and sometimes vomiting, which occur six to forty-eight hours after eating. Infections range from moderate, with recovery in three to four days, to fatal. Salmonella bacteria grow rapidly in cooked foods such as meat, eggs, custards, and salads that have been left unrefrigerated for several hours. It may also be transmitted by infected poultry and by sewage-polluted water. The National Academy of Science's Institute of Medicine estimated that doses of antibiotics in livestock promote growth or prevent infection for less than 2 percent of the human deaths due to food-borne, antibiotic-resistant salmonella. In 1989, according to a "new risks" assessment made for the FDA by the National Academy of Science's Institute of Medicine (IOM), the group "was unable to find data directly implicating subtherapeutic doses of antibiotics in livestock with illnesses in people" or to come up with a "numerical answer" about the risk that animal medication posed to humans. The IOM estimated that the doses of antibiotics given to livestock to promote growth or prevent infection would account for less than 2 percent of the human deaths due to food-borne, antibiotic-resistant salmonella. The committee felt that stopping the use of antibiotics to promote growth in livestock might reduce the total number of human deaths due to salmonella poisoning, but that such results could not be supported scientifically. Since 1989, of course, the incidences of salmonella resistant to antibiotics has been increasing, according to another government agency, the Centers for Disease Control. Salmonella has contaminated almost every chicken sent to market and has led the U.S. government to require warning labels on poultry products.

**SALT** • A compound formed by the interaction of an acid and a base. Sodium chloride, or common table salt, is an example. Sodium is the alkali or base and chloride provides the acidic factor.

**SALTPETER** • Potassium Nitrate. Niter. *See* Nitrate and Potassium. Acute intoxication is unlikely because a large dose causes vomiting and because it is rapidly excreted. Potassium poisoning disturbs the rhythm of the heart, and orally poisoned animals die from respiratory failure. Prolonged exposure to even small amounts may produce anemia, methemoglobinemia (lack of oxygen in the blood), and kidney damage.

**SALT OF STEARIC ACID** • *See* Stearic Acid.

**SALTS OF FATTY ACIDS** • Aluminum, calcium, magnesium, potassium, and sodium salts of capric, caprylic, myristic, oleic, palmitic, and stearic acids *(see all)* manufactured from fats and oils derived from edible sources. Used as anticaking additives, binders, and emulsifiers in various foods. ASP

**SALVIA** • *See* Sage.

**SAMBUCUS EXTRACT** • *See* Elder Flowers.

**SANDALWOOD OIL, EAST INDIAN** • The pale yellow, somewhat viscous volatile oil obtained by steam distillation from the dried ground roots and wood of the plant. A strong, warm, persistent odor; soluble in most fixed oils. Used in floral, fruit, honey, and ginger ale flavorings for beverages, ice cream, ices, candy, baked goods, and chewing gum. May produce skin rash in the hypersensitive, especially if present in high concentrations. EAF

**SANDALWOOD OIL, WEST INDIAN** • Less soluble than the East Indian variety. *See* Amyris Oil. EAF

**SANDALWOOD OIL, YELLOW** • Arheol. Same origin as East Indian sandalwood oil *(see)*. A floral, fruit, honey, and ginger ale flavoring additive for beverages, ice cream, ices, candy, baked goods, and chewing gum. EAF

**SANDARAC** • Used in alcoholic beverages only. Resin from a plant grown in Morocco, *Tetraclinis articulata.* Used in tooth cements, varnishes, and for gloss and adhesion in nail lacquers. NUL

**SANITIZING SOLUTIONS** • For use on food processing equipment followed by adequate draining. The FDA sets limits on uses and concentrations for many compounds. *See,* for example, Quaternary Ammonium Compounds or Butoxy Monoether of mixed (ethylene) prolyalkylene glycol.

**SANTALOL, ALPHA AND BETA** • Alcohols from sandalwood used in fragrances. *See* Sandalwood Oil. ASP

**SANTALUM ALBUM** • *See* Sandalwood Oil.

**SANTALYL ACETATE** • Acetic Acid. A synthetic flavoring additive obtained from sandalwood oils *(see).* Used in floral, pear, and pineapple flavorings for beverages, ice cream, ices, candy, baked goods, and chewing gum. ASP

**SANTALYL PHENYLACETATE** • Phenylacetic Acid. A synthetic flavoring obtained from sandalwood oils *(see).* Used in butter, caramel, fruit, and honey flavorings for beverages, ice cream, ices, candy, and baked goods. NIL

**SANTOQUIN** • Ethoxyquin. A yellow liquid antioxidant and herbicide. It has been found to cause liver tumors in newborn mice. *See* Sodium Acid Pyrophosphate (SAP). A questionable additive. *See* Ethoxyquin.

**SAPONIN** • Any of numerous glycosides—natural or synthetic compounds derived from sugars—that occur in many plants such as soapbark, soapwort, or sarsaparilla. Characterized by their ability to foam in water. Yellowish to white, acrid, hygroscopic. In powder form they can cause sneezing. Extracted from soapbark or soapwort and used chiefly as foaming and emulsifying additives and detergents.

**SARCODACTYLIS OIL** • From the fruit of the dried fruit of *Citrus medica* var. *sarcodactylis* (Fam. Rutaceae). Its volatile oil is an expectorant and antiasthmatic. Used in oil-based sprays to control scale insects. EAF

**SARSAPARILLA EXTRACT** • The dried root from tropical American plants, *Smilax* spp. Used in cola, mint, root beer, sarsaparilla, wintergreen, and birch beer flavorings for beverages, ice cream, ices, candy, and baked goods. Still used for psoriasis; formerly used for syphilis. There is reported use of the chemical, but it has not yet been assigned for toxicology literature. EAF

**SASSAFRAS BARK EXTRACT** • Safrole. Safrole-free. It is the yellow to reddish yellow volatile oil obtained from the roots of the sassafras, *Sassafras albidum.* It is 80 percent safrole *(see)* and has the characteristic odor and taste of sassafras. Used in rum and root beer flavorings for beverages, ice cream, ices, candy, and baked goods. Applied to insect bites and stings to relieve symptoms; also a topical antiseptic and used medicinally to break up intestinal gas. May produce dermatitis in hypersensitive individuals. EAF

**SASSAFRAS LEAVES** • Safrole-free. Same origin as the bark extract. Used in soups (30,000 ppm). There is no reported use of the chemical and no toxicology information is available. *See* Sassafras Bark Extract for toxicity. NIL

**SAT FAT** • Abbreviation for saturated fat on food labels.

**SAT FAT CAL** • Abbreviation for saturated fat calories on food labels.

**SATURATED FATS** • Saturated fats contain only single-bond carbon linkages and are the least active chemically. They are usually solid at room temperature. Most animal fats are saturated. The common saturated fats are acetic, butyric, caproic, caprylic, capric, lauric, myristic, palmitic, stearic, arachidic, and behenic. Butterfat, coconut oil, and peanut oil are high in saturated fats. *See* Fat.

**SAUNDERS WHITE OIL** • *See* Sandalwood Oil.

**SAUSAGE CASINGS, HCL AND CELLULOSE FIBERS** • Tree pulp is used to make sausage casings. *See* also Collagen. ASP

**SAVORY EXTRACT** • An extract of *Satureja hortensis,* an aromatic mint known as summer or winter savory. The dried leaves of summer savory is a spice used in baked goods, condiments, and meats. Summer savory oil is obtained from the dried whole plant. It is used as a spice in condiments, candy, and baked goods. Summer savory oil oleoresin *(see)* is a spice used in candy, baked goods, and condiments. Winter savory *(S. montana)* oil and oleoresin spices are used in candy, baked goods, and condiments. Poisonous by skin contact. Moderately toxic by ingestion. A severe skin irritant. GRAS. ASP

**SAVORY, WINTER** • *Satureja montana. See* Savory Extract. NIL

**SAVORY, WINTER OLEORESIN** • *Satureja montana. See* Savory Extract. NIL

**SCHINUS MOLLE OIL** • A natural flavoring extract from the tropical pepper tree, *Schinus molle.* Used in candy, baked goods, and condiments. GRAS. There is reported use of the chemical, it has not yet been assigned for toxicology literature. EAF

**SCLAREOLIDE** • There is reported use of the chemical; it was not assigned for toxicology literature in 1999 and is still EAF.

**SCURVY GRASS EXTRACT** • The extract of the leaves and flower stalks of *Cochlearia officinalis.* The bright green leaves of this northerly herb were collected and eaten in large quantities by European seamen to prevent scurvy. The plant has the strong odor of horseradish, to which it is related.

**SDA** • FDA's abbreviation for solubilizing and dispersing agent.

**SEBACIC ACID** • Decanedioic acid. Colorless leaflets, sparingly soluble in water and soluble in alcohol. Manufactured by heating castor oil with alkalies or by distillation of oleic acid *(see).* The esters of sebacic acid are used as stabilizers.

**SELENIUM** • Yellow solid or brownish powder, insoluble in water. Discovered in 1807 in the earth's crust. Used as a nutrient. Can severely irritate the eyes if it gets into them while hair is being washed. Occupational exposure causes pallor, nervousness, depression, garlic odor of breath, gastrointestinal disturbances, and skin rash. Liver injury in experimental animals.

**SELENIUM AS SODIUM SELENITE or SELENATE** • Used as a feed additive. The FDA limits it to less than 0.1 ppm in complete feed for chickens, swine, turkeys, sheep, beef cattle, dairy cattle, and ducks.

**SENNA, ALEXANDRIA** • Flavoring from the dried leaves of *Cassia senna* grown in India and Egypt. Has been used as a cathartic. EAF

**SENSITIVITY** • Hypersensitivity. An increased reaction to a substance that may be quite harmless to nonallergic persons.

**SENSITIZE** • To administer or expose to an antigen provoking an immune response so that, on later exposure to that antigen, a more vigorous secondary response will occur.

**SEQ** • FDA's abbreviation for sequestrant.

**SEQUESTERING ADDITIVE** • A preservative that prevents physical or chemical changes affecting color, flavor, texture, or appearance of a product. Ethylenediamine tetraacetic acid (EOTA) is an example. It is used in carbonated beverages.

**SERINE** • L form only. An amino acid *(see),* nonessential, taken as a dietary supplement. It is a constituent of many proteins. *See* Proteins. Was on the FDA list requiring further information from at least 1980 to 1999. Now ASP

**SEROTONIN** • A neurotransmitter thought to play a role in temperature regulation, mood, and sleep. It is believed that it can be raised by eating carbohydrates, and it inhibits secretions in the digestive tract and stimulates smooth muscles. It is an important regulator of both mood and appetite. It may be useful for victims of seasonal depression, people who want to stop smoking, and others.

**SERPENTARIA EXTRACT** • Snakeroot. Snakeweed. Virginia Snakeroot. Extracted from the roots of *Aristolochia serpentaria,* its yellow rods turn red upon drying. Used in the manufacture of resins and as a bitter tonic. It is permitted in alcoholic beverages only. Can affect heart and blood pressure when ingested. Related to black cohosh and echinacea *(see both).* NIL

**SERUM ALBUMIN** • The major protein component of blood plasma derived from bovines. Used as a moisturizing ingredient.

**SERUM PROTEINS** • *See* Serum Albumin.

**SERV SIZE** • Abbreviation on labels for serving size.

**SERVINGS** • Label listing for servings per container.

**SESAME** • Seeds and Oils. The edible seeds of an East Indian herb, *Sesamum indicum,* which has a rosy or white flower. The seeds, which flavor bread, crackers, cakes, confectionery, and other products, is used in the manufacture of margarine as well. The oil has been used as a laxative and skin softener and contains elements active against lice. May cause allergic reactions, primarily contact dermatitis. GRAS. ASP

**SESQUITERPENE LACTONES** • In recent years, more than six hundred plants have been identified as containing these substances, and more than fifty are known to cause allergic contact dermatitis. Among them are arnica, chamomile, and yarrow *(see all)*.

**SHADDOCK EXTRACT** • An extract of *Citrus grandis* and named for a seventeenth-century sea captain who brought the seeds back from the East Indies to Barbados. Shaddock is a large, thick-rinded, pear-shaped citrus fruit related to and largely replaced by the grapefruit.

**SHARK-LIVER OIL** • A rich source of vitamin A, believed to be beneficial to the skin. A brown, fatty oil obtained from the livers of the large predatory fish.

**SHEA BUTTER** • The natural fat obtained from the fruit of the karite tree, *Butyrospermum parkii*. Also called karite butter, it is chiefly used as a food but also in soap and candies.

**SHEA BUTTER UNSAPONIFIABLES** • The fraction of shea butter that is not saponified during processing, that is, not turned into fatty alcohol.

**SHEA NUT OIL** • Obtained as a fractionated "by-product" of shea butter production. The kernels yield an edible oil somewhat similar to olive oil. EAF

**SHELLAC** • A resinous excretion of certain insects feeding on appropriate host trees, usually in India. As processed for marketing, the lac, which is formed by the insects, may be mixed with small amounts of arsenic trisulfide for color and with rosin. White shellac is free of arsenic. Shellac is used as a candy glaze and polish up to 0.4 percent. May cause allergic contact dermatitis. There is reported use of the chemical, but it has not yet been assigned for toxicology literature. ASP. E

**SHELLAC WAX** • Bleached, refined shellac. *See* Shellac. ASP

**SHORTENINGS** • A fat such as butter, lard, or vegetable oil used to make cake, pastry, bread, etc., light and flaky. *See* Salad Oil and Hydrogenated.

**SIBERIAN FIR OIL** • *See* Pine Needle Oil.

**SILICA** • A white powder, slightly soluble in water, that occurs abundantly in nature and is 12 percent of all rocks. Sand is a silica. Used as a coloring additive.

**SILICA AEROGEL** • A fine, white powder, slightly soluble in water, that occurs abundantly in nature and is 12 percent of all rocks. Sand is a silica. Chemically and biologically inert, it is used as an antifoaming additive in beverages and as a surfactant. Used chiefly in the manufacture of glass. Also used as a coloring additive. The final report to the FDA of the Select Committee on GRAS Substances stated in 1980 that it should continue its GRAS status with no limitations other than good manufacturing practices. *See* Silicones. EAF

**SILICATES** • Salts or esters derived from silicic acid *(see)*. Any of numerous insoluble complex metal salts that contain silicon and oxygen that constitute the largest group of minerals and that with quartz make up the greater part of the earth's crust (as rocks, soils, and clays). The simplest silicate is sand, a molecule formed by joining one silicon atom with two oxygen atoms.

**SILICIC ACID** • Silica Gel. White, gelatinous substance obtained by the action of acids on sodium silicate *(see)*. Odorless, tasteless, inert, white, fluffy powder when dried. Insoluble in water and acids. Absorbs water readily.

**SILICON DIOXIDE** • Silica. Transparent, tasteless crystals or powder, practically insoluble in water. Occurs in nature as agate, amethyst, chalcedony, cristobalite, flint, quartz, sand, and tridymite. Used as a defoamer in beer production. Cleared for use as a food additive and as an anticaking additive at a level not to exceed 2 percent in salt and salt substitutes, in BHT *(see* Butylated Hydroxytoluene), in vitamins up to 3 percent, in urea up to 1 percent, and in sodium propionate up to 1 percent *(see all)*. In feed and feed components it is also used as an anticaking or grinding additive and is limited to 1 percent by weight of finished food. In dried egg products with moisture it is limited to less than 5 percent of weight. It is used as an absorbent for some vitamin E and vitamin B in tableted foods for special dietary use. It is also a component of microcapsules for flavoring oil and it migrates to food from paper and paperboard products. Prolonged inhalation of the dust can injure lungs. The final report to the FDA of the Select Committee on GRAS Substances stated in 1980 that it should continue its GRAS status with no limitations other than good manufacturing practices. *See* Silica Aerogel. ASP. E

**SILICONES** • Any of a large group of fluid oils, rubbers, resins, and compounds derived from silica *(see)* that are water repellent, skin adherent, and stable over a wide range of temperatures.

**SILK PROTEIN FOOD POWDER** • Micro-powder type for food additives as a natural emulsifier and special amino acids supplement. Fibroin is the principal form of natural silk. Silk has no fat, no cholesterol, no sugar, and no added ingredients. Turned down for GRAS status 2002 because of insufficient information.

**SILVER** • When small silver balls known as "silver dragées" are sold exclusively for decorating cakes and are used under conditions which preclude their consumption as confectionery, they are not considered to be in the category of a food or confectionery. Silver-colored almonds have been offered for cake decoration. In this regard, the Center for Food Safety and Applied Nutrition has stated: "Although, the articles [silver-colored almonds] may be intended for cake decoration, we do not agree that they are dragées; further, we see no compelling information that the articles are to be used for decorative purposes only and thus would not be eaten. There is no authority under the color additive regulations which permits silver to be used as a color. Neither is there a food additive regulation (or exemption) authorizing silver as a food coating." Silver is permitted as a coloring in the European Union. E

**SILVER FIR, NEEDLES and TWIGS, OIL** • *Abies alba.* Silver Fir Needle. Highly esteemed in Europe for its medicinal virtues and its fragrant scent, the silver fir needle in a relatively small coniferous tree, with a regular pyramidal shape and a silvery white bark. The essential oil is obtained by steam distillation from the needles and young twigs, fir cones, and broken-up pieces. Silver fir needle is used as an ingredient in some cough and cold remedies and rheumatic treatments, and also as a fragrance. NUL

**SILVER DRAGÉES** • Dragées are a modern alternative to almonds, having a sugar shell usually containing chocolate. NUL

**SIMARUBA BARK** • A flavoring for use in alcoholic beverages only. It is from a southern American tree or shrub with a bitter bark, *Simarouba amara.* NIL

**SIMAZINE** • An herbicide. The tolerance is 1 ppm in molasses for animal feed. The tolerance is 0.01 ppm in drinkable water as a result of spray aquatic plants.

**SIMPLESSE** • A fat substitute developed by the same company that brought you NutraSweet. It is made from egg and milk protein. It can be used, according to the company, in margarine, ice cream, salad dressings, and yogurt. It cannot be used in baked food. Its introduction was delayed by the FDA, which said in 1988 that even though Simplesse was made from natural food, it should be premarket-tested for safety.

**SITOSTANOL** • A substance in some Finnish margarines, it cut LDL cholesterol (the bad kind) by 20 percent. It reportedly inhibits cholesterol absorption, while statins, the medications used for that purpose prevent cholesterol manufacture. Researchers speculate that sitostanol may be especially effective in people with high cholesterol-absorption rates who may not respond to statin therapy.

**SKATOLE** • Used in perfumery as a fixative *(see)*. A constituent of beet root, feces, and coal tar. Gives a violet color when mixed with iron and sulfuric acid. ASP

**SKIM MILK or DEXTROSE CULTURED WITH** • Used as an anti-microbial agent in cheeses, sauces, salad dressings, sausages, soups, deli salads, salsas, pasta, tortillas, muffins, cereal bars, sour cream, yogurt, and hash brown potatoes at a maximum level of 2 percent in the finished products. *See also* Milk. GRAS

**SLOE BERRIES** • Blackthorn Berries. The fruit of the common juniper. The extract is a natural flavoring used in berry, plum, and liquor flavorings for beverages, ice cream, ices, candy, baked goods, and cordials (up to 43,000 ppm). Sloe gin is flavored with sloe berries. GRAS. There is reported use of the chemical; it has not yet been assigned for toxicology literature. ASP

**SMALL PLANKTIVOROUS PELAGIC FISH BODY OIL** • *See* Fish Oil. GRAS

**SMALLAGE** • *See* Lovage.

**SMELLAGE** • *See* Lovage.

**SMOKE FLAVORING SOLUTIONS** • Condensates from burning hard-wood in a limited amount of air. The solutions are used to flavor various foods, primarily meats, and as antioxidants to retard bacterial growth. Also permitted in cheese and smoke-flavored fish. The Select Committee of the Federation of American Societies for Experimental Biology (FASEB), under contract to the FDA, concluded that smoke flavorings in general pose no hazard to the public when used at current levels and under present procedures, but uncertainties exist that require further study. The committee also said there are insufficient data upon which to base an evaluation of smoked-yeast flavoring, produced by exposing food-grade yeast to wood smoke. It is used to flavor soups, cheese, crackers, dip, pizza, and seasoning mixes.

**SMOKED SHEET RUBBER** • A chewing-gum base.

**S-METHYL BENZOTHIOATE** • Flavoring. FAO/WHO *(see)* says it has no safety concern. EAF

**S-METHYL HEXANETHIOATE** • Synthetic flavoring. EAF

**S-METHYL 3-METHYLBUTANETHIOATE** • Synthetic flavoring. EAF

**S-METHYL 4-METHYLPENTANETHIOATE** • Synthetic flavoring. EAF

**S-METHYL THIOACETATE** • Synthetic flavoring. EAF

**SNAKEROOT OIL** • Canadian Oil. Wild Ginger. Derived from the roots of the plant *Asarum canadense,* which had a reputation for curing snakebites. Grown from Canada to North Carolina and Kansas. Used in ginger, ginger ale, wintergreen, and birch beer flavorings for beverages, ice cream, ices, candy, baked goods, and condiments. *See* Black Cohosh and Echinacea. EAF

**SOAPBARK** • *See* Quillaja Extract.

**SODIUM** • A metallic element that is soft, silvery, and oxidizes easily in air. It is waxlike at room temperature and brittle at low temperature. It has many uses in combination with other chemicals. Sodium chloride *(see)* is common table salt.

**SODIUM ACETATE** • Sodium Salt of Acetic Acid. Transparent crystals highly soluble in water. Used as a preservative, flavoring, and pH control additive in candy, cereals, fats, grain products, jams, jellies, meat products, oils, pasta, snack foods, soup mixes, soups, and sweet sauces. Also migrates from cotton and cotton fabrics used in dry food packaging. Medicinally it is used as an alkalizer and as a diuretic. Moderately toxic by ingestion. A skin and eye irritant. The final report to the FDA of the Select Committee on GRAS Substances stated in 1980 that it should continue its GRAS status with no limitations other than good manufacturing practices. ASP. E

**SODIUM ACID PHOSPHATE** • Sequestrant in cheeses and frozen desserts. GRAS. ASP

**SODIUM ACID PYROPHOSPHATE (SAP)** • A white mass or free-flowing powder used as a buffer. It is a slow-acting acid constituent of a leavening mixture for self-rising and prepared cakes, doughnuts, waffles, muffins, cupcakes, and other types of flours and mixes. Also used in canned tuna fish. The U.S. Department of Agriculture has proposed that SAP be added to hot dogs and other sausages to accelerate the development of a rose-red color, thus cutting production time by some 25 to 40 percent. It is related to phosphoric acid, which is sometimes used as a gastric acidifier. The final report to the FDA of the Select Committee on GRAS Substances stated in 1980 that it should continue its GRAS status with no limitations other than good manufacturing practices. ASP

**SODIUM ACID SULFITE** • *See* Sodium Bisulfite.

**SODIUM ADIPATE** • *See* Adipates. E

**SODIUM ALGINATE** • Dissolves in water to form a viscous, colloidal solution and is used in cosmetics as a stabilizer, thickener, and emulsifier. Used in frozen desserts, fruit jelly preservatives, and jams. It is the sodium salt of alginic acid extracted from brown seaweed. GRAS. E

**SODIUM N-ALKYLBENZENESULFONATE** • Processing for fruits and vegetables. *See* Surfactants. ASP

**SODIUM ALUM** • *See* Alum.

**SODIUM ALUMINATE** • A strong alkaline employed in the manufacture of lake colors used in foods (*see* FD and C Lakes). Also used in water softening and printing. The final report to the FDA of the Select Committee on GRAS Substances stated in 1980 that it should continue its GRAS status with no limitations other than good manufacturing practices. Migrates to food from paper and paperboard products. NIL

**SODIUM ALUMINOSILICATE** • Sodium Silicoaluminate. Anticaking additive used in dried whole eggs and egg yolks and grated cheese. A chemical substance used in dental compounds, colored lakes (*see* FD and C Lakes) for foods, and in washing compounds. The final report to the FDA of the Select Committee on GRAS Substances stated in 1980 that it should continue its GRAS status with no limitations other than good manufacturing practices.

**SODIUM ALUMINUM PHOSPHATE** • A white, odorless powder, insoluble in water, used as a buffer in self-rising flour. Used with sodium bicarbonate (*see*). Used also in various cheeses. The final report to the FDA of the Select Committee on GRAS Substances stated in 1980 that it should continue its GRAS status with no limitations other than good manufacturing practices. ASP

**SODIUM ALUMINUM PHOSPHATE ACIDIC** • *See* Sodium Aluminum Phosphate and Acid. E

**SODIUM ALUMINUM SILICATE** • Anticaking additive. ASP. E

**SODIUM ALUMINUM SULFATE** • A flour-bleaching additive alone or in combination with potassium aluminum, calcium sulfate, and other compounds. Used in cereal flours. *See* Aluminum. GRAS

**SODIUM ARSANILATE** • Used in animal feed. *See* Arsenic.

**SODIUM ASCORBATE** • Vitamin C. Sodium. Aside from its use in vitamin C preparations, it can serve as an antioxidant in chopped meat and other foods to retard spoiling; also used in curing meat. The final report to the FDA of the Select Committee on GRAS Substances stated in 1980 that it should continue its GRAS status with no limitations other than good manufacturing practices. *See* Ascorbic Acid. ASP. E

**SODIUM BENZOATE** • White, odorless powders or crystals; sweet, antiseptic taste. Works best in slightly acid media. Used as a preservative in margarine, codfish, bottled soft drinks, maraschino cherries, mincemeat, fruit juices, pickles, confections, fruit jelly preserves, and jams. Once used medicinally for rheumatism and tonsillitis. Nontoxic for external use. Moderately toxic by ingestion. Caused birth defects in experimental animals. Larger doses of 8 to 10 grams by mouth may cause nausea and vomiting. Small doses have little or no effect. GRAS. ASP. E

**SODIUM BICARBONATE** • Bicarbonate of Soda. Baking Soda. An alkali prepared by the reaction of soda ash with carbon dioxide and used in prepared pancake, biscuit, and muffin mixes; a leavening additive in baking powders; in various crackers and cookies; to adjust acidity in tomato soup, ices, and sherbets; in pastes and beverages; in syrups for frozen products; in confections and self-rising flours. Also used in cornmeals and canned peas. Its white crystals or powder are used as a gastric antacid, as an alkaline wash, and to treat burns. Used also as a neutralizer for butter, cream, milk, and ice cream. It may alter the urinary excretion of other drugs, thus making those drugs either more toxic or less effective. GRAS. ASP

**SODIUM BISULFATE** • Sodium Acid Sulfite. Sodium Hydrogen Sulfite. Colorless or white crystals fused in water, with a disagreeable taste. It is used as a disinfectant in the manufacture of foods and pickling compounds. *See* Sodium Bisulfite. GRAS

**SODIUM BISULFITE** • Sodium Acid Sulfite. An inorganic salt. It is a white powder with a disagreeable taste, used as a bleaching additive in ale, wine, beer, and other food products. Used as a preservative in canned shrimp but not recognized as a source of vitamin E. Commercial bisulfite consists chiefly of sodium metabisulfite *(see)*. In its aqueous solution, it is an acid. Concentrated solutions are highly irritating to the skin and mucous membranes. Sodium bisulfite can cause changes in the genetic material of bacteria and is a suspect mutagen. Not permitted in meats and other sources of vitamin $B_1$; strong irritant to the skin and tissue. The Select Committee on GRAS Substances found it did not present a hazard at present use levels but that additional data would be needed if higher use occurred. The committee said in 1980 that it should continue as GRAS with limitations on the amounts that can be added to food. *See* Sulfites. ASP

**SODIUM BORATE** • Used as a preservative and emulsifier. Hard, odorless powder insoluble in water, it is a weak antiseptic and astringent for mucous membranes. NIL

**SODIUM BOROHYDRIDE** • Prepared from methyl borate and sodium hydride, it is used as a reducing additive *(see)* for various food-additive chemicals. It scavenges for traces of aldehyde, ketones, and peroxides in organic chemicals. It is used as a modifier for hops extract. ASP

**SODIUM BROMATE** • Inorganic salt. Colorless, odorless crystals that liberate oxygen. Used as a solvent. *See* Potassium Bromate for toxicity.

**SODIUM BROMIDE** • A sanitizing additive that requires adequate drainage, according to the FDA.

**SODIUM CALCIUM ALUMINOSILICATE** • Used to prevent salt and dry mixes from caking. The final report to the FDA of the Select Committee on GRAS Substances stated in 1980 that it should continue its GRAS status with no limitations other than good manufacturing practices. NIL

**SODIUM CAPRATE** • *See* Surfactants. NUL

**SODIUM CAPRYLATE** • *See* Palm Oil. NUL

**SODIUM CARBONATE** • Soda Ash. Small, odorless crystals or powder that occur in nature in ores and in lake brines or seawater. Absorbs water from the air. Used as a neutralizer for butter, cream, fluid milk, and ice cream; in the processing of olives before canning; and in cocoa products. Used in cocoa products and canned peas as an optional ingredient in standardized foods *(see)*. A strong alkali. Ingestion of large quantities may produce corrosion of the gastrointestinal tract, vomiting, diarrhea, circulatory collapse, and death. The final report to the FDA of the Select Committee on GRAS Substances stated in 1980 that it should continue its GRAS status with no limitations other than good manufacturing practices. ASP. E.

**SODIUM CARBOXYMETHYLCELLULOSE** • Made from a cotton by-product. Prepared by treating alkali cellulose with sodium chloroacetate. Used as a stabilizer, thickener, gelling additive, and nonnutritive bulking aid. Used to prevent water loss, make food opaque, and to texturize food. Found in ice cream, beverages, confections, baked goods, icings, toppings, chocolate milk, chocolate-flavored beverages, gassed cream (pressure-dispensed whipped cream), syrup for frozen products, variegated mixtures, cheese spreads, and in certain cheeses. Also used in French dressing, artificially sweetened jellies, preserves, gelling ingredients, and mix-it-yourself and powdered drinks. Medicinally used as a laxative (1.5 grams orally), antacid (15–30 milligrams of 5 percent solution), and in pharmacies for preparing suspensions. Can cause digestive disturbances. *See* Cellulose Gums.

**SODIUM CARRAGEENAN** • Sodium salt of carrageenan *(see)*.

**SODIUM CASEINATE** • Casein. The soluble form of milk protein in which casein is partially neutralized with sodium hydroxide and used as a texturizer in ice cream, frozen custard, ice milk, and sherbet. Cleared by the USDA Meat Inspection Department for use in imitation sausage, soups, and stews. GRAS. The final report to the FDA of the Select Committee on GRAS Substances stated in 1980 that it should continue its GRAS status with no limitations other than good manufacturing practices. ASP

**SODIUM CASTORATE** • The sodium salt of the fatty acids derived from castor oil *(see).*

**SODIUM CHLORIDE** • Common table salt. In addition to seasoning it is used as a pickling additive, a preservative for meats, vegetables, and butter. Prevents browning in cut fruit. Also reported to irritate the roots of the teeth when used for a long time in dentifrices. Not considered toxic but can adversely affect persons with high blood pressure and kidney disease. The final report to the FDA of the Select Committee on GRAS Substances stated in 1980 that it should continue its GRAS status with no limitations other than good manufacturing practices. ASP

**SODIUM CHLORITE** • A powerful oxidizer prepared commercially and used to modify food starch *(see* Modified Starch) up to 0.5 percent. Used as a bleaching additive for textiles and paper pulp and in water purification. Toxicity depends on concentration. ASP

**SODIUM CHOLATE** • *See* Cholic Acid.

**SODIUM CITRATE** • White, odorless crystals, granules, or powder with a cool salty taste. Stable in air. Prevents "cream plug" in cream and "feathering" when cream is used in coffee; an emulsifier in ice cream, processed cheese, and evaporated milk; a buffer to control acidity and retain carbonation in beverages, in frozen fruit drinks, confections, fruit jellies, preserves, and jams. It attaches itself to trace metals present in water and inhibits their entering the living cell. Proposed as a replacement for phosphates in detergents, but also causes algae growth and removes the necessary trace metals from water as well as the toxic ones. Used as a sequestering additive *(see)* to remove trace metals in solutions and as an alkalizer in cosmetic products. Can alter urinary excretion of other drugs, thus making those drugs either less effective or more toxic. The final report to the FDA of the Select Committee on GRAS Substances stated in 1980 that it should continue its GRAS status with no limitations other than good manufacturing practices. E

**SODIUM CLOXACILLIN** • A penicillin antibiotic. FDA tolerance for residues in milk is 0.01 ppm. *See* Cloxacillin.

**SODIUM COCOATE** • *See* Coconut Oil.

**SODIUM COCO-HYDROLYZED ANIMAL PROTEIN** • The sodium salt of the condensation product of coconut acid chloride and hydrolyzed animal protein. *See* Hydrolyzed Protein.

**SODIUM COCOYL GLUTAMATE** • A softener. *See* Glutamate.

**SODIUM DECYLBENZENESULFONATE** • An additive with miscellaneous uses but generally used in coatings for fresh citrus fruits. *See* Benzoic Acid. NIL

**SODIUM DEHYDROACETATE** • Dehydroacetic Acid. A preservative;

white, odorless, powder, with an acrid taste. Used in cut or peeled squash and as a plasticizer, fungicide, and bactericide in antienzyme toothpaste. Can cause impaired kidney function. Large doses can cause vomiting, ataxia, and convulsions. There are no apparent allergic skin reactions. NEW

**SODIUM DIACETATE** • A compound of sodium acetate and acetic acid *(see);* a white, crystalline solid. Smells like vinegar. Used as a preservative. Inhibits molds and rope-forming bacteria in baked goods. The final report to the FDA of the Select Committee on GRAS Substances stated in 1980 that it should continue its GRAS status with no limitations other than good manufacturing practices. ASP

**SODIUM DIALKYLPHENOXYBENZENEDISULFONATE** • Used in lye mixtures for peeling fruits and vegetables.

**SODIUM 2,2-DICHLOROPROPIONATE** • Dalapon. A pesticide. The FDA tolerance is 20 ppm in dehydrated citrus pulp for cattle feed from application to citrus during growing season. It is a strong irritant to the eyes and skin. *See* Propionic Acid.

**SODIUM DIHYDROGEN PHOSPHATE** • White, odorless powder or granules used as a buffer, dietary supplement, emulsifier, nutrient, and in poultry wash. Used in beverages, cheese, meat products, poultry, and soft drinks. In meat food products, where allowed, limited to 5 percent. Mildly toxic by ingestion. A human eye irritant.

**SODIUM N, *n*-DIMETHYLDITHIOCARBAMATE** • Vinstop. Sta-Fresh 615. An antimicrobial additive used on beets and sugarcane. The FDA limits the additive to 3 ppm based on weight of raw product. Moderately toxic by ingestion. Has caused mutations in experimental animals. ASP

**SODIUM DODECYLBENZENESULFONATE** • An anionic detergent, it is used to treat raw food products. It may irritate the skin. Will cause vomiting if swallowed. NIL

**SODIUM ERYTHORBATE** • Sodium Isoascorbate. A white, odorless powder used as an antioxidant in pickling brine up to 7.5 ounces per 100 gallons and in meat products up to three-quarters of an ounce per 100 pounds. Also used in beverages and baked goods; in cured cuts and cured, pulverized products to accelerate color fixing in curing. The final report to the FDA of the Select Committee on GRAS Substances stated in 1980 that it should continue its GRAS status with no limitations other than good manufacturing practices. ASP. E

**SODIUM 2-ETHYL 1-HEXYLSULFATE** • A component of a commercial detergent for washing raw foods. ASP

**SODIUM ETHYL *p*-HYDROXYBENZOATE** • *See* Hydroxybenzoate. E

**SODIUM FERRIC EDTA** • Prepared from disodium ethylenediamine-tetraacetic acid and ferric nitrate. Used as an iron source. The final report to the FDA of the Select Committee on GRAS Substances stated in 1980 that there were insufficient biological and other studies upon which to base an evaluation of it when it is used as a food ingredient. Nothing new apparently has been reported by the FDA since. *See* Iron Salts.

**SODIUM FERRICITROPYROPHOSPHATE** • A white powder used in food enrichment. It is less prone to induce rancidity than other orthophosphates. The final report to the FDA of the Select Committee on GRAS Substances stated in 1980 that there were insufficient biological and other studies upon which to base an evaluation of it when it is used as a food ingredient. *See* Iron Salts. NUL

**SODIUM FERROCYANIDE** • Used as an anticaking additive for table salt and as a processing aid in wine. The FDA limits residue to 1 ppm in finished wine. E

**SODIUM FLUORIDE** • Used in toothpastes to prevent tooth decay and an insecticide, disinfectant, and preservative. It is used to fluoridate municipal water, as a wood preservative, rodenticide, for chemical cleaning, electroplating, and glass manufacture as well as a preservative for adhesives. Can cause nausea and vomiting when ingested, and even death, depending upon the dose. Strong irritant to the tissues. Fluorides added to water to reduce the incidence of dental caries is 1 ppm. The concentration used has been established to be far below the permissible level of toxicity. The program has been in existence for more than thirty years, yet there are still some scientists and citizens who worry about its adverse effects. Chronic endemic fluorosis due to a high concentration of natural fluoride in local water supplies involves mottling of the teeth, bone changes, and, rarely, brain and nerve involvement. Acute fluoride poisoning can cause heart, brain, nerve, and gastrointestinal damage. This is a substance for which a petition has been filed but the FDA has not allowed it as a nutrient additive because "it has not been proven safe." NUL

**SODIUM FORMATE** • White, deliquescent crystals used in paper packaging. Moderately toxic by ingestion. NUL

**SODIUM FUMARATE** • *See* Fumaric Acid. NUL

**SODIUM GLUCOHEPTONATE** • Chelating agent *(see)*. ASP

**SODIUM GLUCONATE** • Gluconic Acid. Sodium Salt. A pleasant-smelling compound, it is used as a sequestering additive *(see)*. The final report to the FDA of the Select Committee on GRAS Substances stated in 1980 that it should continue its GRAS status with no limitations other than good manufacturing practices. ASP. E

**SODIUM GLUTAMATE** • The monosodium salt of the L-form of glutamic acid *(see)*.

**SODIUM GLYCERYL OLEATE PHOSPHATE** • *See* Glyceryl Monostearate.

**SODIUM HEXAMETAPHOSPHATE** • Sodium Polymetaphosphate. Graham's Salt. An emulsifier, sequestering additive *(see)*, and texturizer. Used in breakfast cereals, angel food cake, flaked fish, ice cream, ice milk, beer, bottled beverages, reconstituted lemon juice, puddings, processed cheeses, and artificially sweetened jellies. Used in foods and potable water to prevent scale formation and corrosion. Because it keeps calcium, magnesium, and iron salts in solution, it is an excellent water softener and detergent. Phosphorus is an essential nutrient, but it has to be in balance with other minerals such as calcium in the diet. Too much phosphorus in foods could lead to an imbalance and adversely affect bones, kidney, and heart. Lethal dose in dogs is 140 milligrams per kilogram of body weight. Used in Calgon, Giltex, and other such products. The final report to the FDA of the Select Committee on GRAS Substances stated in 1980 that it should continue its GRAS status for packaging with no limitations other than good manufacturing practices. EAF

**SODIUM HUMATE** • Sodium humate is the salt of humic acids, derived from natural oxidized lignite through extraction. Sodium humate has a wide use in industry such as the removal of toxic metals from wastewater. Used as an emulsifier. ASP

**SODIUM HYALURONATE** • The sodium salt of hyaluronic acid. From the fluid in the eye; it is used as a gelling additive.

**SODIUM HYDROSULFATE** • Sodium Dithionate. A bacterial inhibitor and antifermentative.

**SODIUM HYDROSULFITE** • A bacterial inhibitor and antifermentative in the sugar and syrup industries. Slight odor. The final report to the FDA of the Select Committee on GRAS Substances stated in 1980 that it should continue its GRAS status with no limitations other than good manufacturing practices. There is reported use of the chemical, it has not yet been assigned for toxicology literature. *See* Sulfites. ASP. E

**SODIUM HYDROXIDE** • Caustic Soda. Soda Lye. An alkali and emulsifier. Readily absorbs water. Used as a modifier for food starch, a glazing additive for pretzels, and a peeling additive for tubers and fruits. The FDA banned use of more than 10 percent in household liquid drain cleaners. Its ingestion causes vomiting, prostration, and collapse. Inhalation causes lung damage. The final report to the FDA of the Select Committee on GRAS Substances stated in 1980 that it should continue its GRAS status for packaging with no limitations other than good manufacturing practices. ASP. E

**SODIUM HYDROXIDE GELATINIZED STARCH** • Starch *(see)* that has been gelatinized with sodium hydroxide. The final report to the FDA of the Select Committee on GRAS Substances stated in 1980 that there were insufficient biological and other studies upon which to base an evaluation of it when it is used as a food ingredient. Nothing new has been reported since.

**SODIUM HYPHOSPHITE** • An emulsifier or stabilizer used in food with no limitations other than current good manufacturing practices. The affirmation of this ingredient as generally recognized as safe (GRAS) as a direct human food ingredient is based upon following current good manufacturing practices.

**SODIUM HYPOCHLORITE** • A preservative used in the washing of cottage cheese curd. Also used medically as an antiseptic for wounds. Ingestion may cause corrosion of mucous membranes, esophageal or gastric perforation. The aqueous solutions are Eau de Javelle, Clorox, Dazzle. ASP

**SODIUM HYPOPHOSPHATE** • White crystals, soluble in water, used as a sequestering additive.

**SODIUM IODATE** • A source of iodine in animal feed. *See* Iodine. GRAS

**SODIUM IODIDE** • A source of iodine in animal feed. *See* Iodine. GRAS

**SODIUM INOSINATE** • *See* Inosinate.

**SODIUM IRON EDTA** • A dietary supplement for use in supervised food fortification programs in populations in which iron-deficiency anemia is widespread. The FAO/WHO Expert Committee on Food Additives was asked to comment on this additive that is supposed to be restricted to specific supervised applications. The committee was concerned about overfortification or misuse and did not recommend its availability for general use by individuals. It recommended it be used only as a supervised dietary supplement.

**SODIUM IRON PYROPHOSPHATE** • *See* Sodium Pyrophosphate.

**SODIUM ISCISTEROYL LACTYLATE** • The sodium salt of isostearic acid and lactyl lactate. *See* Stearic Acid and Lactic Acid.

**SODIUM ISOASCORBATE** • *See* Erythrobic Acid.

**SODIUM LACTATE** • Plasticizer substitute for glycerin. Colorless, thick, odorless liquid miscible with water, alcohol, and glycerin. It is used as an antioxidant, bodying additive, and humectant. Solution is neutral. Used medicinally as a systemic and urinary alkalizer. GRAS. ASP. E

**SODIUM LAURATE** • *See* Sodium Lauryl Sulfate. NUL

**SODIUM LAURETH SULFATE** • The sodium salt of sulfated ethoxylated lauryl alcohol, widely used as a water softener. *See also* Surfactants.

**SODIUM LAUROYL GLUTAMATE** • A softener. *See* Glutamate.

**SODIUM LAURYL SULFATE (SLS)** • A detergent, wetting additive, and emulsifier. It is used to treat raw foods, followed by a water rinsing. It is employed as a whipping aid in cake mixes and dried-egg products. In frozen and liquid egg whites the FDA allows up to 125 ppm; in egg white solids, 0.1 percent; 5,000 ppm by weight of gelatin as a whipping additive used in preparing marshmallows; 25 ppm in finished product. It is also used as a surfactant in fumaric acid–acidulated dry beverage base and fruit juice drinks unless precluded by food standards *(see)*. The FDA allows 10 ppm in crude vegetable oils and animal fats. Prepared by sulfation of lauryl alcohol followed by neutralization with sodium carbonate. Faint fatty odor; also emulsifies fats. ASP

**SODIUM LIGNOSULFONATE** • The sodium salt of polysulfonated lignin derived from wood. It is used as a dispersing additive. A tan, free-flowing powder, it is also used as an emulsifier, stabilizer, and cleaning additive.

**SODIUM MAGNESIUM SILICATES** • *See* Silicates.

**SODIUM MALATES** • Food Acids. E

**SODIUM 3-MERCAPTOOXOPROPIONATE** • Synthetic flavoring. EAF

**SODIUM METABISULFITE** • An inorganic salt. A bacterial inhibitor in wine, ale, and beer; an antifermentative in sugar and syrups; a preservative for fruit and vegetable juices; antibrowning additive in cut fruits, frozen apples, dried fruits, prepared fruit pie mix, peeled potatoes, and maraschino cherries. The final report to the FDA of the Select Committee on GRAS Substances stated in 1980 that the additive did not present a hazard when used at present levels but that increased use would require additional safety data. *See* Sulfites. ASP. E

**SODIUM METAPHOSPHATE** • Graham's Salts. A dough conditioner. Used in dental polishing additives, detergents, water softeners, sequestrants, emulsifiers, food additives, and textile laundering. The final report to the FDA of the Select Committee on GRAS Substances stated in 1980 that it should continue its GRAS status with no limitations other than good manufacturing practices. *See* Sodium Hexametaphosphate. ASP

**SODIUM METASILICATE** • Alkali usually prepared from sand and soda ash. Used as a peeling solution for peaches and as a denuder for tripe "in amounts sufficient for the purpose." Used in detergents. Caustic substance, corrosive to the skin, harmful if swallowed, and cause of severe eye irritations. Preserves eggs in shampoos. GRAS. ASP

**SODIUM (4-METHOXYBENZOYLOXY)ACETATE** • Synthetic flavoring that FEMA *(see)* labels GRAS. It is used in cereals and confectionery frostings. EAF

**SODIUM 3-METHOXY-4-HYDROXYCINNAMATE** • Synthetic flavoring. *See* Cinnamic Acid. EAF

**SODIUM 2-(4-METHOXYPHENOXY)PROPANOATE** • Synthetic flavoring. NUL

**SODIUM METHYL COCOYL TAURATE** • *See* Ox Bile.

**SODIUM METHYL OLEYL TAURATE** • *See* Ox Bile.

**SODIUM n-METHYL-n-OLEYL TAURATE** • *See* Ox Bile.

**SODIUM METHYL SULFATE** • Used in processing pectin *(see)*. ASP

**SODIUM MONOALKYLPHENOXYBENZENEDISULFONATE** • Used in lye for peeling fruits and vegetables.

**SODIUM MONO- and DIMETHYL NAPHTHALENE SULFONATE** • Anticaking additive and lye peeling additive used in cured fish and meats, and potable water. Also used in sodium nitrite in cured fish and meat. ASP

**SODIUM MONOHYDROGEN PHOSPHATE** • Dibasic Sodium Phosphate. Used as a buffer, to retain juices, as a dietary supplement, emulsifier, hog wash, poultry wash, and in evaporated milk, poultry, instant pudding, and whipped products. Limited by the FDA to 0.5 percent of total poultry product. Mildly toxic by ingestion. A skin and eye irritant.

**SODIUM MYRISTATE** • *See* Myristic Acid and Fatty Acids. NUL

**SODIUM MYRISTOYL ISETHIONATE** • *See* Myristic Acid

**SODIUM NICOTINATE** • This was used for what the FDA termed "deceptive use in ground meat for color retention." The FDA has banned it despite the request by producers for extension of its use.

**SODIUM NITRATE** • *See* Nitrate. ASP. E

**SODIUM NITRITE** • *See* Nitrite. ASP. E

**SODIUM OLEATE** • Sodium salt of oleic acid. White powder, fatty odor, alkaline. Used in soaps. NUL

**SODIUM ORTHOPHENYL PHENOL** • A preservative in and on citrus fruits. *See* Phenol. E

**SODIUM PALMITATE** • Sodium salt of palmitic acid *(see)*. *See also* Fatty Acids. NUL

**SODIUM PANTOTHENATE** • A member of the B vitamin family. It is important as a constituent of coenzyme A. Its name is derived from the Greek word *pantothen* meaning "everywhere." Used as a dietary supplement. The final report to the FDA of the Select Committee on GRAS Substances stated in 1980 that it should continue its GRAS status with no limitations other than good manufacturing practices. NUL

**SODIUM PECTINATE** • A stabilizer and thickener for syrups for frozen products, ice cream, ice milk, confections, fruit sherbets, French dressing and other salad dressings, fruit jelly, preserves, and jams. Used in quantities that reasonably compensate for the deficiency, if any, of natural pectin content of the fruit ingredients. GRAS. NUL

**SODIUM PHOSPHATE (DIBASIC)** • Disodium Phosphate. Used in frozen desserts, enriched farina, and macaroni and noodle products. *See* Sodium Phosphate. GRAS. ASP. E

**SODIUM PHOSPHATE (MONO-, DI-, and TRIBASIC)** • Buffer and effervescent used in the manufacture of nail enamels and detergents. White crystalline or granular powder, stable in air. Without water, it can be irritating to the skin but has no known skin toxicity. The final report to the FDA of the Select Committee on GRAS Substances stated in 1980 that it should continue its GRAS status with no limitations other than good manufacturing practices. *See* Phosphorous Sources. ASP. E

**SODIUM PHOSPHOALUMINATE** • The acid salt of phosphoric acid. An ingredient of baking powders and other leavening mixtures. GRAS for packaging. *See* Phosphoric Acid for toxicity.

**SODIUM POLYACRYLATE-ACRYLAMIDE RESIN** • A miscellaneous additive used in beet sugar or cane sugar juice to control organic mineral scale. The FDA says it can be up to 2.5 percent by weight of juice or liquor. *See* Acrylates and Acrylamide.

**SODIUM POLYMETHACRYLATE** • Used in boiler water to inhibit mineral scale in beet and cane sugar production. The FDA allows up to 3.6 ppm of raw juice weight. *See* Acrylates. ASP

**SODIUM POTASSIUM TARTRATE** • Rochelle Salt. A buffer for confections, fruit jelly preserves, and jams. For each 100 pounds of saccharin in these products, 3 ounces of sodium potassium tartrate is used. Also used in cheese. Used medicinally as a cathartic. GRAS. NUL. E

**SODIUM PROPIONATE** • Colorless or transparent, odorless crystals that gather water in moist air. Used as a preservative in cosmetics and foodstuffs to prevent mold and fungus. Used in baked goods, frostings, confections, and gelatin. It has been used to treat fungal infections of the skin, but can cause allergic reactions. GRAS. ASP. E

**SODIUM PROPYL *p*-HYDROXYBENZOATE** • Almost odorless, small, colorless crystals or a white crystalline powder. Preservative. *See p*-Hydroxybenzoate. E

**SODIUM PYROPHOSPHATE** • Used to decrease the amount of cooked-out juices in canned hams, pork shoulders, and bacon at 5 percent phosphate in pickle; 0.5 percent phosphate in product (only clear solution may be injected into hams). It is also used in cold-water puddings and processed cheese. It is an emulsifier salt and a texturizer as well as a sequestrant. The FDA labeled it GRAS for use as a sequestrant. ASP

**SODIUM RIBOFLAVIN PHOSPHATE** • A B vitamin containing sodium phosphate *(see).*

**SODIUM SACCHARIN** • An artificial sweetener in dentifrices, mouthwashes, and lipsticks. In use since 1879. Pound for pound it is three hundred times as sweet as natural sugar but leaves a bitter aftertaste. It was used along with cyclamates in the experiments that led to their ban in 1969. The FDA has proposed restricting saccharin to 15 milligrams per day for each kilogram of body weight or 1 gram a day for a 150-pound person. On the FDA's priority list for further safety testing.

**SODIUM SALT** • *See* Sodium Benzoate.

**SODIUM SALTS OF FATTY ACIDS** • *See* Sodium and Fatty Acids. ASP

**SODIUM SESQUICARBONATE** • Lye. White crystals, flakes, or powder produced from sodium carbonate. Soluble in water. Used as a neutralizer for butter, cream, fluid milk, and ice cream, in the processing of olives before canning, cacao products, and canned peas. Used as an alkalizer in bath salts, shampoos, tooth powders, and soaps. Irritating to the skin and mucous membranes. May cause an allergic reaction in the hypersensitive. The final report to the FDA of the Select Committee on GRAS Substances stated in 1980 that it should continue its GRAS status with no limitations other than good manufacturing practices. There is reported use of the chemical; it has not yet been assigned for toxicology literature. ASP

**SODIUM SILICATE** • Water Glass. Soluble Glass. An anticaking additive for preserving eggs, detergents in soaps, depilatories, and protective creams. Consists of colorless to white or grayish white, crystalline pieces or lumps. These silicates are almost insoluble in cold water. Strongly alkaline. As a topical antiseptic can be irritating and caustic to the skin and mucous membranes. If swallowed, it causes vomiting and diarrhea. The final report to the FDA of the Select Committee on GRAS Substances stated in 1980 that it should continue its GRAS status with no limitations other than good manufacturing practices. ASP

**SODIUM SILICOALUMINATE** • Anticaking additive used in table salt up to 2 percent; dried egg yolks up to 2 percent; in sugar up to 1 percent; and in baking powder up to 5 percent. Slightly alkaline. *See* Silicates. GRAS

**SODIUM SOAP** • *See* Sodium Stearate.

**SODIUM SORBATE** • A food preservative used in cheeses alone or in combination with potassium sorbate or sorbic acid *(see both)*. It is also used in fruit butter, artificially sweetened fruit jelly, preserves, jams, and margarines. Also migrates from packaging into food. The final report to the FDA of the Select Committee on GRAS Substances stated in 1980 that it should continue its GRAS status with no limitations other than good manufacturing practices. ASP

**SODIUM STEARATE** • Alkaline; 92.82 percent stearic acid *(see)*. Used as an emulsifier in foods. A fatty acid used as a chewing-gum base. It was approved in 1998 as an anticaking additive in animal feed. Also used in deodorant sticks, stick perfumes, toothpastes, soapless shampoos, and shaving lather. A white powder with a soapy feel and a slight tallowlike odor. Slowly soluble in cold water or cold alcohol. One of the least allergy-causing of the sodium salts of fatty acids. Nonirritating to the skin. ASP

**SODIUM STEAROYL LACTYLATE** • Used as follows unless precluded by food standards *(see):* 0.5 percent by weight of flour as a dough strengthener, emulsifier, or processing aid in baked products, pancakes, waffles, and prepared mixes; 0.2 percent by weight of finished food as surface active additive, emulsifier, or stabilizer in icings, fillings, puddings, and toppings; 0.3 percent by weight of finished emulsion or stabilizer in liquid and solid edible fat–water emulsion used as substitutes for milk and cream in coffee; 0.5 percent of dry weight as formulation aid, processing aid, or surfactant in dehydrated potatoes; 0.2 percent by weight as an emulsifier, stabilizer, or texturizer in snack dips and cheese and cheese product substitutes and imitations; 0.25 percent by weight of finished food as an emulsifier, stabilizer, or texturizer in sauces or gravies, products containing same, and prepared mixes of same. *See* Lactic Acid. ASP. E

**SODIUM STEAROYL-2-LACTYLATE** • The sodium salt of a lactylic ester of fatty acid. Prepared from lactic acid and fatty acids. It is used as an emulsifier, plasticizer, or surfactant in an amount not greater than that required to produce the intended physical or technical effect, and where standards of identity *(see)* do not preclude use, in the following: bakery mixes, baked products, cake icings, fillings and toppings, dehydrated fruits and vegetables, dehydrated fruit and vegetable juices, frozen desserts, liquid shortenings for household use, pancake mixes, precooked instant rice, pudding mixes, solid-state edible vegetable fat–water emulsions used as substitutes for milk or cream in coffee, and with shortening and edible fats and oils when such are required in the foods listed above. *See* Lactic Acid for toxicity. E

**SODIUM STEARYL FUMARATE** • Fine white powder used as a dough conditioner in bakery products, cereals processed for cooking, starch-thickened flour, and dehydrated potatoes. As a stabilizing additive in nonyeast-leavening bakery products up to 1 percent of weight of flour used. FDA limits are 0.5 percent of flour for yeast-leavened baked goods; 1 percent for nonyeast-leavened baked goods; 1 percent of dehydrated potatoes; 1 percent of dry processed cereals for cooking; and 0.2 percent for starch-thickened flour. ASP

**SODIUM SULFACHLOROPYRIDAZINE MONOHYDRATE** • An antibiotic used for chickens. The FDA requires zero residue in uncooked edible tissues of chickens.

**SODIUM SULFATE** • Salt Cake. Occurs in nature as the minerals mirabilite and nardite. Used in chewing-gum base and to preserve tuna fish and biscuits. Used medicinally to reduce body water. Used chiefly in the manufacture of dyes, soaps, and detergents. It is a readditive *(see)* and a precipitant; mildly saline in taste. Usually harmless when applied in toilet preparations. May prove irritating in concentrated solutions if applied to the skin and permitted to dry and then remain. May also enhance the irritant action of certain detergents. Taken by mouth, it stimulates gastric mucous production and sometimes inactivates a natural digestive juice—pepsin. Fatally poisoned animals show only diarrhea and intestinal bloating with no gross lesions outside the intestinal tract. ASP. E

**SODIUM SULFIDE** • Composition in chewing-gum base. Crystals or granules prepared from ammonia that easily absorb water. Also used in dehairing hides and wool pulling, engraving, and cotton printing. NUL

**SODIUM SULFITE** • White to tan-pink, odorless or nearly odorless powder having a cooling, salty, sulfurlike taste. An antiseptic, preservative, and antioxidant used as a bacterial inhibitor in wine-brewing and distilled-beverage industries. Also an antifermentative in the sugar and syrup industries and a browning inhibitor in cut fruits, used in frozen apples, dried fruit, prepared fruit pie mix, peeled potatoes, maraschino cherries, dried fruits, and glacéed fruits. Foods and drinks containing sulfites may release sulfur dioxide. If this is inhaled by people who suffer from asthma, it can trigger an asthmatic attack. Sulfites are known to cause stomach irritation, nausea, diarrhea, skin rash, or swelling in sulfite-sensitive people. People whose kidneys or livers are impaired may not be able to produce the enzymes that break down sulfites in the body. Sulfites may destroy thiamin and consequently are not added to foods that are sources of this B vitamin. The final report to the FDA of the Select Committee on GRAS Substances stated in 1980 that it did not present a hazard when used at present levels but that additional data would be necessary if a significant increase in consumption occurred. *See* Sulfites. ASP. E

**SODIUM SULFO-ACETATE DERIVATIVES** • Used as emulsifiers in margarine. Up to 0.5 percent. *See* Sodium Sulfate.

**SODIUM TARTRATE** • A laxative, sequestrant, chemical reactant, and stabilizer in cheese and artificially sweetened jelly. *See* Tartaric Acid. GRAS. NUL. E

**SODIUM TAUROCHOLATE** • Taurocholic Acid. The chief ingredient of the bile of carnivorous animals. Used as an emulsifier in dried egg white up to 0.1 percent. It is a lipase accelerator. Lipase is a fat-splitting enzyme in the blood, pancreatic secretion, and tissues. NUL

**SODIUM TETRABORATE** • *See* Borax. E

**SODIUM TETRAPHOSPHATE** • Sodium Polyphosphate. Used as a sequestering additive. The final report to the FDA of the Select Committee on GRAS Substances stated in 1980 that it should continue its GRAS status with no limitations other than good manufacturing practices. *See* Phosphate.

**SODIUM THIOSULFATE** • An antioxidant used to protect sliced potatoes and uncooked french fries from browning and as a stabilizer for potassium iodide in iodized salt. Also used to neutralize chlorine and to bleach bone. It is an antidote for cyanide poisoning and has been used in the past to combat blood clots; used to treat ringworm and mange in animals. Poorly absorbed by the bowel. The final report to the FDA of the Select Committee on GRAS Substances stated in 1980 that it should continue its GRAS status with no limitations other than good manufacturing practices. ASP

**SODIUM *p*-TOLUENE-SULFOCHLORAMINE** • Chloramine-T. Water-purifying additive and a deodorant used to remove weed odor in cheese. Suspected of causing rapid allergic reaction in the hypersensitive. Poisoning by chloramine-T is characterized by pain, vomiting, sudden loss of consciousness, circulatory and respiratory collapse, and death.

**SODIUM TOLUENESULFONATE** • Methylbenzenesulfonic Acid, Sodium Salt. An aromatic compound that is used as a solvent. *See* Benzene.

**SODIUM TRIMETAPHOSPHATE** • A starch modifier. *See* Sodium Metaphosphate and Modified Starch.

**SODIUM TRIPOLYPHOSPHATE (STPP)** • A texturizer and sequestrant cleared for use in food-starch modifiers. A water softener. Also cleared by the USDA Meat Inspection Department to preserve meat by decreasing cooked-out juices in canned hams, pork shoulders, chopped ham, and bacon. Also used as a dilutant for Citrus Red No. 2 *(see)*. It is used in angel food cake mix, beef, desserts, gelling juices, goat, canned ham, lamb, lima beans, meat loaf, meat toppings, meringues, mutton, canned peas, pork, poultry, sausage products, and veal. It may deplete the body of calcium if taken in sufficient amounts, and such a case of low calcium was reported in a patient poisoned with water softener. Used in bubble baths and as a texturizer in soaps. It is a crystalline salt, moderately irritating to the skin and mucous membranes. Ingestion can cause violent purging. The final report to the FDA of the Select Committee on GRAS Substances stated in 1980 that it should continue its GRAS status for packaging with no limitations other than good manufacturing practices. *See* Sodium Phosphate. ASP

**SODIUM XYLENESULFONATE** • A composition of sanitizing solutions.

**SODIUM ZINC METASILICATE** • Fusing silica (sand) with sodium carbonate, it is used as a water softener and as an anti-corrosion agent in boiler-water feed. NUL

**SOL FIBER** • Listing on food labels for soluble fiber. *See* Solubilization and Fiber.

**SOLUBILIZATION** • The process of dissolving in water such substances as fats and liquids that are not readily soluble under standard conditions by the action of a detergent or similar additive. Technically, a solubilized product is clear because the particle size in an emulsion is so small that light is not bounced off the particle. Solubilization is used in colognes and clear lotions. Sodium sulfonates are common solubilizing additives.

**SOLUBLE ANIMAL COLLAGEN** • *See* Solubilization and Collagen.

**SOLUBLE COLLAGEN** • The protein derived from the connective tissue of young animals.

**SOLV** • FDA abbreviation for solvent *(see)*.

**SOLVENT** • A liquid capable of dissolving or dispersing one or more substances. Methyl ethyl ketone is an example of a solvent.

**SORBATE, CALCIUM** • *See* Calcium Sorbate.

**SORBIC ACID** • Acetic Acid. Hexadienic Acid. Hexadienoic Acid. Sorbistat. A white, free-flowing powder obtained from the berries of the mountain ash. It is also made from chemicals in the factory. It is used in cosmetics as a preservative and humectant. A mold and yeast inhibitor, it is used in foods, especially cheeses and beverages. It is also used in baked goods, chocolate syrup, fresh fruit cocktail, soda-fountain-type syrups, tangerine puree (sherbet base), salads (potato, macaroni, coleslaw, gelatin), cheesecake, pie fillings, cake, cheese in consumer-size packages, and artificially sweetened jellies and preserves. Percentages range from 0.003 percent in beverages to 0.2 percent in cheeses. Practically nontoxic but may cause skin irritation in susceptible people. When injected under the skin in 2,600-milligram doses per kilogram of body weight, it caused cancer in rodents. The final report to the FDA of the Select Committee on GRAS Substances stated in 1980 that it should continue its GRAS status with no limitations other than good manufacturing practices. ASP. E

**SORBITAN** • A compound from sorbitol that has the water removed.

**SORBITAN DIISOSTEARATE** • The diester of isostearic acid and hexitol (*see* Fatty Acids).

**SORBITAN DIOLEATE** • The diester of oleic acid and hexitol anhydrides derived from sorbitol. *See* Sorbitan Fatty Acid Esters.

**SORBITAN FATTY ACID ESTERS** • Mixture of fatty acids *(see)* and esters of sorbitol *(see)* and sorbitol with the water removed. Widely used in food and the cosmetics industry as an emulsifier and stabilizer.

**SORBITAN ISOSTEARATE** • *See* Sorbitan Fatty Acid Esters.

**SORBITAN LAURATE** • Span 20. Oily liquid used as an emulsifier and stabilizer of essential oils in water.

**SORBITAN MONOLAUREATE** • Emulsifier and stabilizer. *See* Sorbitan and Lauric Acid. E

**SORBITAN MONOOLEATE** • Polysorbate 80. An emulsifying additive for special dietary products and pharmaceuticals, a defoamer in yeast production, and a chewing gum plasticizer. An unintentionally administered daily dose of 19.2 grams per kilogram of body weight for two days to a four-month-old baby caused no harm except loose stools. ASP. E

**SORBITAN MONOPALMITATE** • An emulsifier and flavor-dispersing additive used as an alternate for sorbitan monostearate *(see)* in cake mixes. E

**SORBITAN MONOSTEARATE** • An emulsifier, defoamer, and flavor dispersing additive. Used in cakes and cake mixes, whipped vegetable-oil toppings, cookie coatings, cake icings and fillings, solid-state edible vegetable fat–water emulsions used as substitutes for milk or cream in coffee, coconut spread, beverages, confectionery, baked goods. Percentages range from 1 to 0.66 percent. No single dose is known to be lethal in animals, and man has been fed a daily single dose of 20 grams without harm. ASP. E

**SORBITAN OLEATE** • Sorbitan Monooleate. An emulsifying additive, defoaming additive, and plasticizer.

**SORBITAN PALMITATE** • Span 40. Derived from sorbitol *(see)*. An emulsifier in cosmetic creams and lotions, a solubilizer of essential oils in water.

**SORBITAN SESQUIOLEATE** • An emulsifier. *See* Sorbitol and Oleic Acid.

**SORBITAN SEQUISTEARATE** • *See* Sorbitan Stearate.

**SORBITAN STEARATE** • Sorbitan Monostearate. An emulsifier and a solubilizer of essential oils in water. Manufactured by reacting edible commercial stearic acid with sorbitol *(see both)*. E

**SORBITAN TRIISOSTEARATE** • *See* Stearic Acid.

**SORBITAN TRIOLEATE** • *See* Sorbitol.

**SORBITAN TRISTEARATE** • An emulsifier and alternate for sorbitan stearate *(see)*.

**SORBITOL, D-** • An alcohol first found in the ripe berries of the mountain ash; it also occurs in other berries (except grapes), and in cherries, plums, pears, apples, seaweed, and algae. Consists of white, hygroscopic powder, flakes, or granules with a sweet taste. A sugar substitute for diabetics. Used as a thickener in candy, a sequestrant in vegetable oils, a stabilizer and sweetener in frozen desserts for special dietary purposes, and a humectant and texturizing additive in shredded coconut and dietetic fruits and soft drinks. Used in embalming fluid and mouthwashes. Medicinally used to reduce body water and for intravenous feedings. If ingested in excess, it can cause diarrhea and gastrointestinal disturbances. Eating as little as 10 grams of sorbitol can cause diarrhea in some children. One piece of hard, sugar-free candy contains about 2.6 grams of sorbitol, and one thin, sugar-free chocolate bar contains about 10 grams. In adults and children, sorbitol may alter the absorption of other drugs, making them less effective or more toxic. GRAS. ASP. E

**SORBOSE** • Derived from sorbitol *(see)* by fermentation. Used in the manufacture of vitamin C—accounts for nearly a thousand tons of ascorbic acid *(see)* produced yearly. The final report to the FDA of the Select Committee on GRAS Substances stated in 1980 that it should continue its GRAS status for packaging with no limitations other than good manufacturing practices. NUL

**SORBUS EXTRACT** • Service Tree Extract. The extract of *Sorbus domestica.* An extract was used by the Indians to make a wash for sore and blurred eyes from the sun, as from climbing and hiking or from dust.

**SORGHUM** • The second most widely grown feed grain in the United States. Only 2 to 3 percent of the crop is used for human food in the United States, but it is the reverse in Africa and Asia. However, a new sorghum plant has been developed that is twice as nutritious in protein as the common variety and is 50 percent richer in lysine, an essential amino acid. The syrup, produced by evaporation from the stems and the juice, resembles cane sugar but contains a high proportion of invert sugars *(see)* as well as a starch and dextrin *(see both)*. Very sweet, it is used as a texturizer and sweetener in foods.

**SORGHUM GRAIN SYRUP** • Produced from dried sorghum juice. *See* Sorghum.

**SORREL EXTRACT** • Rumex Extract. An extract of the various species of *Rumex*. The Europeans imported this to America and the Indians adopted it. Originally the root was used as a laxative and as a mild astringent. It was also used for scabs on the skin and as a dentifrice. It was widely used by American medical circles in this century to treat skin diseases.

**SOY EXTRACT** • *See* Soybean Oil.

**SOY FLOUR** • *See* Soybean Oil.

**SOY PROTEIN ISOLATES** • *See* Soybean.

**SOY SAUCE** • Fermented or Hydrolyzed. A hydrolysis product of soybeans. A combination of mold fermentation and acid hydrolysis is used. The molds employed are *Aspergillus flavus, A. niger,* and *A. oryzae.* Soy sauce consists of a mixture of amino acids, peptides, polypeptides, peptones, simple proteins, purines, carbohydrates, and other organic compounds suspended in an 18 percent sodium chloride solution. In 1983, some manufacturers began producing soy sauce with a lower salt content. Used directly on food as a flavoring. The final report to the FDA of the Select Committee on GRAS Substances stated in 1980 that there is no available evidence that it is a hazard to the public when used as it is now and it should continue its GRAS status with limitations on the amounts that can be added to food.

**SOY STEROL** • *See* Soybean Oil.

**SOY STEROL ACETATE** • *See* Soybean Oil and Acetate.

**SOYA FATTY ACIDS HYDROXYLATED** • *See* Soybean and Hydroxylate. ASP

**SOYA HYDROXYETHYL IMIDAZOLINE** • *See* Ethylenediamine and Urea.

**SOYAMIDE DEA** • *See* Soybean Oil.

**SOYAMINE** • *See* Soybean Oil.

**SOYBEAN** • An erect, bushy, hairy legume, *Glycine max,* native to Asia and extensively cultivated in China, Japan, and elsewhere, whose seeds yield valuable products. Contains glycerides of linoleic, oleic, linolenic, and palmitic acids. *See* Soybean Oil.

**SOYBEAN OIL and FLOUR** • Extracted from the seeds of plants grown in eastern Asia, especially Manchuria, and the midwestern United States. The oil is made up of 40 percent protein, 17 percent carbohydrates, 18 percent oil, and 4.6 percent ash. It contains ascorbic acid, vitamin A, and thiamine. Pale yellow to brownish yellow. Also used in the manufacture of margarine. Debittered soybean flour contains practically no starch and is widely used in dietetic foods. Soybean oil is used in defoamers in the production of beet sugar and yeast, and in the manufacture of margarine, shortenings, candy, and soap. Soybean is used in many products including MSG, dough mixes, Lea & Perrins and Heinz's Worcestershire sauces, soy sauce, salad dressings, pork link sausages, luncheon meats, hard candies, nut candies, and milk and coffee substitutes. It is made into soybean milk, soybean curd, and soybean cheese. About 300 million bushels of soybeans are grown yearly in the United States, one-third more than in China. May cause allergic reactions, including hair damage and acnelike pimples. The final report to the FDA of the Select Committee on GRAS Substances stated in 1980 that it should continue its GRAS status with no limitations other than good manufacturing practices. EAF

**SOYBEAN OIL UNSAPONIFIABLES** • The fraction of soybean oil that is not saponified (turned into fatty alcohol) in the refining of soybean oil fatty acids.

**SOY CONCENTRATE, ENZYME ACTIVATED** • Enzymes are used to break down soy into easier to use amino acids and peptides. ASP

**SOY PROTEIN, ISOLATE** • The principle active components are isoflavones, phytochemicals which have been demonstrated antioxidant, antiangiogenetic, and estrogen activity. ASP

**SP** • FDA abbreviation for spices and other natural seasonings and flavorings.

**SP/ADJ** • FDA abbreviation for spray adjuvant.

**SPANISH HOPS** • *See* Ditanny of Crete.

**SPANISH ORIGANUM** • *See* Origanum Oil.

**SPEARMINT** • Garden Mint. Green Mint. It is the essential volatile oil obtained by steam distillation from the fresh aboveground parts of the flowering plant *Mentha spicata,* grown in the United States, Europe, and Asia. It is colorless, yellow, or yellow-green with the characteristic taste and odor of spearmint. The principal active constituent of the oil contains at least 50 percent carvone *(see)*. The fresh ground parts of the aromatic herb are used in spearmint flavoring for beverages, meats, and condiments (1,000 ppm). Widely cultivated in the United States it is used in butter, caramel, citrus, fruit, garlic, soy, and spice flavorings for beverages, ice cream, ices, candy, baked goods, condiments (100,000 ppm), fats, oils, and icings (50,000 ppm). Has been used to break up intestinal gas. May cause allergic reactions such as skin rash. GRAS. ASP

**SPECTINOMYCIN** • A veterinary antibacterial additive. The FDA tolerance for its residue in edible tissues of chicken and in drinking water is 0.1 ppm.

**SPERMACETI** • Cetyl Palmitate. Derived as a wax from the head of the sperm whale. Used to make creams glossy and increase their viscosity. Generally nontoxic but may become rancid and cause irritations.

**SPERM OIL** • Hydrogenated *(see)*. Obtained from the sperm whale. Yellow, thin liquid; slightly fishy odor if not of good quality. Used as a releasing additive or lubricant in baking pans and as a coating on fresh citrus fruits. NIL

**SPICE OLEORESINS** • Derived from spices and contain the total odors and related characteristics. They are produced by extraction of the spice with a solvent or by distillation. Spice oleoresins are frequently used with added food-grade dilutents, preservatives, and antioxidants, and other substances that must be listed on the label in accordance with current U.S. regulations or with the regulations of other countries. *See* Oleoresins.

**SPIKE LAVENDER OIL** • French Lavender. Used in perfumes. A pale yellow, stable oil obtained from a flower grown in the Mediterranean region. A lavenderlike odor. Used in fruit, floral, mint, and spice flavorings for beverages, ice cream, ices, candy, and baked goods. Used also for fumigating to keep moths from clothes. Moderately toxic by ingestion. GRAS

**SPIKENARD EXTRACT** • *Nardostachys jatamansi.* An East Indian aromatic plant. The dried roots and young stems are used as an ingredient in flavorings and perfumes. It was not assigned for toxicology literature in 1999 and is still EAF.

**SPINACH EXTRACT** • An extract of the leaves of spinach, *Spinaciea oleracea.*

**SPIRAEA EXTRACT** • Queen Meadow. Extract from the flowers of *Spiraea ulmaria.* Contains an oil similar to wintergreen oil *(see).* The roots are rich in tannic acid *(see).*

**SPIRAL FLAG OIL** • *See* Costus Root Oil.

**SPIRIT of NITROUS ETHER** • *See* Ethyl Nitrite.

**SPIRO(2,4-DITHIA-1-METHYL-8-OXABICYCLO(3.3.0)OCTANE-3,3′-(1′-OXA-2′-ME)** • Synthetic flavoring. ASP

**SPIRULINA** • The dried biomass of *Athrospira platensis.* Used in foods such as bars, powdered nutritional drink mixes, popcorn, and as a condiment in salads and pasta, at levels ranging from 0.5 to 3 grams per serving size. GRAS

**SPLENDA** • *See* Sucralose.

**SPRUCE NEEDLES and TWIGS** • Extract of *Picea* spp. used in flavorings. *See* Spruce Oil. NUL

**SPRUCE OIL** • Colorless to light yellow, pleasant-smelling oil obtained from the needles and twigs of various spruces and hemlocks. Used chiefly in scenting soaps and cosmetics but also used as a flavoring. *See* Hemlock Oil. EAF

**SQUALENE** • Obtained by hydrogenation of shark-liver oil. Occurs in smaller amounts in olive oil, wheat germ oil, and rice bran oil. A faint agreeable odor, tasteless, miscible with vegetable and mineral oils, organic solvents, and fatty substances. A lubricant and perfume fixative. A bactericide used in surfactants *(see).*

**STABILIZER** • A substance added to a product to give it body and to maintain a desired texture or consistency. Chocolate milk needs a stabilizer to keep the particles of chocolate from settling to the bottom of the container. Calcium *(see* Calcium Acetate) is used as a stabilizer in canned tomatoes to keep them from falling apart. Stabilizers that migrate from food-packaging material include aluminum mono-, di- and tristearate and ammonium citrate.

**STANDARDS OF COMPOSITION** • Regulate the amounts of cooked meat and poultry that processed products must contain. These standards dictate how much chicken goes into a chicken pot pie along with the peas and gravy. When shopping, you can compare foods for overall content. In "beef with noodles," beef is the main ingredient. In "noodles with beef," noodles are the main ingredient.

**STANDARDS OF FILL** • Guarantee that a minimum amount of food is placed in its container and prohibits excessive amounts of air or water.

**STANDARDS OF IDENTITY** • The FDA and USDA previously established a "recipe" for about three hundred foods such as peanut butter and mayonnaise, fixing the ingredients by law. Many of these foods were exempted from the need for ingredient listing. The 1994 labeling law requires manufacturers to give full ingredient listings for all foods.

**STANDARDS OF QUALITY** • Ensure that only those fruits and vegetables of high quality, free of defects, are used. Products of lesser quality might be so labeled (mandarin orange pieces instead of segments, for example).

**STANILO** • Spectinomycin. An antibiotic used on chickens. The FDA limits residues to 0.1 ppm in chickens. Used to treat syphilis in humans. Potential adverse reactions in humans include hives, decreased urine output, fever, and chills.

**STANNIC CHLORIDE** • Tin Tetrachloride. A thin, colorless, fuming, caustic liquid, soluble in water. May be highly irritating to the eyes and mucous membranes. *See* Stannous Chloride. NUL. E

**STANNOUS CHLORIDE** • Tin Dichloride. An antioxidant, soluble in water, and a powerful reducing additive, used in canned asparagus, canned soda (11 ppm), and other foods. Used to revive yeast. Low systemic toxicity but may be irritating to the skin and mucous membranes. On the FDA list for further study of mutagenic, teratogenic, subacute, and reproductive effects since 1980. GRAS. ASP. E

**STAPHYBIOTIC** • Bactopen. Cloxacillin. Tegopen. A penicillin antibiotic used on cattle. The FDA permits residue of 0.01 ppm in uncooked edible tissue of cattle and in milk. Mildly toxic by ingestion but can cause allergic reactions.

**STAR ANISE** • Chinese Anise. Fruit of *Illicium verum* from China, called star because of the fruit's shape. The extract is used in fruit, licorice, anise, liquor, sausage, root beer, sarsaparilla, vanilla, wintergreen, and birch beer flavorings for beverages, ice cream, ices, candy, meats (1,000 ppm), and liqueurs. The oil is used in blackberry, peach, licorice, anise, liquor, meat, root beer, spice, wintergreen, and birch beer flavorings for beverages, ice cream, ices, candy, baked goods, meats, syrups, and liqueurs. The fruit is a source of anise oil (*see* Anise). Star anise has been used as an expectorant and carminative. Japanese star anise is *Illicium anisatum* and contains a toxic lactone called anisatin, unknown in the Chinese variety. The Food and Drug Administration (FDA) released an advisory on September 10, 2003, warning consumers against drinking teas containing star anise. Reportedly, these teas caused illness in approximately forty individuals, including fifteen infants, over the last two years. Symptoms ranged from seizures and vomiting to jitteriness and rapid eye movement. GRAS

**STARCH** • Acid Modified. Pregelatinized and Unmodified. Starch is stored by plants and is taken from grains of wheat, potatoes, rice, corn, beans, and many other vegetable foods. Insoluble in cold water or alcohol but soluble in boiling water. Comparatively resistant to naturally occurring enzymes, and this is why processors "modify" starch to make it more digestible. Starch is modified with propylene oxide, succinic anhydride, 1-octenyl succinic anhydride, aluminum sulfate, or sodium hydroxide *(see all)*. Starch is a major component of cereals and many vegetables. The average U.S. diet has about 180 grams per person daily. Modified starch contributes about a gram per person per day. The source of starch and the type of modification are not usually identified on the label, since the FDA does not require it. The modified starches used in foods are most often bleached starch, acetylated distarch adipate, distarch phosphate, acetylated distarch phosphate, and hydroxypropyl distarch phosphate. The latter three are commonly used in baby foods. Used internally to alleviate diarrhea. The final report to the FDA of the Select Committee on GRAS Substances said there was no information that starch acetate was hazardous to the public when used as it is now and it should continue its GRAS status with limitations on amounts that can be added to food. On the other hand, starch sodium succinate, starch sodium octenyl succinate, and starch sodium hypochlorite oxidized were said not to demonstrate a hazard to the public at current use levels, but uncertainties do exist, requiring additional studies. However, GRAS status continues while tests are being completed and evaluated. Acid-modified and pregelatinized starches were said in the final report to be GRAS to require no limitations other than good manufacturing practices.

**STARCH, ACID MODIFIED** • *See* Acid Modified Starch. ASP

**STARCH/ACRYLATES/ACRYLAMIDE COPOLYMER** • *See* Starch and Acrylic Acid.

**STARCH, ALPH-AMYLASE MODIFIED** • *See* Modified Starch. NUL

**STARCH DIETHYLAMINCIETHYL ETHER** • *See* Starch.

**STARCH, FOOD MODIFIED ACETYLATED DISTARCH ADIPATE** • *See* Modified Starch. ASP

**STARCH, FOOD, MODIFIED ACETYLATED DISTARCH GLYCEROL** • *See* Modified Starch. NIL

**STARCH, FOOD, MODIFIED ACETYLATED DISTARCH OXYPROPANOL** • *See* Modified Starch. EAF

**STARCH, FOOD, MODIFIED BETA-AMYLASE MODIFIED STARCH** • *See* Modified Starch and Enzymes. EAF

**STARCH, FOOD, MODIFIED DISTARCH GLYCEROL** • *See* Modified Starch and Glycerol. NIL

**STARCH, FOOD, MODIFIED: PULLULANASE MODIFIED STARCH** • *See* Modified Starch. EAF

**STARCH, PREGELATININZED** • Pregelatinized starch is starch (vegetable source) which has been processed (cooking starch slurries, drying and grinding, or applying chemicals to modify its properties) to permit swelling in cold water, unlike natural starch which requires heating. ASP

**STARCH SODIUM OCTENYL SUCCINATE** • Emulsifier, stabilizer, thickener. *See* Succinic Acid.

**STARCH, UNMODIFIED** • Refers to the absence of any attempt to alter or influence the raw material's physical properties. ASP

**STARTER DISTILLATE** • Butter Starter Distillate. Steam distillate of *Streptococcus lactis, S. cremoris, S. lactis* subsp. *diacetylactic, Leuconostoc citrovorum,* and *L. dextronicum.* Used as a flavoring additive in margarine. GRAS

**STEARAMIDE** • Emulsifier. Colorless leaflets, insoluble in water. *See* Stearic Acid.

**STEARAMINE** • *See* Stearic Acid.

**STEARAMINE OXIDE** • *See* Stearyl Alcohol.

**STEARATES** • Salts of stearic acid *(see)*.

**STEARETH-2** • A polyoxyethylene *(see)* ether of fatty alcohol. The oily liquid is used as a surfactant *(see)* and emulsifier *(see)*.

**STEARETH-4 THROUGH-100** • The polyethylene glycol esthers of stearyl alcohol. The number indicates the degree of liquidity; the higher, the more solid. *See* Steareth-2.

**STEARIC ACID** • Octadecanoic Acid. Occurs naturally in some vegetable oils, cascarilla bark extract, and as a glyceride *(see)* in tallow and other animal fats and oils. A white, waxy, natural fatty acid, it is the major ingredient used in making bar soap and lubricants. Prepared synthetically by hydrogenation *(see)* of cottonseed and other vegetable oils. Slight tallowlike odor. Used in butter and vanilla flavorings for beverages, baked goods, and candy (4,000 ppm). Also a softener in chewing-gum base. It is also used for suppositories. It is a possible sensitizer for allergic people. Caused tumors in experimental animals. A human skin irritant. The final report to the FDA of the Select Committee on GRAS Substances stated in 1980 that it should continue its GRAS status with no limitations other than good manufacturing practices. In 1988, University of Texas researchers reported in *The New England Journal of Medicine* that it did not raise blood cholesterol levels as much as other saturated fats. *See* Fatty Acids. ASP

**STEARYL ACETATE** • The ester of stearyl alcohol and acetic acid *(see both)*.

**STEARYL ALCOHOL** • Stenol. A mixture of solid alcohols prepared from sperm whale oil. White flakes, insoluble in water, soluble in alcohol and ether. Used as a coating additive, emulsifier, lubricant, solvent, and texturizing additive in baked goods, cake, desserts, fruits, ice cream, nuts, peanut butter, puddings, shortening, and whipped topping. A substitute for cetyl alcohol *(see)* to obtain a firmer product at ordinary temperatures. ASP

**STEARYL ALCOHOL, PLUS BEESWAX** • Emulsifier and thickener. ASP

**STEARYL BETAINE** • *See* Surfactants and Stearic Acid.

**STEARYL CAPRYLATE** • The ester of stearyl alcohol and citric acid *(see both)*.

**STEARYL CITRATE** • The ester of stearyl alcohol and citric acid *(see both)*. A metal scavenger to prevent adverse effects of trace metals in foods and an antioxidant to prevent rancidity in margarine. The final report to the FDA of the Select Committee on GRAS Substances stated in 1980 that it should continue its GRAS status with no limitations other than good manufacturing practices. ASP

**STEARYL DIMETHYLAMINE** • *See* Stearyl Alcohol.

**STEARYL ERUCATE** • *See* Stearyl Alcohol and Erucic Acid.

**STEARYL GLYCYRRHETINATE** • The ester of stearyl alcohol and glycyrrhetinic acid *(see both)*.

**STEARYL HEPTANOATE** • Ester of stearyl alcohol and heptanoic acid *(see both)*. Used as a wax.

**STEARYL LACTATE** • An emulsifier that occurs in tallow and other animal fats as well as vegetable oils. Used to emulsify shortening in nonyeast-leavened bakery products and pancake mixes. Also used to emulsify cakes, icings, and fillings.

**STEARYL MONOGLYCERIDYL CITRATE** • The soft, practically tasteless, off-white, waxy solid used as an emulsion stabilizer in shortening with emulsifiers. Not over 0.15 percent in food. It is prepared by the chemical reaction of citric acid on monoglycerides of fatty acids *(see)*. ASP

**STEARYL OCTANOATE** • The ester of stearyl alcohol and 2-ethylhexanoic acid. *See* Stearyl Alcohol.

**STEARYL STEARATE** • The ester of stearyl alcohol and stearic acid *(see both)*.

**STEARYL STEAROYL STEARATE** • *See* Stearyl Alcohol.

**STEARYL TARTRATE** • The product of the esterification of tartaric acid with commercial stearyl alcohol. Used as a dough strengthening additive.

**S-(TETRAHYDRO-2,5-DIMETHYL-3-FURANYL) ETHANETHIOATE** • Synthetic flavoring. EAF

**STERCULEN** • Sterculia. *See* Karaya Gum.

**STERCULIA GUM** • *See* Karaya Gum. GRAS

**STEROIDS** • Class of compounds that includes certain compounds of hormonal origin, such as cortisone, and used to treat inflammations caused by allergies. Cholesterol, precursors of certain vitamins, bile acids, alcohols, and many plant derivatives such as digitalis are steroids. Steroids can reduce white blood cell production, and reduce prostaglandins and leukotrienes. Natural and synthetic steroids have four rings of carbon atoms but have different actions according to what is attached to the rings. Cortisone and oral contraceptives are steroids.

**STEROL** • Any class of solid complex alcohols from animals and plants. Cholesterol is a sterol.

**STEROYL MONOGLYCERIDYL CITRATE** • A stabilizer in shortenings. *See* Monoglycerides and Citric Acid.

**STEVIA REBAUDIANA** • *See* Stevioside.

**STEVIOSIDE** • Sweetleaf. Candy Leaf. Flavoring ingredient equal in sweetness to sugar. Extract of the leaves of *Stevia rebaudiana,* a South American plant claimed to have antibacterial, antifungal, antiinflammatory, antimicrobial, antiviral, antiyeast, cardiotonic, diuretic, hypoglycemic, hypotensive, tonic, and vasodilator benefits. However, in animal experiments it was found to be toxic to pregnant rodents and to affect the kidneys. Insufficient testing has been conducted on stevioside to support a food additive petition for its use as a sweetener in the United States. In 1999, the Joint Expert Committee on Food Additives of the World Health Organization (JECFA) and the Scientific Committee for Food of the European Union reviewed stevioside and determined that on the basis of the scientific data currently available stevioside is not acceptable as a sweetener. Stevioside is allowed in food for sweetening purposes in ten countries. Since the 1970s, stevioside has been used as a sweetener in Japan where it is used alone or in combination with other sweeteners in beverages, tabletop sweeteners, chewing gums, pickles, dried seafoods, flavorings, and confectioneries. Used in the United States in the 1980s, then banned in 1991 and subsequently allowed in as a dietary supplement but not a food additive. A candidate for approval as an artificial sweetener in the United States at this writing. It would be used as a tabletop sweetener, in soft drinks, gum, sauces, and syrups if approved by the FDA.

**ST. JOHN'S WORT** • *See* Saint John's Wort.

**STONEROOT** • Horse Balm. Used for its constituents of resin, saponin, and tannic acid *(see all).* An erect, smooth perennial; a strong-scented herb of eastern North America with pointed leaves. It produces a chocolate-colored powder with a peculiar odor and bitter, astringent taste. Soluble in alcohol.

**STORAX** • Styrax. Sweet Asian gum from *Liquidambar* spp. Used in perfumes. It is the resin obtained from the bark of an Asiatic tree. Grayish brown, fragrant semiliquid, containing also styrene and cinnamic acid *(see both).* Once used in medicine as a weak antiseptic and as an expectorant. Used in strawberry, fruit, and spice flavorings for beverages, ice cream, ices, candy, baked goods, chewing gum, and toppings. Moderately toxic when ingested. Can cause urinary problems when absorbed through the skin. Can cause skin irritation, welts, and discomfort when applied topically. A common allergen. There was reported use of the chemical in 1999 and it had not been assigned for toxicology literature. It is still EAF.

**STPP** • *See* Sodium Tripolyphosphate.

**STRAWBERRY ALDEHYDE** • Synthetic flavoring. GRAS

**STRAWBERRY EXTRACT** • *See* Strawberry Juice.

**STRAWBERRY JUICE** • Flavoring. Fresh ripe strawberries are reputed to contain ingredients that soften and nourish the skin. Widely used in natural cosmetics today. No scientific evidence of benefit or harm.

**STRAWFLOWER EXTRACT** • The extract of *Helichrysum italicum,* grown for its bright yellow, strawlike flowers. Used in coloring.

**STREPTOMYCIN** • An aminoglycoside antibiotic, it is given by injection and is active against streptococcal endocarditis, an infection of the heart in humans. It is used as an animal antibiotic in chickens, swine, and turkeys. The FDA limits residue to zero in these products, including eggs. EPA Genetic Toxicology Program *(see)*. Potential adverse reactions in humans to streptomycin include ear problems, muscle problems, kidney dysfunction, local pain, irritation, and sterile abscesses at the site of injection and skin disorders. Has been implicated in aplastic anemia.

**STRONTIUM HYDROXIDE** • Used chiefly in making soaps and greases in cosmetics. Colorless, water-absorbing crystals or white powder. Absorbs carbon dioxide from the air. Very alkaline in solution. Also used in refining beet sugar and separating sugar from molasses. Irritating when applied to the skin.

**STRUCTURED TRIGLYCERIDES** • Used in infant formula for term and preterm infants at levels of up to 80 percent total fat intake. GRAS

**STYRACIN** • *See* Cinnamyl Cinnamate.

**STYRAX** • *See* Storax.

**STYRENE** • Obtained from ethylbenzene by taking out the hydrogen. Colorless to yellowish oil with a penetrating odor. Used in the manufacture of paper and paperboard and used as a chewing substance in chewing gum. May be irritating to the eyes and mucous membranes, and in high concentrations it is narcotic. ASP

**STYRYLCARBINOL** • *See* Cinnamyl Alcohol.

**STYRYLPYRIDINIUM CHLORIDE, DIETHYL CARBAMAZINE** • Used in animal feed to combat worms.

**SUBACUTE** • A zone between acute and chronic or the process of a disease that is not overt. Subacute endocarditis, for example, is an infection of the heart. It is usually due to a "strep germ" and may follow temporary infection after a tooth extraction.

**SUBSTITUTE** • Means the product is equivalent to the food it resembles. *See* Imitation.

**SUCCINIC ACID** • Occurs in fossils, fungi, lichens, etc. Prepared from acetic acid *(see)*. Odorless; acid taste. The acid is used as a plant-growth retardant. A buffer and neutralizing additive in food processing. Has been employed medicinally as a laxative. Large amounts injected under the skin of frogs kills them. The final report to the FDA of the Select Committee on GRAS Substances stated in 1980 that it should continue its GRAS status with no limitations other than good manufacturing practices. ASP. E

**SUCCINIC ANHYDRIDE** • A starch modifier up to 4 percent. *See* Succinic Acid. NIL

**SUCCINILSTEARIN** • Stearoyl propylene glycol hydrogen succinate. The additive is the reaction product of succinic anhydride, fully hydrogenated vegetable oil predominantly fatty acids and propylene glycol *(see both)*. An emulsifier in or with shortenings and edible oils intended for use in cakes, cake mixes, fillings, icings, pastries, and toppings, in accordance with good manufacturing practices. NIL *See* Succinic Acid.

**SUCCINYLATED GELATIN** • Used for making microcapsules for flavoring oils. NUL

**SUCCINYLATED MONOGLYCERIDES** • Surfactants *(see)* used as dough conditioners to add loaf volume and firmness. *See* Glycerides and Succinic Acid.

**SUCRALOSE** • Splenda. An artificial sweetener made from sugar. It is about six hundred times sweeter than sugar but does not contain calories. Producers claim it has no aftertaste and is more stable. It can be used in cooking and is already sold in Canada and Latin America. Among its users are Cadbury Beverages and Corby Distilleries in liqueurs. The FDA approved it in April 1998. It is used as a tabletop sweetener, in baked goods, fruit spreads, desserts, and confections, but its biggest use is expected to be in diet drinks. There were early reports of thymus shrinkage in animals and some reports of mutagencity. The EU ordered further studies and in 2000 concluded that at current use, Sucralose is safe. EAF. E

**SUCROGLYCERIDES** • Used as emulsifiers. Sucroglycerides are obtained by reacting sucrose with an edible fat or oil with or without the presence of a solvent. They consist of a mixture of mono- and diesters of sucrose and fatty acids together with mono-, di-, and triglycerides from the fat or oil. E

**SUCROSE** • Sugar. Cane Sugar. Saccharose. A sweetening additive and food, a starting additive in fermentation production, a preservative and antioxidant in pharmaceuticals, a demulcent, and a substitute for glycerin *(see)*. Table sugar can stimulate the production of fat in the body, apart from its calorie content in the diet, and may be particularly fat-producing in women on the "pill." Workers who handle raw sugar often develop rashes and other skin problems. The final report to the FDA of the Select Committee on GRAS Substances stated in 1980 that it should continue its GRAS status with no limitations other than good manufacturing practices. ASP

**SUCROSE ACETATE ISOBUTYRATE** • A mixture of esters *(see)* of sucrose with acetic and isobutyric acids *(see both)*. Sucrose acetate isobutyrate produced liver damage in dogs but not in mice or rats. Three studies involving a total of seventy-one human volunteers did not respond the same way as dogs did and did not seem to have any adverse effects. The committee decided to use the NOEL *(see)* of 2 grams per kg of body weight per day for rats—the lowest obtained in long-term toxicity studies—to allocate a temporary ADI of 0–10 mg per kg of body weight using a safety factor of 200. They also asked for further data that would explain the disparate effects of sucrose acetate isobutyrate on the liver functions in dogs compared to other species, in particular the human. EAF. E

**SUCROSE BENZOATE** • *See* Benzoic Acid.

**SUCROSE DISTEARATE** • A mixture of sucrose and stearic acid *(see both)*.

**SUCROSE FATTY ACID ESTERS** • Sucrose Esters. Derived from sucrose *(see)* and edible tallow, the FDA gave permission in 1982 for their use as components of protective coatings for fruits. They are also used as emulsifiers, stabilizers, and texturizers. The FDA said that there was not a basis for GRAS determination. Application was resubmitted in 2001 for GRAS and it is now GRAS. The FDA is amending the food additive regulations to provide for the safe use of sucrose oligoesters (sucrose esters of fatty acids with an average degree of esterification ranging from four to seven) as an emulsifier or stabilizer, at a level not to exceed 2 percent, in chocolate and in butter-substitute spreads. This action is in response to a petition filed by Mitsubishi Chemical Corp. ASP. E

**SUCROSE LAURATE** • A mixture of sucrose and lauric acid *(see both)*.

**SUCROSE LIQUID** • *See* Sucrose. ASP

**SUCROSE OCTAACETATE** • Prepared from sucrose *(see)*. A synthetic flavoring used in bitters, spice, and ginger ale flavorings for beverages. Used in adhesives; a denaturant for alcohol. ASP

**SUCROSE OLIGOESTERS** • *See* Sucrose Fatty Acid Esters.

**SUCROSE POLYESTER** • *See* Olestra.

**SUCROSE STEARATE** • A mixture of sucrose and stearic acid *(see both)*.

**SUGAR** • A carbohydrate product made up of one, two, or more saccharose groups. The monosaccharide sugars—often called simple sugars—are composed of chains of 207 carbon atoms. Chief among the monosaccharides are glucose, dextrose, fructose, and levulose. Among the disaccharides are sucrose—cane or beet sugar—lactose found in milk, maltose found in starch, and cellobiose from cellulose *(see)*. High polymer sugars occur as water-soluble gums such as arabic and tragacanth. Sugar is an important source of metabolic energy in foods and its formation in plants is an essential factor in the life process. It has many uses as a food additive other than just sweetening. It acts as a tenderizer by absorbing water and inhibiting flour gluten development, as well as slowing down starch gelling. It mixes air into shortening in the creaming process and caramelizes under heat, to provide cooked and baked foods with pleasing color and aroma. It speeds the growth of yeast by providing nourishment and helps to keep beaten eggs whipped. It delays coagulation of egg proteins in custards and helps the gelling of fruit jellies and preserves. It also helps prevent them from spoiling and keeps canned and frozen fruits looking appetizing and tender. It helps to make a wide variety of candies through varying degrees of recrystallization and enhances the smoothness and flavor of ice cream. Most people think of table sugar or sucrose when the word is mentioned. It contains only sixteen calories per teaspoon, something to consider when considering a sugar substitute.

**SUGAR ALC** • Listing on food labels for sugar alcohols *(see)*.

**SUGAR ALCOHOLS** • These are monosaccharides. One of the most important is glycerol *(see)*, while others include inositol, mannitol, sorbitol, and xylitol *(see all)*. Many so-called "dietetic" foods that are labeled "sugar free" or "no sugar added" in fact contain these sugar alcohols. They have less calories than sucrose (table sugar) but they can raise blood sugar levels. Foods containing sugar alcohols can cause stomach problems, including diarrhea if eaten in large quantities.

**SUGAR BEET EXTRACT FLAVOR BASE** • A flavoring in foods. *See* Sucrose. ASP

**SUGAR BEET FIBER** • Beet Fiber. Sugar Beet Pulp. Natural fiber of sugar beets remaining after water extraction of the sugar from the mechanically sliced sugar beets. Exists in various grades from coarse fibrous flakes to fine powders. Used as an anticaking additive, binding additive, bulking additive, dietary supplement, dispersing additive, nutrient, stabilizing additive, texturizing additive, and thickening additive.

**L-SUGARS** • Candidate for artificial sweeteners. No specific use given as yet.

**SUGAR SOLID EXTRACT** • *See* Sucrose.

**SULFA ANTIBIOTICS** • More than fifty compounds that contain both sulfur and nitrogen with a specificity for certain bacteria. Because of their toxicity and often serious side effects, their use in treating disease is limited, at least intentionally in humans. They are widely used, however, in treating animals and animal feeds.

**SULFABROMOMETHAZINE SODIUM** • 5-Bromosulfamethazine. A widely used sulfa antibacterial to treat cattle. The FDA limits residue to 0.1 ppm in uncooked edible tissues of cattle and 0.01 ppm in milk. Sulfa drugs can cause sensitivity to the sun. Mildly toxic by ingestion. Caused tumors and birth defects in experimental animals.

**SULFACHLORPYRIDAZINE** • A veterinary antibiotic. The FDA allows 0.1 ppm as residue in uncooked edible tissue of calves and swine. *See* Sulfa Antibiotics.

**SULFADIMETHOXINE PLUS ORMETOPRIM** • A feed additive, the FDA allows 0.1 ppm sulfa residue in uncooked edible tissues of chickens, turkeys, cattle, ducks, salmon, and catfish. The agency allows 0.01 ppm in milk. Ormetoprim residue is allowed at 0.1 ppm in edible tissues of chickens, turkeys, ducks, salmon, and catfish. *See* Sulfa Antibiotics.

**SULFAETHOXYPYRIDAZINE** • A feed additive. The residues allowed in edible tissues of cattle are 0.1 ppm and zero in milk and uncooked edible tissue of swine. It is used in the drinking water of cattle and swine. *See* Sulfa Antibiotics.

**SULFAMERAZINE** • Used in fish feed on fish farms. FDA tolerance is zero in edible tissues of trout as residue. *See* Sulfa Antibiotics.

**SULFAMETHAZINE** • An antibiotic used in cattle. The FDA permits 0.1 ppm as residue in the edible tissues of cattle, swine, turkeys, and chicken. *See* Sulfa Antibiotics.

**SULFAMETHAZINE A (WITH CHLORTETRACYCLINE and PENICILLIN) or SULFAMETHAZINE B (WITH TYLOSIN)** • Antibiotics used in animal feed. The FDA permits 0.1 ppm in uncooked edible tissues of chickens, turkeys, cattle, and swine. *See* Sulfa Antibiotics, Tetracyclines, Penicillin, and Tylosin.

**SULFAMETHAZINE SODIUM** • *See* Sulfa Antibiotics.

**SULFAMIC ACID** • A strong, white crystalline acid used chiefly as a weed killer, in cleaning metals, and as a softening additive. Used as a plasticizer and fire retardant for paper and other cellulose products; as a stabilizing additive for chlorine and hypochlorite, bleaching paper pulp; and as a catalyst for urea formaldehyde resin. Moderately irritating to the skin and mucous membranes. The final report to the FDA of the Select Committee on GRAS Substances stated in 1980 that it should continue its GRAS status with no limitations other than good manufacturing practices. ASP

**6-SULFANILAMIDO-2,4-DIMETHOXYPYRIMIDINE** • Abcid. Agribon. Albon. Bactrovet. A widely used sulfa antibacterial drug to treat cattle, poultry, and in animal feed. It is also used in catfish farming to prevent infections. The FDA limits residues to 0.1 ppm in chickens, turkeys, cattle, ducks, salmon, and catfish. Caused birth defects in experimental animals. Sulfa drugs can cause sensitivity to sunlight and allergic reactions.

**SULFANITRAN** • A sulfa antibiotic used to treat chickens. FDA residue limit is zero in chickens. Sulfa drugs can cause sensitivity to light and allergic reactions in humans.

**SULFAQUINOXALINE** • A sulfa drug used in animal feed. Moderately toxic by ingestion. Sulfa drugs can cause sensitivity to light and allergic reactions in humans.

**SULFATE** • A salt or ester of sulfuric acid *(see)*. A chemical is "sulfated" to help control the acid-alkali balance.

**SULFATED BUTYL OLEATE** • An emulsion used to dehydrate grapes to raisins. Made from oleic acid with butanol. *See* Oleic Acid and Butyl Alcohol.

**SULFATED GLYCERYL OLEATE** • Produced by adding sulfuric acid to glyceryl oleate. *See* Sulfonated Oils.

**SULFATED OIL** • A compound to which a salt of sulfuric acid has been added to help control the acid-alkali balance.

**SULFATED TALLOW** • Fat from fatty tissues of sheep and cattle that becomes solid at 40 to 46°F. It is a defoaming additive in yeast and beet sugar production in "amounts reasonably required to inhibit foaming." *See* Tallow Flakes for toxicity.

**SULFATHIAZOLE COMBINED WITH CHLORTETRACYCLINE and PENICILLIN** • Antibiotic compound used in animal feeds. *See* Sulfa Antibiotics, Tetracycline, and Penicillin.

**SULFIDES** • Inorganic sulfur compounds that occur free or in combination with minerals. They are salts of weak acid.

**SULFITE DIOXIDE** • *See* Sulfites.

**SULFITES** • Sodium, Potassium, and Ammonium. Preservatives, antioxidants, and antibrowning additives used in foods. Sulfites are also used for bleaching food starches and as a preventive against rust and scale in boiler water used in making steam that will come in contact with food. Some sulfites are used in the production of cellophane for food packaging. The FDA prohibits the use of sulfites in foods that are important sources of thiamine (vitamin $B_1$), such as enriched flour, because sulfites destroy the nutrient. There are six sulfiting additives that are currently listed as GRAS chemical preservatives. They are sulfur dioxide, sodium sulfite, sodium and potassium bisulfite, and sodium and potassium metabisulfite *(see all)*. Under the current listing, sulfiting additives may be used as preservatives in any food except recognized sources of vitamin $B_1$. These additives have been used in many processed foods and in cafeterias and restaurants to prevent fruits, green vegetables, potatoes, and salads from turning brown, as well as to enhance their crispness. The FDA had sulfiting additives under review. As part of this review, a proposal to affirm the GRAS status of sulfur dioxide, sodium bisulfite, and sodium and potassium metabisulfite, with specific use limitations, was published in the Federal Register of July 9, 1982. The agency did not propose to affirm the GRAS status of sodium sulfite and potassium bisulfite because it had no evidence to indicate their current use in food. Reactions to sulfites can include acute asthma attacks, loss of consciousness, anaphylactic shock, diarrhea, and nausea occurring soon after ingesting sulfiting additives. There have been seventeen deaths that the FDA has determined were "probably or possibly" associated with sulfites. The FDA banned the use of the preservative on fresh fruits and vegetables and at this writing is reviewing a proposal to prohibit it on fresh, precut potatoes. The FDA decided in 1988 against extending its ban on the use of sulfites to a variety of foods sold in supermarkets and served in restaurants, including wine, dried fruit, some seafood, and condiments. Sulfites must be declared on the labels of wine and packaged foods sold in supermarkets when they are added in excess of 10 ppm. A citizens' petition was submitted by the Center for Science in the Public Interest, Washington, D.C., on October 28, 1982, that asked the agency to restrict the use of sulfiting additives to a safe residue level in food or require labels on those food products in which sulfiting additives must be used at higher levels to perform essential public health functions. In the meantime, the California Grape and Tree Fruit League recommended that the Food and Drug Administration affirm as GRAS sulfiting additives used in sulfur dioxide fumigation within specific limitations and include its use as an ingredient to treat fresh grapes. Stating that the compound is essential to the marketing, transport, storage, and export of table grapes, the group claimed lack of any known substitute for the gaseous compound effective in preventing mold-rot and other storage fungi and in prolonging storage life. A spokesperson for the Wine Institute, which represents 460 domestic wine makers, said that many of the sulfur compounds in wine are natural parts of fermentation, but they are also added to many wines. Sulfites are still used in processed foods, dried fruits, wines, and beers. When dining in a restaurant, you have to have a lot of faith in your waiter if you are allergic to sulfites. Foods, especially potato products and some canned foods served in restaurants, could contain sulfites. You can ask, but you may not receive an informed answer. You have to be cautious about "prepared" products in general if you are sulfite sensitive. For example, lemon juice from a lemon may be fine, but from a bottle it may contain sodium bisulfite. The FAO/WHO Expert Committee on Food Additives concluded in June 1998 that "the potential exists for high consumers of sulfites to exceed the ADI, but the available data were insufficient to estimate the number of high consumers or the magnitude and duration of intake above the ADI." The committee is reviewing this additive's levels in dried fruits, jams, jellies, marmalades, fruit preparations including pulp and fruit toppings, dried vegetables, vegetables, nut and seed purees and spreads, white and semiwhite sugar, concentrates for fruit juice, wines, and fruit wines. ASP

**SULFOACETATE DERIVATIVES OF MONOGLYCERIDES and DIGLYCERIDES** • Used as emulsifiers. The final report to the FDA of the Select Committee on GRAS Substances stated in 1980 that there were insufficient biological and other studies upon which to base an evaluation of them when they are used as food ingredients.

**SULFOMYXIN** • A sulfa drug used to combat bacteria in chickens and turkeys. The FDA limits residue to zero in uncooked edible tissues of chickens and turkeys. Sulfa drugs can cause sensitivity to light and allergic reactions in humans.

**SULFONATED OILS** • Sulfated. Prepared by reacting oils with sulfuric acid. Used in soapless shampoos and hairsprays as an emulsifier and wetting additive.

**SULFO-*p*-TOLUENE** • Sodium Chloramine. A water-purifying additive and a deodorant used to remove onion and weed odors in cheese. Toluene may cause mild anemia and is narcotic in high concentrations.

**SULFUR DIOXIDE** • A gas formed when sulfur burns. Used to bleach vegetable colors and to preserve fruits and vegetables; a disinfectant in breweries and food factories; a bleaching additive in gelatin, glue, and beet sugars; an antioxidant, preservative, and antibrowning additive in wine, corn syrup, table syrup, jelly, dried fruits, brined fruit, maraschino cherries, beverages, dehydrated potatoes, soups, and condiments. Should not be used on meats or on foods recognized as a source of vitamin A because it destroys the vitamin. Poisonous, highly irritating. Often cited as an air pollutant. EPA Extremely Hazardous Substances List and EPA Genetic Toxicology Program *(see both)*. Inhalation produces respiratory irritation and death when sufficiently concentrated. The final report to the FDA of the Select Committee on GRAS Substances stated in 1980 that there is no available evidence that it is a hazard to the public when used as it is now and it should continue its GRAS status with limitations on amounts that can be added to food. Sulfur dioxide is also a preservative, but not to be used in meats or in foods recognized as a source of vitamin $B_1$. The following are food categories with common levels of sulfur dioxide: baked goods 30 ppm; beer 25 ppm; canned vegetables 30 ppm; condiments and relishes 30 ppm; dehydrated vegetables 200 ppm. ASP. E

**SULFURIC ACID** • Oil of Vitriol. A clear, colorless, odorless, oily acid used to modify starch and to regulate acidity-alkalinity balance in the brewing industry. It is corrosive and produces severe burns on contact with the skin and other body tissues. Inhalation of the vapors can cause serious lung damage. Diluted sulfuric acid has been used to stimulate appetite and to combat overalkaline stomach juices. It is used as a topical caustic in cosmetic products. If ingested undiluted, it can be fatal. The final report to the FDA of the Select Committee on GRAS Substances stated in 1980 that it should continue its GRAS status with no limitations other than good manufacturing practices. ASP. E

**SULFUROUS ACID** • A solution of sulfur dioxide in water. It is toxic by ingestion and inhalation and very irritating to tissue. It is used in bleaching, paper manufacturing, wine manufacturing, brewing, and as a preservative for fruits, nuts, foods, and wines. There is reported use of the chemical; it has not yet been assigned for toxicology literature. EAF

**SUNETTE** • *See* Acesulfame Potassium.

**SUNFLOWER SEED OIL** • Oil obtained by milling the seeds of the large flower produced in Russia, India, Egypt, and Argentina. A bland, pale yellow oil, it contains vitamin E (*see* Tocopherols) and forms a "skin" after drying. Used in food, salad oils, and in resin and soap manufacturing.

**SUNSET YELLOW, ORANGE YELLOW** • See FD and C Yellow No. 6. E

**SUNFLOWER SEED OIL GLYCERIDE** • *See* Sunflower Seed Oil and Glycerides.

**SUPERGLYCERINATED FULLY HYDROGENATED RAPESEED OIL** • Used in some margarines and emulsions. *See* Rapeseed Oil, Glycerin, and Hydrogenation.

**SUPER-OV** • Derived from pig pituitary glands, it is used for the induction of superovulation in cows for procedures requiring the production of multiple eggs at a single estrus. Follicle-stimulating hormone is not orally active; therefore residues of this drug are said to be safe for human consumption, and therefore "no toxicological studies were required" by the U.S. government.

**SURFACE-ACTIVE ADDITIVE** • *See* Surfactants.

**SURFACTANTS** • These are wetting additives. They lower water's surface tension, permitting water to spread out and penetrate more easily. These surface-active additives are classified by whether or not they ionize in solution and by the nature of their electrical charges. There are four major categories—anionic, nonionic, cationic, and amphoteric. Anionic surfactants, which carry a negative charge, have excellent cleaning properties. They are stain and dirt removers in household detergents, powders, and liquids and in toilet soaps. Nonionic surfactants have no electrical charge. Since they are resistant to hard water and dissolve in oil and grease, they are especially effective in spray-on oven cleaners. Cationic surfactants have a positive charge. These are primarily ammonia derivatives and are antistatic and sanitizing additives used as friction reducers in hair rinses and fabric softeners. Amphoteric surfactants may be either negatively charged or positively charged depending on the acidity or alkalinity of the water. They are used for cosmetics where mildness is important, such as in shampoos and lotions. Surfactants may be classified as emulsifiers, dispersants, wetting and foaming additives, detergents, viscosity modifiers, or stabilizers. For example, in peanut butter, a surfactant keeps oil and water mixtures from separating; in cosmetics, it makes lotions more spreadable; salad dressings and cheeses are thickened by surfactants, which make them pour better.

**SWEET BIRCH** • *See* Methyl Salicylate.

**SWEET CLOVER EXTRACT** • Extract of various species of *Melilotus,* grown for hay and soil improvement. It contains coumarin *(see)* and is used as a scent to disguise bad odors.

**SWEET FLAG** • *See* Calamus.

**SWEET MARJORAM OIL** • Pot Marjoram. Used in perfumery and hair preparations. The natural extract of the flowers and leaves of two varieties of the fragrant marjoram. Also a food flavoring.

**SWEETENER 2000** • An artificial sweetener made by the company that brought us NutraSweet. It is not on the market as of this writing. *See* Aspartame.

**SY/FL** • FDA abbreviation for synthetic flavoring.

**SYLVIC ACID** • *See* Abietic Acid.

**SYNDIOTACTIC 1,2-POLYBUTADIENE** • A petition to use this as a one-way disposable food packaging film was put in abeyance *(see)* by the FDA in 2003.

**SYNTHETIC** • Made in the laboratory and not by nature. For example, vanillin, made in the laboratory, may be identical to vanilla extracted from the vanilla bean, but vanillin cannot be called "natural."

**SYNTHETIC BEESWAX** • A mixture of alcohol esters.

**SYNTHETIC FATTY ALCOHOLS** • Made from fatty alcohols *(see)* obtained by distillation. Used as substitutes for naturally derived fatty acids *(see)*.

**SYNTHETIC GLYCERIN** • *See* Glycerin.

**SYNTHETIC IRON OXIDE** • For coloring sausage casings and for cat and dog food. Limited to 0.1 percent of weight of finished human food and 0.25 percent of weight of finished food for dogs and cats. Exempt from color certification.

**SYNTHETIC JOJOBA OIL** • *See* Jojoba Oil.

**SYNTHETIC LYCOPENE** • Coloring made by synthetic lycopene as a crystalline material derived from chemical synthesis. *See* Lycopene. GRAS

**SYNTHETIC PARAFFIN and SUCCINIC DERIVATIVES** • Used as a coating on fresh citrus, muskmelons, and sweet potatoes. *See* Paraffin Wax and Succinic Acid.

**SYNTHETIC SPERMACETI** • *See* Spermaceti.

**SYNTHETIC WAX** • A hydrocarbon wax derived from various oils.

# T

**TAGALOSE, D** • *See* D-Tagalose.

**TAGETES** • Meal, Extract, and Oil. Marigold. The meal is the dried, ground flower petals of the Aztec marigold, a strong-scented, tropical American herb, mixed with no more than 0.3 percent ethoxyquin, an herbicide and antioxidant. The extract is taken from tagetes petals. Both the meal and the extract are used to enhance the yellow color of chicken skin and eggs. They are incorporated in chicken feed, supplemented sufficiently with the yellow coloring xanthophyll. The coloring has been permanently listed since 1963 but is exempt from certification. The oil is extracted from the Aztec flower and used in fruit flavorings for beverages, ice cream, ices, candy, baked goods, gelatin, desserts, and condiments.

**TAGETES OIL** • Flavoring produced from the *Tagetes glandulifera* obtained by steam distillation just after the inflorescence of the crop and has a dark yellow to orange-yellow color and green odor with a sweet-fruity undertone. EAF

**TALC** • French Chalk. Magnesium Silicate. The lumps are known as soapstone of steatite. An anticaking additive added to vitamin supplements to render a free flow; also to chewing-gum base, rice, herbs, spices, seasonings (including salt substitutes), and condiments (e.g., seasoning for instant noodles). Also used in animal feed. Gives a slippery sensation to powders and creams. In olive oil production, as a processing aid to increase yield and improve the clarity of the oil. Prolonged inhalation can cause lung problems because it is similar in chemical composition to asbestos, a known lung irritant and cancer-causing ingredient in its powdered state. There is no known acute toxicity, but there is a question about it being a cancer-causing additive upon ingestion. It is suspected that the high incidence of stomach cancer among the Japanese is due to the fact that the Japanese prefer that their rice be treated with talc. GRAS. ASP. E

**TALLAMIDE DEA** • *See* Tall Oil.

**TALLAMPHOPROPIONATE** • *See* Tall Oil.

**TALL OIL** • Liquid Rosin. A by-product of the wood pulp industry. *Tall* is Swedish for "pine." Dark brown liquid. Acrid odor. A fungicide and cutting oil. It may be a mild irritant and sensitizer. The final report to the FDA of the Select Committee on GRAS Substances stated in 1980 that it should continue its GRAS status with no limitations other than good manufacturing practices. EAF

**TALL OIL BENZYL HYDROXYETHYL IMIDAZOLINIUM CHLORIDE** • *See* Quaternary Ammonium Compounds and Tall Oil.

**TALL OIL ROSIN, GLYCEROL ESTER** • Softener for chewing-gum base. *See* Tall Oil.

**TALLOW ACID** • *See* Tallow Flakes.

**TALLOW ALCOHOL, HYDROGENATED** • *See* Hydrogenated Tallow. NUL

**TALLOW AMIDE** • *See* Tallow Flakes.

**TALLOWAMIDE DEA and MEA** • *See* Tallow Acid.

**TALLOW AMIDOPROPYLAMINE OXIDE** • *See* Tallow Acid.

**TALLOW AMINE** • *See* Tallow Flakes.

**TALLOW AMINE OXIDE** • *See* Tallow Flakes.

**TALLOW, BEEF** • Adds body, aroma, and improves mouth feel in a variety of applications. Used for shortening in some varieties of commercial cookies, and oleo stearine, which is used for the making of some chewing gums. Free fatty acids derived from tallow are also used in the production of candles, fabric softeners, crayons, paper, explosives, and cement blocks. NEW

**TALLOWETH-6** • *See* Tallow Flakes.

**TALLOW FATTY ACIDS** • *See* Tallow Flakes and Fatty Acids.

**TALLOW FLAKES** • Suet. Dripping. The fat from the fatty tissue of bovine cattle and sheep in North America. White, almost tasteless when pure, and generally harder than grease. Used as a defoaming additive in yeast and beet sugar production. In miniature pigs in one year, feeding tallow caused moderate to severe atherosclerosis (clogging of the arteries) similar to that in humans. The final report to the FDA of the Select Committee on GRAS Substances stated in 1980 that it should continue its GRAS status for packaging with no limitations other than good manufacturing practices. EAF

**TALLOW GLYCERIDES** • A mixture of triglycerides (fats) derived from tallow.

**TALLOW, HYDROGENATED, OXIDIZED, or SULFATED** • Antifoaming additive. Used in defoaming additives. *See* Tallow Flakes and Hydrogenation. ASP

**TALLOW HYDROXYETHYL IMIDAZOLINE** • *See* Tallow and Imidazoline.

**TALLOW IMIDAZOLINE** • *See* Tallow Flakes.

**TAMARIND EXTRACT** • The extract of *Tamarindus indica,* a large tropical tree grown in the East Indies and Africa. Preserved in sugar or syrup, it is used as a natural fruit flavoring. The pulp contains about 10 percent tartaric acid *(see).* Has been used as a cooling laxative drink. GRAS. There is reported use of the chemical, but it has not yet been assigned for toxicology literature. ASP

**TANGERINE, ESSENCE** • Uncut, undiluted, and alcohol free. *See* Tangerine Oil. ASP

**TANGERINE EXTRACT** • *Citrus reticulata. See* Tangerine Oil.

**TANGERINE OIL** • The oil obtained by expression from the peels of the ripe fruit from several related tangerine species. Reddish orange, with a pleasant orange aroma. Used in blueberry, mandarin, orange, tangerine, and other fruit flavorings for beverages, ice cream, ices, candy, baked goods, gelatin desserts, and chewing gum. A skin irritant. GRAS. ASP

**TANNIC ACID** • Occurs in the bark and fruit of many plants, notably in the bark of the oak and sumac, and in cherries, coffee, and tea. It is used to clarify beer and wine, and as a refining additive for rendered fats. As a flavoring it is used in butter, caramel, fruit, brandy, maple, and nut flavorings for beverages, ice cream, ices, candy, baked goods, and liquor (1,000 ppm). Used medicinally as a mild astringent and when applied it may turn the skin brown. Low toxicity orally, but large doses may cause gastric distress. Can cause tumors and death by injection, but not, evidently, by ingestion. IARC review and EPA Genetic Toxicology Program *(see both).* The final report to the FDA of the Select Committee on GRAS Substances stated in 1980 that there is no evidence in the available information that it is a hazard to the public when used as it is now and it should continue its GRAS status with limitations on the amount that may be added to food. ASP

**TANNIN** • Used in alcoholic beverages only. *See* Tannic Acid.

**TANSY** • A common herb, *Tanacetum vulgare,* which the Greeks believed prolonged life. Strong aromatic odor and bitter taste. Flavoring used in alcoholic beverages only. NUL

**TANSY OIL** • *Tanacetum vulgare.* NIL

**TAPIOCA STARCH** • A preparation of cassava, the tapioca plant. Used for thickening liquid foods such as puddings, juicy pies, and soups. The final report to the FDA of the Select Committee on GRAS Substances stated in 1980 that it should continue its GRAS status with no limitations other than good manufacturing practices. ASP

**TAR OIL** • The volatile oil distilled from wood tar, generally from the family Pinaceae. Used externally to treat skin diseases, the principle toxic ingredients are phenols (very toxic) and other hydrocarbons such as the naphthalenes. Toxicity estimates are hard to make because even the U.S. Pharmacopoeia does not specify the phenol content of official preparations. However, if ingested, it is estimated that one ounce would kill. *See* Pine Tar Oil, which is a rectified tar oil used as a licorice flavoring.

**TARA GUM** • Peruvian Carob. Obtained by grinding the endosperms of the seeds of an evergreen tree common to Peru. The whitish yellow, nearly odorless powder that is produced is used as a thickening additive and stabilizer. *See* also Locust Bean Gum. E

**TARAXACUM ERYTHROSPERUMUM** • *See* Dandelion Leaf and Root.

**TARRAGON EXTRACT** • *Artemisia dracunculus.* The name is derived from the Arabic word *tharkhoum* and the Latin word *dracunculus* meaning "little dragon," probably because of the way the root seems to coil up like a dragon. The extract is from the dried leaves of this small European perennial wormwood herb. Pale yellow oil extracted for its aromatic, pungent taste. Used in making pickles and vinegar. ASP

**TARRAGON OIL** • Estragon. Russian Tarragon. Little Dragon. Extracted by steam distillation from the leaves and the flowering tops of *Atremisia dracunculus* from the Compositae family. Used in folk medicine as an antirheumatic, appetite stimulant, deodorant, emmenagogue stimulant, and vermifuge. ASP

**TARS** • An antiseptic, deodorant, and bug killer. Any of the various dark brown or black bituminous, usually odorous, viscous liquids or semiliquids obtained by the destructive distillation of wood, coal, peat, shale, and other organic materials. Used as a licorice food flavoring. May cause allergic reactions.

**TARTARIC ACID** • Sodium Tartrate. Sodium Potassium Tartrate. Rochelle Salts. Described in ancient times as being a residual of grape fermentation. Widely distributed in nature in many fruits but usually obtained as a by-product of wine making. Consists of colorless or translucent crystals or a white fine-to-granular crystalline powder, which is odorless and has an acid taste. It is the acidic constituent of some baking powders and is used to adjust acidity in frozen dairy products, jellies, bakery products, beverages, confections, dried egg whites, food colorings, candies, artificially sweetened preserves up to 4 percent. Used as a sequestrant, especially in wines, as an emulsifier, and as a grape and sour flavoring for candies, canned sodas and colas, preserves, baked goods, dried egg white, lemon meringue pie mix, pasteurized processed cheese, cheese food and cheese spread, and some types of baking powder. Large amounts may have a laxative effect. GRAS. E

**TARTRATE, SODIUM POTASSIUM** • Final report to the FDA of the Select Committee on GRAS Substances stated in 1980 it should continue its GRAS status with no limitations other than good manufacturing practices. *See* Sodium Potassium Tartrate.

**TARTRAZINE** • FD and C Yellow No. 5. Bright orange-yellow powder used in foods, drugs, and cosmetics and as a dye for wool and silk. Those allergic to aspirin are often allergic to tartrazine. Allergies have been reported in persons eating sweet corn, soft drinks, and cheese crackers—all colored with Yellow No. 5. It is derived from coal tar. E

**TAURINE** • An amino acid found in almost every tissue of the body and high in human milk. Most infant soy protein formulas are now supplemented with taurine. It is also used as a nutritional supplement in feed for growing chicks. Taurine is almost absent from vegetarian diets. It is believed necessary for healthy eyes and it is an antioxidant. Irregular heartbeat is characteristic of lack of blood to the heart and may be partly due to loss of intracellular taurine, some researchers theorize. Much like magnesium, taurine affects membrane excitability by normalizing potassium flux in and out of the heart muscle cells. Supplementation may prevent digitalis-induced arrhythmias. Taurine may also lower blood pressure. In a group of nineteen young patients with borderline high blood pressure, some received six grams daily of taurine and others a placebo. After seven days, systolic and diastolic blood pressure fell significantly in patients receiving taurine. Epinephrine, which stimulates heartbeat, was blunted by taurine, suggesting that its anti–high blood pressure effect may be mediated by reduction in signals from the nervous system. ASP

**TAUROCHOLIC ACID** • Cholic Acid. Cholyltaurine. Occurs as a sodium salt in bile. It is formed by the combination of the sulfur-containing amino acid, taurine, and cholic acid. It aids digestion and absorption of fats. It is used as an emulsifying additive in foods. The final report to the FDA of the Select Committee on GRAS Substances stated in 1980 that it should continue its GRAS status with no limitations other than good manufacturing practices. NUL

**TBHQ** • *See* Tertiary Butylhydroquinone.

**TBS** • *See* Tribromsalan.

**TCC** • *See* Triclocarban.

**TEA-** • The abbreviation for triethanolamine *(see)*.

**TEA** • The leaves, leaf buds, and internodes of plant and fragrant white flowers prepared and cured to make an aromatic beverage. Tea is a mild stimulant and its tonic properties are due to the alkaloid caffeine; tannic acid *(see)* makes it astringent. There is tremendous interest among researchers worldwide to identify those nutraceuticals in tea that may help prevent malignancies. Cultivated principally in China, Japan, Sri Lanka, and other Asian countries, tea leaves come from an evergreen of the camellia family, *Camellia sinensis,* and are processed in different ways to produce green, black, and oolong tea. Each emerges with different chemical properties. To produce black tea, which most Americans drink, leaves are subjected to warmth for a few hours and heated to 200°F to finish the drying process. Green tea is popular in Asia and is not heated but simply steamed, rolled, and crushed. Oolong tea is less heated than black, but just enough to give it a different character from green. Green tea, which has been used in Japan for more than a thousand years, is now believed to have the most beneficial effects. GRAS. ASP

**TEA-ABIETOYL HYDROLYZED ANIMAL PROTEIN** • The salt of the condensation product of abietic acid and hydrolyzed animal protein *(see both)*.

**TEA-C12-15 ALCOHOLS SULFATE** • *See* Triethanolamine, Alcohol, and Sulfate.

**TEA-COCO-HYDROLYZED ANIMAL PROTEIN** • *See* Hydrolyzed Animal Protein and Surfactants.

**TEA-COCO-HYDROLYZED PROTEIN** • *See* Proteins.

**TEA-COCYL GLUTAMATE** • A softener. *See* Glutamate.

**TEA-EDTA** • *See* Ethylenediamine Tetraacetic Acid.

**TEA EXTRACT** • Essential oil. *See* Tea. GRAS. ASP

**TEA-HYDROGENATED TALLOW GLUTAMATE** • A softener. *See* Glutamate.

**TEA-LAUROYL GLUTAMATE** • A softener. *See* Glutamate.

**TEA-SORBATE** • *See* Triethanolamine and Sorbic Acid.

**TEA-STEARATE** • *See* Triethanolamine and Stearic Acid.

**TEA-SULFATE** • *See* Triethanolamine and Sulfuric Acid.

**TEA TREE OIL** • *Melaleuca alternifolia.* Any of various shrubs or trees so named because their leaves are used as a substitute for tea leaves. The essential oil is obtained from the leaves and used as a germicide. ASP

**TECHNICAL WHITE MINERAL OIL** • A mineral supplement for animals. The ratio is 0.06 percent in total feed.

**TERA JAPONICA** • *See* Catechu Extract.

**TERATOGENIC** • From the Greek *teraf* (monster) and Latin *genesis* (origin): the origin or cause of a monster—or defective fetus.

**TERGITOL** • Tergemist. Sodium Etasulfate. Lye peeling additive, poultry scald additive, washing water additive used on fruits, poultry, and vegetables. The FDA limits residue to 0.2 percent in wash water. Moderately toxic by ingestion and skin contact. A skin and eye irritant.

**TERPENELESS OILS** • An essential oil from which the terpene components have been removed by extraction and fractionation, either alone or in combination. The terpeneless grades are more highly concentrated than the original oil. Removal of the terpenes is necessary to inhibit spoilage, particularly of oils derived from citrus. It also makes the compound more soluble in alcohol. *See* Terpenes.

**TERPENE RESINS** • Moisture barrier on soft gelatin capsules and on powders of ascorbic acid *(see)* or its salts. Also used as a component of chewing-gum bases. *See* Terpenes. ASP

**TERPENE RESINS, SYNTHETIC** • Synthetic resins such as ethylene vinyl acetate and polyethylene are used for chewing-gum bases, adhesives, packing, and many other uses in food processing. ASP

**TERPENES** • A class of unsaturated hydrocarbons *(see)*. Its removal from products improves their flavor and gives them a more stable, stronger odor. However, some perfumers feel that the removal of terpenes destroys some of the original odor. Has been used as an antiseptic.

*a***-TERPINENE** • A terpene *(see)* isolated from oil of marjoram, nutmeg, and tea tree oil and other plants. Flavoring additive. ASP

*g***-TERPINENE** • A terpene *(see)* found in coriander oil, tea tree oil, citrus, bergamot, and many other plants. Flavoring additive. ASP

**TERPINEOL, ALPHA AND BETA** • Colorless, viscous liquid with a lilac-like odor, insoluble in mineral oil and slightly soluble in water. It is primarily used as a flavoring additive but is also employed as a denaturant to make alcohol undrinkable. It has been used as an antiseptic. It can be a sensitizer. ASP

**TERPINOLENE** • A synthetic citrus and fruit flavoring additive for beverages, ice cream, ices, candy, and baked goods. *See* Turpentine for toxicity. ASP

**TERPINYL ACETATE** • Colorless liquid, odor suggestive of bergamot and lavender occurs naturally in cardamom. Slightly soluble in water and glycerol. Derived by heating terpineol with acetic acid *(see both)*. Used in berry, lime, orange, cherry, peach, plum, and meat flavorings for beverages, ice cream, ices, candy, and baked goods. *See* Turpentine for toxicity. ASP

**TERPINYL ANTHRANILATE** • A synthetic fruit flavoring additive. Derived by heating terpineol with anthranilic acid *(see both)*. Used as a synthetic fruit flavoring additive for beverages, ice cream, ices, candy, and baked goods. *See* Turpentine for toxicity.

**TERPINYL BUTYRATE** • A synthetic fruit flavoring additive. Derived by heating terpineol with butyric acid *(see both)*. Used as a synthetic fruit flavoring additive for beverages, ice cream, ices, candy, chewing gum, and baked goods. *See* Turpentine for toxicity. ASP

**TERPINYL CINNAMATE** • A synthetic fruit flavoring additive. Derived by heating terpineol with cinnamic acid *(see both)*. Used as a synthetic fruit flavoring additive for beverages, ice cream, ices, candy, and baked goods. *See* Turpentine for toxicity. ASP

**TERPINYL FORMATE** • Formic Acid. A synthetic fruit flavoring additive. Derived by heating terpineol with formic acid *(see both)*. Used as a synthetic fruit flavoring additive for beverages, ice cream, ices, candy, liqueurs, and baked goods. *See* Turpentine for toxicity. ASP

**TERPINYL ISOBUTYRATE** • A synthetic fruit flavoring additive. Derived by heating terpineol with isobutyric acid *(see both)*. Used as a synthetic fruit flavoring additive for beverages, ice cream, ices, candy, and baked goods. *See* Turpentine for toxicity. ASP

**TERPINYL ISOVALERATE** • A synthetic fruit flavoring additive. Derived by heating terpineol with isovaleric acid *(see both)*. Used as a synthetic fruit flavoring additive for beverages, ice cream, ices, candy, and baked goods. *See* Turpentine for toxicity. NIL

**TERPINYL PROPIONATE** • A synthetic fruit flavoring additive, colorless with a lavender odor. Derived by heating terpineol with propionic acid *(see both)*. Used as a synthetic fruit flavoring additive for beverages, ice cream, ices, candy, and baked goods. *See* Turpentine for toxicity. ASP

**TERTIARY BUTYLHYDROQUINONE (TBHQ)** • This antioxidant was put on the market after years of pushing by food manufacturers to get it approved. It contains petroleum-derived butane and is used either alone or in combination with the preservative-antioxidant butylated hydroxyanisole (BHA) and/or butylated hydroxytoluene (BHT) *(see both)*. Hydroquinone combines with oxygen very rapidly and becomes brown when exposed to air. The FDA said that TBHQ must not exceed 0.02 percent of its oil and fat content. Death has occurred from the ingestion of as little as 5 grams. Ingestion of a single gram (a thirtieth of an ounce) has caused nausea, vomiting, ringing in the ears, delirium, a sense of suffocation, and collapse. Industrial workers exposed to the vapors—without obvious systemic effects—suffered clouding of the eye lens. Application to the skin may cause allergic reactions.

**TESTOSTERONE PROPIONATE** • Agovirin. Androgen. Androsan. Testoviron. TP. Uniteston. Vulvan. The male hormone, a steroid *(see)* produced by cells of the testicles. It is used to increase growth in cattle. The FDA limits residue to 0.60 ppb in muscle, 2.6 ppb in fat, 1.9 ppb in kidney, and 1.3 ppb in liver of heifers. IARC review *(see)* and EPA Genetic Toxicology Program *(see)*. Moderately toxic by ingestion. Given by injection or tablet, it stimulates target tissues to develop normally in androgen-deficient men. It is used to treat eunuchs and male hormonal-change symptoms. It is used for breast engorgement in nonnursing mothers and to treat breast cancer in women one to five years postmenopausal. Potential adverse reactions in women include acne, edema, oily skin, weight gain, hairiness, hoarseness, clitoral enlargement, changes in libido, flushing, sweating, and vaginitis with itching. In males, used to treat in prepuberty, premature epiphyseal closure, priapism, growth of body and facial hair, phallic enlargement; in postpuberty, testicular atrophy, scanty sperm, decreased ejaculatory volume, impotence, enlargement of breasts, and epididymitis. In both sexes, edema, gastroenteritis, nausea, vomiting, diarrhea, constipation, changes in appetite, bladder irritability, jaundice, liver toxicity, and high levels of calcium in the blood.

**2,4,4,4-TETRACHLORODIPHENYL SULFONE •** Tetradifon. Tedion. A pesticide. A white crystalline powder. The FDA allows a residue of 10 ppm in dried figs from use on growing crops; 120 ppm in dried hops; 8 ppm in dried tea.

**TETRACHLOROETHYLENE •** Perchlorethylene. Tetrachloroethane. Ethylene Tetrachloride. 1,1,2,2-Tetrachloroethylene. Perchlor. Carbon Bichloride. A clear, colorless, nonflammable liquid with an etherlike smell, it is the main solvent used in the dry-cleaning process. Used in food packaging. The FDA limits residue to 0.3 percent in finished foamed polyethylene. IARC review *(see).* This chemical enters your body when you breathe its vapors in the air. Liquid "perc" can be absorbed through your skin, to a limited extent. The most common effects of overexposure are irritation of the eyes, nose, throat, or skin. Like most organic solvents, it affects the brain the same way as drinking alcohol does. The symptoms of short-term overexposure usually clear up within hours after exposure stops. The mildest effects may start occurring at exposure levels of about 1,090 ppm. Effects occur more quickly and become more noticeable and serious as the exposure levels increase. Effects of this chemical on the nervous system include feeling "high," dizziness, headache, nausea, vomiting, fatigue, weakness, confusion, slurred speech, loss of balance, and poor coordination. At very high exposure (above 5,000 to 10,000) it can cause loss of consciousness and even death. Some studies, according to the California State Hazard Evaluation and Information System, show that overexposure to organic solvents over months or years may have long-lasting and possibly permanent effects on the nervous system. The symptoms of these long-term effects include fatigue, poor muscle coordination, difficulty in concentrating, loss of short-term memory, and personality changes such as increased anxiety, nervousness, and irritability. Tetrachloroethylene causes cancer in laboratory animals at exposure levels close to the level of what is legally allowed in the workplace. Contamination of drinking water with this chemical in Massachusetts and New Jersey has been implicated in clusters of leukemia and birth defects among residents. In any case, do not use perc around an open flame or intense ultraviolet light. Like most solvents containing chlorine, perc can break down into very hazardous compounds such as phosgene, hydrochloric acid, and chlorine.

**TETRACHLOROISOPHTHALONITRILE** • Bravo. Termil. TCPN. A fungicide used on broccoli, cabbage, cantaloupe, carrots, cauliflower, celery, citrus oil, cucumber, lettuce, onions, potatoes, tomatoes, and watermelon. Fungicide residue tolerance of 10 ppm in citrus oil. IARC review *(see)*. Cyanide products are on the Community Right-To-Know List *(see)* and the EPA Genetic Toxicology Program *(see)*. Causes cancer in experimental animals. Mildly toxic by ingestion.

**TETRACHLORVINPHOS** • A white powder that inhibits the transmission of nerve signals, it is used as an insecticide. Used as a feed additive for cattle and swine. The FDA limits residue to 0.00015 pound per 100 pounds of body weight of cattle and horses when used in animal feed. Limitation of 0.00011 pound per 100 pounds of body weight of swine when used in animal feed. Found to be carcinogenic in feed by the National Cancer Institute. On the Community Right-To-Know List *(see)*. Poisonous by ingestion. Also caused reproductive problems in experimental animals.

**TETRACYCLINE** • Achromycin. Antibiotic introduced in 1953, tetracycline antibiotics are among the most widely prescribed. Used to treat cattle, chickens, lambs, swine, and turkeys. The FDA limits residues to 0.25 ppm in calves, swine, sheep, chickens, and turkeys. In humans, tetracyclines are used to treat acne, bronchitis, pneumonia, syphilis, gonorrhea, inflammation of the tube that carries urine, and to prevent chest infections. Also used to treat Rocky Mountain spotted fever, brucellosis, relapsing fever, cholera, trachoma, and arthritis due to infection, syphilis, gonorrhea, chlamydia, trachoma, shigellosis, rickettsia, and mycoplasma. Tetracyclines are also used to prevent and treat eye infections. Potential adverse effects of oral tetracyclines include nausea, vomiting, and diarrhea, drop in white blood cells, dizziness, headache, pressure on the brain, sore throat, sore tongue, trouble swallowing, loss of appetite, colitis, inflammation around the anus, liver problems, kidney problems, and diarrhea. Tetracyclines may cause sensitivity to sunlight and result in a rash and discoloration of the skin. If tetracycline is taken during pregnancy, a child may have discolored teeth. Oral tetracyclines must be used with extreme caution if kidney or liver problems are present. The effects of antibiotics such as tetracycline in meat eaten by humans is a matter of controversy. It is believed by many scientists that it causes resistance to antibiotics used by humans and may cause allergic reactions in sensitive persons, even in minute amounts.

*d*-**TETRADECALACTONE** • Flavoring with a coconutlike taste. ASP
**TETRADECANAL** • *See* Myristaldehyde.
**TETRADECANOIC ACID** • *See* Ethyl Myristate.
**(Z)-8-TETRADECENAL** • A flavoring for baked goods, gelatins, ices, fish

products, reconstituted vegetables, seasonings, and many other food products. Determined GRAS by FEMA *(see)*.

**TETRADECYL ALDEHYDE** • *See* Myristaldehyde.

**TETRAETHYLENE GLYCOL** • Colorless or pale yellow liquid used as a finishing additive on twine used to tie meat. Mildly toxic by ingestion. *See* Glycols.

**TETRAETHYLENEPENTAMINE CROSSLINKED WITH EPICHLORO-HYDRIN** • Used in processing. *See* Epichlorhydrin. NUL

**1,2,5,6-TETRAHYDROCUMINIC ACID** • Flavoring with a sweaty odor. *See* Cuminic Acid. NIL

**4,5,6,7-TETRAHYDRO-3,6-DIMETHYLBENZOFURAN** • Synthetic flavoring. ASP

**TETRAHYDROFURAN** • Butylene oxide. Oxolane. A colorless liquid with an etherlike odor, it is used as a solvent for packaging materials. The FDA limits it to 1.5 percent of film. Moderately toxic by ingestion. Causes mutations in experimental animals. Human systemic effects by inhalation. Affects consciousness. Irritating to eyes and mucous membranes.

**TETRAHYDROFURFURYL ACETATE** • *See* Furfural. ASP

**TETRAHYDROFURFURYL ALCOHOL** • A liquid that absorbs water and is flammable in air. A solvent for cosmetic fats, waxes, and resins. Mixes with water, ether, and acetone. Mildly irritating to the skin and mucous membranes. *See* Furfural. ASP

**TETRAHYDROFURFURYL BUTYRATE** • Butyric Acid. A synthetic chocolate, honey, and maple flavoring additive for beverages, ice cream, ices, candy, arid baked goods. May be irritating to the skin and mucous membranes. ASP

**TETRAHYDROFURFURYL PROPIONATE** • Propionic Acid. A synthetic chocolate, honey, and maple flavoring additive for beverages, ice cream, ices, candy, and baked goods. Also used as a solvent for intravenous drugs. Moderately irritating to skin and mucous membranes. ASP

**TETRAHYDROGERANYL HYDROXYL STEARATE** • See Stearic Acid and Hydroxylation.

**TETRAHYDROLINALOOL** • Colorless liquid with a floral odor used as a flavoring additive in various foods. *See* Linalool. ASP

**TETRAHYDRO-4-METHYL-2-(2-METHYLPROPEN-1-YL)PYRAN** • Synthetic flavoring. ASP

**TETRAHYDRO-PSEUDO-IONONE** • Synthetic flavoring. ASP

**5,6,7,8-TETRAHYDROQUINOXALINE** • A musty, nutty flavor that occurs naturally in cocoa, coffee, filberts, peanuts, and sesame seed. Used in cheese, chocolate, corn, nut, pecan, and popcorn flavorings. ASP

**TETRAHYDROXYPROPYLETHYLENEDIAMINE** • Clear, colorless, thick liquid, a component of the bacteria-killing substance in sugarcane.

It is strongly alkaline and is used as a solvent and preservative. It may be irritating to the skin and mucous membranes and may cause skin sensitization.

**TETRAIODOFLUORESCEIN SODIUM** • FD and C Red No. 3. Brown powder used as a color additive for candy, cherries, and confections. EPA Genetic Toxicology Program *(see)*. Moderately toxic by ingestion. See FD and C Red No. 3.

**TETRAKIS (HYDROXYMETHYL) PHOSPHONIUM CHLORIDE** • Catalyst, humectant, emulsifier, and plasticizer.

**ALPHA-{P-(1,1,3,3-TETRAMETHYLBUTYL)PHENYL}-OMEGA-HYDROXYPOLY(OXYETHYLE** • Polymer *(see)* on EU list for priority study. EAF

**ALPHA-(P-(1,1,3,3-TETRAMETHYLBUTYL)PHENYL)-OMEGA-HYDROXYPOLY(OXYETHYLENE)(GREATER THAN 1 MOL)** • *See* Polyethylene Glycol. NIL

**TETRAMETHYL DECYNEDIOL** • *See* Fatty Alcohols.

**TETRAMETHYL ETHYLCYCLOHEXENONE (MIXTURE OF ISOMERS)** • Synthetic flavoring. ASP

**1,5,5,9-TETRAMETHYL-13-OXATRICYCLO(8.3.0.0(4,9))TRIDECANE** • Synthetic flavoring used in cigarettes. ASP

**2,3,5,6-TETRAMETHYLPYRAZINE** • Synthetic flavoring with a nutty, musty, chocolate odor; chocolate taste. ASP

**TETRAMETHYL PYRAZINE** • White crystals or powder with a fermented soybean odor. Used as a flavoring additive in various foods. Moderately toxic by ingestion. GRAS

**2,4,5,8-TETRAMETHYL-1,2,5,6-TETROXOCANE** • Metason. SlugTox. A pesticide to kill slugs and other parasites on strawberries. Human poison by ingestion. Can cause convulsions. Causes mutations in experimental animals.

**TETRAMETHYLTHIURAM** • Sprayed on some bananas. Seed disinfectant and fungicide. Can cause contact dermatitis. Irritating to mucous membranes.

**TETRA POTASSIUM PHOSPHATE (TKPP)** • An emulsifier. *See* Tetrasodium Pyrophosphate.

**TETRA POTASSIUM PYROPHOSPHATE** • An emulsifier used in cheese and as a sequestering additive in cheese and ice cream. Also used in cleaning compounds, oil-well drilling, water treatment, and as a general sequestering additive to remove rust stains. Produced by molecular dehydration of dibasic sodium phosphate. It is alkaline and irritating and ingestion can cause nausea, diarrhea, and vomiting. GRAS for packaging. *See* Tetrasodium Pyrophosphate.

**TETRASODIUM EDTA** • Sodium Edetate. Powdered sodium salt that reacts with metals. A sequestering additive and chelating additive *(see both)*.

Can deplete the body of calcium if taken internally. *See* Ethylenediamine Tetraacetic Acid.

**TETRASODIUM PYROPHOSPHATE (TSPP)** • Used in cheese emulsification and as a sequestering additive in cheese and ice cream. Also used in cleansing compounds, oil-well drilling, water treatment, and as a general sequestering additive to remove rust stains. A sequestering additive, clarifying additive, and buffering additive for shampoos. Produced by molecular dehydration of dibasic sodium phosphate. Insoluble in alcohol. It is alkaline and irritating and ingestion can cause nausea, diarrhea, and vomiting. GRAS for packaging.

**TEXTURIZER** • A chemical used to improve the texture of various foods. For instance, canned tomatoes, canned potatoes, and canned apple slices tend to become soft and fall apart unless, for example, the texturizer calcium chloride *(see)* of its salts are added, which keep the product firm.

**TFC** • Abbreviation for tricloflucarban, a disinfectant.

**THALOSE** • A blend of food-grade acidulants *(see)* that contains propylene glycol and citric, lactic, phosphoric, and tartaric acids *(see all)*, and water and salt. Adding this compound to sugar permits a reduction in the amount required to achieve a desired sweetness (1 ounce of liquid Thalose added to 32 pounds of sugar causes the perceived sweetness to be increased by 90 percent). One pint added to sugar will result in a saving of 500 pounds of sugar without reducing sweetness. Thalose itself is not sweet and does not alter the flavor or aroma of the foods to which it is added. It does not contribute calories but will reduce the caloric level of the end product by lowering the amount of carbohydrates in the compound. Thalose can be used in beverages, bakery and confectionery products, and in ice cream, as long as the physical properties of the sugar are not needed (sugar is often used as a thickening additive and texturizer). All of the substances contained in this extender are GRAS and comply with the FDA provision for food-grade ingredients.

**THAMNIDIUM ELEGANS** • A grayish white mold used for aging meat. It is related to the tropical bread mold.

**THAUMATIN** • A mixture of intensely sweet-tasting proteins extracted from the fruit of a West African plant, *Thaumatococcus daniellii*. It has about two thousand to three thousand times the sweetness of sugar. It does contain calories. The fruits of the plant have been used for centuries by the West Africans as a source of sweetness. It is also sold in Japan. Because of problems with stability, taste profile, and compatibility, thaumatin is used primarily as a flavor enhancer at levels below the sweet-taste threshold. EAF. E

**THAUMATIN B, RECOMBINANT** • Genetically altered amino acid. On priority list to be evaluated. EAF

**THBP** • Antioxidant in fats and oils. *See* 2-4-5-Trihydroxybutyrophenone.

**THEASPIRANE** • Intense fresh-fruity flavoring. It is used in essence of rose, haw, litchi, strawberry, and tobacco. NUL

**THEINE** • *See* Caffeine.

**THEOBROMA OIL** • Cacao Butter. Cocoa Butter. Yellowish white solid with chocolatelike taste and odor. Derived from the cacao bean. Widely used in confections. May cause allergic reactions in the sensitive.

**THEOBROMINE** • The alkaloid found in cocoa, cola nuts, tea, and chocolate products, closely related to caffeine. It is used as a diuretic, smooth muscle relaxant, heart stimulant, and blood vessel dilator. In 1992, the FDA proposed a ban on theobromine sodium salicylate in oral menstrual drug products because it has not been shown to be safe and effective for its stated claims. ASP

**THERMALLY OXIDIZED SOYA BEAN OIL INTERACTED WITH MONO and DIGLYCERIDES OF FATTY ACIDS** • *See* Soybean Oil and Fatty Acids. E

**THIABENDAZOLE HYDROCHLORIDE** • A mold retardant used on animal feed, apples, bananas, beef, citrus fruit, lamb, milk, pears, pheasants, pork, potato processing waste, rice hulls. FDA limits are 0.1 ppm in cattle, goats, sheep, pheasant, and swine; 0.05 ppm in milk; 33 ppm in dried apple pomace; 150 ppm in dry or wet grape pomace; 30 ppm in potato processing waste; and 8 ppm in rice hulls when used for animal feed. Moderately toxic by ingestion. E

**THIAMINE** • See Thiamine Hydrochloride. ASP

**THIAMINE HYDROCHLORIDE** • A co-enzyme of vitamin $B_1$. A white crystalline powder used as a dietary supplement in prepared breakfast cereals, peanut butter, poultry, stuffing, baby cereals, skimmed milk, bottled soft drinks, enriched flours, enriched farina, cornmeal, enriched macaroni and noodle products, and enriched bread and rolls. Acts as a helper in important energy-yielding reactions in the body. Practically all $B_1$ sold is synthetic. The vitamin is destroyed by alkalies and alkaline drugs such as phenobarbital. GRAS. ASP

**THIAMINE MONONITRATE** • A co-enzyme of vitamin $B_1$. A white crystalline powder used as a diet supplement and to enrich flour. GRAS. ASP

**THIAMUTILIN** • Tiamulin. Crystals from acetone *(see)* used in animal feed and as an animal drug to combat bacterial infections. Moderately toxic by ingestion and injections under the skin.

**THIAZOLE** • Colorless or pale yellow liquid. Widely used in the manufacture of synthetic flavorings for drinks, frozen food, nuts, meat, and spices Used in organic synthesis of fungicides, dyes, and rubber accelerators. ASP

**2-(THIAZOL-4-YL)BENZIMIDAZOLE** • Thiabendazole. Arbotect. TBDZ. Mycozol. White to tan odorless compound used as a fungicide in animal feed and for citrus fruit and to control fungal diseases in seed potatoes. Used therapeutically in animals to combat worms and fungus infections. EPA Genetic Toxicology Program. Poisonous by ingestion. Caused birth defects in experimental animals.

**THIAZOLYLSULFANILAMIDE** • Sulzol. Thiazamide. An antibiotic used to treat infections in swine. EPA Genetic Toxicology Program. Human poison.

**THIBETOLIDE** • *See* Pentadecalactone.

**THICKENERS** • Many natural gums and starches are used to add body to mixtures. Pectin *(see)*, for instance, which is used in fruits naturally low in this gelling additive, enables manufacturers to produce jams and jellies of a marketable thickness. Algin (*see* Alginates) is used to make salad dressings that will not be runny. Also used to add body to lotions and creams. Those usually employed include such natural gums as sodium alginate and pectins.

**THIDIAZURON** • A pesticide used on cottonseed hulls. The FDA's residue tolerance is 0.05 ppm in milk; 0.1 ppm in eggs; and 0.2 ppm as residue in meat, fat, and meat by-products of cattle, sheep, and poultry.

**2-THIENYL DISULFIDE** • Synthetic flavoring. ASP

**2-THIENYL MERCAPTAN** • A synthetic flavoring additive that occurs naturally in coffee. Used in coffee flavoring for candy and baked goods. ASP

**THIETHYL CITRATE** • An antioxidant used primarily in dried egg whites. *See* Citric Acid. GRAS

**THIOBIS (DODECYL PROPIONATE)** • White crystalline flakes with a sweet odor used as an antioxidant in fats, oils, and packaging materials. FDA regulations limit to 0.005 percent migrating from food packaging. An eye irritant.

**THIOCYANATE** • Colorless or white crystals derived from cyanide. Used in animal feeds as a growth stimulant.

**THIODICARB** • An insecticide used on cottonseed and soybean hulls. The FDA permits 0.8 ppm on cottonseed hulls and 0.4 ppm on soybean hulls. *See* Carbamate.

**2,2′-(THIODIMETHYLENE)-DIFURAN** • Synthetic roastedlike flavoring. ASP

**THIODIPROPIONIC ACID** • An acid freely soluble in hot water, alcohol, and acetone. Used as an antioxidant in general food use. Percent of fat or oil, including essential oil, content of food is up to 0.02. The final report to the FDA of the Select Committee on GRAS Substances stated in 1980 that there is no evidence in the available information that it is a hazard to the public when used as it is now and it should continue its GRAS status with limitations on the amounts that can be added to food. NEW

**THIOGERANIOL** • Synthetic flavoring. *See* Gerianol.

**THIOPHANATE, METHYL** • A fungicide. The FDA residue tolerance in or on dried apple pomace feed to animals is 40 ppm.

**THIOUREA** • A banned antioxidant. BANNED

**THISTLE, BLESSED** • Holy Thistle. Extract of the prickly plant *Cnicus benedictus*. Cleared for use as a natural flavoring in alcoholic beverages only. Also called cardin, it is an annual herb. The plant is a native of southern Europe and is cultivated in gardens all over the world. It has been used in medicine since A.D. 100. Once believed to be a panacea, it has been credited with reducing excess fluid. EAF

**THREONINE** • L form only. An essential amino acid *(see)*; the last to be discovered (1935). Prevents the buildup of fat on the liver. Occurs in whole eggs, skim milk, casein, and gelatin. On the FDA list for further study. GRAS. ASP

**4-THUJANOL** • An alcohol from thuja oil *(see)*. ASP

**THUJA OIL** • A constituent of many essential oils. Usually derived from the needles of white cedar. Colorless liquid, almost insoluble in water. Ingestion may cause convulsions. It is used in flavorings and perfumery.

**THYME EXTRACT** • Natural flavor isolated by physical methods. *See* Thyme Oil. EAF

**THYME OIL** • A seasoning from the dried leaves and flowering tops of the wild creeping thyme grown in Eurasia and throughout the United States, *Thymus vulgaris* and *Thymus zygis*. Colorless, yellow, or red, with a pleasant odor. Used in sausage, spice, and thyme flavorings for beverages, ice cream, ices, candy, baked goods, chewing gum, condiments, meats, and soups. Used as a flavoring in cough medicines. May cause contact dermatitis and hay fever. GRAS. ASP

**THYME OLEORESIN** • Dark greenish brown viscous semisolid that smells like fresh thyme. ASP

**THYME, WHITE OIL** • Obtained from the plant and used in fruit, liquor, and thyme. Used in fruit, peppermint, and spice flavorings for beverages, ice cream, ices, candy, baked goods, and chewing gum. Oral dose as medicine is 0.067 grams. It can cause vomiting, diarrhea, dizziness, and cardiac depression when taken in sufficient amounts. *See* Thyme Oil. GRAS

**THYME, WILD or CREEPING EXTRACT** • *Thymus serpyllum*. NUL

**THYMOL** • Obtained from the essential oil of lavender, origanum oil, and other volatile oils. It destroys mold, preserves anatomical specimens, and is a topical antifungal additive with a pleasant aromatic odor. Used in fruit, peppermint, and spice flavorings for beverages, ice cream, ices, candy, baked goods, and chewing gum. It is omitted from hypoallergenic cosmetics because it can cause allergic reactions. Oral dose as medicine is 0.067 grams. It can cause vomiting, diarrhea, dizziness, and cardiac depression when taken in sufficient amounts. GRAS. ASP

**THYMOL IODIDE** • A dietary supplement. In animal feed a source of trace mineral. GRAS

**THYMUS CAPITATUS** • Spanish Origanum. Flavoring. *See* Origanum Oil.

**THYROID** • The thyroid is a butterfly-shaped gland located in the neck with a "wing" on either side of the windpipe. The gland produces thyroxine, which controls the rates of chemical reactions in the body. Generally, the more thyroxine, the faster the body works. Thyroxine needs iodine to function.

**TIAMULIN** • *See* Thiamutilin.

**TIGLIC ACID** • *See* Allyl Tiglate.

**TIN CHLORIDE** • Colorless crystals used as an antioxidant and reducing additive *(see)* in asparagus and in carbonated beverages. The FDA limits it to 20 ppm in asparagus packed in glass. EPA Genetic Toxicology Program *(see)*. Poison by ingestion.

**TINCTURE** • Solution in alcohol of the flavors derived from plants obtained by mashing or boiling.

**TIPA** • The abbreviation for triisopropanolamine *(see)*.

**TIPA-STEARATE** • *See* Stearic Acid.

**TITANIUM DIOXIDE** • Occurs naturally in minerals. Used chiefly as a white pigment and as an opacifier; also a white pigment for candy, gum, and marker ink. A pound has been ingested without apparent ill effects. In high concentrations the dust may cause lung damage. It has been permanently listed for use as a food color with a limit of 1 percent by weight of finished food since 1966. ASP. E

**TITANIUM HYDROXIDE** • *See* Titanium Dioxide.

**TITANIUM OXIDE** • *See* Titanium Dioxide.

**TOASTED PARTIALLY DEFATTED COOKED COTTONSEED FLOUR** • Used as a food coloring. It is exempt from certification.

**ALPHA TOCOPHEROL ACETATE** • A dietary supplement. *See* Tocopherols. GRAS. NEW

**ALPHA TOCOPHERYL ACID SUCCINATE** • Vitamin E Succinate. Obtained by the distillation of edible vegetable oils and used as a dietary supplement and as an antioxidant for fats and oils. ASP

**TOCOPHEROLS** • Vitamin E. Obtained by the vacuum distillation of edible vegetable oils. Protects fat in the body's tissues from abnormal breakdown. Experimental evidence shows vitamin E may protect the heart and blood vessels and retard aging. Used as a dietary supplement and as an antioxidant for essential oils, rendered animal fats, or a combination of such fats with vegetable oils. Helps form normal red blood cells, muscle, and other tissues. The final report to the FDA of the Select Committee on GRAS Substances stated in 1980 that it should continue its GRAS status with no limitations other than good manufacturing practices. ASP

**TOCOPHEROL-RICH EXTRACT** • *See* Tocopherols. E

**TOLERANCE** • The ability to live with an allergen.

**a-TOLUALDEHYDE** • *See* Phenylacetaldehyde.

**TOLUALDEHYDE GLYCERYL ACETAL** • A synthetic chocolate, fruit, cherry, coconut, and vanilla flavoring additive for beverages, ice cream, ices, candy, and baked goods.

**TOLUALDEHYDES (MIXED o, m, p)** • Synthetic berry, loganberry, fruit, cherry, muscatel, peach, apricot, nut, almond, and vanilla flavorings for beverages, ice cream, ices, candy, baked goods, chewing gum, gelatin desserts, and maraschino cherries. ASP

**TOLU BALSAM** • Extract and Gum. Extract from the Peruvian or Indian plant, *Myroxylon* spp. Contains cinnamic acid and benzoic acid *(see both)*. Used in butter, butterscotch, cherry, and spice flavorings for beverages, ice cream, ices, candy, baked goods, and chewing gum. The gum is used in fruit, maple, and vanilla flavorings for beverages, ice cream, ices, candy, baked goods, and syrups. Mildly antiseptic and may be mildly irritating to the skin. ASP

**TOLUENE** • Toluol. Methyl Benzene. Used in water-purifying additives, to remove odors in cheese, and in a number of food-processing compounds. Also used as a solvent for paints, nail polish, lacquers, thinners, coatings, shellacs, adhesives, metal cleaners, rust preservatives, fuel system antifreezes, asphalt removers, flame retardants, high-octane gasoline blends, rotogravure printing processes, and glue, and is being used to replace more toxic benzene solvents in many products. Obtained from petroleum or by distilling balsam Tolu. May cause mild anemia if ingested, and it is narcotic in high concentrations. Being tested at the Frederick Cancer Research Center for possible cancer-causing effects. It can cause liver damage and is irritating to the skin and respiratory tract.

While halogenated hydrocarbons like toluene are assumed responsible for health risks, the long-term effects of low-level exposure to them in drinking water of at least twenty cities is unknown. There is concern about the role of toluene on the brain and nervous system because symptoms have been observed in workers chronically exposed in jobs such as spray painting. The chronic high-dose exposures seen in toluene abuse such as glue sniffers have been associated epidemiologically with sudden death secondary to irregular heartbeat, liver, and neurologic disorders. The current U.S. standard is 200 ppm in eight hours and maximum peaks up to 500 ppm for ten minutes. NIOSH *(see)* currently recommends that toluene exposures be limited to 100 ppm. Brief exposure to 100 ppm causes statistical impairment of reflexes and thinking. Exposure to 800 ppm causes severe fatigue, confusion, and staggering that may persist for several days. Exposure to 10,000 ppm can cause loss of consciousness and death.

**o-TOLUENETHIOL** • Thiocresol. Cream to white, moist crystals with a musty odor. A skin irritant. Used as an intermediate *(see)* and as a germicide. ASP

**p-TOLYLACETALDEHYDE** • Synthetic flavoring. See Tolyl Acetate. ASP

**TOLYL ACETATE** • Acetic Acid. A synthetic butter, caramel, fruit, honey, nut, and spice flavoring for beverages, ice cream, ices, candy, baked goods, chewing gum, and gelatin desserts.

*o*-**TOLYL ACETATE** • Acetic Acid. A synthetic butter, caramel, fruit, honey, and cherry flavoring for beverages, ice cream, ices, candy, baked goods, chewing gum, and gelatin desserts. ASP

*p*-**TOLYL ACETATE** • Acetic Acid. A synthetic butter, caramel, fruit, honey, nut, and spice flavoring for beverages, ice cream, ices, candy, baked goods, chewing gum, and condiments. ASP

**4-(*p*-TOLYL)-2-BUTANONE** • A synthetic fruit flavoring for beverages, ice cream, ices, candy, and baked goods. ASP

*p*-**TOLYL ISOBUTYRATE** • A synthetic fruit flavoring for beverages, ice cream, ices, candy, and baked goods. ASP

*p*-**TOLYL LAURATE** • Dodecanoic Acid. A synthetic butter, caramel, fruit, honey, and nut flavoring for beverages, ice cream, ices, candy, and baked goods. NIL

*p*-**TOLYL PHENYLACETATE** • A synthetic butter, caramel, fruit, honey, and nut flavoring for beverages, ice cream, ices, candy, and baked goods. ASP

**TOLYLACETALDEHYDE** • A synthetic berry, loganberry, fruit, cherry, muscatel, peach, apricot, nut, almond, and vanilla flavoring additive for beverages, ice cream, ices, candy, baked goods, gelatin desserts, chewing gum, and maraschino cherries.

*p*-**TOLYALDEHYDE** • Colorless liquid derived from benzene. Used in perfumes and flavoring additives.

**2-(*p*-TOLYL) PROPIONALDEHYDE** • A synthetic caraway flavoring additive for beverages, ice cream, ices, candy, baked goods, and liqueurs. ASP

**O-TOLYL SALICYLATE** • Synthetic flavoring. NIL

**TOMATO EXTRACT** • Tomatine. Extract from the fruit of the tomato, *Lycopersicon esculentum.* Used as a fungicide and as a precipitating additive. Nontoxic.

**TONKA** • Tonka Bean. Coumarouna Bean. Black-brown seeds with a wrinkled surface and brittle, shining or fatty skins. A vanillalike odor and a bitter taste. Used in the production of natural coumarin *(see)* in flavoring extracts. Food containing any added coumarin as such or as a constituent of tonka beans or tonka extract is deemed to be adulterated. Banned from food in United States because of its coumarin content. *See* Coumarin.

**TORMENTIL EXTRACT** • The extract of the roots of *Potentilla erecta.*

**TORULA YEAST** • Dried *Candida utils.* Flavoring in food. *See* Yeast.

**TOTAL CARB** • Label listing for total carbohydrates. *See* Carbohydrates.

**TOUCH OF NATURE** • A sweetener made from both sap extracts and crushed leaves of nature's taste tree, grown in the Brazilian rain forest.

**TOXAPHENE** • Chlorinated camphene containing 67–69 percent chlorine. Yellow waxy solid with a pleasant pine odor, it is used as an insecticide in soybean oil. FDA regulations set a residue tolerance of 6 ppm in soybean oil from use on growing crop. Human poison by ingestion. Can be absorbed through the skin. Causes cancer and birth defects in experimental animals. Lethal amounts of toxaphene can enter the body through the mouth, lungs, and skin.

**TRAGACANTH** • *See* Gum Tragacanth. GRAS. ASP. E

**TRAILBLAZER** • A fat-based replacer for fat. It is a microparticulated protein product (MPP) similar to Simplesse *(see)*. It is made from whey protein or milk and egg protein. It has about 1 to 4 calories per gram and is approved for use in frozen dessert-type foods. The FDA says that whey-based MPP conforms to the definition of whey protein concentrate *(see)* such as the fat replacer Dairy-Lo, a GRAS substance. Therefore, it can be used in other foods including reduced-fat versions of butter, sour cream, cheese, yogurt, salad dressing, margarine, mayonnaise, baked goods, coffee creamers, soups, and sauces.

**TRALOMETHRIN** • An insecticide. FDA residue tolerance in or on cottonseed oil 0.2 ppm; on or in cottonseed, 0.02 ppm; on or in soybeans 0.05 ppm.

**TRANS FATS** • "Trans" means "across" in Latin. *See* Trans Fatty Acids.

**TRANS FATTY ACIDS** • A polyunsaturated *(see)* fatty acid in which some of the missing hydrogen atoms have been put back by hydrogenation. Trans fatty acids are the building blocks of hydrogenated fats. Trans fatty acids, also known as trans fats, are found naturally in small quantities in some foods, including beef, pork, lamb, butter, and milk. But most trans fatty acids in the diet come from hydrogenated foods. Oils are hydrogenated to give a more desirable quality to food or make foods last longer. Hydrogenation enables some types of peanut butter to have a creamier consistency and is used to make stick margarine from vegetable oil. In the 1960s, doctors told us to eat margarine instead of butter to lower our cholesterol levels and protect our hearts. The amount of butter consumed by Americans is now half of what it was in 1961. In 1992, reports from the U.S. Department of Agriculture researchers and scientific institutions in Europe stated that margarines, which develop trans fatty acids during the processing to form "sticks," may be as bad or worse for our cholesterol levels and our hearts. The sale of margarine immediately plummeted after publicity about the research. In the body, trans fatty acids act like saturated fats and tend to raise blood cholesterol levels. It's wise to be prudent in how much you consume, especially if you have high cholesterol levels already. What types of foods contain trans fatty acids? Look on the label for the phrase "partially hydrogenated vegetable oil," which is found in stick margarine, vegetable shortening, and some prepared foods like cakes, cookies, crackers, and commercially fried foods. Scientific reports have confirmed the relationship between trans fat and an increased risk of coronary heart disease. On July 11, 2003, the FDA published a final rule requiring manufacturers to list trans fatty acids, or trans fat, on the label. Manufacturers have until January 1, 2006, to list trans fat on the nutrition label. The FDA estimates that by three years after that date, trans fat labeling will have prevented from 600 to 1,200 cases of coronary heart disease and 250 to 500 deaths each year. *See also* Polyunsaturated Fats and Monounsaturated Fats.

**TREFOIL, SWEET** • *Meliotus caerulea. Trigonella caerulea.* Powdered leaves and flowers used in Switzerland to flavor and color cheese, also to flavor breads, soups, potato dishes, greens. Grown as a fodder crop and spice in most Mediterranean countries. Related to fenugreek. NUL

**TRENBOLONE** • A synthetic anabolic steroid. A male sex hormone given to cattle to "build up," to stimulate growth, weight gain, strength, and appetite. Abuse of these drugs has caused problems, especially among young athletes who wish to build muscle and strength. Uncontrolled use can cause liver damage and cancer. On February 27, 1991, anabolic steroids became controlled drugs requiring security ordering and record keeping for humans. Increased tumors were evident in long-term studies of rats fed trenbolone. The FDA limits residues to 50 ppb in the muscle of beef, 100 ppb in liver, 300 ppb in kidney, and 400 ppb in fat in cattle. The FAO/WHO *(see)* set a marginal no-effect level at 0.1 mg/kg diet equal to approximately 2 mg/kg of body weight. The committee set an ADI *(see)* of 0–0.02 mg/kg of body weight. The European Union will not permit United States red meat to be imported with this growth promoter.

**TRENBOLONE ACETATE and ESTRADIOL** • Hormones used as implants in feedlot cattle. As residues in cattle, *see* Trenbolone and Estradiol.

**TRIACETIN** • Glyceryl Triacetate. Primarily a solvent for hair dyes. Also a fixative in perfume and used in toothpaste. A colorless, somewhat oily liquid with a slight fatty odor and a bitter taste. Obtained from adding acetate to glycerin *(see both)*. Soluble in water and miscible with alcohol. Large subcutaneous injections are lethal to rats. GRAS. ASP

**TRIACETYL GLYCERIN** • Colorless, oily liquid with a fatty odor and taste, it is used as a flavoring additive, a humectant *(see)*, plasticizer, solvent, and carrier for food additives. Used in baked goods, baking mixes, beverages, candy, chewing gum, confections, fillings, frostings, frozen dairy desserts, dessert mixes, gelatins, and puddings. Poison by ingestion. An eye irritant.

**TRIAMMONIUM CITRATE** • Citric acid triammonium salt. Buffering agent. E

**TRIBASIC CALCIUM PHOSPHATE** • Tricalcium Diorthophosphate. Tricalcium Phosphate. An anticaking additive and calcium supplement in grain products used in packaged cake mixes, candy, baked goods, gelatin desserts, powdered beverage mixes, seasoning mixes, powdered soups, and sugar. Too much phosphorus in the form of phosphates from processed foods could upset the body's mineral balance, particularly calcium, and could adversely affect teeth, bones, and kidneys.

**TRIBROMSALAN** • TBS. 3,4',5-Tribromosalicylanilide. Used in medicated cosmetics; an antiseptic and fungicide. Irritating to the skin and may cause allergic reaction when skin is exposed to the sun. Salicylanilide is an antifungal compound used to treat ringworm. TBS is in the most popular soaps to kill skin bacteria. Used as a germicide, frequently replacing hexachlorophene.

**TRIBUTYL ACETYLCITRATE** • Synthetic fruit flavoring additive for beverages. NIL

**TRIBUTYL CITRATE** • The triester of butyl alcohol and citric acid *(see both)*, it is a pale yellow, odorless liquid used as a plasticizer, antifoam additive, and solvent for nitrocellulose. Low toxicity.

**TRIBUTYLCRESYLBUTANE** • Used as a stabilizer. *See* Phenol.

**TRIBUTYRIN** • Glyceryl Tributyrate. A colorless, somewhat oily liquid that occurs naturally in butter. It has a characteristic odor and bitter taste. It is soluble in alcohol. Used as a flavoring additive in beverages, ice cream, candy, baked goods, margarine, and puddings. Moderately toxic by ingestion. *See* Glycerol and Butyric Acid. GRAS.

**TRICALCIUM PHOSPHATE** • The calcium salt of phosphate *(see)*. An anticaking additive in table salt and vanilla powder, and a dietary supplement. Used as a bleaching additive in flour at not more than 6 ppm by weight alone or in combination with potassium alum, calcium sulfate *(see)*, and other compounds. Also used as a polishing additive in dentifrices. *See* Calcium Phosphate. GRAS

**TRICALCIUM SILICATE** • Used in table salt and baking powder as an anticaking additive up to 2 percent. On the FDA list to be studied for subacute, mutagenic, teratogenic, and reproductive effects. GRAS

**TRICETETH-5 PHOSPHATE** • *See* Phosphoric Acid and Cetyl Alcohol.

**TRICHLOROETHYLENE (TCE)** • Residue in decaffeinated coffee powder. Used in spice oleoresins as a solvent. Moderate exposure can cause symptoms similar to alcohol inebriation, and its analgesic and anesthetic properties make it useful for short operations. High concentrations have a narcotic effect. Deaths have been attributed to irregular heart rhythm. Tests conducted by the National Cancer Institute showed that this chlorinated hydrocarbon caused cancer of the liver in mice. Rats failed to show significant response, a fact which may be attributed to the cancer-resistance of the strain used. Despite the species difference in cancer response, the NCI concluded that the TCE test clearly showed the compound caused liver cancer in mice. The findings are considered definitive for animal studies and serve as a warning of possible carcinogenicity in humans. IARC review *(see)*. However, the extent of the possible human risk cannot be predicted reliably on the basis of these studies alone. A related compound vinyl, chloride *(see)*, does cause liver cancer in humans. FDA residue tolerance in decaffeinated ground coffee, 25 ppm (0.0025 percent); decaffeinated soluble (instant) coffee extract, 10 ppm (0.001 percent); spice oleoresins, 30 ppm. In 1997, the NTP *(see)* put it on the list for review as a carcinogen. NUL

**(2,2,2-TRICHLORO-1-HYDROXYETHYL)DIMETHYL PHOSPHO-NATE** • Anthon. Chloroftalm. Chlorophos. Chlorofos. Dimetox. Dipterax. Dipterex. Trichlorfon. Widely used insecticide for the control of flies and roaches and also to fight worms in animals. Used in animal feed and on citrus pulp. FDA limits it to 2.5 ppm in dried citrus pulp when used for animal feed. Inhibits nerve signals. Poison by ingestion, inhalation, and other routes except skin.

**TRICHLOROMETAFOS** • Dermaphos. Ronnel. Fenchlorphos. White powder widely used as an insecticide in animal feed. Chlorophenol compounds are on the Community Right-To-Know List *(see)*. Poisonous by ingestion. Causes birth defects in experimental animals. Inhibits nerve transmission.

***n*-TRICHLOROMETHYLMERCAPTO-4-CYCLOHEXENE-1,2-DICARBOXIMIDE** • A fumigant. *See* Captan.

**TRICLOCARBAN** • Prepared from aniline and chlorophenyl isocyanate, it is used as an antiseptic in soaps and other cleaning products. *See* Aniline and Phenol.

**TRICLOPYR** • A preemergent herbicide. FDA residue tolerance is 0.01 ppm in milk; 0.05 ppm in meat, fat, and meat by-products of cattle, goats, hogs, and sheep; and 0.5 ppm in liver and kidneys of cattle, goats, hogs, and sheep.

**TRICYCLAZOLE** • A fungicide used on rice. The FDA tolerance for residues are 30 ppm in rice bran, rice hulls, and rice polishings.

**TRICYCLOHEXYLTIN HYDROXIDE (TCTH)** • Cyhexatin. A pesticide used on animal feed. FDA residue tolerance is 8 ppm in dried apple pomace, and dried citrus pulp resulting from application to growing crops; 90 ppm in dried hops; 4 ppm in dried prunes. Irritating to the eyes.

**2-TRIDECANONE** • Pesticide found in tomatoes. ASP

**2-TRIDECENAL** • A synthetic citrus and flavoring for beverages, ice cream, ices, candy, baked goods, and chewing gum. ASP

**TRIDECYL ALCOHOL** • Derived from tridecane, a paraffin hydrocarbon obtained from petroleum. Used as an emulsifier in cosmetic creams, lotions, and lipsticks.

**TRIETHANOLAMINE** • A coating additive for fresh fruit and vegetables and widely used in surfactants *(see)*. Used in flume water for washing sugar beets prior to slicing operation. Its principal toxic effect in animals has been attributed to overalkalinity. Gross pathology has been found in the gastrointestinal tract in fatally poisoned guinea pigs. It is an irritant. ASP

**TRIETHANOLAMINE STEARATE** • Made from ethylene oxide. A moisture absorber, viscous, used in making emulsions. May be irritating to the skin and mucous membranes, but less so than many other amines *(see)*.

**TRIETHYL CITRATE** • Citric Acid. Ethyl Citrate. Odorless, practically colorless, bitter; also used in dried egg as a sequestering additive *(see)* and to prevent rancidity. Citrates may interfere with laboratory tests for blood, liver, and pancreatic function, but no known skin toxicity. The final report to the FDA of the Select Committee on GRAS Substances stated in 1980 that it should continue its GRAS status with no limitations other than good manufacturing practices. E

**TRIETHYLENETETRAMINE CROSS-LINKED WITH EPICHLOROHYDRIN** • Processing additive. *See* Epichlorohydrin. NUL

**TRIETHYLENE GLYCOL** • Prepared from ethylene oxide and ethylene glycol *(see both)*. Used as a solvent. *See* Polyethylene Glycol for toxicity. ASP

**TRIFLUMIZOLE** • Fungicide used in animal feed. FDA residue tolerances are 2 ppm in apple pomace; 25 ppm in grape pomace; and 8 ppm in raisin waste.

**TRIFLUOROMETHANE SULFONIC ACID** • A catalyst used in the production of cocoa butter substitute. Toxic by inhalation. Slightly irritating to the skin. NIL

**TRIFORINE** • White crystals used as a fungicide for animal feed and hops. FDA limits residue to 60 ppm in dried hops and in spent hops when used for animal feed.

**TRIFURAN** • A pesticide used in peppermint and spearmint oil. FDA residue tolerance is 2 ppm.

**2-4-5-TRIHYDROXYBUTYROPHENONE (THBP)** • An antioxidant used alone or in combination with other antioxidants. Total antioxidant not to exceed 0.02 percent of the oil or fat content of any product. Also used in the manufacture of food packaging materials, with a limit of 0.005 percent in food. On the FDA list for further study of this widely used additive. May not be listed on labels. NIL

**TRIHYDROXY STEARIN** • Isolated from cork and used as a thickener.

**TRILAURYL CITRATE** • *See* Lauryl Alcohol and Citric Acid.

**TRIISOPROPANOLAMINE (TIPA)** • A crystalline, white solid. A mild base used as an emulsifying additive. A component of a coating used for fresh fruits and vegetables.

**TRIISOSTEARIN** • *See* Glycerin and Isostearic Acid.

**TRILAURIN** • *See* Lauric Acid.

**TRIMETHYLAMINE** • Miscellaneous uses. Colorless gas at room temperature easily liquefied. Derived from the interaction of methanol and ammonia. Used in insecticides, quaternary ammonium compounds *(see),* and plastics. ASP

**p,a,a-TRIMETHYLBENZYL ALCOHOL** • Synthetic flavoring. ASP

**4-(2,6,6-TRIMETHYLCYCLOHEXA-1,3-DIENYL)BUT-2-EN-4-ONE** • Flavoring additive for which FAO/WHO *(see)* said in 1998 there was no safety concern. ASP

**2,6,6-TRIMETHYLCYCLOHEXA-1,3-DIENYL METHANAL** • Synthetic flavoring.

**2,6,6-TRIMETHYL-2-CYCLOHEXANE-1-ONE CARBOXALDEHYDE** • Nicomol. Crystals from diluted acetic acid. Odorless and tasteless. Breaks down fats. ASP

**3,3,5-TRIMETHYLCYCLOHEXANOL** • Synthetic flavoring.

**2,2,6-TRIMETHYLCYCLOHEXANONE** • Synthetic flavoring.

**2,6,6-TRIMETHYL-1-CYCLOHEXEN-1-ACETALDEHYDE** • Synthetic flavoring.

**2,6,6-TRIMETHYLCYCLOHEX-2-ENE-1,4-DIONE** • Synthetic flavoring.

**4-(2,6,6-TRIMETHYLCYCLOHEX-1-ENYL)BUT-2-EN-4-ONE** • Synthetic flavoring.

**2,2,3-TRIMETHYLCYCLOPENT-3-EN-1-YL ACETALDEHYDE** • Synthetic flavoring.

**2,4,5-TRIMETHYL DELTA-3-OXAZOLINE** • Yellow to orange liquid with a strong, nutlike odor. Used as a synthetic flavoring additive in various foods. GRAS

**2,4,6-TRIMETHYL-4H-1,3,5-DITHIAZINE** • Synthetic flavoring in baked goods beverages, breakfast cereal, fats, oils, and gravies, meat products, grains, processed vegetables, snack foods, and soups. Declared GRAS by FEMA *(see)*.

**3,7-11-TRIMETHYL-2,6,10-DODECTRIENAL** • Synthetic flavoring in baked goods, beverages, breakfast cereal, chewing gum, confectionery frostings, fats and oils, fruit ices, gelatins, gravies, instant coffee, jams, milk products, seasonings, soft candy, and soups. Declared GRAS by FEMA *(see)*.

**3,5,5-TRIMETHYLHEXANAL** • Synthetic flavoring. ASP

**3,5,5-TRIMETHYL-1-HEXANOL** • Synthetic flavoring. ASP

**(2,6,6-TRIMETHYL-2-HYDROXYCYCLOHEXYLIDENE)ACETIC ACID GAMMA-LACTONE** • Antioxidant. EAF

**1,3,3-TRIMETHYL-2-NORBORNANYL ACETATE** • Antioxidant. ASP

**2,2,4-TRIMETHYL-1,3-OXACYCLOPENTANE** • Synthetic flavoring. ASP

**2,6,10-TRIMETHYL-2,6,10-PENTADECATRIEN-14-ONE** • Synthetic flavoring. ASP

**2,3,4-TRIMETHYL-3-PENTANOL** • Synthetic flavoring. EAF

**2,3,6-TRIMETHYLPHENOL** • *See* Phenol. EAF

**2,3,5-TRIMETHYLPYRAZINE** • Synthetic nutty flavoring. ASP

**2,4,5-TRIMETHYLTHIAZOLE** • Synthetic earthy flavoring. ASP

**2,2,6-TRIMETHYL-6-VINYLTETRAHYDROPYRAN** • Synthetic lime flavoring. NIL

**TRIPHOSPHATES** • Emulsifyers and stabilizers. *See* Phosphates. E

**TRIPOLYPHOSPHATE** • A phosphorus salt. A sequestering additive *(see)*

in foods and a food additive. Can be irritating because of its alkalinity. May cause esophageal stricture if swallowed. Moderately irritating to the skin and mucous membranes. Ingestion can cause violent vomiting. GRAS

**TRISODIUM-3-CARBOXY-5-HYDROXY-1-*p*-SULFOPHENYL-4-*p*-SULFOPHENYLAZOPYRAZOLE** • See FD and C Yellow No. 5.

**TRISODIUM CITRATE** • Antioxidant, emulsifier, sequestrant, stabilizer. ASP

**TRISODIUM EDTA** • *See* Tetrasodium EDTA.

**TRISODIUM HEDTA** • Mineral suspending additives. *See* Sequestering Additive.

**TRISODIUM HYDROXY EDTA** • *See* Tetrasodium EDTA.

**TRISODIUM HYDROXYETHYL ETHLENEDIAMINETRIACETATE** • *See* Tetrasodium EDTA.

**TRISODIUM NITRILOTRIACETATE** • Sodium salt of nitrilotriacetic acid. A sequestering additive *(see)*. NIL

**TRISODIUM NTA** • *See* Sequestering Additive.

**TRISODIUM PHOSPHATE** • Obtained from phosphate rock. Highly alkaline. An emulsifier in cheese; the FDA allows residue in cheese less than 3 percent of weight. It is also used in fruit jellies. Phosphorus was formerly used to treat rickets and degenerative disorders and is now used as a mineral supplement for foods; also in incendiary bombs and tracer bullets. Can cause skin irritation from alkalinity. GRAS

**TRISTEARIN** • In many animal and vegetable fats, especially hard ones like tallow and cocoa butter, it is used in surfactants and quaternary ammonium compounds.

**TRISTEARYL CITRATE** • The triester of stearyl alcohol and citric acid *(see both)*.

**2,3,5-TRITHIA-HEXAMINE** • Synthetic flavoring in baked goods, beverages, breakfast cereal, chewing gum, confectionery frostings, fats and oils, fruit ices, gelatins, gravies, instant coffee, jams, milk products, seasonings, soft candy, and soups. Declared GRAS by FEMA *(see)*

**TRITHIAHEXANE** • A flavoring used in baked goods, beverages, cheese, gravies, snack foods, and many other food products. Determined GRAS by FEMA *(see)*.

**TRITHIOACETONE** • Synthetic flavoring with a musty note commonly found in fruit flavors. Used in black currant, grapefruit, peach, and tropical fruit flavorings. ASP

**TRITHION** • Acarithion. Akarithion. Endyl. Trithion Miticide. Insecticide and miticide used in animal feed, grapefruit, lemons, limes, oranges, tangelos, tangerines, and dried tea. The FDA's insecticide residue tolerance is 20 ppm on dried tea and 10 ppm in dehydrated citrus pulp and citrus meal when used for cattle feed. EPA Extremely Hazardous Substances List *(see)*. Poisonous by ingestion and skin contact. Inhibits nerve transmission.

**TRITICALE** • A man-made cross between wheat (*see* Dog Grass) and rye (secale), but more nutritious than wheat. The protein content of bread made with it is 10 percent higher and its essential amino acid, lysrne (*see*), exceeds wheat bread by 50 percent. A number of novel products are being made from it, including ethnic breads. Triticale is intended for baked goods, ready-to-eat cereals, and malt products; also used as a thickener, emulsifier, fortifier, and supplement. Once accepted, triticale can be an important nutritious addition to the food supply.

**TRITICUM** • *See* Dog Grass. GRAS

**TROMETHAMINE** • Made by the reduction (*see*) of nitro compounds, it is a crystalline mass used in the manufacture of surfactants (*see*). Used medicinally to correct an overabundance of acid in the body.

**TRUE FIXATIVE** • This holds back the evaporation of the other materials. Benzoin is an example. *See* Fixatives.

**TRYPSIN FROM ANIMAL TISSUE** • An enzyme formed in the intestine. It is administered as a drug in the treatment of indigestion. GRAS. NUL

**TRYPTOPHAN** • L form only. A tremendous amount of research is now in progress with this amino acid (*see*). First isolated in milk in 1901, it is now being studied as a means to calm hyperactive children, induce sleep, and fight depression and pain. It is not believed to be completely harmless and has been suspected of being a co-carcinogen and to affect the liver when taken in high doses. Like niacin, it is capable of preventing and curing pellagra. It is a partial precursor of the brain hormone serotonin and is indispensable for the manufacture of certain cell proteins. In cosmetics, it is used to increase the protein content of creams and lotions. Causes cancer in experimental animals. The FDA called for further study of this additive. BANNED

**TUBEROSE OIL** • Derived from a Mexican bulbous herb, *Polianthes tuberosa,* commonly cultivated for its spike of fragrant white single or double flowers that resemble small lilies. Used in peach flavorings for beverages, ice cream, ices, candy, and baked goods. Tuberose is used in perfumes. Can cause allergic reactions. GRAS. ASP

**TUBEROSE LACTONE** • Flavoring used in baked goods, instant coffee and tea, jams, jellies, meat products, nut products, snack foods, soft candy, soups, sugar substitutes, and many other food productrs. Determined GRAS by the Expert Panel of the Flavor and Extract Manufacturers Association.

**TUMERIC** • *See* Turmeric.

**TUNA OIL** • Rich in omega-3 polyunsaturated fatty acids (omega-3 PUFAs), especially eicosapentaenoic acid (EPA) and docosahexaenoic acid (DHA) which have various physiological functions. GRAS

**TUNG NUT OIL** • Chinawood Oil. Drying oil used to waterproof packaging materials. Toxic by ingestion. Causes contact dermatitis (skin rash). Ingestion causes nausea, vomiting, cramps, diarrhea, thirst, dizziness, lethargy, and disorientation. Large doses can cause fever, irregular heartbeat, and respiratory effects.

**TUNU EXTRACT** • Tuno. From a Central American tree, *Castilla fallax,* closely related to the rubber tree. Cleared for use as a natural masticatory substance of vegetable origin in chewing-gum base. ASP

**TURMERIC** • Tumeric. Derived from an East Indian herb, *Curcuma longa.* Aromatic, with a pepperlike but somewhat bitter taste. The cleaned, boiled, sun-dried, pulverized root is used in coconut, ginger ale, and curry flavorings for puddings, condiments, meats, soups, and pickles; also for yellow coloring used to color sausage casings, oleomargarine, shortening, and marker ink. The extract is used in fruit, meat, and cheese flavorings for beverages, condiments, meats, soup bases, and pickles. The oleoresin *(see)* is obtained by extraction with one or more of the solvents acetone, ethyl alcohol, ethylene dichloride *(see all),* and others. It is used in spice flavorings for condiments, meats, pickles, and brine. Both turmeric and its oleoresin have been permanently listed for coloring food since 1966. It is exempt from certification. GRAS. There is reported use of the chemical, it has not yet been assigned for toxicology literature. ASP

**TURMERIC OLEORESIN** • The color additive turmeric oleoresin is the combination of flavor and color principles obtained from turmeric *(Curcuma longa)* by extraction using any one or a combination of solvents. In two-year animal studies, turmeric oleoresin ingestion was also associated with increased incidences of ulcers, hyperplasia, and inflammation of the forestomach, cecum, and colon in male rats and of the cecum in female rats. In female mice, ingestion of diets containing turmeric oleoresin was also associated with an increased incidence of thyroid gland follicular cell hyperplasia. The induction of cancer by the additive was equivocal. ASP

**TURPENTINE** • Gum and Steam Distilled. Any of the various resins obtained from coniferous trees. A yellowish, viscous exudate with a characteristic smell, both forms are used in spice flavorings for baked goods. Steam-distilled turpentine is also used in candy. It is the oleoresin from a species of pines. Readily absorbed through the skin. Irritating to the skin and mucous membranes. In addition to being a local skin irritant, it can cause allergic reactions. It is also a central nervous system depressant. Death is usually due to respiratory failure. As little as 15 milliliters has killed children. NIL. EAF

**TVP** • Textured vegetable protein. Made from soy. A dry product it requires rehydration.

**(TWO) 2 PERCENT MILK** • *See* Milk.

**TYLOSIN** • Tylon. Tylan. Antibiotic from *Streptomycetes fradiae* used for beef, chicken, eggs, milk, pork, and turkey. FDA limitations are 0.2 ppm in chickens, turkeys, cattle, swine, and eggs; 0.05 ppm in milk. Moderately toxic by ingestion.

**TYLOSIN and SULFAMETHAZINE** • Used in swine feeds. Residues of tylosin *(see)* in edible tissue of swine is tolerated by the FDA at 0.2 ppm and residues of sulfamethazine is 0.1 ppm. Both are antibiotics.

**TYRAMINE** • A derivative of tyrosine *(see)*, it is a chemical present in mistletoe and many common foods and beverages. It raises blood pressure but usually causes no problem because enzymes in the body hold it in check. When drugs are used that inhibit the major enzyme that restrains its actions, monoamine oxidase (MAO) *(see)*, the blood pressure can shoot up to dangerous levels when foods and beverages containing significant levels of tyramine are ingested. Among the foods that are high in tyramine are cheese, beer, wines, pickled herring, chicken livers, yeast extract, canned figs, raisins, bananas, avocados, chocolate, soy sauce, fava beans, meat tenderizers, eggplant, tea, cola, beef liver, and yogurt. Among the drugs that inhibit the enzyme and may lead to a serious rise in blood pressure are the MAO-inhibitors, anti-TB drugs, such as isoniazid, and anticancer drugs, such as procarbazine.

**TYROSINE** • L form. Widely distributed amino acid *(see)*, termed nonessential because it does not seem to be necessary for growth. It is used as a dietary supplement. It is a building block of protein and is used in cosmetics to help creams penetrate the skin. The FDA has asked for further study of this additive. GRAS. ASP

**TYROSINE ETHYL ESTER HYDROCHLORIDE** • Derived from an amino acid. *See* Tyrosine and Ester. NUL

# U

**U** • Symbol meaning "kosher" *(see)*.

**UL** • Abbreviation for tolerable upper (intake) level. The highest level of daily nutrient intake that can be consumed by individuals in the general population without posing a risk of adverse health effects.

**ULTRAMARINE BLUE** • A color additive occurring naturally in the mineral lapis lazuli. Used for packaging material and a salt for animal feed only. FDA limitation of 0.5 percent of salt. It is used for external use only. No longer permitted for use as a drug coloring. NUL

**2,4-UNDECADIENAL** • Synthetic flavoring. ASP

**2,5-UNDECADIENAL** • Synthetic flavoring. NIL

**2,3-UNDECADIONE** • A synthetic butter flavoring additive for beverages, ice cream, ices, candy, and baked goods. ASP

***γ*-UNDECALACTONE** • Peach Aldehyde. Colorless to light yellow liquid with a peachy odor. Derived from undecylenic acid with sulfuric acid. A synthetic fruit flavoring, colorless or yellow, with a strong peach odor. Used for beverages, ice cream, ices, candy, baked goods, gelatin desserts, and chewing gum. Used also in perfumery. ASP

**UNDECANAL** • A synthetic flavoring additive. Colorless to slightly yellow, with a sweet, fatty odor. Used in lemon, orange, rose, fruit, and honey flavorings for beverages, ice cream, ices, candy, baked goods, and chewing gum. ASP

**9-UNDECANAL** • A synthetic citrus and fruit flavoring for beverages, ice cream, ices, candy, baked goods, and chewing gum.

**10-UNDECANAL** • A synthetic citrus, floral, and fruit flavoring additive for beverages, ice cream, ices, and candy.

**3-UNDECANONE** • A synthetic flavoring additive that occurs naturally in rue and hops oil. Used in citrus, coconut, peach, and cheese flavorings for beverages, ice cream, ices, candy, baked goods, and puddings. ASP

**1-UNDECANOL** • Colorless liquid with a citrus odor used in perfumery and as a flavoring in baked goods, beverages, chewing gum, frozen dairy, hard candy, and imitation dairy. ASP

**2-UNDECANOL** • Essential oil from *Ruta chalapensis*. Antifoaming additive, perfume fixative, and plasticizer. NIL

**10-UNDECENOIC ACID** • Occurs in sweat. Obtained from ricinoleic acid *(see)*. Used as an antifungal additive. ASP

**2-UNDECENOL** • White to slightly yellow liquid with a sweet floral odor used as a flavoring additive in beverages, soups, and various foods. GRAS. NIL

**10-UNDECEN-1-YL ACETATE** • A synthetic citrus and fruit flavoring additive for beverages, ice cream, ices, candy, and baked goods. ASP

**UNDECYL ALCOHOL** • A synthetic lemon, lime, orange, and rose flavoring additive for beverages, ice cream, ices, candy, and baked goods. ASP

**N-UNDECYLBENZENESULFONIC ACID** • *See* Castor Oil and Sulfonated Oils. ASP

**UNDECYLPENTADECANOL** • *See* Fatty Alcohols.

**UNSAPONIFIABLE OLIVE OILS** • The oil fraction that is not broken down in the refining of olive fatty acids.

**UNSAPONIFIABLE RAPESEED OIL** • The oil fraction that is not broken down in the refining of rapeseed oil fatty acids. *See* Rapeseed Oil.

**UNSAPONIFIABLE SHEA BUTTER** • The fraction of shea butter that is not broken down during processing.

**UNSAPONIFIABLE SOYBEAN OIL** • The fraction of soybean oil that is not broken down in the refining recovery of soybean oil fatty acids.

**UPC** • Abbreviation for Universal Product Code.

**UNSATURATED FATS** • Unsaturated fats contain one or more double-bond carbon linkages and are usually liquid at room temperature. Vegetable oils and fish oils most frequently contain unsaturated fats. Among the unsaturated fats are caproleic, lauroleic, myristoleic, palmitoleic, oleic, petroselinic, vaccenic, linoleic, linolenic, eleaostearic, gadoleic, arachidonic, and erucic. *See also* Fat and Monounsaturated Fat.

**UREA** • Carbamide. A product of protein metabolism and excreted from human urine. Used in yeast food and wine production up to 2 pounds per gallon. It is used to "brown" baked goods such as pretzels, and consists of colorless or white odorless crystals that have a cool salty taste. Medicinally, urea is used as a topical antiseptic and as a diuretic to reduce body water. Its largest use, however, is as a fertilizer, and only a small part of its production goes into the manufacture of other urea products. The FAO/WHO Expert Committee on Food Additives considered urea for evaluation only in relation to its use in chewing gum. Chewing gum may contain up to 3 percent urea, and intake from this source could be up to 300 mg of urea per day. Since urea is a natural end product of amino acid metabolism in humans and approximately 20 grams per day are excreted in the urine in adults (proportionately less in children), the committee concluded that the use of urea levels of up to 3 percent in chewing gum was of no toxicological concern. The final report to the FDA of the Select Committee on GRAS Substances stated in 1980 that urea should continue its GRAS status with no limitations other than good manufacturing practices. ASP

**UREASE** • An enzyme from *Lactobacillius fermentum.* Used to inhibit urethane formation in wine. Urethane is used in pesticides and fungicides and is toxic by ingestion. Urethane was also the first cancer-causing additive demonstrated to pass through the placenta and affect the fetus. GRAS. NUL

**URETHANE** • A known carcinogen for several species of animals, and, as such, must be viewed as a potential carcinogen for humans as well. The degree of risk to humans, though, is not known. The FDA says scientific data are simply too limited to assess the risk posed by low levels of the chemical in alcoholic beverages. Concern in this country over urethane (also called ethyl carbamate) began in November 1985 with news reports that Canadian authorities had detected the chemical in certain wines and distilled spirits. At that time, the FDA and the Bureau of Alcohol, Tobacco, and Firearms (ATF) began looking for ways to reduce or eliminate urethane in alcoholic beverages. Levels of urethane may be affected not only by temperature, but by other conditions as well, including the type of soil and fertilizer used to grow the raw products, such as grapes, the type of grape used in wine making, and even by the weather. These conditions may cause significant differences in the level of urethane even from one production lot to another of the same brand. After production, levels can still be increased substantially in some products—particularly wines—by shipping, storage, and handling practices. *See also* Polyurethane.

**UROCANIC ACID** • Prepared from Histidine *(see).*

**URSOLIC ACID** • Bearberry. Privet Fruit. Found in leaves and berries of *Arctostaphylos uva-ursi.* Used as an emulsifying additive in foods and pharmaceuticals.

**USDA** • Abbreviation for the United States Department of Agriculture.

**USNIC ACID** • Antibacterial compound found in lichens. Pale yellow, slightly soluble in water.

**UVA-URSI** • *Arctostaphylos uva-ursi* • Bearberry. An astringent used to treat bladder problems, it is believed that its action is due to the high concentration of the antiseptic arbutin. In passing through the system, arbutin yields hydroquinone, a urinary disinfectant. Leaves from the plant uva-ursi also contain anesthetic principles that numb pain in the urinary system and the herb has been shown to have antibiotic activity. Crude extracts of uva-ursi reportedly possess some anticancer property. In 1992, the FDA proposed a ban on uva-ursi in oral menstrual drug products because it had not been shown to be safe and effective for its stated claims.

# V

**VALBAZEN** • Albendazole. Zental. A worm medicine for animals. Moderately toxic by ingestion. Causes birth defects in experimental animals.

**VALENCENE WOODY** • Colorless to pale yellow synthetic flavoring with an orange, citrus odor. ASP

**VALERAL** • *See* Valeraldehyde.

**VALERALDEHYDE** • Pentanal. A synthetic flavoring additive which occurs naturally in coffee extract. Used in fruit and nut flavorings for beverages, ice cream, ices, candy, and baked goods. Has narcotic properties and is a mild irritant. ASP

**VALERIAN** • *Valeriana officinalis.* A perennial native to Europe and the United States, it was reputed as a love potion. Used as a flavoring. Its vapor was found to kill the bacillus of typhoid fever after forty-five minutes. The herb has been widely studied in Europe and Russia, and the major constituents, the valepotriate, have been reported to have marked sedative, anticonvulsive, blood pressure lowering, and tranquilizing effects. It has been used for centuries to treat panic attacks. In Germany, valerian preparations have been used for more than a decade to treat childhood behavioral disorders, supposedly without the side effects experienced with pharmaceuticals for that purpose. It has been reported that it also helps concentration and energy. Prolonged use of valerian may result in side effects such as irregular heartbeat, headaches, uneasiness, nervousness, and insomnia. Very large doses may cause paralysis. ASP

**VALERIC ACID** • Occurs naturally in apples, cocoa, coffee, oil of lavender, peaches, and strawberries. A synthetic flavoring additive used in butter, butterscotch, fruit, rum, and cheese flavorings for beverages, ice cream, ices, candy, and baked goods. Colorless, with an unpleasant odor. Usually distilled from valerian root. Some of its salts are used in medicine. Also used in peeling solutions for fruits and vegetables. Moderately toxic by ingestion. A corrosive irritant to skin, eyes, and mucous membranes. ASP

**VALERIC ALDEHYDE** • *See* Valeraldehyde.

**VALEROLACTONE, GAMMA** • A synthetic vanilla flavoring additive for beverages, ice cream, ices, candy, and baked goods. Moderately toxic by ingestion. A skin irritant. ASP

**VALINE** • L form. An essential amino acid *(see)*. Occurs in the largest quantities in fibrous protein. It is indispensable for growth and nitrogen balance. The FDA had asked for further study of this ingredient as a food additive in 1980. GRAS. ASP

**VANADIUM TETRACHLORIDE** • Derived from chlorination of ferrovanadium. Catalyst. Toxic by ingestion, inhalation, and skin absorption.

**VANAY** • *See* Triacetin.

**VANILLA, ABSOLUTE** • *Vanilla* spp. Vanilla Absolute. A perennial herbaceous climbing vine up to eighty-two feet high, with green stems and large white flowers that have deep narrow trumpets. Vanilla absolute is produced by further extraction from the resin, which is obtained by solvent extraction from the "cured" vanilla bean. Vanilla is native to Central America and Mexico and cultivated mainly in Madagascar and Mexico. Vanilla is also cultivated in Tahiti, the Comoro Islands, East Africa, and Indonesia, although the pods are often processed in Europe or the United States. EAF

**VANILLA EXTRACT** • Extracted from the full-grown unripe fruit of the vanilla plant of Mexico and the West Indies. Contains not less than 35 percent aqueous ethyl alcohol *(see)* and one or more of the following ingredients: glycerin, propylene glycol, sugar (including invert sugar), and corn syrup. Used in many foods and beverages as a flavoring. GRAS. ASP

**VANILLAL** • *See* Ethyl Vanillin.

**VANILLIC ACID** • 4-hydroxy-3-methoxybenzoic acid. An odorless crystalline phenolic acid. Found in some varieties of vanilla, formed by oxidation of vanillin, and used chiefly in the form of esters as food preservatives. EAF

**VANILLIN** • Occurs naturally in vanilla *(see)* and potato parings but is an artificial flavoring. Odor and taste of vanilla. Made synthetically from eugenol *(see);* also from the waste of the wood pulp industry. One part vanillin equals 400 parts vanilla pods. Used in butter, chocolate, fruit, root beer, and vanilla flavorings for beverages, ice cream, ices, candy, baked goods, gelatin desserts, puddings, syrups (30,000 ppm), toppings, margarine, chocolate products, and liqueurs. May migrate from paper and paperboard to food. The lethal dose in mice is 3 grams (30 grams to the ounce) per kilogram of body weight. A skin irritant that produces a burning sensation and eczema. May also cause pigmentation of the skin. GRAS. ASP

**VANILLIN ACETATE** • Vanillin. A synthetic spice and vanilla flavoring additive for beverages, ice cream, ices, candy, and baked goods. *See* Vanillin. ASP

**VANILLIN 1,2-BUTYLENE GLYCOL ACETAL** • Synthetic flavoring. *See* Vanillin. EAF

**VANILLIN ISOBUTYRATE** • Synthetic flavoring. *See* Vanillin. EAF

**VANILLYL BUTYL ETHER** • Synthetic flavoring. *See* Vanillin. ASP

**VANILLYL ETHYL ETHER** • *See* Vanillin. EAF

**VANILLYLIDENE ACETONE** • Synthetic flavoring. *See* Vanillin. ASP

**VEGETABLE CARBON** • Produced by the carbonization of vegetable material such as wood, cellulose residues, peat and coconut and other shells. The raw material is carbonized at high temperatures and consists essentially of finely divided carbon. It may contain minor amounts of nitrogen, hydrogen, and oxygen. Some moisture may be absorbed on the product after manufacture. It may be activated at high temperature in the presence of steam or carbon dioxide. The FAO/WHO says that when used in accordance with good manufacturing practice as a filtrating and clarifying agent no residues should result in food. E

**VEGETABLE GUMS** • Includes derivatives from quince seed, karaya, acacia, tragacanth, Irish moss, guar, sodium alginate, potassium alginate, ammonium alginate, and propylene glycol alginate. All are subject to deterioration and always need a preservative. They are mostly used as thickeners. May cause allergic reactions in hypersensitive persons. ASP

**VEGETABLE JUICE** • Used in food colorings consistent with good manufacturing practices. Permanently listed for coloring since 1966. Does not require certification. ASP

**VEGETABLE OILS** • Peanut, sesame, olive, and cottonseed oil obtained from plants and used in many food additives. *See* Vegetable Oils, Brominated.

**VEGETABLE OILS, BROMINATED** • Peanut, sesame, and cottonseed oil obtained from plants. Used in fruit-flavored beverages where not prohibited by standards. FDA tolerance is less than 15 ppm. *See* Bromates.

**VEGETARIAN** • According to the Vegetarian Resource Group, less than 1 percent of Americans are true vegetarians. Such people never eat meat, fish, or poultry, although they may eat foods derived from animals such as dairy products and eggs. There are even fewer vegans, strict vegetarians who avoid all animal-derived foods—even honey.

**VERATRALDEHYDE** • A synthetic fruit, nut, and vanilla flavoring additive for beverages, ice cream, ices, candy, baked goods, and puddings. Derived from vanillin. May have narcotic and irritant effects but no specific data. ASP

**VERATRIC ALDEHYDE** • *See* Veratraldehye.

**VERBENOL** • An alcohol made from *Verbena officinalis.* NIL

**VERONICA** • Extract of *Veronica qfficinalis,* a small herb of wide distribution that has pink or white flowers. Flavoring in alcoholic beverages only. EAF

**VERVAIN, EUROPEAN** • *Verbena officinalis.* A class of medicinal plants used as a flavoring in alcoholic beverages only. NIL

**VERXITE GRANULES and FLAKES** • Hydrated magnesium-aluminum iron silicate. Soft and resilient. Used as an anticaking and blending additive in ruminant feeds.

**VERXITE GRITS** • Used as a roughage replacement in ruminant feeds.

**VERY LOW SODIUM** • Less than 35 mg per serving.

**VET** • FDA abbreviation for veterinary drug which may leave residue in edible tissues of animals or in edible animal products.

**VETIVER OIL** • Vetiverol. Khus-Khus. Stable brown to reddish brown oil from the roots of a fragrant grass. It has an aromatic to harsh woodsy odor. Used as a flavoring in alcoholic beverages only. EAF

**VETIVERYL ACETATE** • Slightly viscous pale green-yellow liquid. Odor resembles vetiver although much milder and having a sweet fresh note. GRAS. ASP

**VIBURNUM EXTRACT** • Haw Bark. Black Extract. Extract of the fruit of a hawthorn shrub or tree. Used in fragrances and in butter, caramel, cola, maple, and walnut flavorings for beverages. Has been used as a uterine antispasmodic.

**VIBURNUM PRUNIFOLIUM** • *See* Viburnum Extract.

**VINEGAR** • Used for hundreds of years to remove lime soap after shampooing. It is a solvent for cosmetic oils and resins. Vinegar is about 4 to 6 percent acetic acid. Acetic acid occurs naturally in apples, cheese, grapes, milk, and other foods, but may cause an allergic reaction in those allergic to corn.

**VINEGAR NAPHTHA** • *See* Ethyl Acetate.

**VINYL** • Made from acetylene with various other substances to form plastics.

**VINYL ACETATE** • Used as film former and as a starch modifier not to exceed 2.5 percent in modified starch *(see)*. Vapors in high concentration may be narcotic; animal experiments show low toxicity. NUL

***o*-VINYLANISOLE** • *See* Anisole and Vinyl. ASP

**VINYL CHLORIDE** • Chloroethylene. Prepared from ethylene dichloride and alcoholic potassium, it is a colorless gas that becomes liquid upon freezing. It is one of the most frequently used vinyl compounds and is a very hazardous chemical by all avenues of exposure. It may be narcotic in high concentrations. If spilled on the skin, rapid evaporation causes local frostbite. It is a known cancer-causing additive, and because of that it has been banned from aerosol sprays. It is used for many polyvinyl compounds in paper coating, adhesives, and refrigerants. It is permitted by the FDA for use in adhesives, and in food-contact coatings.

**VINYL CHLORIDE-VINYLIDENE CHLORIDE COPOLYMER** • Used as a coating on fresh citrus fruits. Vinyl chloride was banned in hairsprays because it is a cancer-causing additive. It is a proven liver cancer-causing additive in people who work with the compound. Vinylidene chloride is an irritant to mucous membranes, narcotic in high concentrations, and has caused liver and kidney injury in experimental animals. NUL

**P-VINYLPHENOL** • Synthetic flavoring. In 2000, FAO/WHO said it had no safety concern at current levels of intake when used as a flavoring agent. NIL

***VIOLA ODORATA*** • *See* Violet Extract and Violet Leaves.

**VIOLAXANTHIN** • Natural orange-red coloring isolated from yellow pansies and Valencia orange peel. Soluble in alcohol. *See* Xanthophyll.

**VIOLET EXTRACT** • Flowers and Leaves. Green liquid with typical odor of violet. It is taken from the plant widely grown in the United States. Used in berry, violet, and fruit flavorings for beverages, ice cream, ices, candy, and baked goods. Also used in face powders and for coloring inorganic pigments. May produce skin rash in the allergic. GRAS

**VIOLET LEAVES, ABSOLUTE** • Essential Oil of *Viola odorata*. There is reported use of the chemical; it has not yet been assigned for toxicology literature. *See* Violet Extract. GRAS. EAF

**VIOLET, SWISS** • *Viola calcarata. See* Violet Extract. NIL

**VIRGINIAMYCIN** • Eskalin. Pristinamycin. Staphlyomycin. White powder used as an antibiotic from *Streptomyces* for chickens and swine. FDA limits residue in swine of 0.4 ppm in kidney, skin, and fat, 0.3 ppm in liver, 0.1 ppm in muscle. In broiler chickens, the limit is 0.5 ppm in kidney, 0.3 ppm in liver, 0.2 ppm in skin and fat, 0.1 ppm in muscle. Moderately toxic by ingestion.

**VIRIDINE** • *See* Phenylacetaldehyde Dimethyl Acetal.

**VITAMINS** • Vitamins are organic compounds that are nutritionally essential in small amounts to control metabolic processes and cannot be synthesized by the body. Vitamins are usually classified by their solubility, which to some degree determines their stability, occurrence in foodstuffs, distribution in body fluids, and tissue storage capacity. Each of the fat-soluble vitamins A, D, E, and K has a distinct and separate physiological role. Several are among those supporting antioxidant efforts to depress the effects of metabolic by-products called free radicals, which are thought to cause degenerative changes related to aging. Most of the water-soluble vitamins are components of essential enzyme systems. Many are involved in the reactions supporting energy metabolism. These vitamins are not normally stored in the body in appreciable amounts and are normally excreted in small quantities in the urine. Thus, a daily supply is desirable to avoid depletion and interruption of normal physiological functions.

**VITAMIN A** • Acetate and Palmitate. A yellow viscous liquid insoluble in water. An antiinfective, antixerophthahnic vitamin, essential to growth and development. Deficiency leads to retarded growth in the young, diminished visual acuity, night blindness, and skin problems. Insoluble in water. Toxic when children or adults receive more than 100,000 units daily over several months. Recommended daily dietary allowance is 1,500 units for infants and 4,500 units for adults and 2,000–3,500 units for children. It is used to fortify mellorine (vegetable-fat imitation ice cream), skim milk, dietary infant formula, blue cheese, Gorgonzola cheese, milk, and oleomargarine (1 pound of margarine contains 15,000 USP units of vitamin A). Vitamin A is also used in lubricating creams and oils for its alleged skin-healing properties. Can be absorbed through the skin. The final report to the FDA of the Select Committee on GRAS Substances stated in 1980 that it should continue its GRAS status with no limitations other than good manufacturing practices.

**VITAMIN A ACETATE** • Pale yellow crystals from methanol. *See* Vitamin A. ASP

**VITAMIN A PALMITATE** • Predominate storage of vitamin A in the liver. ASP

**VITAMIN B₁** • *See* Thiamine Hydrochloride. ASP

**VITAMIN B₂** • Riboflavin. Lactoflavin. Formerly called vitamin G. Riboflavin is a factor in the vitamin B complex and is used in emollients. Every plant and animal cell contains a minute amount. Helps to metabolize protein, carbohydrate, and fat; maintains healthy skin, eyes; aids formation of red blood cells and antibodies. Symptoms of deficiency include sores or cracking around the mouth, skin problems, and eye disorders. It is necessary for healthy skin and respiration, protects the eyes from sensitivity to light, and is used for building and maintaining human body tissues. A deficiency leads to lesions at the corner of the mouth and to changes in the cornea. Recommended daily allowances for infants to six months, 0.4 mg; children one to three years, 0.8 mg; children four to six years, 1.1 mg; children seven to ten years, 1.2 mg. Males eleven to fourteen years, 1.5 mg; males fifteen to eighteen years, 1.8 mg; males nineteen to fifty years, 1.7 mg; Males fifty-one years and over, 1.4 mg. Females eleven to fifty years, 1.3 mg; females fifty-one years and over 1.4 mg; pregnant women 1.6 mg; lactating women 1.7–18 mg. It is used to treat riboflavin deficiency or as an adjunct to thiamine treatment for nerve inflammation of lips secondary to pellagra. In 1992, the FDA proposed a ban on riboflavin in oral menstrual drug products because it has not been shown to be safe and effective for its stated claims.

**VITAMIN B₃** • *See* Niacin.

**VITAMIN B₅** • *See* Pantothenic Acid.

**VITAMIN B₆** • Pyridoxine. Beesix. Hexa-Betalin. Hexacrest. Nestrex. Rodex. Vitabee 6. Metabolizes protein; helps produce red blood cells; maintains proper functioning of nervous system tissue. Vitamin B₆ is believed to act as a partner for more than one hundred different enzymes. A number of the brain chemicals that send messages back and forth between nerves depend upon it for formation. A deficiency in this vitamin is known to cause depression and mental confusion. The occurrence of seizures in experimental animals in response to vitamin B₆ antagonists has been observed by many. Similar seizures observed in human infants made vitamin B₆ deficient inadvertently when they were fed a commercial infant formula in which the vitamin had not been properly preserved. Certain substances that deplete B$_6$ also produce deficiency seizures. Vitamin B$_6$ also reportedly helps rid the body tissues of excess fluid that causes some of the symptoms of premenstrual tension. Estrogen and cortisone deplete B$_6$. Storage over a long period of time diminishes the vitamin. Recommended daily allowance for newborns and infants to six months is 0.3 mg. Children four to six years, 1.1 mg. Children seven to ten years, 1.4 mg. Males eleven to fourteen years, 1.7 mg. Males fifteen years and over, 2 mg. Females eleven to fourteen years, 1.4 mg. Females fifteen to eighteen years, 1.5 mg. Females nineteen years and over 1.6 mg. Pregnant women, 2.2 mg. Lactating women, 2.1 mg. Used to treat vitamin B$_6$ deficiency and responsive anemias. Also prevents vitamin B$_6$ deficiency during isoniazid therapy to treat tuberculosis. Patients are likely to have a deficiency of B$_6$ if they are alcoholics, or have burns, diarrhea, heart disease, intestinal problems, liver disease, overactive thyroid, or are suffering the stress of long-term illness or serious injury. Patients on dialysis or who have their stomachs removed are also probably deficient in the vitamin. Current research seems to indicate that B$_6$ enhances the immune response in the elderly and may alleviate some signs of carpal tunnel syndrome, a wrist problem. Overdosing on B$_6$ is unwise. A study reported in the *New England Journal of Medicine* in 1983 described the loss of balance and numbness suffered by seven young adults who took from two to six grams of pyridoxine daily for several months to a year. Other potential adverse reactions include drowsiness and a feeling of pins and needles in limbs. In 1992, the FDA proposed a ban on pyridoxine in fever blister and cold sore treatment products because it has not been shown to be safe and effective for its stated claims.

**VITAMIN B$_9$** • *See* Folic Acid.

**VITAMIN B$_{12}$** • Cyanocobalamin. Anacobin. Bedoce. Betalin 12. Bioglan B$_{12}$. Crystamine. Cyano-Gel. Dodex. Kaybovite. Poyamin. Redisol. Rubesol-1000. Rubramin. Sigamine. Alpha-Ruvite. Codroxomin. Droxomin. Helps form red blood cells; maintains healthy nervous system. Deficiency symptoms include anemia, brain damage, and nervousness. More than one in five older Americans may need to take vitamin B$_{12}$ by injection to prevent neurological disorders, because their stomach acid does not enable them to absorb the vitamin from foods. The condition, known as atrophic gastritis, affects at least 20 percent of people over the age of sixty. Recommended daily allowance: neonates and infants to six months, 0.3 mcg. Infants six months to one year, 0.5 mcg. Children over one year to three years, 0.7 mcg. Children four to six years, 1 mcg. Adults and children eleven years and over, 2 mcg. Pregnant women, 2.2 mcg. Lactating women, 2.6 mcg. Potential adverse reactions include blood clots in veins, transient diarrhea, itching, hives, and severe allergic reactions with IV or injection. Aminoglycosides, colchicine, para-aminosalicylic acid, and chloramphenicol *(see all)* cause malabsorption of Vitamin $B_{12}$. Cobalt and its compounds are on the Community Right-To-Know List *(see)* and on EPA Genetic Toxicology Program *(see)*. Causes adverse reproductive effects in experimental animals. ASP

**VITAMIN B COMPLEX FACTOR** • *See* Panthenol. ASP

**VITAMIN C** • *See* Ascorbic Acid.

**VITAMIN $D_2$** • Calciferol. A pale yellow, oily liquid, odorless, tasteless, insoluble in water. Nutritional factor added to prepared breakfast cereals. Mellorine (vegetable fat imitation ice cream), vitamin D milk, evaporated and skim milks, margarine, infant dietary formulas, enriched flour, self-rising flour, enriched cornmeal and grits, enriched macaroni and noodle products (250–1,000 USP units), enriched farina and enriched bread, rolls, etc. Vitamin D speeds the body's production of calcium and has been found to cause calcium deposits and facial deformities and subnormal IQs in children of mothers given too much vitamin D. Nutritionists recommend 400 units per day for pregnant women. Some women taking vitamin pills and vitamin-enriched milk and foods consume as much as 2,000 to 3,000 units daily. Used for its alleged skin-healing properties in lubricating creams and lotions. The absence of vitamin D in the food of young animals can lead to rickets, a bone-affecting condition. It is soluble in fats and fat solvents and is present in animal fats. Absorbed through the skin. Its value in cosmetics has not been proven. The final report to the FDA of the Select Committee on GRAS Substances stated in 1980 that there is no evidence in the available information that it is a hazard to the public when used as it is now and it should continue its GRAS status with limitations on amounts that can be added to food.

**VITAMIN $D_3$** • Activated 7-dehydrocholesterol. Approximately as effective as vitamin $D_2$ *(see)*. The final report to the FDA of the Select Committee on GRAS Substances stated in 1980 that there is no evidence in the available information that it is a hazard to the public when used as it is now and it should continue its GRAS status with limitations on the amounts that can be added to food. Unilever United States, Inc., filed a petition in August 2003 proposing that the food additive regulations be amended to provide for the safe use of vitamin $D_3$ as a nutrient supplement in certain foods for special dietary use, such as meal replacement products and snack replacement products..

**VITAMIN E** • *See* Tocopherols. ASP

**VITAMIN E ACETATE** • *See* Tocopherols.

**VITAMIN E SUCCINATE** • *See* Tocopherols.

**VITAMIN G** • *See* Riboflavin.

**VITAMIN H** • *See* Biotin.

**VITAMIN K** • Recommended daily allowance for adults has not been established, but the safety and adequate daily dietary intake level is listed at 0.07

to 0.14 mg. It is necessary for blood clotting. Current research seems to indicate it helps maintain bone mass in the elderly and prevents osteoporosis *(see)*. Vitamin K antagonizes the action of anticoagulants and has been used as an antidote in managing overdosages or excessive responses to the latter. The excessive use of vitamin K–containing substances—drugs or dietary items such as green leafy vegetables—should be avoided in patients receiving anticoagulants. ASP

**VIVERRA CIVETTA SCHREBER** • *See* Civet, Absolute.

**VIVERRA ZIBETHA SCHREBER** • *See* Civet, Absolute.

**VOLATILE FATTY ACIDS INCLUDING ISOBUTYRIC ACID; ISO-VALERIC ACID; METHYL BUTYRIC ACID; M-VALERIC ACID** • Used in dairy cattle feeds as a source of energy. *See all.*

**VOLATILE OILS** • The volatility in oils is the tendency to give off vapors, usually at room temperature. The volatile oils in plants such as peppermint or rose produce the aroma. The volatile oils in plants stimulate the tissue with which they come in contact whether they are inhaled, ingested, or placed on the skin. They can relax or stimulate, irritate or soothe, depending upon the treatment and concentration.

# W

**WALNUT HULL EXTRACT** • An extract of the husk of the nut of *Juglans* spp. The English walnut tree, *Juglans regia* (fam. Juglandaceae), also known as European walnut, has been used medicinally for thousands of years, particularly for treating skin disorders. English walnut is native to southeastern Europe, Asia Minor, India, and China. The leaves, bark, and husks of black walnut, *Juglans nigra,* native to North America, have also been used traditionally as medicines by American Indians and later by European settlers. The bark of black walnut was chewed for toothaches and the inner bark was used as a laxative. The fruit husk was chewed for colic, the juice used on ringworm, and poulticed for inflammation. The leaves are considered astringent, and an insecticidal against bedbugs and mites (i.e., scabies). Used in walnut flavorings for beverages, ice cream, ices, candy, and baked goods. Also used for brown coloring. ASP

**WALNUT LEAVES, EXTRACT** • Flavoring. Black walnut has long been used in European folk herbalism for internal cleansing and detoxifying. The leaves of black walnut are most often used to treat hemorrhoids as well as liver and gallbladder problems. In folk medicine, black walnut leaf was also given to relieve headache, hepatitis, and skin conditions. Black walnut juice is believed to cure herpes, eczema, and worms. The compound, juglone, isolated from black walnut, has been shown to be a laxative, fight worms, and have strong activity against bacteria and abnormal growths. Walnuts are used to treat various glandular disorders including thyroid problems and studies have shown the fresh juice of green walnuts boosted thyroxine at least 30 percent. Its most prominent use today is as vermifuge to expel parasites (worms) from the body. *See* Walnut Hull Extract. ASP

**WALNUT SHELL POWDER** • The ground shell of English walnuts, *Juglans regia. See* Walnut Hull Extract.

**WASHES FOR FRUITS AND VEGETABLES** • Potassium bromide; sodium dodecylbenzenesulfonate; sodium hypochlorite; sodium 2-ethyl-1-hexylsulfate; sodium *n*-alkylbenzene sulfonate; sodium mono- and dimethyl-naphthalenesulfonates; alkylene oxide extracts of alkyl alcohols and phosphate esters of alkylene oxides. The chemicals are rinsed off by water although some residues may remain after rinsing.

**WATER** • Although deficiencies of other nutrients can be sustained for months or even years, a person can survive only a few days without water. Experts rank water second only to oxygen as essential for life. In addition to offering true refreshment for the thirsty, water plays a vital role in all bodily processes. It supplies the medium in which various chemical changes of the body occur, aiding in digestion, absorption, circulation, and lubrication of body joints. For example, as a major component of blood, water helps deliver nutrients to body cells and removes waste to the kidneys for excretion. Average adults need about sixty-four ounces of fluid each day for optimal health. Although experts generally advise drinking several glasses of water a day, the need for fluid can also be met by consuming a variety of foods and beverages.

**WATERCRESS EXTRACT** • Extract obtained from *Nasturtium officinale.*

**WAX, PARAFFIN** • Component of chewing-gum base and of certain cheeses. *See* Paraffin Wax.

**WAXES** • Obtained from insects, animals, petroleum, and plants. Waxes made in the United States are vegetable, petroleum, or bug based. One of the most common vegetable waxes, carnauba *(see),* is made from a palm leaf. Waxes from petroleum are the same as those used as chewing-gum bases. The shellac used on some products is made from the secretion of the lac bug, native to Pakistan and India. More than twenty varieties of fruits and vegetables, including cantaloupe, eggplant, oranges, peaches, grapefruit, rutabagas, persimmons, squash, cucumbers, sweet potatoes, and tomatoes are waxed. Waxing reduces the loss of moisture and keeps produce from dehydration. Some waxes are cosmetic. For example, oranges are waxed because consumers prefer a shiny surface rather than the natural dull matte of the rind. Beeswax is a substance secreted by the bee's special glands on the underside of its abdomen. The wax is glossy and hard but plastic when warm. Insoluble in water but partially soluble in boiling alcohol. Used in candy and vegetable coatings as well as for packaging. Waxes are generally nontoxic but may cause allergic reactions in the hypersensitive depending upon the source of the wax. It is also difficult to know which items have been waxed. Some foreign imports may use beef tallow, for example, which is undesirable in vegetarian or kosher diets. In many cases, pesticides and fungicides are added to waxes to help prevent decay. The wax is mainly used to keep produce fresh longer by sealing in moisture. The FDA does have regulations requiring all waxed products at the supermarket to be labeled as such, either with a card listing the specific ingredients in the wax above the bin or on the bin or container itself. (Have you seen such a listing?) Some companies, according to the Cornell University professor of food science Joseph Regenstein, Ph.D., switch waxes three times a day depending on environmental conditions. If you want to reduce the waxes on fruit and vegetables, wash them with warm water, and when appropriate scrub with a brush.

**WAXY MAIZE** • Corn Starch. The soft, sticky material from the inside of the corn kernel. The final report to the FDA of the Select Committee on GRAS Substances stated in 1980 that it should continue its GRAS status with no limitations other than good manufacturing practices.

**WETTING ADDITIVE** • Any of numerous water-soluble additives that promote spreading of a liquid on a surface or penetration into a material such as skin. It lowers surface tension for better contact and absorption. *See* Surfactants.

**WHEAT** • A cereal grain that yields a fine white powder. Wheat is avoided by some allergic people. Bread, cakes, crackers, cookies, pretzels, pastries, and noodles are made of wheat; also breakfast foods such as Cream of Wheat, pablum, Grapenuts, Wheaties, puffed wheat, shredded wheat, and bran; sauces, soups, gravies; Postum, Ovaltine, malted milk; sausages, hamburger, and meat loaf. Nontoxic.

**WHEAT BRAN** • The broken coat of *Triticum aestivum*. About 14.5 percent of the kernel. In addition to indigestible cellulose, it contains 86 percent of niacin, 73 percent of pyridoxine, 50 percent of pantothenic acid, 42 percent of riboflavin, 33 percent of thiamine, and 19 percent of protein. *See* Wheat Germ.

**WHEAT BRAN LIPIDS** • An extract of the coat of wheat. *See* Wheat Germ.

**WHEAT FLOUR** • Milled from the kernels of wheat, *Triticum aestivum*. *See* Wheat Starch.

**WHEAT GERM** • The golden germ of the wheat is high in vitamin E. About 2.5 percent of the whole wheat kernel. The germ contains about 64 percent of thiamine, 26 percent of riboflavin, and 21 percent of pyridoxine. *See* Tocopherols.

**WHEAT GERMAMIDOPROPYLAMINE** • *See* Tocopherols.

**WHEAT GERMAMIDOPROPYL BETAINE** • *See* Surfactants.

**WHEAT GERMAMIDOPROPYL DIMETHYLAMINE LACTATE** • *See* Tocopherols.

**WHEAT GERM EXTRACT** • *See* Tocopherols.

**WHEAT GERM GLYCERIDES** • *See* Tocopherols.

**WHEAT GERM OIL** • *See* Tocopherols.

**WHEAT GLUTEN** • A mixture of proteins present in wheat flour and obtained as an extremely sticky, yellowish gray mass by making a dough and then washing out the starch. It consists almost entirely of two proteins, gliadin and glutenin. It contributes to the porous and spongy structure of bread. Used in powders and creams as a base. ASP

**WHEAT STARCH** • A product of cereal grain. Swells when water is added. A minor part of starch production in the United States. May migrate from cotton and cotton fabrics used in dry food packaging. May cause allergic reactions such as red eyes and stuffy nose. The final report to the FDA of the Select Committee on GRAS Substances stated in 1980 that it should continue its GRAS status with no limitations other than good manufacturing practices. ASP

**WHEY** • The serum that remains after removal of fat and casein *(see)* from milk. Used as a texturizer, processing aid, and nutritional extender. Fermented whey is used as a dietary source of protein and nitrogen for cattle. GRAS. ASP

**WHEY, DELACTOSED** • The whey product that results from condensed whey after lactose has been crystallized and harvested from it. Delactosed whey, which is also referred to as "mother liquor" is composed of whey proteins, residual lactose, and minerals. ASP

**WHEY, DEMINERALIZED** • Formulation of physiologically suitable infant foods necessitates reduction of protein and mineral levels from bovine milk, rich in lactose and whey proteins and containing appropriately low levels of essential minerals. Demineralized whey is an ideal ingredient for infant formula. Demineralization of whey permits formulation of infant foods with a gross composition closest to mother's milk To manufacture this product, a top-quality raw whey is selected, then demineralized and spray-dried. This operation suppresses the salted flavor and it contains proteins with nutritional and functional properties. It is used in confectionery, chocolate, and ice cream. It can be substituted for skim milk powder. ASP

**WHEY, FERMENTED, AMMONIATED, CONDENSED** • Thirty percent of dietary crude protein in animal feed for cattle. Provides source of protein and nonprotein nitrogen.

**WHEY, PARTIALLY DEMINERALIZED AND PARTIALLY DELAC-TOSED** • Dried whey and dried skim milk are by-products of the cheese and fluid milk industry. Whey contains most of the water-soluble components of milk, including lactose, lactalbumin, and lactoglobulin protein, minerals, and water-soluble vitamins. Dried whey contains approximately

70 percent lactose (milk sugar), whereas dried skim milk contains 50 percent. The mineral and lactose *(see)* components are reduced by processing. GRAS. NIL

**WHEY PROTEIN CONCENTRATE** • Milk Serum. Serum Lactis. The water part of milk remaining after the separation of casein *(see)*. Cleared by the U.S. Department of Agriculture's Meat Inspection Department to bind and extend imitation sausage, and for use in soups and stews. Also used as source of protein and nonprotein nitrogen for cattle. GRAS

**WHEY, REDUCED LACTOSE** • Used in frozen desserts. GRAS

**WHITE CEDAR LEAF OIL** • Oil of Arborvitae. Stable, pale yellow volatile oil obtained by steam distillation from the fresh leaves and branch ends of the eastern arborvitae. Has a strong camphoraceous and sagelike scent. Used as a flavoring additive. *See* Cedar for toxicity.

**WHITE FLAG EXTRACT** • *See* Orris.

**WHITE LILY EXTRACT** • Extract of the bulbs of *Lilium candidum*. Edible bulbs that were made into soup by the Indians, the lily is used in perfumery.

**WHITE MINERAL OIL** • Obtained from petroleum and used in baked goods. *See* Mineral Oil.

**WHITE NETTLE EXTRACT** • Obtained from the flowers of *Lamium album*. *See* Nettles.

**WHOLE FISH PROTEIN CONCENTRATE** • Dietary supplement for household use only. FDA tolerance is less than 20 mg per day when consumed regularly by children up to eight years of age. When used in manufactured food, less than 8 ppm total fluoride content of finished food. For household use only. Package size, less than one pound. Less than 8 ppm total fluoride content of finished food when used in manufactured food.

**WILD CHERRY** • *See* Cherry, Wild Bark.

**WILD GINGER** • Canadian Oil. *See* Snakeroot Oil.

**WILD MARJORAM EXTRACT** • Extract of the flowering ends of *Origanum vulgare*. Yellow or greenish yellow liquid containing about 40 percent terpenes *(see)*. Used in flavoring and perfumery. *See* Marjoram Oil.

**WILD MINT EXTRACT** • Extract of the leaves and tender twigs of *Mentha arvensis*. The Cheyenne Indians prepared a decoction of the ground leaves and stems of wild mint and drank the liquid to check nausea. Pulegone and thymol *(see)* are derived from an oil of wild mint. Its odor resembles peppermint. Used in flavoring. *See* Peppermint.

**WILD THYME EXTRACT** • The flowering tops of a plant grown in Eurasia and throughout the United States. The dried leaves are used as a seasoning in foods. Has also been used as a muscle relaxant. GRAS

**WILLOW LEAF EXTRACT** • The extract of the leaves of the willow tree species *Salix*. The willow has been used for pain-relieving and fever-lowering properties since ancient Greece. The American Indians used willow baths to cool fevers, and indeed, the extract of willows contain salicylic acid, a close cousin of aspirin.

**WINTERGREEN EXTRACT** • *Gaultheria procumbens.* Flavoring. EAF

**WINTERGREEN OIL** • Extract and Oil. Menthyl Salicylate. Checkerberry Extract. Obtained naturally from betula, sweet birch, or teaberry oil. Present in certain leaves and bark but usually prepared by treating salicylic acid with methanol *(see both)*. Wintergreen extract is used in root beer and wintergreen flavorings for beverages and candy (5,000 ppm). The oil is used for checkerberry, raspberry, teaberry, fruit, nut, root beer, sassafras, spice, and wintergreen flavorings for beverages, ice cream, ices, candy, baked goods (1,500 ppm), and chewing gum (3,900 ppm). Wintergreen is a strong irritant. Ingestion of relatively small amounts may cause severe poisoning and death. Average lethal dose in children is 10 milliliters and in adults 30 milliliters. It is very irritating to the mucous membranes and skin and can be absorbed rapidly through the skin. Like other salicylates, it has a wide range of interaction with other drugs, including alcohol, antidiabetic medications, vitamin C, and tranquilizers. There is reported use of the chemical; it was not assigned for toxicology literature in 1999. It is still EAF.

**WOOD ROSIN** • The exudate from a living Southern pine tree. Pale yellow to amber, slight turpentine odor. Used as a coating for fresh citrus fruits.

**WOODRUFF** • Master of the Woods. Used as a flavoring in alcoholic beverages only. Made of the leaves of an herb grown in Europe, Siberia, North Africa, and Australia, *Asperula odorata.* It is a symbol of spring, and has a clean, fresh smell. EAF

**WORMWOOD** • Absinthium. A European woody herb with a bitter taste, used in bitters and as a liquor flavoring for beverages and liquors. The extract is used in bitters, liquor, and vermouth flavorings for beverages, ice cream, candy, and liquors, and in making absinthe. The oil is a dark green to brown and a narcotic substance. Used in bitters, apple, vermouth, and wine flavorings for beverages, ice cream, ices, candy, baked goods, and liquors. In large doses or frequently repeated doses, it is a narcotic poison, causing headache, trembling, and convulsions. Ingestion of the volatile oil or of the liquor, absinthe, may cause gastrointestinal symptoms, nervousness, stupor, coma, and death.

# X

**XANTHAN GUM** • A gum produced by a pure culture fermentation of a carbohydrate with *Xanthomonas campestris.* Also called corn sugar gum. The U.S. Department of Agriculture has asked for the use of xanthan gum as a necessary ingredient in packaging meat and poultry products. It is now used to thicken, suspend, emulsify, and stabilize water-based foods, such as dairy products and salad dressings. It is also used as a "pseudo plasticizer" in salad dressings to help them pour well. In animal feeds it is used as a stabilizer, thickener, and suspending additive. FDA tolerance is 0.25 percent in liquid feeds for ruminants; 0.1 percent in calf milk replacer. GRAS. ASP. E

**XANTHENE** • Colorants are divided into acid and basic groups. They are the second-largest category of certified colors. The acids are derived from fluorescein. The quinoid acid type is represented by FD and C Red No. 3, erythrosine, used frequently in lipsticks. The phenolic formulations, often called "bromo acids," are represented by D and C Red No. 2, used to "stain" lips. The only basic type certified is D and C Red No. 19, also called rhodamine B.

**XANTHOPHYLL** • Vegetable Lutein. A yellow coloring originally isolated from egg yolk, now isolated from petals of flowers. Occurs also in colored feathers of birds. One of the most widespread carotinoid alcohols (a group of red and yellow pigments) in nature. Provisionally listed for use in food. Although carotinoids can usually be turned into vitamin A, xanthophyll has no vitamin A activity. EAF

***XANTHOXYLUM AMERICANUM*** • Zanthoxylum. Ash Bark. Toothache Tree. Angelica Tree. The dried bark or berries of this tree, which grows in Canada south to Virginia and Missouri, is used to ease the pain of toothaches, to soothe stomachs, and as an antidiarrheal medicine.

**XYLANASE DERIVED FROM FUSARIUM VENENATUM** • Enzyme used for fermentation. GRAS

**XYLENOL** • A white crystalline solid that is derived from coal tar and is toxic by ingestion and skin absorption. It is used as a disinfectant and as a solvent. It caused cancer when painted on the skin of mice. ASP

**XYLITOL** • Formerly made from birch wood, but now made from waste products from the pulp industry. Xylitol has been reported to have diuretic effect but this has not been substantiated. It is used in chewing gum and as an artificial sweetener. It has been reported to sharply reduce cavities in teeth but costs more than sugar. The reason is that, unlike sugar, it doesn't ferment in the mouth. Therefore, it is sold for foods that stay in the mouth for some time, such as gum, toffee, and mints. FDA preliminary reports cited it as a possible cancer-causing additive. Xylitol is now used in eleven European countries and the United States and Canada. It is also used in large amounts in the former Soviet Union as a diabetic sweetener. Xylitol was evaluated by FAO/WHO *(see)* in Geneva, April 11–20, 1983. On the basis of submitted data, the committee accepted that the adverse effects observed in British studies, in which cancer-prone rats were fed large doses of xylitol, were species-specific and could not be extrapolated to humans. Therefore, no limit on daily intake was set and, no additional toxicological studies were recommended. It can cause stomach upsets when taken in large amounts. It may be of benefit to diabetics since xylitol metabolization does not involve insulin. NIL. E

**D-XYLOSE** • Xylo-Pfan. Wood Sugar. Used for evaluating intestinal absorption and diagnosing malabsorptive states. ASP

# Y

**YARA YARA** • See *b*-Naphthyl Methyl Ether.

**YARROW** • Milfoil. A strong-scented, spicy, wild herb, *Achillea millefolium,* used in liquor, root beer, and spice flavorings for beverages and liquor. Also used in shampoos. Its astringent qualities have caused it to be recommended by herbalists for greasy skin. According to old herbal recipes, it prevents baldness when the hair is washed regularly with it. Used medicinally as an astringent, tonic, and stimulant. May cause a sensitivity to sunlight and artificial light, in which the skin breaks out and swells. EAF

**YEAST** • A fungi that is a dietary source of folic acid. It produces enzymes that will convert sugar to alcohol and carbon dioxide. It is used in enriched farina, enriched cornmeal and corn grits, and in bakery products. It is employed as a flavoring additive and flavor enhancer. It is used in hot dogs, hamburger, and frankfurter buns and rolls, pretzels, milk fortified with vitamins, meat fried in cracker crumbs, mushrooms, truffles, cheeses of all kinds, vinegars, ketchup, barbecue sauce, fermented brews, and all dried fruits. Any yeast is a type of one-celled fungus. Ordinary yeast produces the enzymes invertase and zymase, which eventually convert cane sugar to alcohol and carbon dioxide in the fermentation process. Some of the living organisms pressed into damp starch, or other absorbent material, give a product known as "baker's yeast," which is not as potent as brewer's yeast. GRAS

**YEAST AUTOLYZATES** • Concentrated soluble components of hydrolyzed brewer's or baker's yeasts, a by-product of brewing. They provide a good source of B vitamins. The final report to the FDA of the Select Committee on GRAS Substances stated in 1980 that while no evidence in the available information on it demonstrates a hazard to the public at current use levels, uncertainties exist, requiring that additional studies be conducted. The FDA said GRAS status should continue while tests were being completed and evaluated. ASP

**YEAST, DRIED** • The dry cells of any suitable strain of *Saccharomyces cerevisiae* or *Candida utilis.* It can be obtained as a by-product from the brewing of beer or by growing on media not suitable for beer production. Dried yeast serves as a source of protein and vitamin B complex. ASP

**YEAST, DRIED IRRADIATED** • Dietary supplement used in enriched farina as source of Vitamin D. NUL

**YEAST EXTRACT** • *See* Yeast.

**YEAST, MALT SPROUT EXTRACT** • Used as a flavor enhancer. *See* Yeast. ASP

**YEAST and TORULA YEAST, DRIED** • Dietary supplement used in food to provide total folic acid content. *See* Yeast.

**YELLOW BEESWAX** • Obtained from bee honeycombs, it is brittle with a honeylike odor and a balsamic taste. It is used in the manufacture of wax paper, candles, cosmetics, shoe polish, and in pharmaceutical ointments and plasters. May cause allergic reactions. GRAS

**YELLOW NO. 5** • All foods containing this coloring, which is the most widely used color additive in foods, drugs, and cosmetics, are supposed to identify it on the label. The FDA ordered this so that those allergic to it could avoid it. *See also* Tartrazine and Salicylates.

**YELLOW PRUSSIATE OF SODA** • Sodium Ferrocyanide. An anticaking additive, it is used in table salt to prevent the formation of clumps and keep it free-flowing. The additive is produced by heating sodium carbonate and iron with organic materials. The average daily diet in the United States contains 0.6 milligrams of sodium ferrocyanide per person. FAO/WHO *(see)* considers 1.5 milligrams daily an acceptable and safe intake for a 132-pound human. ASP

**YELLOW WAX** • *See* Beeswax.

**YERBA SANTA FLUID EXTRACT** • Holy Herb. Fruit flavoring derived from evergreen shrubs, *Eriodictyon californicum,* grown in California. Used in beverages, ice cream, ices, candy, and baked goods, and to mask the bitter taste of drugs. Also used as an expectorant.

**YLANG-YLANG OIL** • A light yellow, very fragrant liquid obtained in the Philippines from flowers of *Cananga odorata.* Used in raspberry, cola, violet, cherry, rum, and ginger ale flavorings for beverages, ice cream, ices, candy, baked goods, chewing gum, and icing. Used in perfumes, cosmetics, and soap. GRAS. EAF

**YOGURT** • A dairy product produced by the action of bacteria or yeast on milk.

**YUCCA EXTRACT** • Mohave Extract. Joshua Tree. Adam's Needle. Derived from a southwestern U.S. plant, *Yucca* spp., and used as a root beer flavoring for beverages, ices, and ice cream. ASP

# Z

**ZANTHOXYLUM** • Xanthoxylum. Ash Bark. Toothache Tree. Angelica Tree. The dried bark or berries of this tree, which grows in Canada south to Virginia, and Missouri, is used to ease the pain of toothaches, to soothe stomachaches, and as an antidiarrheal medicine. A member of the rue family.

**ZEDOARY** • A bark extract from the East Indies, *Curcuma zedoaria,* used as a bitters and ginger ale flavoring for beverages. GRAS. There is reported use of the chemical, but it has not yet been assigned for toxicology literature.

**ZEIN** • It is the principal protein in corn. Contains seventeen amino acids. A by-product of corn processing, it is used to coat food and in label varnishes and microencapsulation fibers. Also used in face masks, nail polishes, and as a plasticizer. Obtained as a yellowish powder by extracting corn gluten with an alcohol; also used to make textile fibers, plastics, printing inks, varnishes, and other coatings and adhesives. GRAS. There was reported use of the chemical; it was not assigned for toxicology literature in 1999. It is still EAF.

**ZEIN POWDER** • The water-insoluble protein gluten, manufactured initially as a concentrated powder. It has the ability to form odorless, tasteless, clear, hard and almost invisible edible films. Since zein films are safe to ingest, it is a coating for foods and pharmaceutical ingredients. Zein is extracted from gluten by physical rather than chemical means and is natural. Zein is resistant to bacterial attack, which frequently decomposes other proteins GRAS. ASP

**(Z)-2-HEXEN-1-OL** • Synthetic flavoring. FEMA *(see)* declared it GRAS. *See* Aldehyde. EAF

**(Z)-3-HEXENYL ANTHRANILATE** • Synthetic flavoring with a sweet, fruity odor. FEMA *(see)* has declared it GRAS. EAF

**(Z)-3-HEXENYL (E)-2-HEXENOATE** • Synthetic plumlike odor. Declared GRAS by FEMA. EAF

**(Z)-3-HEXENYL(E)-2-METHYL-2-BUTENOATE** • Synthetic flavoring declared GRAS by FEMA *(see)* and said to be of no safety concern to FAO/WHO *(see)*. EAF

**(Z)-3-HEXENYL ISOBUTYRATE** • Synthetic flavoring declared GRAS by FEMA *(see)* and of no safety concern to FAO/WHO *(see)*. EAF

**(Z)-3-HEXENYL PROPIONATE** • Synthetic flavoring declared GRAS by FEMA *(see)* and of no safety concern to FAO/WHO *(see)*. ASP

**(Z)-3-HEXENYL PYRUVATE** • Synthetic flavoring declared GRAS by FEMA *(see)* and of no safety concern to FAO/WHO *(see)*. EAF

**(Z)-3-HEXENYL VALERATE** • Synthetic flavoring. EAF

**ZERANOL** • Zearalanol. A hormone used to increase growth in animals. The FDA allows zero residues in uncooked edible tissues of sheep; 150 ppb in uncooked edible muscle tissue of cattle; 300 ppb as residue in uncooked kidney of cattle; 450 ppb as residues in uncooked fat of cattle; 600 ppb as an implant.

**ZINC** • Acetate, Carbonate, Chloride, Oxide, Sulfate. A white brittle metal insoluble in water and soluble in acids or hot solutions of alkalies. It is a mineral source and added as a nutrient to food. Widely used as an astringent for mouthwashes and as a reducing additive *(see)* and readditive *(see)*. Ingestion of the salts can cause nausea and vomiting. It can cause contact dermatitis. The FDA says some studies appeared to show zinc supplements improved immunity to disease in older people. But the studies were flawed. In larger, well-designed studies, the FDA says, in which older patients received either zinc or placebos in addition to multivitamins and mineral preparations, the greatest immune function improvements were among those taking placebos. Zinc supplementation, the FDA says, not only did not improve immune system function in the elderly at 100 mg or more a day, it actually suppressed immunity. *See* Zinc Chloride. GRAS

**ZINC ACETATE** • The zinc salt of acetic acid *(see)* used in medicine as a dietary supplement and as a cross-linking additive for polymers *(see)*. For toxicity, *see* Zinc. GRAS. NIL

**ZINC BACITRACIN** • Used in animal feed. *See* Bacitracin.

**ZINC BORATE** • The inorganic salt of zinc oxide and boric oxide, it is used as a fungistat and mildew inhibitor. *See* Zinc.

**ZINC CARBONATE** • A cosmetic coloring additive, it is a crystalline salt of zinc occurring in nature as smithsonite. *See* Zinc for toxicity. GRAS. NUL

**ZINC CHLORIDE** • Butter of Zinc. A zinc salt used as an antiseptic and astringent in shaving creams, dentifrices, and mouthwashes. Odorless and water absorbing; also a deodorant and disinfectant. Can cause contact dermatitis and is mildly irritating to the skin. Can be absorbed through the skin. GRAS. ASP

**ZINC GLUCONATE** • A dietary supplement. *See* Zinc. GRAS. ASP

**ZINC GLUTAMATE** • The zinc salt of glutamic acid *(see)*.

**ZINC ION and MANEB** • A pesticide used on raisins, flours of barley, oats, rye, and wheat. Maneb is a fungicide. FDA residue tolerances: 28 ppm in raisins; 1 ppm in flours of barley, oats, rye, and wheat; 20 ppm in bran of barley, oats, rye, and wheat as well as milled feed fractions of those grains.

**ZINC METHIONINE SULFATE** • A nutrient. *See* Zinc and Methionine.

**ZINC OXIDE** • A nutrient supplement. *See* Zinc. GRAS. ASP

**ZINC RESINATE** • The zinc salt of rosin *(see)*.

**ZINC RICINOLEATE** • The zinc salt of ricinoleate *(see)*. Used as a fungicide, emulsifier, and stabilizer

**ZINC ROSINATE** • The zinc salt of rosin *(see)*.

**ZINC STEARATE** • Nutrient. Should be free from chick edema factor. *See* Zinc. GRAS. ASP

**ZINC SULFATE** • White Vitriol. The reaction of sulfuric acid with zinc. Mild crystalline zinc salt used as a nutrient. Migrates to food from paperboard products. Used medicinally as an emetic. Irritating to the skin and mucous membranes. May cause an allergic reaction. Injection under the skin of 2.5 milligrams per kilogram of body weight caused tumors in rabbits. *See* Zinc. GRAS. ASP

**ZINGERONE** • A synthetic flavoring occurring naturally in ginger. Used in fruit, root beer, sarsaparilla, spice, ginger ale, wintergreen, and birch beer flavorings for beverages, ice cream, ices, candy, baked goods, and chewing gum. ASP

**ZINGIBER OFFICINALE** • *See* Ginger.

**ZINGIBER ONE** • *See* Zingerone.

**ZOALENE** • Dinitolmide. Used in chicken and turkey feed to combat parasites. FDA tolerance residue is 2 ppm in uncooked fat of chickens; 3 ppm in uncooked muscle meat of chickens; 3 ppm in uncooked muscle meat and liver of turkeys; 6 ppm in uncooked liver and kidneys of chickens.

# APPENDIX A
# WHAT COUNTS AS A SERVING?

Americans have gotten fatter. The National Institutes of Health reported for the first time in history in 2003, the majority of us—an estimated 55 percent—are clinically overweight, while one in every four is severely overweight. The USDA statistics show that our daily caloric intake has risen from 1,854 kcal to 2,002 kcal over the last twenty years. Many believe this is in part due to the steady increase in U.S. portion sizes over the past few decades. A European muffin, for example, is about an ounce and a half while ours is as much as eight ounces. Table-service restaurants have increased the plate size from a ten-inch to a twelve-inch size since our parents dined out. If you have been on a diet—and most of us have—portion size is almost always emphasized. One of the problems that occurs with the amount of ingredients listed on package labels is what makes a serving. For instance, one low sodium soy sauce appears to be lower in sodium than a second but when you check the bottles, the serving size of the first is smaller, accounting for the decrease in sodium listed on the label. The second may actually contain less salt although the serving size is larger. So you have to check the serving size as well as the ingredients. The following are common serving sizes:

*Grain Products Group (bread, cereal, rice, and pasta)*
1 slice of bread
1 ounce of ready-to-eat cereal
½ cup of cooked cereal, rice, or pasta

*Vegetable Group*
1 cup of raw leafy vegetables
½ cup of other vegetables—cooked or chopped raw
¾ cup of vegetable juice

*Fruit Group*
1 medium apple, banana, orange
½ cup of chopped, cooked, or canned fruit
¾ cup of fruit juice

*Milk Group (milk, yogurt, and cheese)*
1 cup of milk or yogurt
1½ ounces of natural cheese
2 ounces of processed cheese

*Meat and Beans Group*
*(meat, poultry, fish, dry beans, eggs, and nuts)*
2 to 3 ounces of cooked lean meat, poultry, or fish
$1/2$ cup of cooked dry beans or 1 egg counts as 1 ounce of lean meat
2 tablespoons of peanut butter or $1/3$ cup of nuts count as 1 ounce of meat

# APPENDIX B
# MAKING SURE
# YOUR FOOD HASN'T EXPIRED

A large percentage of food additives are preservatives meant to extend shelf life but even "embalmed" foods may spoil or become less appetizing.

Want a date? You can use the dates that are given on food packaging if the manufacturer is using "open dating." On the other hand, "code dating" is not useful to the consumer. In open dating, dates are stated alphanumerically, such as Oct. 15, or numerically, such as 10-15 or 1015. In code dating, the information is coded in letters, numbers, and symbols so that usually only the manufacturer can translate it.

Open dating may be used for:

**Pull date.** This is the last day that the manufacturer recommends that the product remain for sale. This date takes into consideration additional time for storage and use at home. If the food is bought on the pull date, it still can be eaten at a later date. How long the product should be offered for sale and how much home storage is allowed are determined by the manufacturer, based on knowledge of the product and the product's shelf life.

**Quality assurance or freshness date.** This date shows how long the manufacturer thinks a food will be of optimal quality. On the label, it often appears as: "Best if used by March 2, 2000." This doesn't mean, however, that the product can't be used after the suggested date.

**Pack date.** This is the date the food was packaged or processed. It may enable you to determine how old a product really is.

**Expiration date.** This is the last day on which a product should be eaten. State governments regulate these dates for perishable items, such as milk and eggs. The FDA regulates only the expiration dates of infant formula.

**Code date** is of considerably less use to you. A common type of code dating is the product code. This code enables the manufacturer to convey a relatively large amount of information with a few small letters, numbers, and symbols. It tells when and where a product was packaged. In the case of a recall, this makes it easier for the grocer and manufacturer to quickly identify and track down the product and take it off the market. The FDA encourages manufacturers to put product codes on packaging, especially for products with a long shelf life. Food processors are often masters at making codes inconspicuous. On frozen-food packages, the dates are usually indented on the wrapper or the carton. These colorless indentations are most often found at one end of the package. Another method of dating frozen food involves putting a small letter or number on the food wrapper. It is not stamped, but is part of the printing on the wrapper. Cans have the code numbers embossed on one end of the can, usually the bottom or now digitally printed on the end. Boxes have either stamped or indented codes on one end of the package.

It is impractical to give all the codes here, but most supermarkets keep a thick book of master codes in their offices. If you have no success in breaking the code of a particular product, ask the store manager to see the codebook.

# APPENDIX C
# FOOD STORAGE INFORMATION*

Supermarkets today have an amazing array of fresh, frozen, and prepared foods. Your store maintains rigid quality assurance and sanitation standards to make sure you always receive fresh, wholesome, and safe food products.

After selecting food items, though, it's up to you to take care of them properly. The Food Keeper contains valuable food safety and storage advice to help you maintain the freshness and quality of foods that you purchase.

*Reprinted by permission of The Food Marketing Institute

| Food | Refrigerator | Pantry | Freezer | Special |
|------|-------------|--------|---------|---------|
| Apples | 1 to 3 weeks | | | Do not wash. Store in crisper or moisture-resistant wrap. Wash individual apples before eating. |
| Asparagus | 1 to 2 days | | 8 months | Keep in crisper |
| Bacon (opened) | 5 to 7 days | | Not recommended | Keep wrapped. Store in coldest part of refrigerator or in meat keeper. |
| Bacon (unopened) | 2 weeks | | If frozen, 1 month | Keep wrapped. Store in coldest part of the refrigerator or in meat keeper. |
| Bananas | Only when fully ripe | | | |

| Food | Refrigerator | Pantry | Freezer | Special |
|------|--------------|--------|---------|---------|
| Dried beans | | 12 months | | Keep in crisper or moisture-proof wrap. |
| Green or wax beans | 1 to 2 days | | 8 months | Keep in crisper or moisture-proof wrap |
| Lima beans (unshelled) | 3 to 5 days | | 8 months | Keep in crisper or moisture-proof wrap. |
| Beef casseroles | | | 3 months | Freeze 2 weeks in original wrapper. Use suitable wrap for longer periods. |
| Beef chops | 2 to 3 days | | 6 to 9 months | Freeze 2 weeks in original wrapper. Use suitable wrap for longer periods. |
| Corned beef | 5 to 7 days | | Not recommended | Freeze 2 weeks in original wrapper. Use suitable wrap for longer periods. |
| Dried beef | 10 to 12 days | | | Freeze 2 weeks in original wrapper. Use suitable wrap for longer periods. |
| Ground Beef | 1 to 2 days | | 2 to 3 months | Freeze 2 weeks in original wrapper. Use suitable wrap for longer periods. |

| Food | Refrigerator | Pantry | Freezer | Special |
|---|---|---|---|---|
| Roast beef | 2 to 4 days | | 6 to 12 months | Freeze 2 weeks in original wrapper. Use suitable wrap for longer periods. |
| Beef sausage | 2 to 3 days | | 1 to 2 months | Freeze 2 weeks in original wrapper. Use suitable wrap for longer periods. |
| Beef steaks | 2 to 3 days | | 1 to 2 months | Freeze 2 weeks in original wrapper. Use suitable wrap for longer periods. |
| Beef stew meat | 1 to 2 days | | 6 to 9 months | Freeze 2 weeks in original wrapper. Use suitable wrap for longer periods. |
| TV dinners with beef | | | 6 months | Freeze 2 weeks in original wrapper. Use suitable wrap for longer periods. |
| Varieties of beef (heart, liver, etc.) | | | 1 to 2 months | Freeze 2 weeks in original wrapper. Use suitable wrap for longer periods. |
| Beets | 1 to 2 weeks | | | Remove leafy tops. Keep in crisper. |
| Berries | 1 to 2 days | | 12 months | Store opened. |

| Food | Refrigerator | Pantry | Freezer | Special |
|------|------------|--------|---------|---------|
| Biscuit mix | | 9 months | | Keep cool and dry. |
| Bread, commercial | | | 2 to 3 months | |
| Quick baked bread | | | 3 to 6 months | |
| Yeast bread (baked) | | | 1 month | |
| Yeast bread (unbaked) | Check expiration date on label. | | | |
| Broth (leftover) | 2 days | | 1 month | |
| Brownie mix | | 9 months | | Keep cool and dry. |
| Butter | 1 to 2 weeks | | 6 to 9 months | |
| Buttermilk | 10 to 30 days | | No | |
| Cabbage | 1 to 2 weeks | | No | |
| Cakes, purchased | | 1 to 2 days | | If buttercream, whipped cream, cream, or custard frosting filling, refrigerate. |
| Angel food cake | | | 2 months | If buttercream, whipped cream, cream, or custard frosting filling, refrigerate. |

| Food | Refrigerator | Pantry | Freezer | Special |
|------|--------------|--------|---------|---------|
| Chiffon sponge cake | | | 2 months | If buttercream, whipped cream, cream, or custard frosting filling, refrigerate. |
| Cheesecake | | | 2 to 3 months | If buttercream, whipped cream, cream, or custard frosting filling, refrigerate. |
| Chocolate cake | | | 4 months | If buttercream, whipped cream, cream, or custard frosting filling, refrigerate. |
| Fruit cake | | | 12 months | If buttercream, whipped cream, cream, or custard frosting filling, refrigerate. |
| Yellow pound cake | | | 6 months | If buttercream, whipped cream, cream, or custard frosting filling, refrigerate. |
| Cakes, frosted | | | 8 to 12 months | If buttercream, whipped cream, cream, or custard frosting filling, refrigerate. |
| Home-frozen cake | | | 3 months | If buttercream, whipped cream, cream, or custard frosting filling, refrigerate. |

| Food | Refrigerator | Pantry | Freezer | Special |
|------|--------------|--------|---------|---------|
| Canned food, all types (unopened) | | | | Transfer all opened canned foods to plastic or glass containers before refrigerating. |
| Canned food (opened) | | | | Transfer all opened canned foods to plastic or glass containers before refrigerating. |
| Canned baby foods | 2 to 3 days | | | Transfer all opened canned foods to plastic or glass containers before refrigerating. |
| Canned fish and shellfish | 2 days | | | Transfer all opened canned foods to plastic or glass containers before refrigerating. |
| Canned fruit | 1 week | | | Transfer all opened canned foods to plastic or glass containers before refrigerating. |
| Canned meats | 2 days | | | Transfer all opened canned foods to plastic or glass containers before refrigerating. |

| Food | Refrigerator | Pantry | Freezer | Special |
|---|---|---|---|---|
| Canned pickles | 1 to 2 months | | | Transfer all opened canned foods to plastic or glass containers before refrigerating. |
| Canned poultry | 2 days | | | Transfer all opened canned foods to plastic or glass containers before refrigerating. |
| Canned sauce (tomato) | 5 days | | | Transfer all opened canned foods to plastic or glass containers before refrigerating. |
| Canned vegetables | 3 days | | | Transfer all opened canned foods to plastic or glass containers before refrigerating. |
| Carrots | 1 to 2 weeks | | 8 months | |
| Chili or cocktail sauce (unopened) | | 12 months | | Refrigeration recommended after opening. |
| Celery | 1 to 2 weeks | | Does not freeze successfully. | Keep in crisper or moisture-proof wrapper. |

| Food | Refrigerator | Pantry | Freezer | Special |
|------|--------------|--------|---------|---------|
| Ready-to-eat cereals (unopened) | | 6 to 12 months | | |
| Ready-to-eat cereals (opened) | | 2 to 3 months | | Refold package liner tightly. |
| Hot cereals (require cooking) | | 6 months | | |
| Cottage cheese | 10 to 30 days | | | |
| Cream cheese (opened) | 2 weeks | | | Keep all cheese tightly packaged in moisture-proof wrap. |
| Neufchâtel (opened) | 2 weeks | | | Keep all cheese tightly packaged in moisture-proof wrap. |
| Hard and wax-coated cheese, cheddar, Edam, Gouda, Swiss, brick, etc. (unopened) | 3 to 6 months | | | Moisture-proof wrap. If outside gets somewhat moldy, trim off ½ inch. The cheese may become crumbly after freezing. |

| Food | Refrigerator | Pantry | Freezer | Special |
|------|--------------|--------|---------|---------|
| Hard and wax-coated cheese, cheddar, Edam, Gouda, Swiss, brick, etc. (opened) | 3 to 4 weeks | | | Keep all cheese tightly packaged in moisture-proof wrap. If outside gets somewhat moldy, trim off ½ inch. The cheese may become crumbly after freezing. |
| Hard and wax-coated cheese, cheddar, Edam, Gouda, Swiss, brick, etc. (sliced) | 2 weeks | | | Keep all cheese tightly packaged in moisture-proof wrap. If outside gets somewhat moldy, trim off ½ inch. The cheese may become crumbly after freezing. |
| Parmesan, Romano cheese (opened) | | 2 months | | If it picks up moisture, it will develop mold. |
| Parmesan, Romano cheese (unopened) | 2 months | 10 months | | If it picks up moisture, it will develop mold. |
| Ricotta cheese | 5 days | | No | |
| Processed cheese products | 3 to 4 weeks | | 4 months | Refrigerate after opening. Keep tightly closed. |

| Food | Refrigerator | Pantry | Freezer | Special |
|------|--------------|--------|---------|---------|
| Cherries | 1 to 2 days | | 12 months | Do not wash. Store in crisper or moisture-resistant wrap. Wash before eating. |
| Chicken | 2 to 3 days | | 12 months | |
| Chicken livers | 1 to 2 days | | 3 months | |
| Chicken TV dinners | | | 6 months | |
| Premelted chocolate | | 12 months | | Keep cool. |
| Semisweet chocolate | | 2 years | | Keep cool. |
| Unsweetened chocolate | | 18 months | | Keep cool. |
| Chocolate syrup (unopened) | | 2 years | | |
| Chocolate syrup (opened) | | 6 months | | Cover tightly and refrigerate. |
| Corn | 1 to 2 days in husks | | 8 months | |
| Shucked clams | 1 day | | 3 months | |
| Cocoa mixes | | 8 months | | Cover tightly. |
| Coffee, cans (unopened) | | 2 years | | Refrigerate after opening. Keep tightly closed. Use dry measuring spoon. |

| Food | Refrigerator | Pantry | Freezer | Special |
|------|--------------|--------|---------|---------|
| Coffee, cans (opened) | 2 weeks | | | Refrigerate after opening. Keep tightly closed. Use dry measuring spoon. |
| Coffee lightener, dry (unopened) | | 6 months | | Keep tightly closed. |
| Coffee lightener, dry (opened) | | 6 months | | Keep tightly closed. |
| Cookies, homemade | | 2 to 3 weeks | 8 to 12 months | Put in air-tight container. |
| Cookies, packaged | | 2 months | 8 to 12 months | Keep box tightly closed. |
| Cornmeal | | 12 months | | Keep tightly closed (in refrigerator, especially in summer). |
| Cornstarch | | 18 months | | Keep tightly closed. |
| King crab | | | 10 months | Keep in original wrap. |
| Crab, in shell | 2 days | | | |
| Crackers (unopened) | | 8 months | | Keep box tightly closed. |
| Cream, half & half | 10 days | | No | Cover tightly. To prevent bacteria from spreading to left-over cream, don't return unused cream to original container. Keep covered. |

| Food | Refrigerator | Pantry | Freezer | Special |
|------|-------------|--------|---------|---------|
| Light heavy cream | 10 days | | No | Cover tightly. To prevent bacteria from spreading to leftover cream, don't return unused cream to original container. Keep covered. |
| Cream, coffee lightener (liquid) | 10 days | | No | Cover tightly. To prevent bacteria from spreading to leftover cream, don't return unused cream to original container. Keep covered. |
| Sour cream | 2 to 4 weeks | | | Cover tightly. To prevent bacteria from spreading to leftover cream, don't return unused cream to original container. Keep covered. |

| Food | Refrigerator | Pantry | Freezer | Special |
|------|-------------|--------|---------|---------|
| Whipped cream topping in aerosol can | 3 months | | | Cover tightly. To prevent bacteria from spreading to leftover cream, don't return unused cream to original container. Keep covered. |
| Cream prepared from mix | 3 days | | | Cover tightly. To prevent bacteria from spreading to leftover cream, don't return unused cream to original container. Keep covered. |
| Dry cream | | 12 months | | |
| Frozen cream topping (after thawed) | 2 weeks | | | Cover tightly. To prevent bacteria from spreading to leftover cream, don't return unused cream to original container. Keep covered. |
| Duck | 2 days | | 6 months | |
| Eggs, in shell | 4 to 5 weeks | | No | |
| Egg whites | 1 week | | 12 months | |

| Food | Refrigerator | Pantry | Freezer | Special |
|------|-------------|--------|---------|---------|
| Egg yolks | 3 days | | 12 months | Yolks will thicken when frozen. |
| Hardcooked eggs | 1 week | | | |
| Lean fish (cod, flounder, haddock, sole) | 1 to 2 days | | 6 months | Freeze in original wrap for up to 2 weeks. For longer periods wrap with suitable freezer wrap. |
| Fatty fish (bluefish, perch, mackerel, salmon) | 1 to 2 days | | 2 to 3 months | Freeze in original wrap for up to 2 weeks. For longer periods wrap with suitable freezer wrap. |
| Breaded fish | | | 3 months | Keep purchased frozen fish in original wrap, thaw, and follow cooking directions on package. |
| White flour | | 6 to 8 months | | Keep in airtight container. |
| Whole-wheat flour | 6 to 8 months | | | Keep in airtight container. |
| Frosting, canned | | 3 months | | Store leftover in refrigerator. |
| Frosting, mix | | | 8 months | Store leftover in refrigerator. |
| Citrus fruit | 1 week | | | |

| Food | Refrigerator | Pantry | Freezer | Special |
|------|-------------|--------|---------|---------|
| Citrus fruit (dried) | | | 6 months | Keep cool in airtight container. |
| Citrus fruit (sections) | | | | 6 months |
| Gelatin (all types) | | 18 months | | |
| Gravy (leftover) | 2 days | | 1 month | |
| Greens | 1 to 2 days | | | |
| Whole ham | 1 week | | | Freezing cured meat not recommended. |
| Canned ham (unopened) | 6 months | | | Freezing cured meat not recommended. |
| Ham TV dinner | | | 3 months | |
| Honey | | 12 months | | If crystals form, heat in pan of water. |
| Hot roll mix | | 18 months | | |
| Ice cream, ice milk | | | 2 to 4 months | |
| Jellies (unopened) | | 12 months | | Cover tightly. Storage life lengthened if refrigerated after opening. |
| Canned juices | | 9 months | | |
| Citrus juices | 6 days | | 6 months | |
| Concentrated juices | 6 days | | 12 months | |

| Food | Refrigerator | Pantry | Freezer | Special |
|------|-------------|--------|---------|---------|
| Ketchup | | 12 months | | Refrigeration recommended after opening. |
| Ground lamb | 1 to 2 days | | 2 to 3 months | |
| Lamb steak and chops | 2 to 3 days | | 3 to 4 months | |
| Lamb roasts | 2 to 4 days | | 3 to 4 months | |
| Lamb stew meat | 1 to 2 days | | 3 to 4 months | |
| Varieties of lamb meats | 1 day | | 2 to 3 months | |
| Lettuce head (unwashed) | 5 to 7 days | | | |
| Lettuce head (washed, thoroughly drained) | 3 to 5 days | | | |
| Bibb lettuce | 1 to 2 days | | | |
| Lobster tails | 2 days in the shell | | 3 months | |
| Lunch meats | 4 to 6 days | No | Freezing not recommended. | |
| Margarine | | 2 to 3 months | | Keep in airtight container. |
| Marshmallows | | 2 to 3 months | | Keep in airtight container. |
| Marshmallow cream | | 3 to 4 months | | Cover tightly. Refrigerate after opening to extend storage life. Use at room temperature. |

| Food | Refrigerator | Pantry | Freezer | Special |
|------|-------------|--------|---------|---------|
| Mayonnaise (opened) | | 2 to 3 months | | Refrigerate after opening. |
| Meat substitutes, textured protein products (e.g., imitation bacon bits) | | 4 months | | Keep tightly closed. For longer storage, refrigerate. |
| Melon | 1 week | | | |
| Metered-caloric products, instant breakfast | | 6 months | | Keep in can, closed jars, or original packets. |
| Condensed or evaporated milk (unopened) | | 9 months | | Invert can every 2 months. |
| Condensed or evaporated milk (opened) | 4 to 5 days | | | |
| Fresh milk | 5 days | | 1 month | |
| Molasses (unopened) | | 12 months | | |
| Molasses (opened) | | 6 months | | Keep tightly closed. Refrigerate to extend storage life. |
| Nuts in shell (unopened) | | 4 months | | Refrigerate after opening. Freeze for longer life. Unsalted and blanched nuts keep longer than salted. |

| Food | Refrigerator | Pantry | Freezer | Special |
|------|-------------|--------|---------|---------|
| Nutmeats, packaged in vacuum can (unopened) | | 1 year | | Refrigerate after opening. Freeze for longer life. Unsalted and blanched nuts keep longer than salted. |
| Nutmeats, packaged in vacuum can (opened) | | 3 months | | Refrigerate after opening. Freeze for longer life. Unsalted and blanched nuts keep longer than salted. |
| Salted nuts | | | 6 to 8 months | Package tightly in suitable freezer wrap. |
| Unsalted nuts | | | 9 to 12 months | Package tightly in suitable freezer wrap. |
| Onions | | 3 to 4 weeks | | Keep dry and away from sun. |
| Oysters | 1 day | | 4 months | |
| Pancake mix | | 6 to 9 months | | Once opened, store in airtight container. |
| Pasta (spaghetti, pasta, etc.) | | 2 years | | |
| Peaches (ripe) | | 1 to 2 weeks | | 12 months |
| Peanut butter (unopened) | | 6 to 9 months | | |

| Food | Refrigerator | Pantry | Freezer | Special |
|------|--------------|--------|---------|---------|
| Peanut butter (opened) | | 2 to 3 months | | Keeps longer if refrigerated. |
| Pears (ripe) | | 1 week | 12 months | |
| Peas | | | 8 months | |
| Dried peas | | 12 months | | Store in a cool, dry place in air-tight container. |
| Unshelled peas | 3 to 5 days | | | Store in cool, dry place in air-tight container. |
| Pectin, liquid (opened) | | | 1 month | Recap and refrigerate. |
| Pies and pastries | | 2 to 3 days | | Refrigerate whipped cream, custard, and chiffon fillings. |
| Pies and pastries, baked | | | 1 to 2 months | Refrigerate whipped cream, custard, and chiffon fillings. |
| Pies and pastries, unbaked | | | 8 months | Refrigerate whipped cream, custard, and chiffon fillings. |
| Pineapple | 1 week | | 12 months | |
| Popcorn (unpopped) | | 2 years | | Store in airtight container. |
| Pork chops | 2 to 3 days | | 2 to 3 months | Original wrap up to 2 weeks. For longer period rewrap in suitable freezer wrap. |

| Food | Refrigerator | Pantry | Freezer | Special |
|------|-------------|--------|---------|---------|
| Ground pork | 1 to 2 days | | 1 to 2 months | Original wrap up to 2 weeks. For longer period rewrap in suitable freezer wrap. |
| Pork roast | 2 to 4 days | | 3 to 6 months | Original wrap up to 2 weeks. For longer period rewrap in suitable freezer wrap. |
| Pork steaks | 2 to 3 days | | 2 to 3 months | Original wrap up to 2 weeks. For longer period rewrap in suitable freezer wrap. |
| Pork TV dinners | | | 3 months | Original wrap up to 2 weeks. For longer period rewrap in suitable freezer wrap. |
| Fresh, white potatoes | | 2 to 3 months | | Keep dry and away from sun. For longer storage keep about 50°F. Don't refrigerate potatoes. |
| Sweet potatoes | | 2 to 3 weeks | | Keep dry and away from sun. For longer storage keep about 50°F. Don't refrigerate potatoes. |

| Food | Refrigerator | Pantry | Freezer | Special |
|------|-------------|--------|---------|---------|
| Instant potatoes | | 6 to 12 months | | Keep in airtight package. |
| Pudding | 1 to 2 days | | | |
| Pudding mixes | | 12 months | | Keep cool and dry. |
| Radishes | 1 to 2 weeks | | | |
| White rice | | 2 years | | Keep tightly closed, cool, and dry. |
| Flavored or herb rice | | 6 months | | Keep tightly closed, cool, and dry. |
| Rice mixes | | 6 months | | Keep tightly closed, cool, and dry. |
| Rolls, yeast, baked | | | 3 to 6 months | |
| Rolls, partially baked | Expiration date on label | | 2 to 3 months | Do not store in refrigerator door; temperature fluctuation and jarring lowers quality. |
| Salad dressings, bottled (unopened) | | 10 to 12 months | | |
| Salad dressings, bottled (opened) | | 3 months | | Refrigerate after opening or preparing. |
| Salad dressings made from mix | | 2 weeks | | |
| Salad oils (unopened) | | 6 months | | |

| Food | Refrigerator | Pantry | Freezer | Special |
|------|--------------|--------|---------|---------|
| Salad oils (opened) | | 1 to 3 months | | |
| Sauces and gravy mixes | | 6 to 12 months | | Keep cool and dry. |
| Scallops | 1 day | | 3 months | |
| Sherbet | | | 2 months | |
| Shortenings, solid | | 8 months | | Refrigeration not needed. |
| Shrimp TV dinners | | | 3 months | |
| Frozen shrimp | | | 12 months | |
| Fresh shrimp (uncooked) | 1 day | | | |
| Soup mixes | | 12 months | | Keep cool and dry. |
| Whole spices | | 1 to 2 years | | Spices and herbs keep longer if refrigerated or frozen. Store in airtight containers in a dry place away from sunlight and heat. |
| Ground spices | | 6 months | | Spices and herbs keep longer if refrigerated or frozen. Store in airtight containers in a dry place away from sunlight and heat. |

| Food | Refrigerator | Pantry | Freezer | Special |
|------|--------------|--------|---------|---------|
| Herbs | | 6 months | | Spices and herbs keep longer if refrigerated or frozen. Store in airtight containers in a dry place away from sunlight and heat. |
| Herb/spice blends | | 6 months | | Spices and herbs keep longer if refrigerated or frozen. Store in airtight containers in a dry place away from sunlight and heat. |
| Paprika, red pepper | | | 6 months | Best stored in refrigerator. |
| Chili powder | | 6 months | | |
| Spinach | 3 to 5 days | | 8 months | |
| Brown sugar | | 4 months | | Put in airtight container. |
| Confectioners' sugar | | 18 months | | Put in airtight container. |
| Granulated sugar | | 2 years | | Close tightly. |
| Artificial sweetener | | 2 years | | Close tightly. |
| Syrup | | 12 months | | Keep tightly closed. Refrigerate to extend life. |

| Food | Refrigerator | Pantry | Freezer | Special |
|------|-------------|--------|---------|---------|
| Tea bags | | 18 months | | Put in airtight container. |
| Instant tea | | 3 years | | Cover tightly. |
| Loose tea | | 2 years | | Put in airtight container. |
| Toaster pastries | | 2 to 3 months | | Keep in airtight packet. |
| Tomatoes | 1 to 2 days | | No | |
| Turkey | 2 days | | 6 months | |
| Vanilla (unopened) | | 2 years | | |
| Vanilla (opened) | | 12 months | | Keep tightly closed; volatile oils escape. |
| Other vanilla-type extracts (opened) | | 12 months | | Keep tightly closed; volatile oils escape. |
| Ground veal | 1 to 2 days | | 2 to 3 months | Check for holes in trays and plastic wrap of fresh meat. If none, freeze in this wrap up to 2 weeks. For longer storage, wrap with suitable freezer wrap. |

| Food | Refrigerator | Pantry | Freezer | Special |
|------|-------------|--------|---------|---------|
| Veal steaks | 2 to 3 days | | 3 to 4 months | Check for holes in trays and plastic wrap of fresh meat. If none, freeze in this wrap up to 2 weeks. For longer storage, wrap with suitable freezer wrap. |
| Veal chops | 2 to 3 days | | 3 to 4 months | Check for holes in trays and plastic wrap of fresh meat. If none, freeze in this wrap up to 2 weeks. For longer storage, wrap with suitable freezer wrap. |
| Veal stew meat | 1 to 2 days | | | Check for holes in trays and plastic wrap of fresh meat. If none, freeze in this wrap up to 2 weeks. For longer storage, wrap with suitable freezer wrap. |

| Food | Refrigerator | Pantry | Freezer | Special |
|------|--------------|--------|---------|---------|
| Veal roasts | 2 to 4 days | | | Check for holes in trays and plastic wrap of fresh meat. If none, freeze in this wrap up to 2 weeks. For longer storage, wrap with suitable freezer wrap. |
| Varieties of veal meat | 1 day | | | Check for holes in trays and plastic wrap of fresh meat. If none, freeze in this wrap up to 2 weeks. For longer storage, wrap with suitable freezer wrap. |
| Home frozen vegetables | | | 10 months | |
| Purchased frozen vegetables | | | 8 months | |
| Dehydrated vegetables, flakes | | 6 months | | |
| Dried vegetables | | 1 year | | If possible, refrigerate. |

| Food | Refrigerator | Pantry | Freezer | Special |
|------|-------------|--------|---------|---------|
| Venison and game birds | | | 8 to 12 months | Check for holes in trays and plastic wrap of fresh meat. If none, freeze in this wrap up to 2 weeks. For longer storage, wrap with suitable freezer wrap. |
| Vinegar (unopened) | | 2 years | | |
| Vinegar (opened) | | 12 months | | Keep tightly closed. Slightly cloudy appearance doesn't affect quality. Distilled vinegar keeps longer. |
| Yeast, dry | | Expiration date on package | | Keep cool and dry. |
| Yogurt | 7 to 10 days. Check date on package | | No | |

# BIBLIOGRAPHY

Adams, Catherine F. *Nutritive Value of American Foods in Common Units.* Washington, D.C.: Agriculture Handbook No. 456, U.S. Department of Agriculture, 1975.

Bowes, Helen N., and Charles F. Church. *Food Values of Portions Commonly Used,* 11th ed., rev. Philadelphia: J.B. Lippincott Co., 1970.

Center for Food Safety and Applied Nutrition, U.S. Food and Drug Administration, *CFSAN 2002 Program Priorities,* January 29, 2002.

*Chemicals Used in Food Processing.* Washington, D.C.: National Academy of Sciences, Publication 1274, 1965.

*Code of Federal Regulations: Food and Drugs,* Parts 100 to 169, Revised April 1, 1993.

Done, Alan. *Toxic Reactions to Common Household Products.* Paper read at the Symposium on Adverse Reactions Sponsored by the Drug Service Center for Disease Control, San Francisco, December 1976.

*EAFUS: A Food Additive Database.* U.S. Food and Drug Administration Center for Food Safety, May 16, 2003.

Ensminger, Audrey, M. E. Ensminger, James Konlande, and John R. K. Robson, eds. *Concise Encyclopedia of Foods & Nutrition.* Boca Raton, Fla.: CRC Press, 1994.

European Parliament Committee on the Environment, *Public Health and Consumer Policy Ammendment 12–37,* May 8, 2003.

*Evaluation of Certain Veterinary Drug Residues in Food. Thirty-fourth Report of the Joint FAO/WHO Expert Committee on Food Additives.* WHO Technical Report Series, No. 800, 1991.

*Evaluation of Certain Food Additives and Contaminants: Forty-first Report of the Joint FAO/WHO Expert Committee on Food Additives, World Health Organization, Geneva 1993.* WHO Technical Report Series 837.

Fisher, Alexander A. *Contact Dermatitis,* 3rd ed., Philadelphia: Lea & Febiger, 1986.

*Food Additive Status List, Investigations Operations Manual.* U.S. Food and Drug Administration, corrected to January 30, 1998.

*Food Allergy and Intolerances.* Bethesda, Md.: NIAD Publications, 1997.

*Food Labeling: Questions and Answers for Guidance to Facilitate the Process of Developing or Revision Labels for Foods Other than Dietary Supplements.* Office of Food Labeling Center for Food Safety and Applied Nutrition, U.S. Food and Drug Administration, August 1993.

*Food Chemicals Codex.* Washington D.C.: National Academy of Sciences Publication 1406, 1966, Third Supplement to the Fourth Edition, 2001.

Food Standards Agency, Board meeting, London September 11, 2003. "A List of Additives Currently Permitted in Food in the European Union and their E Numbers."

Gleason, Marion N., et al. *Clinical Toxicology of Commercial Products.* Baltimore: Williams & Wilkins, 1969.

Furia, Thomas E., ed. *Handbook of Food Additives.* Cleveland: The Chemical Rubber Co., 1971.

Gordon, Lesley. *A Country Herbal.* New York: Mayflower Books, 1980.

*GRAS Flavoring Substances, the 20th Publication by the Expert Panel of the Flavor and Extract Manufacturers Association on Recent Progress in the Consideration of Flavoring Ingredients Generally Recognized as Safe Under the Food Additives Ammendment. Food Technology,* December 2001. Vol 55, no. 12.

Lewis, Richard, Sr. *Food Additives Handbook.* New York: Van Nostrand Reinhold, 1991.

"List of Substances Scheduled for Evaluation and Request for Data." Joint FAO/WHO Expert Committee on Food Additives, 61st meeting. *Food Additives and Contaminants.* Rome, 10–19, June 2003.

Martin, Eric W., et al. *Hazards of Medications.* Philadelphia: J.B. Lippincott Co., 1971.

*The Merck Index,* 8th, 9th, 10th, and 13th ed. Rahway, N.J.: Merck, Sharp and Dohme Research Laboratories, 1997.

*The Merck Manual,* 16th edition. Edited by Robert Berkow, M.D. Rahway, N.J.: Merck, Sharp and Dohme Research Laboratories, 1992.

Edited by Metcalfe, Dean D., M.D., Hugh Sampson, M.D., and Ronald A. Simon, M.D., eds. *Food Allergy: Adverse Reactions to Foods and Food Additives.* Boston: Blackwell Scientific Publications, 1991.

Miall, L. Mackenzie, and D. W. A. Sharp. *A New Dictionary of Chemistry,* 4th ed. New York: John Wiley & Sons, Inc., 1968.

*Physicians' Desk Reference.* Oradell, N.J.: Medical Economics, 2002.

*Present Knowledge in Nutrition,* 5th ed. Washington, D.C.: The Nutrition Foundation, Inc., 1984.

*Recommended Dietary Allowances,* rev. ed. Washington, D.C.: National Academy of Sciences, 1980.

"Reports on Meetings of Expert Committees and Study Groups: Evaluation of Certain Food Additives." Geneva, Switzerland: World Health Organization, April 10, 2000.

Sax, N. Irving, and Richard J. Lewis, Sr., eds. *Condensed Chemical Dictionary,* 11th rev. ed. New York: Van Nostrand Reinhold, 1987.

Sax, N. Irving, and Richard J. Lewis, Sr., eds. *Hawley's Condensed Chemical Dictionary,* 11th ed. New York: Van Nostrand Reinhold, 1987.

Scarpa, Joannis, Ph.D., Helen Kiefer, Ph.D., and Rita Tatum, eds. *Sourcebook on Food and Nutrition,* 3rd ed. Chicago: Marquis Academic Media, 1982.

Smith, Jim. *Food Additives User's Handbook.* New York: Van Nostrand Reinhold, 1991.

*Steadman's Medical Dictionary,* 27th ed. Baltimore: Williams & Wilkins, 2000.

*"Summary of All GRAS Notices, July 2003."* Food and Drug Administration Office of Food Additive Safety.

*Suspected Carcinogens: A Subfile of the NIOSH Toxic Substance List.* Rockville, Md.: Tracor Jitco, Inc., U.S. Department of Health, Education and Welfare, 1975.

*Suspected Carcinogens: A Subfile of The Registry of Toxic Effects of Chemical Substances.* Cincinnati: U.S. Department of Health, Education and Welfare, Public Health Services, Centers for Disease Control, 1976.

*Tenth Report on Carcinogens.* U.S. Department of Health and Human Services, Public Health Service, National Toxicology Program, December 2002.

*Toxicants Occurring Naturally in Foods,* 2nd ed. Washington, D.C.: National Academy of Sciences, 1973.

*Toxicity Testing: Strategies to Determine Needs and Priorities.* Washington, D.C.: National Research Council; National Academy Press, 1984.

Watt, Bernice, and Annabel Merrill, et al. *Composition of Foods: Raw, Processed, Prepared.* Washington, D.C.: Agriculture Handbook No. 8, U.S. Department of Agriculture, 1963.

White, John Henry. *A Reference Book of Chemistry,* 3rd ed. New York: Philosophical Library, 1965.

Winter, Ruth. *Cancer-Causing Agents: A Preventive Guide.* New York: Crown, 1979.

Winter, Ruth. *A Consumer's Dictionary of Household, Yard, and Office Chemicals.* New York: Crown, 1992.

Winter, Ruth. *A Consumer's Dictionary of Medicines: Prescription, Over-the-Counter, Homeopathic, and Herbal Plus Medical Definitions.* New York: Crown, 1996.

Winter, Ruth. *A Consumer's Guide to Medicines in Food: Nutraceuticals That Help Prevent and Treat Physical and Emotional Illnesses.* New York: Crown, 1995.

Winter, Ruth. *Poisons in Your Food, New, Revised, Updated Edition.* New York: Crown, 1991.

## About the Author

RUTH WINTER is an award-winning science writer and author of more than thirty books on food additives, cosmetic ingredients, and environmental issues. She lives in New Jersey.

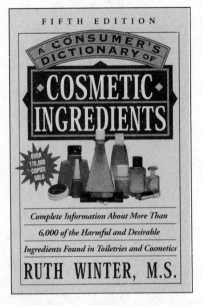
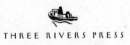